PSYCHOPATHOLOGY

PSYCHOPATHOLOGY

Foundations for a Contemporary Understanding

3rd Edition

Edited by

James E. Maddux and Barbara A. Winstead

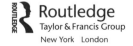

Routledge
Taylor & Francis Group
New York   London

Routledge
Taylor & Francis Group
711 Third Avenue
New York, NY 10017

Routledge
Taylor & Francis Group
2 Park Square
Milton Park, Abingdon
Oxon OX14 4RN

International Standard Book Number: 978-0-415-88790-8 (Hardback)

Library of Congress Cataloging-in-Publication Data

Psychopathology : foundations for a contemporary understanding / edited by James E. Maddux,
   Barbara A. Winstead. -- 3rd ed.
      p. cm.
   Includes bibliographical references and index.
   ISBN 978-0-415-88790-8 (hardback)
   1. Psychology, Pathological. I. Maddux, James E. II. Winstead, Barbara A. III. Title.

RC454.P786 2012
616.89--dc23   2011033326

Visit the Taylor & Francis Web site at
http://www.taylorandfrancis.com

and the Routledge Web site at
http://www.routledgementalhealth.com

Contents

Editors

James E. Maddux, PhD, is University Professor Emeritus in the Department of Psychology at George Mason University in Fairfax, Virginia and former director of its clinical doctoral program. He is also Editor Emeritus of the *Journal of Social and Clinical Psychology*. He is a Fellow of the American Psychological Association's Divisions of General, Clinical, and Health Psychology and a Fellow of the Association for Psychological Science. Maddux is also the co-editor, with Barbara A. Winstead, of *Psychopathology: Foundations for a Contemporary Understanding*.

Barbara A. Winstead received her PhD in Personality and Developmental Psychology from Harvard University. She completed a clinical internship at Harvard University Mental Health Services. She has been a faculty member at Old Dominion University, Norfolk, Virginia, since 1979. She is currently Professor and Chair of the Department of Psychology. She is also a clinical faculty member with the Virginia Consortium Program in Clinical Psychology. Her research focuses on gender and friendships, including friendships in the workplace; the effects of relationships and self-disclosure on coping with illness; and, most recently, the predictors of unwanted pursuit and stalking and coping with unwanted pursuit. Her research has resulted in more than 70 journal articles, chapters, and books and numerous conference presentations.

Contributors

Lauren B. Alloy, PhD
Department of Psychology
Temple University
Philadelphia, Pennsylvania

Jessica Arsenault, BSc
University of Toronto
Toronto, Ontario, Canada

Shimrit K. Black, MA
Temple University
Philadelphia, Pennsylvania

Michele Boivin, PhD
Royal Ottawa Mental Health Centre
Ottawa, Ontario, Canada

Elaine Boland, MA
Temple University
Philadelphia, Pennsylvania

Annie Bollini, PhD
Atlanta Veteran Affairs Medical Center
Atlanta, Georgia

Dianne L. Chambless, PhD
Department of Psychology
University of Pennsylvania
Philadelphia, Pennsylvania

Caroline M. Ciliberti, MS
West Virginia University
Morgantown, West Virginia

Megan M. Clegg-Kraynok, PhD
Ohio Northern University
Ada, Ohio

Georg H. Eifert, PhD
Schmid College of Science and Technology
Chapman University
Orange, California

Amy Fiske, PhD
Department of Psychology
West Virginia University
Morgantown, West Virginia

Paul J. Frick, PhD
Department of Psychology
University of New Orleans
New Orleans, Louisiana

Katherine A. Fowler, PhD
National Institutes of Health
Silver Spring, Maryland

Howard N. Garb, PhD
Lackland Air Force Base
San Antonio, Texas

Kim Goldstein, MA
Temple University
Philadelphia, Pennsylvania

Jennifer T. Gosselin, PhD
Center for Women's Reproductive Care
Columbia University
New York, New York

Christine E. Gould, PhD
West Virginia University
Morgantown, West Virginia

Peter J. Guarnaccia, PhD
Institute for Health, Health Care Policy, and
    Aging Research
Rutgers The State University of New Jersey
New Brunswick, New Jersey

C. Peter Herman, PhD
Department of Psychology
University of Toronto
Toronto, Ontario, Canada

Karen Hochman, MD
Department of Psychiatry and Behavioral
    Science
Emory University
Atlanta, Georgia

Abigail Jenkins, MA
Temple University
Philadelphia, Pennsylvania

Michelle L. Jochim, BS
Indiana University
Bloomington, Indiana

Michelle L. Kelley, PhD
Department of Psychology
Old Dominion University
Norfolk, Virginia

Lisa Kestler, PhD
MedAvante, Inc.
Hamilton, New Jersey

Eva R. Kimonis, PhD
Department of Mental Health Law and
    Policy
Louis de la Parte Florida Mental Health
    Institute
University of South Florida
Tampa, Florida

Keith Klostermann, PhD
Department of Psychology
Old Dominion University
Norfolk, Virginia

Denise LaBelle, MA
Temple University
Philadelphia, Pennsylvania

Scott O. Lilienfeld, PhD
Department of Psychology
Emory University
Atlanta, Georgia

Steven Regeser López, PhD
Department of Psychology
University of Southern California
Los Angeles, California

James E. Maddux, PhD
Department of Psychology
George Mason University
Fairfax, Virginia

Rebecca S. Martinez, PhD
Department of Counseling and Educational
    Psychology
Indiana University
Bloomington, Indiana

Ellen McCormack, MA
Schmid College of Science
Chapman University
Orange, California

Traci McFarlane, PhD
University of Toronto and Toronto General
    Hospital
Toronto, Ontario, Canada

Vijay A. Mittal, PhD
Department of Psychology and
    Neuroscience
University of Colorado at Boulder
Boulder, Colorado

Danielle K. Nadorff, PhD
West Virginia University
Morgantown, West Virginia

Michael R. Nadorff, MS
West Virginia University
Morgantown, West Virginia

Sarra Nazem, MS
West Virginia University
Morgantown, West Virginia

Leah M. Nellis, PhD
Blumberg Center for Interdisciplinary
    Studies
Indiana State University
Terre Haute, Indiana

Olga Obraztsova, MA
Temple University
Philadelphia, Pennsylvania

Thomas H. Ollendick, PhD
Child Study Center, Department of
    Psychology
Virginia Polytechnic Institute and State
    University
Blacksburg, Virginia

Janet Polivy, PhD
Department of Psychology
University of Toronto
Toronto, Ontario, Canada

Jennifer Ruth Presnall, MS
Department of Psychology
University of Kentucky
Lexington, Kentucky

Janis Sanchez, PhD
Department of Psychology
Old Dominion University
Norfolk, Virginia

Janay B. Sander, PhD
Department of Educational Psychology
The University of Texas at Austin
Austin, Texas

Benjamin Shapero, MA
Temple University
Philadelphia, Pennsylvania

Robert F. Smith, PhD
Department of Psychology
George Mason University
Farifax, Virginia

Sarah T. Stahl, PhD
West Virginia University
Morgantown, West Virginia

Rebecca E. Stewart, MA
Department of Psychology
University of Pennsylvania
Philadelphia, Pennsylvania

Cynthia Suveg, PhD
Department of Psychology
University of Georgia
Athens, Georgia

Kathryn Trottier, PhD
Eating Disorders Program
University of Toronto and Toronto General
    Hospital
Toronto, Ontario, Canada

Elaine Walker, PhD
Department of Psychology
Emory University
Atlanta, Georgia

Stacy E. White, BS
Department of Counseling and Educational
    Psychology
Indiana University
Bloomington, Indiana

Thomas A. Widiger, PhD
Department of Psychology
University of Kentucky
Lexington, Kentucky

S. Lloyd Williams, PhD
Ruhr-Universität Bochum
Bochum, Germany

Barbara A. Winstead, PhD
Department of Psychology
Old Dominion University
Norfolk, Virginia

Janice Zeman, PhD
Department of Psychology
College of William and Mary
Williamsburg, Virginia

Michael J. Zvolensky, PhD
Department of Psychology
University of Houston
Houston, Texas

Part I
Thinking About Psychopathology

1

Conceptions of Psychopathology

A Social Constructionist Perspective

JAMES E. MADDUX

George Mason University
Fairfax, Virginia

JENNIFER T. GOSSELIN

Sacred Heart University
Fairfield, Connecticut

BARBARA A. WINSTEAD

Old Dominion University
Norfolk, Virginia

A textbook about a topic should begin with a clear definition of that topic. Unfortunately, for a textbook on psychopathology, this is a difficult, if not impossible, task. The definitions or conceptions of psychopathology and such related terms as *mental disorder* have been the subject of heated debate throughout the history of psychology and psychiatry, and the debate is not over (Gorenstein, 1984; Horwitz, 2002; Widiger, 1997, this volume). Despite its many variations, this debate has centered on a single overriding question: Are psychopathology and related terms such as mental disorder and mental illness scientific terms that can be defined objectively and by scientific criteria, or are they social constructions (Gergen, 1985) that are defined largely or entirely by societal and cultural values? The goal of this chapter is to address this issue. Addressing this issue in this opening chapter is important because the reader's view of everything else in the rest of this book will be influenced by his or her view on this issue.

This chapter deals with *conceptions* of psychopathology. A conception of psychopathology is not a *theory* of psychopathology (Wakefield, 1992a). A conception of psychopathology attempts to define the term—to delineate which human experiences are considered psychopathological and which are not. A conception of psychopathology does not try to explain the psychological phenomena that are considered pathological, but instead tells us which psychological phenomena are considered pathological and thus need to be explained. A theory of psychopathology, however, *is* an attempt to explain those psychological phenomena and experiences that have been identified by the conception as pathological. Theories and explanations for what is currently considered to be psychopathological human experience can be found in a number of other chapters, including all of those in Part II of this book.

Understanding various conceptions of psychopathology is important for a number of reasons. As medical philosopher Lawrie Reznek (1987) said, "Concepts carry consequences—classifying things one way rather than another has important implications for the way we behave towards such things" (p. 1). In speaking of the importance of the conception of disease, Reznek wrote:

The classification of a condition as a disease carries many important consequences. We inform medical scientists that they should try to discover a cure for the condition. We inform benefactors that they should support such research. We direct medical care towards the condition, making it appropriate to treat the condition by medical means such as drug therapy, surgery, and so on. We inform our courts that it is inappropriate to hold people responsible for the manifestations of the condition. We set up early warning detection services aimed at detecting the condition in its early stages when it is still amenable to successful treatment. We serve notice to health insurance companies and national health services that they are liable to pay for the treatment of such a condition. Classifying a condition as a disease is no idle matter. (p. 1)

If we substitute *psychopathology* or *mental disorder* for the word *disease* in this paragraph, its message still holds true. How we conceive of psychopathology and related terms has wide-ranging implications for individuals, medical and mental health professionals, government agencies and programs, and society at large.

Conceptions of Psychopathology

A variety of conceptions of psychopathology have been offered over the years. Each has its merits and its deficiencies, but none suffices as a truly scientific definition.

Psychopathology as Statistical Deviance

A common and "commonsense" conception of psychopathology is that pathological psychological phenomena are those that are *abnormal*—statistically deviant or infrequent. Abnormal literally means "away from the norm." The word "norm" refers to what is typical or average. Thus, this conception views psychopathology as deviation from statistical psychological normality.

One of the merits of this conception is its commonsense appeal. It makes sense to most people to use words such as psychopathology and mental disorder to refer only to behaviors or experiences that are infrequent (e.g., paranoid delusions, hearing voices) and not to those that are relatively common (e.g., shyness, a stressful day at work, grief following the death of a loved one).

A second merit to this conception is that it lends itself to accepted methods of measurement that give it at least a semblance of scientific respectability. The first step in employing this conception scientifically is to determine what is statistically normal (typical, average). The second step is to determine how far a particular psychological phenomenon or condition deviates from statistical normality. This is often done by developing an instrument or measure that attempts to quantify the phenomenon and then assigning numbers or scores to people's experiences or manifestations of the phenomenon. Once the measure is developed, norms are typically established so that an individual's score can be compared to the mean or average score of some group of people. Scores that are sufficiently far from average are considered to be indicative of abnormal or pathological psychological phenomena. This process describes most tests of intelligence and cognitive ability and many commonly used measures of personality and emotion (e.g., the Minnesota Multiphasic Personality Inventory).

Despite its commonsense appeal and its scientific merits, this conception presents problems. It sounds relatively objective and scientific because it relies on well-established psychometric methods for developing measures of psychological phenomena and developing norms. Yet, this approach leaves much room for subjectivity.

The first point at which subjectivity comes into play is in the conceptual definition of the construct for which a measure is developed. A measure of any psychological construct, such as intelligence, must begin with a conceptual definition. We have to ask ourselves "What is 'intelligence'?" Of course, different people (including different psychologists) will come up with different answers to this question. How then can we scientifically and objectively determine which definition or conception is "true" or "correct"? The answer is that we cannot. Although we have tried-and-true methods for developing a reliable and valid (i.e., it consistently predicts what we want to predict) measure of a psychological construct once we have agreed on its conception or definition, we cannot use these same methods to determine which conception or definition is true or correct. The bottom line is that there is no "true" definition of intelligence and no objective, scientific way of determining one. Intelligence is not a thing that exists inside people and makes them behave in certain ways and that awaits our discovery of its true nature. Instead, it is an abstract idea that is defined by people as they use the words *intelligence* and "intelligent" to describe certain kinds of human behavior and the covert mental processes that supposedly precede or are at least concurrent with the behavior.

We usually can observe and describe patterns in the way most people use the words *intelligence* and *intelligent* to describe the behavior of themselves and others. The descriptions of the patterns then comprise the definitions of the words. If we examine the patterns of the use of the words *intelligence* and *intelligent*, we find that at the most basic level, they describe a variety of specific behaviors and abilities that society values and thus encourages; unintelligent behavior is a variety of behaviors that society does not value and thus discourages. The fact that the definition of intelligence is grounded in societal values explains the recent expansion of the concept to include good interpersonal skills (i.e., social and emotional intelligence), self-regulatory skills, artistic and musical abilities, and other abilities not measured by traditional tests of intelligence (e.g., Gardner, 1999). The meaning of intelligence has broadened because society has come to place increasing value on these other attributes and abilities, and this change in societal values has been the result of a dialogue or discourse among the people in society, both professionals and laypersons. One measure of intelligence may prove more reliable and more useful than another measure in predicting what we want to predict (e.g., academic achievement, income), but what we want to predict reflects what we value, and values are not derived scientifically.

Another point for the influence of subjectivity is in the determination of how deviant a psychological phenomenon must be from the norm to be considered abnormal or pathological. We can use objective, scientific methods to construct a measure, such as an intelligence test, and develop norms for the measure, but we are still left with the question of how far from normal an individual's score must be to be considered abnormal. This question cannot be answered by the science of psychometrics because the distance from the average that a person's score must be to be considered abnormal is a matter of debate, not a matter of fact. It is true that we often answer this question by relying on statistical conventions, such as using one or two standard deviations from the average score as the line of division between normal and abnormal. Yet the decision to use that convention is itself subjective because a convention (from the Latin *convenire*, meaning "to come together") is an agreement or contract made by people, not a truth or fact about the world. Why should one standard deviation from the norm designate abnormality? Why not two standard deviations? Why not half a standard deviation? Why not use percentages? The lines between normal and abnormal can be drawn at many different points using many different strategies. Each line of demarcation may be more or less useful for certain purposes, such as determining the criteria for eligibility for limited services and resources. Where the line is set also determines the prevalence of abnormality or mental disorder among the general population (Kutchens & Kirk, 1997), so it has great practical significance. But no such line is more or less "true" than the others, even when those others are based on statistical conventions.

We cannot use the procedures and methods of science to draw a definitive line of demarcation between normal and abnormal psychological functioning, just as we cannot use them to draw definitive lines of demarcation between short and tall people or hot and cold on a thermometer. No such lines exist in nature.

Psychopathology as Maladaptive (Dysfunctional) Behavior

Most of us think of psychopathology as behaviors and experiences that are not just statistically abnormal but also maladaptive (dysfunctional). *Normal* and *abnormal* are statistical terms, but *adaptive* and *maladaptive* refer not to statistical norms and deviations but to the effectiveness or ineffectiveness of a person's behavior. If a behavior "works" for the person—if the behavior helps the person deal with challenges, cope with stress, and accomplish his or her goals—then we say the behavior is more or less effective and adaptive. If the behavior does not work for the person in these ways, or if the behavior makes the problem or situation worse, we say it is more or less ineffective and maladaptive. The *Diagnostic and Statistical Manual of Mental Disorders* (4th ed., text rev.; *DSM–IV–TR*; American Psychiatric Association, 2000) incorporates this notion in its definition of mental disorder by stating that a mental disorder "is associated with present distress (e.g., a painful symptom) or disability (i.e., impairment in one or more areas of functioning) or with significantly increased risk of suffering pain, death, disability, or an important loss of freedom" (p. xxxi).

Like the statistical deviance conception, this conception has commonsense appeal and is consistent with the way most laypersons use words such as *pathology, disorder*, and *illness*. Most people would find it odd to use these words to describe statistically infrequent high levels of intelligence, happiness, or psychological well-being. To say that someone is "pathologically intelligent" or "pathologically well adjusted" seems contradictory because it flies in the face of the commonsense use of these words.

The major problem with the conception of psychopathology as maladaptive behavior is its inherent subjectivity. Like the distinction between normal and abnormal, the distinction between adaptive and maladaptive is fuzzy and arbitrary. We have no objective, scientific way of making a clear distinction. Very few human behaviors are in and of themselves either adaptive or maladaptive; instead, their adaptiveness or maladaptiveness depends on the situations in which the behavior is enacted and on the judgment and values of the actor and the observers. Even behaviors that are statistically rare and therefore abnormal will be more or less adaptive under different conditions and more or less adaptive in the opinion of different observers and relative to different cultural norms. The extent to which a behavior or behavior pattern is viewed as more or less adaptive or maladaptive depends on a number of factors, such as the goals the person is trying to accomplish and the social norms and expectations in a given situation. What works in one situation might not work in another. What appears adaptive to one person might not appear so to another. What is usually adaptive in one culture might not be so in another (see López & Guarnaccia, this volume). Even so-called normal personality involves a good deal of occasionally maladaptive behavior, which you can find evidence for in your own life and the lives of friends and relatives. In addition, people given official "personality disorder" diagnoses by clinical psychologists and psychiatrists often can manage their lives effectively and do not always behave in maladaptive ways.

Another problem with the "psychopathological equals maladaptive" conception is that judgments of adaptiveness and maladaptiveness are logically unrelated to measures of statistical deviation. Of course, we often do find a strong relationship between the statistical abnormality of a behavior and its maladaptiveness. Many of the problems described in the *DSM–IV–TR* and in this textbook are both maladaptive and statistically rare. There are, however, major exceptions to this relationship.

First, psychological phenomena that deviate from the norm or the average are not all maladaptive. In fact, sometimes deviation from the norm is adaptive and healthy. For example, IQ scores of 130 and 70 are equally deviant from norm, but abnormally high intelligence is much more adaptive than abnormally low intelligence. Likewise, people who consistently score abnormally low on measures of anxiety and depression are probably happier and better adjusted than people who consistently score equally abnormally high on such measures.

Second, not all maladaptive psychological phenomena are statistically infrequent and vice versa. For example, shyness is almost always maladaptive to some extent because it almost always interferes with a person's ability to accomplish what he or she wants to accomplish in life and relationships, but shyness is very common and therefore is statistically frequent. The same is true of many of the problems with sexual functioning that are included in the *DSM* as mental disorders—they are almost always maladaptive to some extent because they create distress and problems in relationships, but they are relatively common (see Gosselin, this volume).

Psychopathology as Distress and Disability

Some conceptions of psychopathology invoke the notions of *subjective distress* and *disability*. Subjective distress refers to unpleasant and unwanted feelings such as anxiety, sadness, and anger. Disability refers to a restriction in ability (Ossorio, 1985). People who seek mental health treatment usually are not getting what they want to out of life, and many feel that they are unable to do what they need to do to accomplish their valued goals. They may feel inhibited or restricted by their situation, their fears or emotional turmoil, or by physical or other limitations. Individuals may lack the necessary self-efficacy beliefs (beliefs about personal abilities), physiological or biological components, self-regulatory skills, or situational opportunities to make positive changes (Bergner, 1997).

As noted previously, the *DSM* incorporates the notions of distress and disability into its definition of mental disorder. In fact, subjective distress and disability are simply two different but related ways of thinking about adaptiveness and maladaptiveness rather than alternative conceptions of psychopathology. Although the notions of subjective distress and disability may help refine our notion of maladaptiveness, they do nothing to resolve the subjectivity problem. Different people will define personal distress and personal disability in vastly different ways, as will different mental health professionals and different cultures. Likewise, people differ in their thresholds for how much distress or disability they can tolerate before seeking professional help. Thus, we are still left with the problem of how to determine normal and abnormal levels of distress and disability. As noted previously, the question "How much is too much?" cannot be answered using the objective methods of science.

Another problem is that some conditions or patterns of behavior (e.g., pedophilia, antisocial personality disorder) that are considered psychopathological (at least officially, according to the *DSM*) are *not* characterized by subjective distress, other than the temporary distress that might result from social condemnation or conflicts with the law.

Psychopathology as Social Deviance

Psychopathology has also been conceived as behavior that deviates from social or cultural norms. This conception is simply a variation of the conception of psychopathology as statistical abnormality, only in this case judgments about deviations from normality are made informally by people using social and cultural rules and conventions rather than formally by psychological tests or measures.

This conception also is consistent to some extent with common sense and common parlance. We tend to view psychopathological or mentally disordered people as thinking, feeling, and doing things that most other people do not do (or do not want to do) and that are inconsistent with socially accepted and culturally sanctioned ways of thinking, feeling, and behaving.

The problem with this conception, as with the others, is its subjectivity. Norms for socially normal or acceptable behavior are not derived scientifically but instead are based on the values, beliefs, and historical practices of the culture, which determine who is accepted or rejected by a society or culture. Cultural values develop not through the implementation of scientific methods but through numerous informal conversations and negotiations among the people and institutions of that culture. Social norms differ from one culture to another, and therefore what is psychologically abnormal in one culture may not be so in another (see López & Guarnaccia, this volume). Also, norms of a given culture change over time; therefore, conceptions of psychopathology will change over time, often very dramatically, as evidenced by American society's changes over the past several decades in attitudes toward sex, race, and gender. For example, psychiatrists in the 1800s classified masturbation, especially in children and women, as a disease, and it was treated in some cases by clitoridectomy (removal of the clitoris), which Western society today would consider barbaric (Reznek, 1987). Homosexuality was an official mental disorder in the *DSM* until 1973 (see Gosselin, this volume).

In addition, the conception of psychopathology as a social norm violation is at times in conflict with the conception of psychopathology as a maladaptive behavior. Sometimes violating social norms is healthy and adaptive for the individual and beneficial to society. In the 19th century, women and African Americans in the United States who sought the right to vote were trying to change well-established social norms. Their actions were uncommon and therefore considered abnormal, but these people were far from psychologically unhealthy, at least not by today's standards. Earlier in the 19th century, slaves who desired to escape from their owners were said to have drapetomania. Although still practiced in some parts of the world, slavery is almost universally viewed as socially deviant and pathological, and the desire to escape enslavement is considered to be as normal and healthy as the desire to live and breathe.

Psychopathology as Dyscontrol or Dysregulation

Some have argued that only those maladaptive patterns of behaving, thinking, and feeling that are not within the person's ability to control or self-regulate should be considered psychopathologies or mental disorders (Klein, 1999; see also Widiger, this volume, for detailed discussion). The basic notion here is that if a person voluntarily behaves in maladaptive or self-destructive ways, then that person's behavior should not be viewed as in indication or result of a mental disorder. Indeed, as does the notion of a physical or medical disorder, the term mental disorder seems to incorporate the notion that what is happening to the person is not within the person's control. The basic problem with this conception is that its draws an artificial line between "within control" (voluntary) and "out of control" (involuntary) that simply cannot be drawn. There may be some behaviors that person might engage in that most of us would agree are completely voluntary, deliberate, and intentional and other behaviors that a person might engage in that most of us would agree are completely involuntary, nondeliberate, and unintentional. Such behaviors, however, are probably few and far between. The causes of human behavior are complex, to say the least, and environmental events can have such a powerful influence on any behavior that concluding that anything a person does is completely or even mostly voluntary and intentional may be a stretch. In fact, considerable research suggests that most behaviors most of the time are automatic and therefore involuntary (Weinberger, Siefier, & Haggerty, 2010). Determining the degree to which a behavior is voluntary and within a person's control or involuntary and beyond a person's control is difficult, if not impossible. We also are left, once again, with the question of who gets to make this determination. The actor? The observer? The patient? The mental health professional?

Psychopathology as Harmful Dysfunction

A more recent attempt at defining psychopathology is Wakefield's (1992a, 1992b, 1993, 1997, 1999) *harmful dysfunction* (HD) conception. Presumably grounded in evolutionary psychology (Cosmides, Tooby, & Barkow, 1992), the HD conception acknowledges that the conception of mental disorder is influenced strongly by social and cultural values. It also proposes, however, a supposedly scientific, factual, and objective core that is not dependent on social and cultural values. In Wakefield's (1992a) words:

> [A mental] disorder is a harmful dysfunction wherein *harmful* is a value term based on social norms, and *dysfunction* is a scientific term referring to the failure of a mental mechanism to perform a natural function for which it was designed by evolution … a disorder exists when the failure of a person's internal mechanisms to perform their function as designed by nature impinges harmfully on the person's well-being as defined by social values and meanings. (p. 373)

One of the merits of this conception is that it acknowledges that the conception of mental disorders must include a reference to social norms; however, this conception also tries to anchor the concept of mental disorder in a scientific theory—the theory of evolution.

Wakefield (2006) reiterated this definition in writing that a mental disorder "satisfies two requirements: (1) it is negative or harmful according to cultural values; and (2) it is caused by a dysfunction (i.e., by a failure of some psychological mechanism to perform a natural function for which it was evolutionarily designed)" (p. 157). He and his colleagues also stated: "Problematic mismatches between designed human nature and current social desirability are not disorders … [such as] adulterous longings, taste for fat and sugar, and male aggressiveness" (Wakefield, Horwitz, & Schmitz, 2006, p. 317).

However, the claim that identifying a failure of a "designed function" is a scientific judgment and not a value judgment is open to question. Wakefield's claim that dysfunction can be defined in "purely factual scientific" (Wakefield, 1992a, p. 383) terms rests on the assumption that the "designed functions" of human "mental mechanisms" have an objective and observable reality and, thus, that failure of the mechanism to execute its designed function can be objectively assessed. A basic problem with this notion is that although the physical inner workings of the body and brain can be observed and measured, mental mechanisms have no objective reality and thus cannot be observed directly—no more so than the unconscious forces that provide the foundation for Freudian psychoanalytic theory.

Evolutionary theory provides a basis for explaining human behavior in terms of its contribution to reproductive fitness. A behavior is considered more functional if it increases the survival of those who share your genes in the next generation, and the next, and less functional if it does not. Evolutionary psychology cannot, however, provide a catalog of mental mechanisms and their natural functions. Wakefield stated that "discovering what in fact is natural or dysfunctional may be extraordinarily difficult" (1992b, p. 236). The problem with this statement is that, when applied to human behavior, "natural" and "dysfunctional" are not properties that can be "discovered"; they are value judgments. The judgment that a behavior represents a dysfunction relies on the observation that the behavior is excessive or inappropriate under certain conditions. Arguing that these behaviors represent failures of evolutionarily designed "mental mechanisms" (itself an untestable hypothesis because of the occult nature of mental mechanisms) does not absolve us of the need to make value judgments about what is excessive, inappropriate, or harmful and under what circumstances (Leising, Rogers, & Ostner, 2009). These are value judgments based on social norms, not scientific facts, an issue that we will explore in greater detail later in this chapter (see Widiger, this volume).

Another problem with the HD conception is that it is a moving target. For example, Wakefield modified his original HD conception by saying that it is concerned not with what a mental disorder *is* but only with what most scientists *think* it is. For example, he stated, "My comments were intended to argue, not that PTSD [posttraumatic stress disorder] is a disorder, but that the HD analysis is capable of explaining why the symptom picture in PTSD is *commonly judged* to be a disorder" (1999, p. 390, emphasis added). Wakefield's original goal was to "define mental disorders *prescriptively*" (Sadler, 1999, p. 433, emphasis added) and to "help us decide whether someone is mentally disordered or not" (Sadler, 1999, p. 434). His more recent view, however, "avoids making any prescriptive claims, instead focusing on explaining the conventional clinical use of the disorder concept" (Sadler, 1999, p. 433). Wakefield "has abandoned his original task to be prescriptive and has now settled for being *descriptive* only, for example, telling us why a disorder is judged to be one" (Sadler, 1999, p. 434, emphasis added).

Describing how people have agreed to define a concept is not the same as defining the concept in scientific terms, even if those people are scientists. Thus, Wakefield's revised HD conception simply offers another criterion that people (clinicians, scientists, and laypersons) might use to judge whether or not some behavior constitutes a mental disorder. But consensus of opinion, even among scientists, is not scientific evidence. Therefore, no matter how accurately this criterion might describe how some or most people define mental disorder, it is no more or no less scientific than other conceptions that are also based on how some people *agree* to define mental disorder. It is no more scientific than the conceptions involving statistical infrequency, maladaptiveness, or social norm violations (see Widiger, this volume).

The DSM Definition of Mental Disorder

Any discussion of conceptions of psychopathology has to include a discussion of the most influential conception of all—that of the *DSM*. First published in 1952 and revised and expanded five times since, the *DSM* provides the organizational structure for virtually every textbook (including this one) on abnormal psychology and psychopathology, as well as almost every professional book on the assessment and treatment of psychological problems. (See Widiger, this volume, for a more detailed history of psychiatric classification and the *DSM*.)

Just as a textbook on psychopathology should begin by defining its key term, so should a taxonomy of mental disorders. To their credit, the authors of the *DSM* attempted to do that. The difficulties inherent in attempting to define psychopathology and related terms are clearly illustrated by the definition of mental disorder found in the latest edition of the *DSM*, the *DSM–IV–TR* (American Psychiatric Association, 2000):

> In DSM-IV, each of the mental disorders is conceptualized as a clinically significant behavioral or psychological syndrome or pattern that occurs in an individual and that is associated with present distress (e.g., a painful symptom) or disability (i.e., impairment in one or more important areas of functioning) or with a significantly increased risk of suffering death, pain, disability, or an important loss of freedom. In addition, this syndrome or pattern must not be merely an expectable and culturally sanctioned response to a particular event, for example, the death of a loved one. Whatever its cause, it must currently be considered a manifestation of a behavioral, psychological, or biological dysfunction in the individual. Neither deviant behavior (e.g., political, religious, or sexual) nor conflicts that are primarily between the individual and society are mental disorders unless the deviance or conflict is a symptom of a dysfunction in the individual, as described above. (p. xxxi)

All of the conceptions of psychopathology described previously can be found to some extent in this definition—statistical deviation (i.e., not "expectable"); maladaptiveness, including distress and disability; social norms violations; and some elements of the harmful dysfunction conception ("a dysfunction in the individual") although without the flavor of evolutionary theory. For this reason, it is a comprehensive, inclusive, and sophisticated conception and probably as good, if not better, than any proposed so far.

Nonetheless, it falls prey to the same problems with subjectivity as other conceptions. For example, what is the meaning of "clinically significant," and how should clinical significance be measured? Does clinical significance refer to statistical infrequency, maladaptiveness, or both? How much distress must a person experience or how much disability must a person exhibit before he or she is said to have a mental disorder? Who gets to judge the person's degree of distress or disability? How do we determine whether a particular response to an event is "expectable" or "culturally sanctioned"? Who gets to determine this? How does one determine whether deviant behavior or conflicts "are primarily between the individual and society"? What exactly does this mean? What does it mean for a dysfunction to exist or occur "in the individual"? Certainly a biological dysfunction might be said to be literally "in the individual," but does it make sense to say the same of psychological and behavioral dysfunctions? Is it possible to say that a psychological or behavioral dysfunction can occur "in the individual" apart from the social, cultural, and interpersonal milieu in which the person is acting and being judged? Clearly, the *DSM*'s conception of mental disorder raises as many questions as do the conceptions it was meant to supplant.

Categories Versus Dimensions

The difficulty inherent in the *DSM* conception of psychopathology and other attempts to distinguish between normal and abnormal or adaptive and maladaptive is that they are *categorical models* that attempt to describe guidelines for clearly distinguishing between individuals who are normal or abnormal and for determining which specific abnormality or "disorder" a person has to the exclusion of other disorders. An alternative model, overwhelmingly supported by research, is the *dimensional model*. In the dimensional model, normality and abnormality, as well as effective and ineffective psychological functioning, lie along a continuum; so-called psychological disorders are simply extreme variants of normal psychological phenomena and ordinary problems in living (Keyes & Lopez, 2002; Widiger, this volume). The dimensional model is concerned not with classifying people or disorders, but with identifying and measuring individual differences in psychological phenomena such as emotion, mood, intelligence, and personal styles (Lubinski, 2000). Great differences among individuals on the dimensions of interest are expected, such as the differences we find on standardized tests of intelligence. As with intelligence, divisions between normality and abnormality may be demarcated for convenience or efficiency but are not to be viewed as indicative of true discontinuity among "types" of phenomena or "types" of people. Also, statistical deviation is not viewed as necessarily pathological, although extreme variants on either end of a dimension (e.g., introversion/extraversion, neuroticism, intelligence) may be maladaptive if they lead to inflexibility in functioning.

This notion is not new. As early as 1860, Henry Maudsley commented that "there is no boundary line between sanity and insanity; and the slightly exaggerated feeling which renders a man 'peculiar' in the world differs only in degree from that which places hundreds in asylums" (1860, p. 14, quoted in Millon, 2010, p. 33).

Empirical evidence for the validity of a dimensional approach to psychological adjustment is strongest in the area of personality and personality disorders (Maddux & Mudell, 1999; Widiger & Trull, 2007; Widiger, this volume). Factor analytic studies of personality problems among the general population and clinical populations with "personality disorders" demonstrate striking similarity between the two groups. In addition, these factor structures are not consistent with the *DSM*'s system of classifying disorders of personality into categories and support a dimensional view rather than a categorical view. For example, the most recent evidence strongly suggests that psychopathic personality (or antisocial personality) and other externalizing disorders of adulthood display a dimensional structure, not a categorical structure (Edens, Marcus, Lilienfeld, & Poythress, 2006; Krueger, Markon, Patrick, & Iacono, 2005; Larsson, Andershed, & Lichtenstein, 2006). The same is true of narcissism and narcissistic personality disorder (Brown, Budzek, & Tamborski, 2009). In addition, the recent Emotional Cascade

Model of borderline personality disorder, although not presented explicitly as a dimensional model, is in almost every respect consistent with a dimension model (Selby & Joiner, 2009). The dimensional view of personality disorders is also supported by cross-cultural research (Alarcon, Foulks, & Vakkur, 1998).

Research on other problems supports the dimensional view. Studies of the varieties of normal emotional experiences (e.g., Carver, 2001; Oatley & Jenkins, 1992; Oatley, Keltner, & Jenkins, 2006) indicate that "clinical" emotional disorders are not discrete classes of emotional experience that are discontinuous from everyday emotional upsets and problems. Research on adult attachment patterns in relationships strongly suggests that dimensions are more accurate descriptions of such patterns than are categories (Fossati, 2003; Fraley & Waller, 1998; Hankin, Kassel, Abela, 2005). Research on self-defeating behaviors has shown that they are extremely common and are not by themselves signs of abnormality or symptoms of disorders (Baumeister & Scher, 1988). Research on children's reading problems indicates that dyslexia is not an all-or-none condition that children either have or do not have but occurs in degrees without a natural break between dyslexic and nondyslexic children (Shaywitz, Escobar, Shaywitz, Fletcher, & Makuch, 1992; Shaywitz, Morris, & Shaywitz, 2008; Snowling, 2006). Research on attention deficit hyperactivity (Barkley, 2005), posttraumatic stress disorder (Anthony, Lonigan, & Hecht, 1999; Rosen & Lilienfeld, 2008; Ruscio, Ruscio, & Keane, 2002), and panic disorder (Eaton, Kessler, Wittchen, & Magee, 1994) demonstrates this same dimensionality. Research on depression and schizophrenia indicates that these "disorders" are best viewed as loosely related clusters of dimensions of individual differences, not as disease-like syndromes (Claridge, 1995; Costello, 1993a, 1993b; Eisenberg et al., 2009; Flett, Vredenburg, & Krames, 1997). For example, a recent study on depressive symptoms among children and adolescents found a dimensional structure for all of the *DSM–IV* symptoms of major depression (Hankin, Fraley, Lahey, & Waldman, 2005).

The inventor of the term "schizophrenia," Eugene Bleuler, viewed so-called pathological conditions as continuous with so-called normal conditions and noted the occurrence of "schizophrenic" symptoms among normal individuals (Gilman, 1988). In fact, Bleuler referred to the major symptom of "schizophrenia" (thought disorder) as simply "ungewonlich," which in German means "unusual," not "bizarre," as it was translated in the first English version of Bleuler's classic monograph (Gilman, 1988). Essentially, the creation of schizophrenia as a classification was "an artifact of the ideologies implicit in nineteenth century European and American medical nosologies" (Gilman, 1988, p. 204). Indeed, research indicates that the hallucinations and delusions exhibited by people diagnosed with a schizophrenic disorder are continuous with experiences and behaviors among the general population (Johns & van Os, 2001; Kestler, Bollini, Hochman, Mittal, & Walker, this volume van Os, Verdoux, Maurice-Tison, Gay, Liarud, Salamon, & Bourgeois, 1999). Recent research also suggests that dimensional measures of psychosis are better predictors of dysfunctional behavior, social adaptation, and occupational functioning than are categorical diagnoses (Rosenman, Korten, Medway, & Evans, 2003). Finally, biological researchers continue to discover continuities between so-called normal and abnormal (or pathological) psychological conditions (Claridge, 1995; Livesley, Jang, & Vernon, 1998; Nettle, 2001; Smith, this volume).

Dimensional approaches, of course, are not without their limitations, including the greater difficulties they present in communication among professionals compared to categories and their greater complexity for clinical use (Simonsen, 2010). In addition, researchers and clinicians have not reached a consensus on which dimensions to use (Simonsen, 2010). Finally, dimensional approaches do not solve the subjectivity problem, noted previously, because the decision regarding how far from the mean a person's thoughts, feelings, or behavior must be to be considered abnormal remains a subjective one. Nonetheless, dimensional approaches have been gradually gaining great acceptance and will inevitably be integrated more and more into the traditional categorical schemes. (An extensive discussion of the pros and cons of categorical approaches are beyond the scope of this chapter. Detailed and information discussions can be found in other recent sources [e.g., Grove & Vrieze, 2010; Simonsen, 2010].)

Social Constructionism and Conceptions of Psychopathology

If we cannot come up with an objective and scientific conception of psychopathology and mental disorder, then is there some way left for to us to understand these terms? How then are we to conceive of psychopathology? The solution to this problem is not to develop yet another definition of psychopathology, but rather to accept the fact that the problem has no solution—at least not a solution that can be arrived at by scientific means. We have to give up the goal of developing a scientific definition and accept the idea that psychopathology and related terms are not the kind of terms that can be defined through the processes we usually think of as scientific. We have to stop struggling to develop a scientific conception of psychopathology and attempt instead to try to understand the struggle itself—why it occurs and what it means. We need to better understand how people go about trying to conceive of and define psychopathology, what they are trying to accomplish when they do this, and how and why these conceptions are the topic of continual debate and undergo continual revision.

We start by accepting the idea that psychopathology and related concepts are abstract ideas that are not scientifically constructed but *socially* constructed. *Social constructionism* involves "elucidating the process by which people come to describe, explain, or otherwise account for the world in which they live" (Gergen, 1985, pp. 3–4). Social constructionism is concerned with "examining ways in which people understand the world, the social and political processes that influence how people define words and explain events, and the implications of these definitions and explanations—who benefits and who loses because of how we describe and understand the world" (Muehlenhard & Kimes, 1999, p. 234). From this point of view, words and concepts such as psychopathology and mental disorder "are products of particular historical and cultural understandings rather than … universal and immutable categories of human experience" (Bohan, 1996, p. xvi). Universal or "true" definitions of concepts do not exist because these definitions depend primarily on who gets to do the defining. The people who define them are usually people with power, and so these definitions reflect and promote their interests and values (Muehlenhard & Kimes, 1999, p. 234). Therefore, "when less powerful people attempt to challenge existing power relationships and to promote social change, an initial battleground is often the words used to discuss these problems" (Muehlenhard & Kimes, 1999, p. 234). Because the interests of people and institutions are based on their values, debates over the definition of concepts often become clashes between deeply and implicitly held beliefs about the way the world works or should work and about the difference between right and wrong. Such clashes are evident in the debates over the definitions of terms such as *domestic violence* (Muehlenhard & Kimes, 1999), *child sexual abuse* (Holmes & Slapp, 1998; Rind, Tromovich, & Bauserman, 1998), and other such terms.

The social constructionist perspective can be contrasted with the *essentialist* perspective. Essentialism assumes that there are natural categories and that all members of a given category share important characteristics (Rosenblum & Travis, 1996). For example, the essentialist perspective views our categories of race, sexual orientation, and social class as objective categories that are independent of social or cultural processes. It views these categories as representing "empirically verifiable similarities among and differences between people" (Rosenblum & Travis, 1996, p. 2) and as "depict[ing] the inherent structure of the world in itself" (Zachar & Kendler, 2010, p. 128). In the social constructionist view, however, "reality cannot be separated from the way that a culture makes sense of it" (Rosenblum & Travis, 1996, p. 3). In social constructionism, such categories represent not what people *are*, but rather the ways that people think about and attempt to make sense of differences among people. Social processes also determine what differences among people are more important than other differences (Rosenblum & Travis, 1996).

Thus, from the essentialist perspective, psychopathologies and mental disorders are natural entities whose true nature can be discovered and described. From the social constructionist perspective, however, they are but abstract ideas that are defined by people and thus reflect their values—cultural, professional, and personal. The meanings of these and other concepts are not *revealed* by the methods of science but are *negotiated* among the people and institutions of society who have an interest in their definitions. In fact, we typically refer to psychological terms as *constructs* for this very reason—that their meanings are constructed and negotiated rather that discovered or revealed. The ways in which conceptions of so basic a psychological construct as the self (Baumeister, 1987) and self-esteem (Hewitt, 2002) have changed over time and the different ways they are conceived by different cultures (Cross & Markus, 1999; Cushman, 1995; Hewitt, 2002) provide an example of this process at work. Thus, "all categories of disorder, even physical disorder categories convincingly explored scientifically, are the product of human beings constructing meaningful systems for understanding their world" (Raskin & Lewandowski, 2000, p. 21). In addition, because "what it means to be a person is determined by cultural ways of talking about and conceptualizing personhood ... identity and disorder are socially constructed, and there are as many disorder constructions as there are cultures" (Neimeyer & Raskin, 2000, pp. 6–7; see also López & Guarnaccia, this volume). Finally, "if people cannot reach the objective truth about what disorder really is, then viable constructions of disorder must compete with one another on the basis of their use and meaningfulness in particular clinical situations" (Raskin & Lewandowski, 2000, p. 26).

From the social constructionist perspective, sociocultural, political, professional, and economic forces influence professional and lay conceptions of psychopathology. Our conceptions of psychological normality and abnormality are not facts about people but abstract ideas that are constructed through the implicit and explicit collaborations of theorists, researchers, professionals, their clients, and the culture in which all are embedded and that represent a shared view of the world and human nature. For this reason, mental disorders and the numerous diagnostic categories of the *DSM* were not "discovered" in the same manner that an archaeologist discovers a buried artifact or a medical researcher discovers a virus. Instead, they were invented (Raskin & Lewandowski, 2000). By saying that mental disorders are invented, however, we do not mean that they are "myths" (Szasz, 1974) or that the distress of people who are labeled as mentally disordered is not real. Instead, we mean that these disorders do not exist and have properties in the same manner that artifacts and viruses do. Therefore, a conception of psychopathology "does not simply describe and classify characteristics of groups of individuals, but ... actively constructs a version of both normal and abnormal ... which is then applied to individuals who end up being classified as normal or abnormal" (Parker, Georgaca, Harper, McLaughlin, & Stowell-Smith, 1995, p. 93).

Conceptions of psychopathology and the various categories of psychopathology are not mappings of psychological facts about people. Instead, they are social artifacts that serve the same sociocultural goals as do our conceptions of race, gender, social class, and sexual orientation—those of maintaining and expanding the power of certain individuals and institutions and maintaining social order, as defined by those in power (Beall, 1993; Parker et al., 1995; Rosenblum & Travis, 1996). As are these other social constructions, our concepts of psychological normality and abnormality are tied ultimately to social values—in particular, the values of society's most powerful individuals, groups, and institutions—and the contextual rules for behavior are derived from these values (Becker, 1963; Kirmeyer, 2005; Parker et al., 1995; Rosenblum & Travis, 1996). As McNamee and Gergen (1992) stated: "The mental health profession is not politically, morally, or valuationally neutral. Their practices typically operate to sustain certain values, political arrangements, and hierarchies of privilege" (p. 2). Thus, the debate over the definition of psychopathology, the struggle over who gets to define it, and the continual revisions of the *DSM* are not aspects of a search for "truth." Rather, they are debates over the definition of socially constructed abstractions and struggles for the personal, political, and economic power that derives from the authority to define these abstractions and thus to determine what and whom society views as normal and abnormal.

Millon (2010) has even suggested that the development of the *DSM–IV* was hampered by the reluctance of work groups to give up their rights over certain disorders once they were assigned them, even when it became clear that some disorders fit better with other work groups. In addition, over half of the members of the *DSM–IV* work groups (including every member of the work groups responsible for mood disorders and schizophrenia/psychotic disorders) had received financial support from pharmaceutical companies (Cosgrove, Krimsky, Vijayaragahavan, & Schneider, 2006).

As David Patrick (2005) concluded about a definition of mental disorder offered by the British government in a recent mental health bill, "The concept of mental disorder is of dubious scientific value but it has substantial political utility for several groups who are sane by mutual consent" (p. 435).

These debates and struggles are described in detail by Allan Horwitz (2000) in *Creating Mental Illness*. According to Horwitz:

> The emergence and persistence of an overly expansive disease model of mental illness was not accidental or arbitrary. The widespread creation of distinct mental diseases developed in specific historical circumstances and because of the interests of specific social groups.... By the time the *DSM-III* was developed in 1980, thinking of mental illnesses as discrete disease entities ... offered mental health professionals many social, economic, and political advantages. In addition, applying disease frameworks to a wide variety of behaviors and to a large number of people benefited a number of specific social groups including not only clinicians but also research scientists, advocacy groups, and pharmaceutical companies, among others. The disease entities of diagnostic psychiatry arose because they were useful for the social practices of various groups, not because they provided a more accurate way of viewing mental disorders. (p. 16)

Psychiatrist Mitchell Wilson (1993) has offered a similar position. He has argued that the dimensional/continuity view of psychological wellness and illness posed a basic problem for psychiatry because it "did not demarcate clearly the well from the sick" and that "if conceived of psychosocially, psychiatric illness is not the province of medicine, because psychiatric problems are not truly medical but social, political, and legal" (p. 402). The purpose of *DSM–III*, according to Wilson, was to allow psychiatry a means of marking out its professional territory. Kirk and Kutchins (1992) reached the same conclusion following their thorough review of the papers, letters, and memos of the various *DSM* working groups.

The social construction of psychopathology works something like this. Someone observes a pattern of behaving, thinking, feeling, or desiring that deviates from some social norm or ideal or identifies a human weakness or imperfection that, as expected, is displayed with greater frequency or severity by some people more than others. A group with influence and power decides that control, prevention, or "treatment" of this problem is desirable or profitable. The pattern is then given a scientific-sounding name, preferably of Greek or Latin origin. The new scientific name is capitalized. Eventually, the new term may be reduced to an acronym, such as OCD (obsessive-compulsive disorder), ADHD (attention-deficit/hyperactivity disorder), and BDD (body dysmorphic disorder). The new disorder then takes on an existence all its own and becomes a disease-like entity. As news about "it" spreads; people begin thinking they have "it";

medical and mental health professionals begin diagnosing and treating "it"; and clinicians and clients begin demanding that health insurance policies cover the "treatment" of "it." Once the "disorder" has been socially constructed and defined, the methods of science can be employed to study it, but the construction itself is a social process, not a scientific one. In fact, the more "it" is studied, the more everyone becomes convinced that "it" really is "something."

Medical philosopher Lawrie Reznek (1987) has demonstrated that even our definition of physical disease is socially constructed. He stated:

> Judging that some condition is a disease is to judge that the person with that condition is less able to lead a good or worthwhile life. And since this latter judgment is a normative one, to judge that some condition is a disease is to make a normative judgment.... This normative view of the concept of disease explains why cultures holding different values disagree over what are diseases.... Whether some condition is a disease depends on where we choose to draw the line of normality, and this is not a line that we can discover ... disease judgments, like moral judgments, are not factual ones. (pp. 211–212)

Likewise, Sedgwick (1982) points out that human diseases are natural processes. They may harm humans, but they actually promote the "life" of other organisms. For example, a virus's reproductive strategy may include spreading from human to human. Sedgwick stated:

> There are no illnesses or diseases in nature. The fracture of a septuagenarian's femur has, within the world of nature, no more significance than the snapping of an autumn leaf from its twig; and the invasion of a human organism by cholera-germs carries with it no more the stamp of "illness" than does the souring of milk by other forms of bacteria. Out of his anthropocentric self-interest, man has chosen to consider as "illnesses" or "diseases" those natural circumstances which precipitate death (or the failure to function according to certain values). (p. 30)

If these statements are true of physical disease, they are certainly true of psychological disease or psychopathology. Like our conception of physical disease, our conceptions of psychopathology are social constructions that are grounded in sociocultural goals and values, particularly our assumptions about how people should live their lives and about what makes life worth living. This truth is illustrated clearly in the American Psychiatric Association's 1952 decision to include homosexuality in the first edition of the *DSM* and its 1973 decision to revoke its "disease" status (Kutchins & Kirk, 1997; Shorter, 1997). As stated by Wilson (1993), "The homosexuality controversy seemed to show that psychiatric diagnoses were clearly wrapped up in social constructions of deviance" (p. 404). This issue also was in the forefront of the debates over posttraumatic stress disorder, paraphilic rapism, and masochistic personality disorder (Kutchins & Kirk, 1997), as well as caffeine dependence, sexual compulsivity, low-intensity orgasm, sibling rivalry, self-defeating personality, jet lag, pathological spending, and impaired sleep-related painful erections, all of which were proposed for inclusion in *DSM–IV* (Widiger & Trull, 1991). Others have argued convincingly that schizophrenia (Gilman, 1988), addiction (Peele, 1995), posttraumatic stress disorder (Herbert & Forman, 2010), personality disorder (Alarcon et al., 1998), dissociative identity disorder (formerly multiple personality disorder; Spanos, 1996), intellectual disability (Rapley, 2004), and both conduct disorder and oppositional defiant disorder (Mallet, 2007) also are socially constructed categories rather than disease entities.

With each revision, our most powerful professional conception of psychopathology, the *DSM*, has had more and more to say about how people should live their lives. Between 1952 and 2000, the number of pages in the *DSM* increased from 86 to 943, and the number of mental disorders listed increased from 106 to 385. As the scope of "mental disorder" has expanded with each *DSM* revision, life has become increasingly pathologized, and the sheer number of people with diagnosable mental disorders has continued to grow. Moreover, mental health professionals have not been content to label only obviously and blatantly dysfunctional patterns of behaving, thinking, and feeling as mental disorders. Instead, we have defined the scope of psychopathology to include many common problems in living.

Consider some of the mental disorders listed in the *DSM–IV* (American Psychiatric Association, 1996). Cigarette smokers have "nicotine dependence." If you drink large quantities of coffee, you may develop "caffeine intoxication" or "caffeine-induced sleep disorder." If you have "a preoccupation with a defect in appearance" that causes "significant distress or impairment in ... functioning" (p. 466), you have "body dysmorphic disorder." A child whose academic achievement is "substantially below that expected for age, schooling, and level of intelligence" (p. 46) has a "learning disorder." Toddlers who throw tantrums have "oppositional defiant disorder." Not wanting sex often enough is "hypoactive sexual desire disorder." Not wanting sex at all is "sexual aversion disorder." Having sex but not having orgasms or having them too late or too soon is an "orgasmic disorder." Failure (for men) to maintain "an adequate erection ... that causes marked distress or interpersonal difficulty" (p. 504) is "male erectile disorder." Failure (for women) to attain or maintain "an adequate lubrication or swelling response of sexual excitement" (p. 502) accompanied by distress is "female sexual arousal disorder."

Consider also some of the new disorders proposed for DSM–5 (expected publication, May, 2013): hypersexual disorder, temper dysregulation disorders of childhood, hoarding disorder, skin picking disorder, psychosis risk syndrome, among others. Psychiatrist Allen Frances (2010), the chair of the *DSM–IV* task force, argued that these new "disorders" and other changes represent a further encroachment of the *DSM* into the realm of common problems in living. (See Widiger and the chapters in Part II of this volume for a more detailed discussion of the proposed changes for DSM–5.)

The past few years have witnessed media reports of epidemics of Internet addiction, road rage, and "shopaholism." Discussions of these new disorders have turned up at scientific meetings and in courtrooms. They are likely to find a home in a future revision of the *DSM* if the media, mental health professions, and society at large continue to collaborate in their construction and if "treating" them and writing books about them become lucrative (Beato, 2010).

The social constructionist perspective does not deny that human beings experience behavioral and emotional difficulties—sometimes very serious ones. It insists, however, that such experiences are not evidence for the existence of entities called "mental disorders" that can then be invoked as causes of those behavioral and emotional difficulties. The belief in the existence of these entities is the product of the all too human tendency to socially construct categories in an attempt to make sense of a confusing world.

Summary and Conclusions

The debate over the conception or definition of psychopathology and related terms has been going on for decades, if not centuries, and will continue, just as we will always have debates over the definitions of truth, beauty, justice, and art. Our position is that psychopathology and mental disorder are not the kinds of terms whose "true" meanings can be discovered or defined objectively by employing the methods of science. They are social constructions—abstract ideas whose meanings are negotiated among the people and institutions of a culture and that reflect the values and power structure of that culture at a given time. Thus, the conception and definition of psychopathology always has been and always will be debated and continually changing. It is not a static and concrete thing whose true nature can be discovered and described once and for all.

By saying that conceptions of psychopathology are socially constructed rather than scientifically derived, we are not proposing, however, that human psychological distress and suffering are not real or that the patterns of thinking, feeling, and behaving that society decides to label psychopathology cannot be studied objectively and scientifically. Instead, we are saying that it is time to acknowledge that science can no more determine the "proper" or "correct" conception of psychopathology and mental disorder than it can determine the "proper" and "correct" conception of other social constructions, such as beauty, justice, race, and social class. We can nonetheless use science to study the phenomena that our culture refers to as psychopathological. We can use the methods of science to understand a culture's conception of mental or psychological health and disorder, how this conception has evolved, and how it affects individuals and society. We also can use the methods of science to understand the origins of the patterns of thinking, feeling, and behaving that a culture considers psychopathological and to develop and test ways of modifying those patterns.

Psychology and psychiatry will not be diminished by acknowledging that their basic concepts are socially and not scientifically constructed—no more than medicine is diminished by acknowledging that the notions of health and illness are socially constructed (Reznek, 1987), nor economics by acknowledging that the notions of poverty and wealth are socially constructed. Likewise, the recent controversy in astronomy over how to define the term *planet* (Zachar & Kendler, 2010) does not make astronomy any less scientific. Science cannot provide us with purely factual, scientific definitions of these concepts. They are fluid and negotiated constructs, not fixed matters of fact.

As Lilienfeld and Marino (1995) stated:

> Removing the imprimatur of science … would simply make the value judgments underlying these decisions more explicit and open to criticism … heated disputes would almost surely arise concerning which conditions are deserving of attention from mental health professionals. Such disputes, however, would at least be settled on the legitimate basis of social values and exigencies, rather than on the basis of ill-defined criteria of doubtful scientific status. (pp. 418–419)

References

Alarcon, R. D., Foulks, E. F., & Vakkur, M. (1998). *Personality disorders and culture: Clinical and conceptual interactions.* New York: Wiley.

American Psychiatric Association. (1996). *Diagnostic and statistical manual of mental disorders* (4th ed.). Washington, DC: Author.

American Psychiatric Association. (2000). *Diagnostic and statistical manual of mental disorders* (4th ed., text revision). Washington, DC: Author.

Anthony, J. L., Lonigan, C. J., & Hecht, S. A. (1999). Dimensionality of post-traumatic stress disorder symptoms in children exposed to disaster: Results from a confirmatory factor analysis. *Journal of Abnormal Psychology, 108*, 315–325.

Barkley, R. A. (2005). *Attention-deficit hyperactivity disorder: A handbook for diagnosis and treatment* (3rd ed.). New York: Guilford.

Baumeister, R. F. (1987). How the self became a problem: A psychological review of historical research. *Journal of Personality and Social Psychology, 52*, 163–176.

Baumeister, R. F., & Scher, S. J. (1988). Self-defeating behavior patterns among normal individuals: Review and analysis of common self-destructive tendencies. *Psychological Bulletin, 104*(1), 3–22.

Beall, A. E. (1993). A social constructionist view of gender. In A. E. Beall & R. J. Sternberg (Eds.), *The psychology of gender* (pp. 127–147). New York: Guilford.

Beato, G. (2010, August–September). Internet addiction: What once was parody may soon be diagnosis. *Reason,* 16–17.

Becker, H. S. (1963). *Outsiders.* New York: Free Press.

Bergner, R. M. (1997). What is psychopathology? And so what? *Clinical Psychology: Science and Practice, 4*, 235–248.

Bohan, J. (1996). *The psychology of sexual orientation: Coming to terms.* New York: Routledge.

Brown, R. P., Budzek, K., & Tamborski, M. (2009). On the meaning and measure of narcissism. *Personality and Social Psychology Bulletin, 35*, 951–964.

Carver, C. S. (2001). Affect and the functional bases of behavior: On the dimensional structure of affective experience. *Personality and Social Psychology Review, 5,* 345–356.

Cosgrove, L., Krimsky, S., Vijayaraghaven, M., & Schneider, L. (2006). Financial ties between DSM-IV panel members and the pharmaceutical industry. *Psychotherapy and Psychosomatics, 75,* 154–160.

Claridge, G. (1995). *Origins of mental illness.* Cambridge, MA: Malor Books/ISHK.

Cosmides, L., Tooby, J., & Barkow, J. H. (1992). Introduction: Evolutionary psychology and conceptual integration. In J. H. Barkow, L. Cosmides, & J. Tooby (Eds.), *The adapted mind: Evolutionary psychology and the generation of culture* (pp. 3–17). New York: Oxford University Press.

Costello, C. G. (1993a). *Symptoms of depression.* New York: Wiley.

Costello, C. G. (1993b). *Symptoms of schizophrenia.* New York: Wiley.

Cross, S. E., & Markus, H. R. (1999). The cultural constitution of personality. In L. A. Pervin & O. P. John (Eds.), *Handbook of personality: Theory and Research* (2nd ed., pp. 378–396). New York: Guilford.

Cushman, P. (1995). *Constructing the self, constructing America.* New York: Addison-Wesley.

Eaton, W. W., Kessler, R. C., Wittchen, H. U., & Magee, W. J. (1994). Panic and panic disorder in the United States. *American Journal of Psychiatry, 51,* 413–420.

Edens, J. F., Marcus, D. K., Lilienfeld, S. O., & Poythress, N. G. (2006). Psychopathic, not psychopath: Taxometric evidence for the dimensional structure of psychopathy. *Journal of Abnormal Psychology, 115,* 131–144.

Eisenberg, D. P., Aniskin, D. B., White, L., Stein, J. A., Harvey, P. D., & Galynker, I. I. (2009). Structural differences within negative and depressive syndrome dimensions in schizophrenia, organic brain disease, and major depression: A confirmatory factor analysis of the positive and negative syndrome scale. *Psychopathology, 42,* 242–248.

Flett, G. L., Vredenburg, K., & Krames, L. (1997). The continuity of depression in clinical and nonclinical samples. *Psychological Bulletin, 121,* 395–416.

Fossati, A. (2003). Personality disorders and adult attachment dimensions in a mixed psychiatric sample: A multivariate study. *Journal of Nervous and Mental Disease, 191,* 30–37.

Fraley, R. C., & Waller, N. G. (1998). Adult attachment patterns: A test of the typological model. In J. A. Simpson & W. S. Rholes (Eds.), *Attachment theory and close relationships* (pp. 77–114). New York: Guilford.

Frances, A. (2010). Opening Pandora's Box: The 19 worst suggestions for DSM5. *Psychiatric Times,* February 11, 2010.

Gardner, H. (1999). *Intelligence reframed: Multiple intelligences for the 21st century.* Cambridge, MA: Basic Books.

Gergen, K. J. (1985). The social constructionist movement in modern psychology. *American Psychologist, 40*(3), 266–275.

Gilman, S. L. (1988). *Disease and representation: Images of illness from madness to AIDS.* Ithaca, NY: Cornell University Press.

Gorenstein, E. E. (1984). Debating mental illness: Implications for science, medicine, and social policy. *American Psychologist, 39,* 50–56.

Grove, W. M., & Vrieze, S. I. (2010). On the substantive grounding and clinical utility of categories versus dimensions. In T. Millon, R. F. Krueger, & E. Simonsen (Eds.), *Contemporary directions in psychopathology: Scientific foundations of the DSM-V and ICD-11* (pp. 303–323). New York: Guilford.

Hankin, B. L., Fraley, R. C., Lahey, B. B., & Waldman, I. D. (2005). Is depression best viewed as a continuum or a discrete category? A taxonomic analysis of childhood and adolescent depression in a population-based sample. *Journal of Abnormal Psychology, 114,* 96–110.

Hankin, B. L., Kassel, J. D., & Abela, J. R. Z. (2005). Adult attachment dimensions and specificity of emotional distress symptoms: Prospective investigations of cognitive risk and interpersonal stress generation as mediating mechanisms. *Personality and Social Psychology Bulletin, 31,* 136–151.

Herbert, J. D., & Forman, E. M. (2010). Cross-cultural perspectives on posttraumatic stress. In G. M. Rosen & B. C. Frueh (Eds.), *Clinician's guide to posttraumatic stress disorder* (pp. 235–262). New York: Wiley.

Hewitt, J. P. (2002). The social construction of self-esteem. In C. R. Snyder & S. J. Lopez (Eds.), *Handbook of positive psychology* (pp. 135–147). New York: University Press.

Holmes, W. C., & Slapp, G. B. (1998). Sexual abuse of boys: Definition, prevalence, correlates, sequelae, and management. *Journal of the American Medical Association, 280,* 1855–1862.

Horwitz, A. V. (2002). *Creating mental illness.* Chicago: University of Chicago Press.

Johns, L. C., & van Os, J. (2001). The continuity of psychotic experiences in the general population. *Clinical Psychology Review, 21,* 1125–1141.

Keyes, C. L., & Lopez, S. J. (2002). Toward a science of mental health: Positive directions in diagnosis and interventions. In C. R. Snyder & S. J. Lopez (Eds.), *Handbook of positive psychology* (pp. 45–59). London: Oxford University Press.

Kirk, S. A., & Kutchins, H. (1992). *The selling of DSM: The rhetoric of science in psychiatry.* New York: Aldine de Gruyter.

Kirmeyer, L. J. (2005). Culture, context and experience in psychiatric diagnosis. *Psychopathology, 38,* 192–196.

Krueger, R. F., Markon, K. E., Patrick, C. J., & Iacono, W. G. (2005). Externalizing psychopathology in adulthood: A dimensional-spectrum conceptualization and its implications for *DSM-V. Journal of Abnormal Psychology, 114,* 537–550.

Kutchins, H., & Kirk, S. A. (1997). *Making us crazy: DSM: The psychiatric bible and the creation of mental disorder.* New York: Free Press.

Larsson, H., Andershed, H., & Lichtenstein, P. (2006). A genetic factor explains most of the variation in the psychopathic personality. *Journal of Abnormal Psychology, 115,* 221–230.

Leising, D., Rogers, K., & Ostner, J. (2009). The undisordered personality: Assumptions underlying personality disorder diagnoses. *Review of General Psychology, 13,* 230–241.

Lilienfeld, S. O., & Marino, L. (1995). Mental disorder as a Roschian concept: A critique of Wakefield's "harmful dysfunction" analysis. *Journal of Abnormal Psychology, 104*(3), 411–420.

Livesley, W. J., Jang, K. L., & Vernon, P. A. (1998). Phenotypic and genotypic structure of traits delineating personality disorder. *Archives of General Psychiatry, 55,* 941–948.

Lubinski, D. (2000). Scientific and social significance of assessing individual differences: "Sinking shafts at a few critical points." *Annual Review of Psychology, 51,* 405–444.

Maddux, J. E., & Mundell, C. E. (1999). Disorders of personality: Diseases or individual differences? In V. J. Derlega, B. A. Winstead, & W. H. Jones (Eds.), *Personality: Contemporary theory and research* (2nd ed., pp. 541–571). Chicago: Nelson-Hall.

Mallett, C. A. (2007). Behaviorally-based disorders: The social construction of youths' most prevalent psychiatric diagnoses. *History of Psychiatry, 18,* 435–457.

McNamee, S., & Gergen, K. J. (1992). *Therapy as social construction.* Thousand Oaks, CA: Sage.

Millon, T., & Simonsen, E. (2010). A precis of psychopathological history. In T. Millon, R. F. Krueger, & E. Simonsen (Eds.), *Contemporary directions in psychopathology: Scientific foundations of the DSM IV and ICD-11* (pp. 3–52). New York: Guilford.

Muehlenhard, C. L., & Kimes, L. A. (1999). The social construction of violence: The case of sexual and domestic violence. *Personality and Social Psychology Review, 3,* 234–245.

Neimeyer, R. A., & Raskin, J. D. (2000). On practicing postmodern therapy in modern times. In R. A. Neimeyer & J. D. Raskin (Eds.), *Constructions of disorder: Meaning-making frameworks for psychotherapy* (pp. 3–14). Washington, DC: American Psychological Association.

Nettle, D. (2001). *Strong imagination: Madness, creativity, and human nature.* Oxford: Oxford University Press.

Oatley, K., & Jenkins, J. M. (1992). Human emotions: Function and dysfunction. *Annual Review of Psychology, 43,* 55–85.

Oatley, K., Keltner, D., & Jenkins, J. M. (2006). *Understanding emotions.* Oxford: Blackwell.

Ossorio, P. G. (1985). Pathology. *Advances in Descriptive Psychology, 4,* 151–201.

Parker, I., Georgaca, E., Harper, D., McLaughlin, T., & Stowell-Smith, M. (1995). *Deconstructing psychopathology.* London: Sage.

Patrick, D. (2005). Defining mental disorder: Tautology in the service of sanity in British mental health legislation. *Journal of Mental Health, 14,* 435–443.

Peele, S. (1995). *Diseasing of America: How we allowed recovery zealots and the treatment industry to convince us we are out of control.* San Francisco: Lexington Books.

Rapley, M. (2004). *The social construction of intellectual disability.* Cambridge: Cambridge University Press.

Raskin, J. D., & Lewandowski, A. M. (2000). The construction of disorder as human enterprise. In R. A. Neimeyer & J. D. Raskin (Eds.), *Constructions of disorder: Meaning-making frameworks for psychotherapy* (pp. 15–40). Washington, DC: American Psychological Association.

Reznek, L. (1987). *The nature of disease.* London: Routledge and Kegan Paul.

Rind, B., Tromovich, P., & Bauserman, R. (1998). A meta-analytic examination of assumed properties of child sexual abuse using college samples. *Psychological Bulletin, 124,* 22–53.

Rosen, G. M., & Lilienfeld, S. O. (2008). Posttraumatic stress disorder: An empirical evaluation of core assumptions. *Clinical Psychology Review, 28,* 837–868.

Rosenblum, K. E., & Travis, T. C. (1996). Constructing categories of difference: Framework essay. In K. E. Rosenblum & T. C. Travis (Eds.), *The meaning of difference: American constructions of race, sex and gender, social class, and sexual orientation* (pp. 1–34). New York: McGraw-Hill.

Rosenman, S., Korten, A., Medway, J., & Evans, M. (2003). Dimensional vs. categorical diagnosis in psychosis. *Acta Psychiatrica Scandinavica, 107*, 378–384.

Ruscio, A. M., Ruscio, J., & Keane, T. M. (2002). The latent structure of posttraumatic stress disorder: A taxometric investigation of reactions to extreme stress. *Journal of Abnormal Psychology, 111*, 290–301.

Sadler, J. Z. (1999). Horsefeathers: A commentary on "Evolutionary versus prototype analyses of the concept of disorder." *Journal of Abnormal Psychology, 108*, 433–437.

Sedgwick, P. (1982). *Psycho politics: Laing, Foucault, Goffman, Szasz, and the future of mass psychiatry.* New York: Harper and Row.

Selby, E. A., & Joiner, T. E. (2009). Cascades of emotion: The emergence of borderline personality disorder from emotional and behavioral dysregulation. *Review of General Psychology, 13*, 219–229.

Shaywitz, S. E., Escobar, M. D., Shaywitz, B. A., Fletcher, J. M., & Makuch, R. (1992). Evidence that dyslexia may represent the lower tail of a normal distribution of reading ability. *New England Journal of Medicine, 326*(3), 145–150.

Shaywitz, S. E., Morris, R., & Shaywitz, B. A. (2008). The education of dyslexic children from childhood to young adulthood. *Annual Review of Psychology, 59*, 451–475.

Shorter, E. (1997). *A history of psychiatry: From the era of the asylum to the age of Prozac.* New York: Wiley.

Simonsen, E. (2010). The integration of categorical and dimensional approaches to psychopathology. In T. Millon, R. F. Krueger, & E. Simonsen (Eds.). *Contemporary directions in psychopathology: Scientific foundations of the DSM-V and ICD-11* (pp. 350–361). New York: Guilford.

Snowling, M. J. (2006). Language and learning to read: The dyslexic spectrum. In M. J. Snowling & J. Stackhouse (Eds.), *Dyslexia, speech and language: A practitioner's handbook* (pp. 1–15). Hoboken, NJ: Wiley.

Spanos, N. P. (1996). *Multiple identities and false memories: A sociocognitive perspective.* Washington, DC: American Psychological Association.

Szasz, T. S. (1974). *The myth of mental illness.* New York: Harper and Row.

van Os, J., Verdoux, H., Maurice-Tison, S., Gay, B., Liarud, F., Salamon, R., … Bourgeois, M. (1999). Self-reported psychosis-like symptoms and the continuum of psychosis. *Social Psychiatry and Psychiatric Epidemiology, 34*, 459–463.

Wakefield, J. C. (1992a). The concept of mental disorder: On the boundary between biological facts and social values. *American Psychologist, 47*(3), 373–388.

Wakefield, J. C. (1992b). Disorder as harmful dysfunction: A conceptual critique of DSM-III-R's definition of mental disorder. *Psychological Review, 99*, 232–247.

Wakefield, J. C. (1993). Limits of operationalization: A critique of Spitzer and Endicott's (1978) proposed operational criteria for mental disorder. *Journal of Abnormal Psychology, 102*, 160–172.

Wakefield, J. C. (1997). Normal inability versus pathological inability: Why Ossorio's definition of mental disorder is not sufficient. *Clinical Psychology: Science and Practice, 4*, 249–258.

Wakefield, J. C. (1999). Evolutionary versus prototype analyses of the concept of disorder. *Journal of Abnormal Psychology, 108*, 374–399.

Wakefield, J. C. (2006). Personality disorder as harmful dysfunction: DSM's cultural deviance criterion reconsidered. *Journal of Personality Disorders, 20*(2), 157–169.

Wakefield, J. C., Horwitz, A. V., & Schmitz, M. F. (2006). Are we overpathologizing the socially anxious? Social phobia from a harmful dysfunction perspective. *Canadian Journal of Psychiatry, 50*(6), 317–427.

Widiger, T. A. (1997). The construct of mental disorder. *Clinical Psychology: Science and Practice, 4*, 262–266.

Weinberger, J., Siefert, C., & Haggerty, G. (2010). Implicit processes in social and clinical psychology. In J. E. Maddux & J. P. Tangney (Eds.). *Social psychological foundations of clinical psychology.* New York: Guilford.

Widiger, T. A., & Trull, T. J. (1991). Diagnosis and clinical assessment. *Annual Review of Psychology, 42*, 109–134.

Widiger, T. A., & Trull, T. J. (2007). Plate tectonics in the classification of personality disorder. *American Psychologist, 62*, 71–83.

Wilson, M. (1993). DSM-III and the transformation of American psychiatry: A history. *American Journal of Psychiatry, 150*, 399–410.

Zachar, P., & Kendler, K. S. (2010). Philosophical issues in the classification of psychopathology. In T. Millon, R. F. Krueger, & E. Simonsen (Eds.) *Contemporary directions in psychopathology: Scientific foundations of the DSM-V adn ICD-11* (pp. 127–148). New York: Guilford.

2

Biological Bases of Psychopathology

ROBERT F. SMITH

George Mason University
Fairfax, Virginia

Behavior, including pathological behavior, has its origin in brain functioning. Many of our current treatments for pathological behavior are biological in nature (e.g., drugs altering neurotransmitter systems), and, more and more, noninvasive imaging techniques are being used to study and diagnose brain abnormalities associated with some forms of psychopathology. Understanding psychopathology ultimately must include an understanding of its biological bases. This chapter introduces some important issues in understanding the biology of psychopathology, including recent work that holds promise of a deeper explanation of the nature nurture interaction.

Introduction to the Human Brain

The human brain is the most complex organ known to science, and this chapter cannot do justice to its complexity. The purpose of this chapter is to introduce the brain and its functioning to students who have never had a course in biological psychology. The bulk of the chapter, however, will focus on our evolving understanding of the role of the brain and related systems in psychopathology, including chemical underpinnings of disorders, developmental origins of those disorders, the role of brain connectivity in normal and abnormal information processing, and emerging knowledge of what guides brain development in normal and abnormal directions.

Box 2.1 presents a minitutorial on brain terminology. It is intended to impart a minimal command of some important concepts and terminology; readers interested in more in-depth information are referred to textbooks on biological psychology (Carlson, 2007; Meyer & Quenzer, 2005).

Box 2.2 summarizes just a few of the important neurotransmitters and the concept of second messenger systems involved in brain function and some aspects of psychopathology. As this chapter will emphasize, this summary only reflects the current understanding of the role of particular neurotransmitters; that understanding is certain to evolve as research reveals new information.

The brain is far more complex than these boxes outline. As an indicator of its complexity, it probably consists of about 100 billion neurons, each with up to 10,000 connections to other neurons. Any particular function or behavior typically involves thousands to millions of these neurons, usually in several different brain areas. Neurons interact in ways that influence other neurons; a simple perception such as an odor may be initially processed in the olfactory system, but a connection to another area of brain may also trigger a distant memory of an experience associated with that odor, and that area may then trigger emotional reactions—fear or pleasure—associated with the earlier experience. Our experiences rely on, and our behavior is a product of, shifting patterns of electrochemical activity wafting across loosely connected networks of neurons, influenced by current events; yet they are also a product of past experiences,

BOX 2.1.   A MINITUTORIAL ON BRAIN TERMINOLOGY

Neuron: nerve cell. Neurons usually have distinctive projections from the cell body, which process information. A human brain has around 100 billion neurons.

Dendrite: projection from a nerve cell that is specialized for receiving incoming signals from other neurons. Dendrites have large numbers of receptors for *neurotransmitters*.

Axon: projection from a neuron that is specialized for sending signals, sometimes over very long distances; motor neurons in the spinal cord have axons that reach all the way to the toes. An electrical signal (*action potential*) reaching the end of an axon releases chemicals called *neurotransmitters*, which then chemically interact with receptors on dendrites of the next neurons, which may result in a signal in that neuron.

Action potential: an electrical signal conducted down an axon. Action potentials are biological signals that involve both chemicals (movement of ions, or charged particles of sodium and potassium) and the voltage shifts that accompany ion movement. A full review of it is beyond the scope here, but note that both chemical changes and electrical activity can influence signaling, as signaling involves both.

Synapse: the junction between axon and dendrite, where neurotransmitters transmit information between neurons. Interactions at the synapse are so complex that it is difficult to express that complexity adequately. Each neuron may have hundreds to thousands of synaptic inputs, and whether that neuron fires (has an *action potential*) typically depends on the sum of *excitatory* and *inhibitory* input from a large subset of those inputs.

Neurotransmitters: the chemicals that convey information between neurons. This is not the same as electrical action. Neurotransmitters may chemically *excite* the next neuron (making it more likely to conduct an electrical signal) or *inhibit* it (making it less likely), and thousands of excitatory and inhibitory synapses may interact on a given neuron. Neurotransmitters may act by opening or closing ion channels (thus altering the electrical charge of the neuron) and by activating chains of chemical events called *second messenger systems*, which may alter electrical activity and metabolic activity, protein synthesis, and gene expression. It is believed there are about 200 chemicals that serve as neurotransmitters, with just a few of them listed in Box 2.2.

Learning and memory: to the best of our current knowledge, learning consists of changes in synapses. Changes can include strengthening the connections at a group of synapses, controlling a particular aspect of behavior, and even growing new synapses. Even the adult brain is a very dynamic organism, and formation of new connections, breaking of old and less-used ones, and generation and loss of nerve cells seem to be common events. Most of these changes seem to involve the chemical sequences known as second messenger systems. Changes in the brain during development, which have similar mechanisms of change, will be discussed later in the chapter.

Connectivity: the sequence of activation patterns between major brain areas. In an individual who reads, activity is evoked in visual, language, and thought areas of brain. In an illiterate individual who looks at the same text, activity occurs only in visual areas; we say that the connectivity of the literate and illiterate brain are different.

BOX 2.2.   NEUROTRANSMITTERS AND BEHAVIOR

Complex chemical processes are used to synthesize neurotransmitters and their *receptors*, which are also complex molecules. Drugs that alter neurotransmitters can act in a variety of ways. They can increase *synthesis* of a transmitter, increase its *release*, slow down its *chemical breakdown* so that it can act for a longer period of time, imitate it to *stimulate receptors*, or *block receptors* to block the transmitter action. Only a small fraction of the 200 or so chemicals thought to be transmitters have been connected to various forms of psychopathology. Although the following list is oversimplified, here are some associations between a few transmitters and the functions and malfunctions they are thought to be involved in:

Dopamine: part of the brain's reinforcement system. Involved in addictions (it is a critical transmitter for perceptions of pleasure), in schizophrenia (antipsychotic drugs block dopamine receptors), and in control of movement, it is the main transmitter associated with Parkinson's disease, which is accompanied by loss of many dopamine-producing cells and treated by therapies to increase dopamine availability.

Serotonin: first associated with sleep, now also thought to be involved in depression.

Glutamate: first associated with neural bases of learning, now also thought to be involved in growth and development processes (the processes of growing the brain and forming new connections during learning are fairly similar). Glutamate is a widespread neurotransmitter, and it appears to be involved in many forms of learning, from simple associations to complex learning.

GABA: an acronym for gamma-aminobutyric acid, this transmitter inhibits or slows down firing of nerve cells. Antianxiety drugs act mainly to increase GABA activity.

Cannabinoids: receptors for chemicals, resembling those in marijuana, have recently been found in the brain, as have naturally occurring chemicals that normally interact with those receptors. A major function of cannabinoid systems seems to be modulating release of other transmitters, including those in the dopamine reinforcement system. Cannabinoids are currently targets of several kinds of research on potential therapeutic agents.

Second messenger systems: many neurotransmitters, not just the few listed above, act through second messenger systems. Typically, a neurotransmitter (the "first messenger") binds to a receptor, usually located on a dendrite. That receptor then activates an enzyme (the "second messenger") within the dendrite, and the enzyme then chemically changes the shape of one or several proteins within the dendrite. Those changed proteins can do several things, such as activate gene expression to stimulate changes such as growth or production of more receptors, change existing receptors (to make them more sensitive or less sensitive), open or close channels that permit passage of ions and thus directly affect the likelihood of an action potential, activate microRNAs, or enable a variety of other chemical events in the postsynaptic dendrite. Second messenger systems enable neurotransmitters to have a remarkable range of effects, not just to trigger an action potential.

with some experiences having only transient effects and others processed and repeated to the point where they become persistent parts of us.

With such a staggering degree of complexity, it is hardly surprising that we do not yet fully understand the brain. Work is actively continuing on such topics as determining transmitter bases of cue learning in drug addiction, biological signaling systems that lead to progressive loss of brain tissue in early-onset schizophrenia, gene expression abnormalities that produce brain malformations characteristic of autism, transmitter basis of individual differences in aspects of personality such as temperament and sensation seeking, mechanisms underlying effects of prenatal drugs and chemicals on brain growth, mechanisms underlying environmental effects on brain growth and development, and many others. Despite the complexity, however, research has already revealed much about different aspects of the brain that function abnormally in several types of psychopathology and the neurotransmitter basis of some disorders and their drug therapies.

The brain also has more far-reaching effects than one might guess. The brain is situated within, and interacts extensively with, the entire body. The brain not only controls behavior, it also controls most hormones by controlling the pituitary gland, including hormones associated with sexual behavior, thyroid function, and reactions to stress (Carlson, 2007). Control of hormones is often influenced by psychological processes such as perceptions of stress and of the degree of personal control over stress, and, as explained later, by events that influence the development of the stress response system. Through hormones and through direct nerve connections, the brain also strongly influences the immune system (Wrona, 2006). Both hormones and immune signals can signal the brain. The brain has receptors for most or all hormones and immune signals, through which they can influence brain activity and therefore behavior. Literally, the state of our health and hormonal systems can influence behavior, and our mental health can influence our hormones and our physical health, acting through now-established biological mechanisms. So, when a person suffering from a psychiatric disorder also has a depressed immune system or abnormal levels of stress hormones, the association of psychopathology with disorders of these other systems might go in either direction—pathology in brain function might cause disorders in other systems, or disorders in other systems can trigger psychopathology, as later chapters discuss for depression and schizophrenia. This interaction is an underlying mechanism behind the observation that some psychiatric disorders also result in higher levels of physical illness, and it is the reason that a thorough physical examination is important for individuals with psychopathology. Many times antidepressant medication will be prescribed, while the person is really suffering from a low thyroid hormone level. In general, treating the cause of a disorder is more effective than treating a symptom.

Brain Abnormalities Associated With Psychopathology

In recent years, advances have been made in understanding and treating many psychological disorders using biological techniques. The early, and often accidental, findings that some drugs alleviated psychiatric symptoms led to the development of modern psychotherapeutic drugs and to the hypotheses of the 1950s and 1960s that many psychiatric disorders were a result of imbalances in neurotransmitter systems. Early attempts to verify this through postmortem studies found a number of transmitter differences associated with particular disorders (e.g., between individuals with schizophrenia and normal controls), although we now regard problems associated with these early drug studies (i.e., a lapse of many hours between death and tissue preservation, sometimes coupled with sketchy diagnostic information) as problematic for interpretation of the information obtained. In the 1990s, newly available noninvasive imaging technology largely confirmed, and considerably refined and extended, those early hypotheses, and continuing pharmaceutical development allowed us to refine, revise, and focus our hypotheses concerning the neurochemical bases of many disorders. What exactly do we know today about the neural bases of psychological disorders?

Inferences From Psychiatric Drug Effects

First, we have learned that there are fairly effective treatments for many disorders. Commonly used treatments for schizophrenia, depression, attention-deficit/hyperactivity disorder (ADHD) and anxiety are listed in Table 2.1. Several other disorders have recently been treated successfully with drugs in some individuals, including obsessive-compulsive disorder and some types of addiction. Generally (but see below), the drug treatments tend to be fairly effective, which is good news for professionals treating these disorders and for their clients. How much information this gives us about each disorder's cause, however, is a different story. Why?

For some disorders, the mode of action of the drugs is rather well established. For schizophrenia, for example, it is well accepted that antipsychotic drugs are dopamine receptor blockers—their therapeutic effect is closely related to their effectiveness in reducing activity in the dopamine neurotransmitter system (Seeman, 1987). That does not, however, necessarily imply that schizophrenia *is* an overactivity in the dopamine system. Why? Treating a symptom effectively does not imply that one is treating a cause of the symptom. As an example, if you treat an infection-induced fever with aspirin instead of antibiotics, you can reduce the fever without getting rid of the infection. This also holds true for the brain: early treatments for the motor disorder Parkinson's disease (marked by tremor, postural and motor changes, and loss of brain dopamine neurons) included fairly effective use of drugs that block another transmitter, acetylcholine. More modern treatments increase levels of dopamine, but the early treatments had apparent effects by bringing an acetylcholine/dopamine balance closer to normal. Even dopamine-based treatments do not address the cause, which is a progressive loss of dopamine neurons due to one of several agents or processes that can kill them. So, finding that a drug alleviates a disorder does not necessarily tell us the actual cause of that disorder.

For other effective drugs, the mode of clinical action remains in dispute. For treating depression, several classes of drugs are listed in Table 2.1. Each of them has been found to alleviate depression in some people (but note that placebos are also effective in many people). None of them is effective in every person suffering from depression. Each drug, however, has a number

Table 2.1 Examples of Drugs Used for Treating Psychological Disorders

Disorder	Drug Action	Generic Name	Trade Name
Depression	MAO inhibition	Phenelzine	Nardil
	Tricyclic	Amitriptyline	Elavil
		Imipramine	Tofranil
	SSRI	Fluoxetine	Prozac
		Sertraline	Zoloft
		Paroxetine	Paxil
Anxiety Disorders	GABA agonist	Diazepam	Valium
Schizophrenia	DA receptor blocker	Haloperidol	Haldol
		Chlorpromazine	Thorazine
		Thioridazine	Mellaril
		Trifluoperazine	Stelazine
		Clozapine	Clozaril
ADHD	Various stimulants	Methylphenidate	Ritalin
		Amphetamine	Adderall

MAO, monoamine oxidase; SSRI, selective serotonin reuptake inhibitor; DA, dopaminergic.

of direct and indirect effects on the brain, and determining which of those effects actually is the therapeutic mechanism has been difficult. There is some consensus, mostly based on improved effectiveness of the selective serotonin reuptake inhibitors (SSRIs) such as Prozac, that depression is a serotonin-based phenomenon, but that is not yet a universally accepted conclusion. Recent research suggests that antidepressants also stimulate neurogenesis (formation of new neurons, even in adult brains; Malberg, Eisch, Nestler, & Duman, 2000) and increase levels of a transmitter involved in neural and dendritic growth, called brain-derived neurotrophic factor (BDNF; Levinson, 2006; Molteni et al., 2006). There is growing opinion that, although drugs may alleviate depression, the underlying cause may be a long-lasting change in neural circuitry, possibly triggered by stress interacting with particular gene systems (Lee, Jeong, Kwak, & Park, 2010). However, this has not yet been proven. Clearly, when a drug has several chemical and even anatomical effects and helps depression, it is difficult to determine which of those effects is the reason for the antidepressant action of the drug.

No single drug is universally effective for depression. Pharmaceutical treatment of depression is largely a matter of conducting experiments on a patient until one finds the best treatment. Family history (Was there a depressed family member treated successfully with a drug?), particular symptoms, and research findings can inform that decision, but it is still an individual experiment. This frequent observation may imply that depression can have different underlying mechanisms in different individuals.

With these cautions in mind, we can make some statements about what drug therapies suggest about the causes of various disorders. It is moderately clear that effective therapies for schizophrenia reduce activity in the dopamine system, that drugs for anxiety stimulate GABA receptors, that stimulants for ADHD activate catecholamine (dopamine and norepinephrine) systems, but we do not know exactly the basis for treatment for depression. But a caution for the future remains: *what we now think about the underlying chemical bases of mental disorders may prove in the future to be in error.*

Noninvasive Imaging Studies

Are psychiatric disorders merely chemical imbalances in the brain? In recent years, techniques for studying the chemistry and blood flow of a living brain have allowed us to study brain structure and activity in the live individual and thus to compare brains in normal individuals to brains of individuals with specific disorders. Brain areas have long been linked to specific aspects of normal and pathological behavior, and new techniques have emerged to largely confirm earlier research and considerably amplify our knowledge. Noninvasive techniques include magnetic resonance imaging (MRI) and its offspring functional MRI (fMRI; the former is like an enhanced X-ray in that it gives a static picture, the latter reflects dynamic changes over time, and both primarily look at blood flow to various brain areas), positron emission tomography (PET, which uses tiny amounts of radioactively labeled chemicals to identify locations of particular neurotransmitter receptors), and a variety of other techniques to spy on the chemistry, metabolism, and electrical activity of the living brain (Otte & Halsband, 2006).

Studies using these techniques have largely confirmed some hypotheses about the neurochemical bases of some disorders. For example, D_2 dopamine receptors are more numerous in several brain areas of many, but not all, schizophrenics (Huizink & Mulder, 2006; Wong et al., 1986), and dopamine release is elevated in many, but not all, individuals with schizophrenia (Laruelle et al., 1996), which fits well with the inference from drug studies that schizophrenia might be an overactivity of some aspect of the dopamine system. Schizophrenic individuals also have a well-documented underactivity of areas of prefrontal cortex, which seems to be related to attentional deficits (MacDonald & Carter, 2003). But the picture of the biological bases of schizophrenia is complicated by a number of apparent discrepancies between different individuals. Some schizophrenics have elevated D_2 dopamine receptors, while others do not. Some have loss of brain tissue, but some do not; some respond to antipsychotic drugs, but some do not. Some have acute onset in early adulthood, while some begin deteriorating in middle childhood. Further complicating the picture is that recent work has shown that severe early-onset schizophrenia is accompanied by progressive loss of cortical tissue throughout adolescence; literally, children with schizophrenia progressively lose cortical tissue at a rate that far exceeds normal developmental changes (Thompson et al., 2001). In addition to these changes, individuals with schizophrenia have different patterns of brain connectivity—the sequencing, timing, and strength of activation in brain areas—in a substantial number of brain systems, ranging from attentional to language processing systems (Henseler, Falkai, & Gruber, 2010; Lynall et al., 2010). Schizophrenics with negative symptoms, such as emotional and social withdrawal, show larger connectivity differences than positive symptom individuals, such as hearing voices (Shaw, Gogtay, & Rapoport, 2010). These findings suggest that the brains of schizophrenics are substantially maldeveloped, which leads to different patterns of information processing than in normal individuals. Although there is no real current consensus on the cause(s) of schizophrenia, it appears that it is a neurodevelopmental disorder in many cases (Rapoport, Addington, Frangou, & Psych, 2005), that is, a genetic predisposition exacerbated by unknown developmental influences. Prenatal viruses and stress are among the possible causes that have been suggested, and there may be different triggers for different individuals. In particular, it is thought that progressive brain maldevelopment results in abnormal connections between the frontal lobes and dopamine neurons, altering the normal control of thoughts and behaviors.

Noninvasive techniques are revolutionizing our understanding of the neural basis of psychopathology, but even with noninvasives, the experimental design, method of analysis, and choice of dependent measures can influence what one might find. For example, in evaluating gross levels of blood flow, one can conclude that schizophrenics have an underactive frontal lobe and hypothesize that this is related to poor attentional control. But if we look at sequential changes in blood flow during an ongoing task (one can do this with fMRI), we find that the *sequence of activation* of many different brain regions is changed. This is what we mean by differences in connectivity, and it probably reflects physical differences in the synaptic connections between brain regions. Although the choice of design does not determine what one *does* find, it can influence what one *might* find. If you are not looking at a particular variable such as connectivity, you are unlikely to notice if it differs between individuals or between groups.

In recent years, the use of noninvasive imaging to study brains of individuals with various disorders has increased so rapidly that any summary would be quickly out of date. But it is clear that brains of individuals with many kinds of disorders have various kinds of abnormalities of structure and function. The following is a sample of recent findings.

- Dyslexic individuals have lower activity in several brain regions (especially posterior occipital/temporal and parietal/temporal areas) associated with reading (Shaywitz, Lyon, & Shaywitz, 2006).
- Autistic children have malformed brains in a variety of areas, with overgrowth of anterior areas and undergrowth of posterior areas especially common (Courchesne, Redcay, Morgan, & Kennedy, 2005). For autistic individuals, these findings from noninvasive imaging studies have been substantially confirmed by autopsy studies on brain showing widespread malformations (Wegiel et al., 2010).
- Children with ADHD have less activity in frontal areas associated with response inhibition than normal children (Booth et al., 2005; Konrad, Neufang, Hanisch, Fink, &

Herpertz-Dahlmann, 2006; Turkeltaub, Gareau, Flowers, Zeffiro, & Eden, 2003). They also show developmental delays in reaching adult-like patterns of brain connectivity, and improvement is associated with normalization in connectivity (Shaw et al., 2010).

• Although the picture for depression is complicated, there is evidence that unipolar depression is associated with increased metabolic activity in amygdala and areas of prefrontal cortex, areas associated with emotional processing (Drevets, 2003).

A caution for interpreting noninvasive imaging techniques is that, while the techniques are essential for identifying changes in activity and connectivity in various disorders, it is sometimes difficult to identify exactly what those differences mean. For example, overactivity of some parts of the frontal lobe during effortful tasks has been reported in depression (Ebmeier, Rose, & Burman, 2006). Does that mean that these areas are *performing better* than in normal individuals, as intuition would suggest, or that successful performance on the task *requires more effort* than in normal individuals? Evidence suggests the latter, indicating that the most intuitive explanation for differences may not always be the correct explanation.

As discussed below in the section on brain development, the theory that connectivity differences in the brains of individuals with various disorders is consistent with the notion of developmental origins of psychopathology, as development of brain typically involves processing of more and more complex information with maturation. It is also consistent with the notion that events or processes that occur during development can alter the trajectory of development, the ways in which connections grow, strengthen, or weaken to produce an adult brain. Early errors in development can continue to cascade, as brain development, like cognitive development, is characterized by later development building on earlier development; early errors can trigger additional errors later in the cascade. Shaw et al. (2010) have recently stressed that many childhood psychiatric disorders, including ADHD and childhood schizophrenia, may very well be the result of deviations from normal patterns of brain development.

Noninvasive imaging has increased both our awareness that many disorders have associated brain changes and the specificity of our knowledge of how those brain changes might affect a person's behavior, but there are still some limitations to what noninvasive techniques can reveal. In particular, imaging studies done after diagnosis cannot fully explain how brain abnormalities might come to exist. For that, we turn to a brief discussion of brain development.

Developmental Antecedents of Neurological Disorders

Like the brain itself, the development of the central nervous system is a topic far too complex to adequately discuss in this chapter. Prenatal growth proceeds from a single fertilized egg to differentiation into definable organ systems to growth of the most complex organ known (the brain) in a remarkably short time. After birth, brain growth is associated with rapid increases in information processing, such as rapid acquisition of complex language. We only partially understand the processes involved in that growth and development. In general, however, development of brain is a complicated interaction of genes, prenatal environment, and postnatal environment.

Genes

Genes largely seem to determine the general pattern of brain development that a given organism may undergo. Genes influence such factors as segmentation of the developing brain (initial division into regions that will eventually become forebrain, hindbrain, spinal cord, etc.), types of nerve cells and types of transmitters, and patterns of interconnections that grow between brain areas (Sanes, Reh, & Harris, 2006). Generally, a human embryo will grow a typically *organized* human brain, which will then *function* like a typical human brain; but the process of developing a typical human brain is complex enough that there are many possibilities for deviations from normal development to occur.

A large number of studies indicate that there are genetic risk factors for disorders such as schizophrenia, depression, and substance abuse disorders. With very few exceptions, such as Huntington's disease, genes do not directly determine who develops a particular disorder, they only influence the probability of that disorder. For example, if a person diagnosed with schizophrenia happens to have an identical twin, the probability of the twin also having the disease is as high as 50% (estimates differ in different studies; McGue & Gottesman, 1991). That is a much higher risk than that for the general population, but an overlooked part of the meaning of the statistic is that 50% or more of people who have genes identical to a schizophrenic's genes (by definition, identical twins have identical genes) do not develop schizophrenia. So, whatever genes are associated with schizophrenia do not directly *cause* schizophrenia, although they can make its development much more likely. (Please note the distinction between *being a twin*, which does not increase the risk of schizophrenia, and being the *twin of a schizophrenic*, which does.)

Gene Expression

Genes are not simply "there"—they are expressed (become active and synthesize their respective proteins) in response to signals that can activate or silence them. The degree to which a gene is expressed determines how much of its protein is produced, which in turn determines the magnitude of effect of that gene. For example, D_2 dopamine receptors are involved in several behavioral roles, one of which is reinforcement, including perceptions of pleasure in response to addictive drugs. Literally, all addictive drugs activate D_2 receptors, and that activation is an important part of the euphoria that can lead to repeated use and addiction (Volkow et al., 2006). Internal chemical conditions that activate the gene that produces the D_2 receptor increase sensitivity to addictive drugs. Chemical conditions (such as neurotransmitter activity) that increase expression of the D_2 receptor gene include activation of the dopamine pathways by addictive drugs. Literally, administration of an addictive drug can change the chemistry of the part of the brain that controls reaction to addictive drugs (Volkow et al., 2006), and this change involves both changes in dopamine release and in D_2 receptor expression. Although direct gene expression studies are relatively new, evidence indicates that addictive drugs such as nicotine can induce expression of a variety of genes involved not only with the dopamine receptors, but also with growth and development processes (Polesskaya, Smith, & Fryxell, 2007). Thus, the chemical environment can control expression of particular genes, and, in the case of addiction, the genes activated by drug consumption lead to brain changes cuing additional drug consumption. Probably, disorders with a partial genetic basis such as schizophrenia are induced by a combination of events: having the gene or gene combination necessary for schizophrenia (this is determined by heredity), in conjunction with developmental events that cause a particular level of expression of those genes (this is environmental).

Regulation of Gene Expression

How might genes and environment interact? We are just beginning to learn what factors are involved in regulating gene expression, and our knowledge is rapidly developing. Two factors that have been identified are DNA methylation and microRNAs. Referred to as "epigenetic," processes such as DNA methylation (attaching a methyl group to a segment of DNA to inactivate it) serve as "controllers" of activity of various genes, both during development and into adulthood. DNA methylation can apparently be triggered in at least two ways: production of methylating chemicals by other genes, and the internal chemical environment of the organism. In turn, the internal chemical environment can be influenced by various drugs and by nutrition.

Another type of controller has also been recently discovered. MicroRNAs are noncoding (i.e., they do not produce proteins like regular RNAs do) short segments of RNA, which serve mainly to regulate expression of other genes. They are triggered by neurotransmitters in some cases, showing how intricate the regulation of gene expression can become. Literally, synaptic transmission can activate microRNAs (Wibrand et al., 2010), which then regulate the expression of particular genes, influencing processes such as cell metabolism, cell growth, and formation of new synapses. The growing connections can then shape the "connectivity" of brain regions. This is likely to be an important part of how environment can alter gene expression to produce pathology in both brain and behavior.

Epigenetic regulation of brain development has very recently become of interest in understanding neurodevelopmental disorders, such as schizophrenia. Although the study of epigenetic mechanisms is still in its infancy, studies are beginning to emerge suggesting, for example, that hypermethylation of reelin, a gene important in neural development, may contribute to faulty neural development in schizophrenia (Gräff & Mansuy, 2009). We may soon find that environmentally induced changes in expression of genes, acting through mechanisms such as DNA methylation or microRNAs, are the determining factors for those at risk who actually develop schizophrenia, versus those at risk who do not.

In most cases, we do not yet know what specific genes are risk factors for specific disorders, and a historical caution is that many past theories of the biological cause of particular disorders have proven to be incorrect. Recent research suggests some possibilities for the genetic basis for depression and schizophrenia. For depression, recent research suggests that many depressed individuals have a different allele (form) of a gene that produces a protein involved in transport of serotonin (Caspi et al., 2003); this can result in less efficient activity in the serotonin system. For schizophrenia, research has recently focused on a particular chromosome region (22q11; Shifman et al., 2006), although many other potentially influential genes are being studied. The precise meaning of the possible involvement of the 22q11 region has yet to be determined, and future research will be required to determine whether and which of these possibilities are actually correct. It is important to know that it is not just the presence of a particular gene or genes that produces most forms of psychopathology, but the presence *and* expression, with the latter possibly controlled by epigenetic processes.

Prenatal Development

During the prenatal period, exposure to a variety of drugs and toxins can influence brain development. Rapid, sequential growth of brain cells renders the fetal brain especially susceptible to chemicals that can alter its growth. For example, fetal alcohol syndrome, seen in children born to women who drink heavily during pregnancy, includes distinctive facial malformations, bone and joint abnormalities, and reduction in brain growth and organization, which causes moderate to severe mental retardation (Mattson, Schoenfeld, & Riley, 2001). Many studies have documented that prenatal exposure to other drugs as varied as cocaine, anticonvulsants, and nicotine can induce abnormal brain development, suggesting a general rule that *any drug that can affect brain function or behavior in the adult has the potential to alter prenatal brain development.* Even very short binge consumption of alcohol (the equivalent of as little as getting intoxicated on two occasions) may have striking effects on prenatal physical development in mice (Sulik, Johnston, & Webb, 1981). As a general rule, little can be done to alleviate brain growth problems caused by prenatal conditions, and studies have documented that many problems stemming from alcohol or drug abuse during pregnancy persist at least into adulthood of the offspring. Because effects of prenatal drugs tend to be enduring, prevention (avoid addictive drugs and toxic chemicals altogether, minimize use of medically required drugs that alter brain or behavior) is very important. Avoiding drugs and alcohol is especially important during very early pregnancy, when organ systems such as brain first begin to develop. Because fetal brain damage from drugs or alcohol can occur during very early pregnancy, before most women are aware they are pregnant, it is important to avoid drugs or alcohol if a woman *might become* pregnant. We emphasize that even "minor" drugs, such as cigarettes or some prescription drugs, can affect brain growth during the prenatal period, and these effects are then permanent, negatively affecting the child for his or her entire life.

Although data are still sketchy, it appears that many conditions that affect prenatal brain development do so by influencing a signaling system (retinoic acid, also recently found to be a neurotransmitter), controlling expression of genes that control the overall shape and form of the growing brain, the total number of cells produced, the organization of the basic columnar units of cortex, or signals that guide axons and synaptic connections (Sanes et al., 2006). Drugs as varied as alcohol, some acne medications, and an overdose of vitamin A can affect the level of retinoic acid and hence induce brain defects.

Disorders most often associated with prenatal drugs use include mental retardation, and there is evidence that some types of learning and attentional disorders are more likely in children whose mothers used alcohol or various drugs during pregnancy (Huizink & Mulder, 2006). Other severe disorders, such as autism, seem to have their origins in early pregnancy, but the specific reason for brain malformations in autism are not yet clear (Courchesne et al., 2005).

Postnatal Development

Although most brain cells are formed prior to birth in humans, a tremendous amount of growth in dendrites and in synaptic connections continues for years. Growth lasts for a particularly long time in frontal areas of the brain involved in inhibitory control of behavior and other complex functions (Cunningham, Bhattacharyya, & Benes, 2002). Growth is not always progressive; around the time of puberty, for example, there is a large reduction in synapses through a "pruning" process (Teicher, Andersen, & Hostetter, 1995). Presumably these are excess synapses, and the pruning may be associated with better focusing ability as a child matures. It now appears that there is a lifelong process of forming and breaking synaptic connections (see "Learning and memory" in Box 2.1), and this process is more robust during childhood and adolescence than it is later in adulthood; that is, the young brain is more "plastic" than the fully adult brain. In the child and adolescent, most growth in connections seems to be in reaction to neural activity in brain systems, which in turn is usually induced by sensory input from the environment. Experimental data in animals (Blakemore & Cooper, 1970) and anecdotal evidence in humans indicate that lack of experience with a particular type of visual stimulation in early childhood severely restricts the ability to perceive that kind of stimulation later in life. The brain has to learn to perceive, and if it lacks opportunities to learn some types of perception, its ability to process those kinds of information later in life is severely limited.

Work by Sapolsky, Meaney (2001), and others have found that the quality of maternal care for infant rats can affect development of the pituitary/adrenal stress response system. Rat pups that receive more intensive mothering develop stress response systems that produce lower levels of adrenal hormones in response to stress (Caldji et al., 1998). Interestingly, this can affect the offspring in adulthood and old age. In adulthood, they are calmer, more attentive mothers, thus giving their own offspring the same attention that kept them calm. Thus, there is mother–daughter transmission of behavior, acting through a nongenetic mechanism (Meaney, 2001). In old age, poorly mothered animals have high levels of stress hormones, which are toxic to brain cells, and they lose brain cells and spatial memory relatively rapidly. Well-mothered animals do not have the premature loss of brain cells seen in poorly mothered animals and preserve their spatial memory capability farther into old age (Meaney, Aitken, van Berkel, Bhatnagar, & Sapolsky, 1988). Thus, the quality of maternal care has important biological impacts on brain development. Good maternal care biases a mother toward providing good maternal care to her own young and affects both genders on other aspects of behavior, because good maternal care reduces stress responses and preserves brain capabilities longer into old age.

Enrichment can influence brain development far past the early postnatal period. Recent research indicates that sensory aspects of development normally include an element of recruitment: that is, activity in basic sensory systems "recruits" higher-order systems to process the information in a more sophisticated manner (Chou et al., 2006; Gogtay et al., 2004), which then becomes part of the connectivity of the brain. For example, noninvasive imaging studies have found that presentation of words as stimuli to infants induces activity only in the primary visual cortex. In young children who can recognize the lines as combining to produce letters, they induce activity in secondary visual cortex. In elementary school children who recognize that letters combine into words, activity is induced in areas involved in more complex processing (Schlaggar et al., 2002). Recruitment of additional brain areas eventually extends into areas associated with semantic associations of a word, not just its immediate meaning (Chou et al., 2006). This is a developmental trend in many systems—early on, input gets basic processing from primary systems, and input that gets a lot of basic processing recruits other systems to pay attention to it, and they conduct more sophisticated analysis of the input. That more sophisticated analysis leads a 12-year-old to understand more from the visual stimulus AARDVARK than a 3-year-old can understand. This recruitment becomes semihardwired later in development, and the connections formed by it are a part of what we referred to as connectivity earlier in the chapter. That is, AARDVARK triggers patterns of connectivity in an adult that do not occur in a 3-year-old, with the associated increase in meaningfulness of the stimulus.

A fascinating recent finding is that patterns of connectivity can be changed by developmental or life events. Although it is hard to ascribe connectivity differences observed between schizophrenic or ADHD individuals and normal individuals to a particular life event, it is much easier when connectivity differences are associated with specific instances of abuse during childhood (Miskovic, Schmidt, Georgiades, Boyle, & Macmillan, 2010).

For many individuals, mood and anxiety disorders, schizophrenia, and addictions first become evident in adolescence. Most addictions, for example, originate in experimenting with drugs during early adolescence. For nicotine addiction, the 11- to 14-year age range seems to be a sensitive time period. This seems to be due to a combination of factors involved in brain maturation, including heightened sensitivity to the reinforcing effects of nicotine (Torres, Tejeda, Natividad, & O'Dell, 2008), heightened sensitivity to changes in brain growth (dendritic branching patterns) in several brain areas (Bergstrom, McDonald, French, & Smith, 2008; McDonald et al., 2007), and immature executive function and decision making (Stansfield & Kirstein, 2006). Thus, adolescent animals form a preference for nicotine in as little as a single exposure, and nicotine induces changes in the developmental trajectory of brain systems, which ultimately sculpts an adult brain that is more prone to addiction.

Adolescence is also a period of heightened responsiveness to stress (Spear, 2009). Animal studies have already demonstrated that adolescent stress increases later reactivity to addictive drugs (McCormick, Robarts, Gleason, & Kelsey, 2004). Stress has long been a suspected trigger for depression and schizophrenia, both of which often first become evident during the adolescent period. Because of this increased sensitivity at a time of continued brain plasticity, adolescent stress is a prime candidate for a trigger mechanism that could combine with genetic risks and an earlier developmental event to induce psychopathology of several types.

Understanding the origins of mental disorders has significant implications for treating them. One cannot reverse major brain growth errors, and therapies for disorders that do not involve brain growth errors may be very different if the disorder primarily has inappropriate learned behaviors (overt or covert, including emotions) as its basis, as opposed to a chemical aberration.

The extent to which some disorders may be influenced by early experiences is difficult to determine and can vary from person to person. Although it requires some extrapolation from our current knowledge, patterns of thinking (fearful or negative thoughts, recurring unwanted thoughts, etc.) or particular behavioral experiences (trauma or abuse, enjoyable experiences) that occur during child or adolescent brain development have the potential to sculpt that development in ways that perpetuate problems (or strengths) originating during development. That is, childhood fears and obsessions may become persistent ways of thinking in adulthood for that individual; favorite childhood activities may become lifelong interests; and adolescent drug use may become a continuing pattern of addiction. These can become more than just habits of thinking; they may involve lasting changes in connectivity of different brain areas. Although it is not clear that all behavior pathology originates in development, the tendency of experiences to sculpt the development of brain systems suggests that early interventions are more likely to treat successfully and prevent various disorders than are interventions at later points in time.

Pharmacological Treatment of Psychiatric Disorders

Antipsychotic Drugs

Antipsychotic drugs are most often used to treat symptoms of schizophrenia. As a group, they are dopamine receptor blockers (Wong et al., 1986), although they differ from one another in clinical potency and in relative specificity for the various dopamine receptor types. Table 2.1 lists a few of the many antipsychotic drugs available. Antipsychotic drugs differ in the likelihood of severe side effects, such as tardive dyskinesia (a syndrome of persistent and involuntary motor movements seen after years of antipsychotic drug treatment), immediate motor effects such as tremors, and several others. As with antidepressants, fitting the drug and dosage to the individual may be a process of repeated experimentation.

Antidepressant Drugs

Several pharmacologically different types of drugs are effective in treating depression. The earliest group of drugs inhibit monoamine oxidase (MAO). MAO is an enzyme involved in the breakdown of several different transmitters that regulate the amounts of these transmitters within nerve cells. Inhibiting MAO makes those transmitters more available. The effectiveness of MAO inhibitors (MAOIs) was discovered accidentally when patients given an MAOI for treatment of tuberculosis experienced increased mood beyond that accounted for by improvement seen on chest X-rays. A couple of MAOIs are still used in this country for treatment of depression in patients responding poorly to other medications, but dietary restrictions and hazards (ingesting some dairy proteins, or fermentation products such as beers in conjunction with MAOIs, which can produce life-threatening blood pressure spikes) have reduced their use.

Tricyclic antidepressants reduce reuptake of several neurotransmitters. Individual tricyclics have slightly different actions. Some focus on serotonergic neurons, while others focus on noradrenergic neurons. By slowing reuptake, they make more of the transmitter available to the postsynaptic neuron, effectively increasing the availability of the transmitter. This process, however, is probably not the basis for their antidepressant action, as the reuptake effect is immediate, while clinical antidepressant action typically takes 2 weeks or more to develop. The actual mechanism of symptom improvement is not known.

Selective serotonin reuptake inhibitors, as the name implies, are more selective for serotonergic neurons and have largely become the drug class of choice for treating symptoms of depression.

While the above constitute the principal pharmacological treatments for depression, Drevets and Furey (2010) recently confirmed that several repeated intravenous scopolamine treatments, which target the acetylcholine system, have persisting antidepressant effects. Couple this information with the variety of other treatments that are effective in some depressed individuals (sleep deprivation, rapid eye movement [REM] sleep deprivation, nonpharmacological treatments such as cognitive psychotherapy), and it becomes clear why there is not yet a consensus on the underlying cause of depression or even whether there is a single cause.

Lee et al. (2010) recently reviewed research on depression, emphasizing that multiple factors that can alter brain function have been implicated in depression. These include (at least) the epigenetic modification of gene expression (discussed earlier), changes in stress response systems, systems regulating neurogenesis (growth of new nerve cells), effects of substance abuse, circadian rhythms, and changes in brain connectivity. It is not yet known how these several mechanisms interact to regulate mood, but the complexity of the interacting variables emphasizes that a simple prescription of an antidepressant drug is not likely to be a panacea.

Antianxiety Drugs

Diazepam (Valium) and its relatives have become the drugs of choice for treating anxiety disorders. These drugs largely act to stimulate receptors for the neurotransmitter GABA (gamma-aminobutyric acid). GABA is an inhibitory transmitter (large intravenous doses of diazepam can even stop an ongoing epileptic seizure). Unlike earlier tranquilizing drugs, such as barbiturates, diazepam effectively reduces anxiety in doses too small to sedate the client or to negatively affect cognitive functioning. As noted below, antianxiety drugs can have fatal interactions with other drugs, such as alcohol.

ADHD

Attentional disorders are typically treated with stimulants such as methylphenidate (Ritalin) or closely related compounds. Although it sounds counterintuitive to treat a hyperactive child with a stimulant drug, it appears that stimulants increase activity in anterior brain regions associated with attention by increasing activity in catecholamine systems, and thus partly normalize neural connectivity. It appears that they work in normal individuals, as well as in individuals with ADHD. Concern has been raised that stimulants are overprescribed (Mayes, Bagwell, & Erkulwater, 2008), which is disturbing for any psychiatric drug administered during a time when synaptic connections are still developing. In recent years, it has become apparent that, while hyperactivity abates during the adolescent and postadolescent years, attentional problems persist, and more adults remain on stimulants to treat this disorder (Kooij et al., 2010).

Treatment of Bipolar Disorder

On the surface, it would seem that manic and depressive phases of bipolar disorders should be due to different causes and thus treated with different drugs. The underlying mechanism of bipolar disorder is largely unknown, although noninvasive imaging studies have found that there are large differences in metabolism in brain between manic and depressive episodes. Lithium has proven a fairly effective modulator of both phases of the disorder. The reason for this has yet to be found.

Other Drug Treatments

In recent years, we have seen an increase in the number of disorders for which some drug therapy has become available. Successful reduction of obsessive-compulsive symptoms with SSRIs has been reported, some pharmacotherapy for posttraumatic stress disorder is being used, and increasing emphasis of pharmacotherapy for treatment of substance abuse disorders is ongoing. In general, drug treatments address symptoms of some disorders, but they do not actually cure the disorder. In a few cases (see below), symptom improvement is associated with

Table 2.2 Examples of Side Effects of Drugs

Drug	Common Side Effects
Antipsychotics	Tardive dyskinesia, liver impairment, hypotension
MAO inhibitors	In combination with tyramine in diet (dairy products and yeasts) can produce life-threatening blood pressure spikes
Tricyclic antidepressants SSRIs	Sedation, cardiovascular effects
	Insomnia, gastrointestinal problems, sexual dysfunction; possible association with elevated suicide risk under investigation
Antianxiety drugs	Life-threatening synergism if taken with other depressant drugs, such as alcohol
Stimulants, such as methylphenidate	Growth retardation

normalizing brain function, suggesting that the treatment may be addressing the cause, not just the symptoms.

Side Effects

Most psychoactive drugs can have side effects, as the signaling systems they affect can also regulate other behaviors and other body tissues. Some common side effects are listed in Table 2.2. Side effects can be severe in some cases. For example, tardive dyskinesia is a motor control disorder that can develop after years of antipsychotic treatment, and it often does not abate when the drug is stopped or altered. Liver damage is a common side effect of many drugs taken long term. Some precautions to avoid drug interactions are important. Combining antianxiety drugs with other depressants (especially alcohol) can be fatal in surprisingly small doses. Overdose of many drugs, even some vitamins, can make side effects much more severe. And these are side effects of drugs appropriately prescribed; a misdiagnosis and resulting inappropriate prescription may actually worsen some disorders. In general, drugs for psychiatric disorders are sometimes effective, but they also have some risks. They should be taken only when there is a clear diagnosis and good monitoring to detect side effects, with clear instructions to the client regarding the drug's use. The client's compliance with dose instructions, use of other medications, and sometimes with diet restrictions can dramatically affect the risk–benefit ratio of psychiatric drugs, so much so that the issue of noncompliance with medication instructions has recently been described as a major risk factor for a large number of drugs (Rummel-Kluge et al., 2008). Finally, we should caution that many psychiatric drugs are best used in conjunction with complementary therapies—antidepressant medications with cognitive therapies, for example (see Alloy et al., this volume). In addition, drugs administered to children have generally received little or no testing to determine whether there are effects on brain growth and development.

Brain Plasticity and Nonpharmacological Treatments

Much of what we now know about the ever-changing circuitry of the brain simplifies to one statement: Increasing use of a particular brain area or brain system strengthens and increases synaptic connections. We can add appropriate caveats: Too much activity can trigger activity-induced cell death, but there are exceptions. But the general statement seems to hold across a variety of brain systems. Use of (addictive) drugs that activate the mesolimbic dopamine (reinforcement) system strengthens connections of that system and increases addiction liability, and this is true for a variety of behaviors ranging from drug abuse to gambling to sex addiction (Volkow et al., 2006). Environmental cues repeatedly associated with drug use (or internal cues such as thoughts of drug use) have effects on the brain system similar to those of actual drug administration (Volkow et al., 2006). A focus on one sensory system (i.e., hearing) after loss of another (i.e., vision) leads to expansion of areas of the cortex that respond to and process auditory stimuli (Ptito & Kupers, 2005). Particular types of sensory stimuli, ranging from restricting patterns during development to increasing overall stimulation levels in adulthood, affect the sensitivity of neural systems to those stimuli and can trigger growth in systems being used more extensively and regression in systems not being used (Blakemore & Cooper, 1970; Ptito & Kupers, 2005).

In addition, at the behavioral level, we see that repetition of behaviors leads to their strengthening—repetition of unwelcome thoughts strengthens that pattern of thought, beliefs about control over the situation tend to be self-perpetuating and self-strengthening. All of these behavioral changes probably have underlying neural changes that sustain them. Although it is no doubt surprising to see gambling addiction and sex addiction included in disorders with abnormal brain connections underlying them, recent evidence supports this (Frascella, Potenza, Brown, & Childress, 2010).

These effects of neural activation on brain connectivity patterns probably involve the epigenetic mechanisms, discussed earlier. The important point, however, is that *activity can change connectivity*. What can be developed through behavioral or cognitive processes can often be undone using similar processes. There is reason to believe, for example, that therapies targeting information processing can change beliefs, attitudes, and perceptions, almost certainly by altering the neural substrates that produced those mental phenomena in the first place. Walter, Berger, and Schnell (2009) have recently reviewed the potential for developing therapies based on emerging biological knowledge and suggest that the potential is substantial. Although describing those approaches to therapy is beyond the scope of this chapter, recent research suggests that many types of therapies that are effective derive that effectiveness from their ability to resculpt patterns of synapses in the brain. A clear example of this comes from the work of Shaywitz et al. (2004), who showed that intensive phonological therapy (reading training) for dyslexia can not only improve reading skills, but also improve recruitment of higher level comprehension areas of brain, that is, normalize brain connectivity.

Although research has not confirmed other applications, Shaywitz's work suggests some intriguing possibilities for early intervention in other types of early-onset disorders. For example, children with high levels of anxiety might benefit from parental modeling of calmness or age-appropriate training in coping skills. Children with milder forms of ADHD might benefit from attentional training, ranging from formal therapy to repeated encouragement to pay attention, or simply by limiting exposure to highly attention-getting environments (perhaps video games) and encouraging attention to less sensational aspects of the environment. Therapies designed to modify memories, such as reconsolidation, might aid those suffering from posttraumatic stress disorder. Walter et al. (2009) described some preliminary approaches that suggest an affirmative answer to this latter question.

These are interesting possibilities. Our emerging knowledge of brain development suggests that they may be worth pursuing. Even pharmacological therapies, however, may improve connectivity in the short term—Rubia et al. (2009) found that methylphenidate normalizes activation and connectivity patterns in brains of children with ADHD.

Other work has indicated that psychotherapies can improve fMRI indices of brain abnormalities associated with anxiety, for example (Roffman, Marci, Glick, Dougherty, & Rauch, 2005), and that treatment of obsessive-compulsive disorder with either medication or psychotherapy improves fMRI indices of frontal lobe hyperactivation that accompanies this disorder (Nakao et al., 2005). These are just a few examples of the emerging research suggesting that treatments that improve aspects of behavior can also improve brain functioning related to that behavior. LeDoux's (2002) speculation that therapies essentially "rewire" the brain is gathering some support from emerging evidence.

As behavior has the brain as its underlying substrate, so does behavior pathology. Pathologies can be developed from many different factors affecting brain function: genes or gene expression, patterns of behavior, developmental or environmental events, drug use, among others. Although some pathologies, particularly those of early developmental origin, may be resistant to therapies simply because they have produced irreversible changes in brain organization and brain functioning, others are reversible with medication or effective psycho- or behavior therapy. Even those of early developmental origin may eventually prove to be partly or wholly preventable, as we understand the origins better and develop diagnostic methods for earlier identification.

Pathology, like normal behavior, often involves a confluence of several different influences. In many cases, the interaction of genetic susceptibility with specific environmental conditions that, in turn, elicit changes in brain connectivity, contributes to the development of a disorder. That interaction probably results in a wiring of the brain to produce a particular pattern of behavior that is labeled as abnormal or maladaptive. But our understanding of the processes resulting from the convergence of genes and environment suggests that a potential for better understanding and better treatment in the future already exists. Genetic screening to tell us who is at risk, controlling maternal exposure to drugs and other toxins during pregnancy, and remedial work during early brain development all offer some promise of reducing psychopathology. But our emerging understanding of the plasticity of the brain suggests that even when psychopathology has already developed, altering behavior patterns or patterns of thought, and perhaps even drug therapies in a limited number of cases, may effect change by rewiring some areas of brain not functioning optimally.

Biologically, what causes a psychological disorder? There is no single answer to this question. The old notion that behavior is determined both by heredity and environment is still true, but we can now add some detail to that statement, and the contributions of environment are becoming better understood. Certainly a few specific disorders, such as Huntington's disease, can be directly inherited. In many other cases, chemicals such as alcohol, drugs, or stress hormones may alter the expression of genes, thus altering brain and behavioral development. In still other cases, the sensory stimuli and thoughts an individual processes during early development sculpt the growth of brain systems, which interpret those kinds of stimuli, and this can lead to more complex development of systems stimulated during brain growth and less complete development of systems deprived of normal stimulation. In addition, the causes for a similar set of symptoms may vary from one individual to another. For one person, it may be an inherited trait; for another, an early life experience; for a third, maternal drug use; for a fourth, an experience in adolescence or young adulthood; for a fifth, a combination of some of these factors. All of these can modify the brain and lead to altered emotions, information processing, vigilance, and so forth, which continue to drive behavior and perceptions. This diversity of possibilities may also underlie the observation that a treatment that works for one person may be ineffective for another; if the cause of apparently similar symptoms is really different, a treatment that works for one may be ineffective for another. Although the processes that produce psychopathology may be complex, a better understanding of the biological bases of psychopathology increases our ability to understand, prevent, and treat such disorders.

Emerging Trends

Twenty-five years ago, a doctoral student made the statement that schizophrenia has no biological basis to it (which now seems woefully naive). In the ensuing years, we have discovered that signaling systems other than dopamine are apparently involved (glutamate, DNA methylation, microRNAs), that schizophrenia involves substantial changes in activity and connectivity of brain areas, that developmental events are risk factors, that there are differences in adolescent cortical growth/regression rates in some types of schizophrenia as compared to normal individuals, that there are differences in neural connectivity between subtypes of schizophrenia, that widespread neuronal changes accompany schizophrenia, and many others. In the process, the neurodevelopmental hypothesis of schizophrenia emerged and remains in its broadest form the dominant theory of the origins of schizophrenia (and is being adapted to other disorders with developmental components). At present, however, we do not know the full extent of involvement of epigenetic processes in the etiology of schizophrenia; connectivity changes are being actively studied and interpreted, and we just do not know what, if anything, advances, such as better temporal and spatial resolution in imaging techniques, the discovery of new neurotransmitters, or processes we cannot yet envision, may contribute to our understanding and treatment of this and many other forms of psychopathology. The rapidity of recent increases in knowledge illustrates how far we have come, but suggests how far we may yet have to go.

Chapter Summary

1. Many different types of disorders are associated with brain differences. These can include differences in neurotransmitters and other signaling systems, maldevelopment or overdevelopment of specific parts of brain, or differences in connectivity between different brain regions. Any of these can lead to disturbances in thoughts, emotions, perceptions, and behavior.

2. Brain differences often derive from developmental influences. Prenatal and postnatal environmental variables can influence brain development, apparently by acting through mechanisms such as DNA methylation and microRNA systems, to influence gene expression. These epigenetic mechanisms provide a means for environmental events to alter gene expression, brain development, and behavior.

3. Environment influences development at least from the prenatal period through adolescence. A normal environment is highly important for development of brain and behavior. "Normal" includes avoiding drugs and chemicals that can alter development—throughout the *entire* period of development—and provision of positive experiences such as parental care, enriched sensory environment, and opportunities to learn all essential life skills. Deviations from normal can result in altered brain growth and development, with consequent (usually negative) effects on many aspects of behavior. Our current understanding emphasizes the importance of prevention, early detection, and early treatment of disorders with any developmental basis.

4. Even when connectivity changes have already occurred during development, it may be possible in some cases to largely reverse those using training-like methods such as cognitive psychotherapy.

5. Understanding the biological bases of mental disorders requires careful attention to study design, capabilities and limitations of the research techniques, and a critical interpretation of the data; it is all too easy to skew interpretation of data to support a particular viewpoint. Advances in research are virtually guaranteed to advance our understanding of mental disorders, but rigorous design, conduct, and analysis of studies is crucial to that effort.

References

Bergstrom, H. C., McDonald, C. G., French, H. T., & Smith, R. F. (2008). Continuous nicotine administration produces selective, age-dependent structural alteration of pyramidal neurons from prelimbic cortex. *Synapse (New York), 62*(1), 31–39.

Blakemore, C., & Cooper, G. F. (1970). Development of the brain depends on the visual environment. *Nature, 228*(5270), 477–478.

Booth, J. R., Burman, D. D., Meyer, J. R., Lei, Z., Trommer, B. L., Davenport, N. D., ... Mesulam, M. M. (2005). Larger deficits in brain networks for response inhibition than for visual selective attention in attention deficit hyperactivity disorder (ADHD). *Journal of Child Psychology and Psychiatry and Allied Disciplines, 46*(1), 94–111.

Caldji, C., Tannenbaum, B., Sharma, S., Francis, D., Plotsky, P. M., & Meaney, M. J. (1998). Maternal care during infancy regulates the development of neural systems mediating the expression of fearfulness in the rat. *Proceedings of the National Academy of Sciences of the United States of America, 95*(9), 5335–5340.

Carlson, N. (2007). *Physiology of behavior.* Boston, MA: Allyn and Bacon.

Caspi, A., Sugden, K., Moffitt, T. E., Taylor, A., Craig, I. W., Harrington, H., ... Poulton R. (2003). Influence of life stress on depression: moderation by a polymorphism in the 5-HTT gene. *Science (New York), 301*(5631), 386–389.

Chou, T., Booth, J. R., Burman, D. D., Bitan, T., Bigio, J. D., Lu, D., & Cone, N. E. (2006). Developmental changes in the neural correlates of semantic processing. *Neuroimage, 29*(4), 1141–1149.

Courchesne, E., Redcay, E., Morgan, J. T., & Kennedy, D. P. (2005). Autism at the beginning: microstructural and growth abnormalities underlying the cognitive and behavioral phenotype of autism. *Development and Psychopathology, 17*(3), 577–597.

Cunningham, M. G., Bhattacharyya, S., & Benes, F. M. (2002). Amygdalo-cortical sprouting continues into early adulthood: implications for the development of normal and abnormal function during adolescence. *Journal of Comparative Neurology, 453*(2), 116–130.

Drevets, W. C. (2003). Neuroimaging abnormalities in the amygdala in mood disorders. *Annals of the New York Academy of Sciences, 985,* 420–444.

Drevets, W. C., & Furey, M. L. (2010). Replication of scopolamine's antidepressant efficacy in major depressive disorder: a randomized, placebo-controlled clinical trial. *Biological Psychiatry, 67*(5), 432–438.

Driscoll, C. D., Streissguth, A. P., & Riley, E. P. (1990). Prenatal alcohol exposure: comparability of effects in humans and animal models. *Neurotoxicology and Teratology, 12*(3), 231–237.

Frascella J., Potenza, M. N., Brown, L. L., & Childress, A. R. (2010). Shared brain vulnerabilities open the way for nonsubstance addictions: Carving addiction at a new joint? *Annals of the New York Academy of Sciences, 1187,* 294–315.

Gogtay, N., Giedd, J. N., Lusk, L., Hayashi, K. M., Greenstein, D., Vaituzis, A. C., ... Thompson, P. M. (2004). Dynamic mapping of human cortical development during childhood through early adulthood. *Proceedings of the National Academy of Sciences of the United States of America, 101*(21), 8174–8179.

Gräff, J., & Mansuy, I. M. (2009). Epigenetic dysregulation in cognitive disorders. *European Journal of Neuroscience, 30*(1), 1–8.

Henseler, I., Falkai, P., & Gruber, O. (2010). Disturbed functional connectivity within brain networks subserving domain-specific subcomponents of working memory in schizophrenia: relation to performance and clinical symptoms. *Journal of Psychiatric Research, 44*(6), 364–372.

Huizink, A. C., & Mulder, E. J. H. (2006). Maternal smoking, drinking or cannabis use during pregnancy and neurobehavioral and cognitive functioning in human offspring. *Neuroscience and Biobehavioral Reviews, 30*(1), 24–41.

Konrad, K., Neufang, S., Hanisch, C., Fink, G. R., & Herpertz-Dahlmann, B. (2006). Dysfunctional attentional networks in children with attention deficit/hyperactivity disorder: Evidence from an event-related functional magnetic resonance imaging study. *Biological Psychiatry, 59*(7), 643–651.

Kooij, S. J., Bejerot, S., Blackwell, A., Caci, H., Casas-Brugué, M., Carpentier, P. J., ... Asherson, P. (2010). European consensus statement on diagnosis and treatment of adult ADHD. *BMC Psychiatry, 10,* 67.

Laruelle, M., Abi-Dargham, A., van Dyck, C. H., Gil, R., D'Souza, C. D., Erdos, J., ... Innis, R. B. (1996). Single photon emission computerized tomography imaging of amphetamine-induced dopamine release in drug-free schizophrenic subjects. *Proceedings of the National Academy of Sciences of the United States of America, 93*(17), 9235–9240.

LeDoux, J. (2002). *Synaptic self: How our brains become who we are.* New York: Viking Penguin.

Lee, S., Jeong, J., Kwak, Y., & Park, S. K. (2010). Depression research: where are we now? *Molecular Brain, 3,* 8.

Levinson, D. F. (2006). The genetics of depression: A review. *Biological Psychiatry, 60*(2), 84–92.

Lynall, M., Bassett, D. S., Kerwin, R., McKenna, P. J., Kitzbichler, M., Muller, U., & Bullmore, E. (2010). Functional connectivity and brain networks in schizophrenia. *Journal of Neuroscience: The Official Journal of the Society for Neuroscience, 30*(28), 9477–9487.

MacDonald, A. W., & Carter, C. S. (2003). Event-related FMRI study of context processing in dorsolateral prefrontal cortex of patients with schizophrenia. *Journal of Abnormal Psychology, 112*(4), 689–697.

Malberg, J. E., Eisch, A. J., Nestler, E. J., & Duman, R. S. (2000). Chronic antidepressant treatment increases neurogenesis in adult rat hippocampus. *Journal of Neuroscience: The Official Journal of the Society for Neuroscience, 20*(24), 9104–9110.

Mattson, S. N., Schoenfeld, A. M., & Riley, E. P. (2001). Teratogenic effects of alcohol on brain and behavior. *Alcohol Research and Health: The Journal of the National Institute on Alcohol Abuse and Alcoholism, 25*(3), 185–191.

Mayes, R., Bagwell, C., & Erkulwater, J. (2008). ADHA and the rise in stimulant use among children. *Harvard Review of Psychiatry, 16*(3), 151–166.

McCormick, C. M., Robarts, D., Gleason, E., & Kelsey, J. E. (2004). Stress during adolescence enhances locomotor sensitization to nicotine in adulthood in female, but not male, rats. *Hormones and Behavior, 46*(4), 458–466.

McDonald, C. G., Eppolito, A. K., Brielmaier, J. M., Smith, L. N., Bergstrom, H. C., Lawhead, M. R., & Smith, R. F. (2007). Evidence for elevated nicotine-induced structural plasticity in nucleus accumbens of adolescent rats. *Brain Research, 1151*, 211–218.

McGue, M., & Gottesman, I. I. (1991). The genetic epidemiology of schizophrenia and the design of linkage studies. *European Archives of Psychiatry and Clinical Neuroscience, 240*(3), 174–181.

Meaney, M. J. (2001). Maternal care, gene expression, and the transmission of individual differences in stress reactivity across generations. *Annual Review of Neuroscience, 24*, 1161–1192.

Meaney, M. J., Aitken, D. H., van Berkel, C., Bhatnagar, S., & Sapolsky, R. M. (1988). Effect of neonatal handling on age-related impairments associated with the hippocampus. *Science (New York), 239*(4841, Pt. 1), 766–768.

Meyer, J., & Quenzer, L. (2005). *Psychopharmacology: Drugs, the brain, and behavior.* Sunderland, MA: Sinauer.

Miskovic, V., Schmidt, L. A., Georgiades, K., Boyle, M., & Macmillan, H. L. (2010). Adolescent females exposed to child maltreatment exhibit atypical EEG coherence and psychiatric impairment: linking early adversity, the brain, and psychopathology. *Development and Psychopathology, 22*(2), 419–432.

Molteni, R., Calabrese, F., Bedogni, F., Tongiorgi, E., Fumagalli, F., Racagni, G., & Riva, M. A. (2006). Chronic treatment with fluoxetine up-regulates cellular BDNF mRNA expression in rat dopaminergic regions. *International Journal of Neuropsychopharmacology: Official Scientific Journal of the Collegium Internationale Neuropsychopharmacologicum (CINP), 9*(3), 307–317.

Nakao, T., Nakagawa, A., Yoshiura, T., Nakatani, E., Nabeyama, M., Yoshizato, C., ... Kanba, S. (2005). Brain activation of patients with obsessive-compulsive disorder during neuropsychological and symptom provocation tasks before and after symptom improvement: A functional magnetic resonance imaging study. *Biological Psychiatry, 57*(8), 901–910.

Otte, A., & Halsband, U. (2006). Brain imaging tools in neurosciences. *Journal of Physiology, Paris, 99*(4–6), 281–292.

Polesskaya, O. O., Smith, R. F., & Fryxell, K. J. (2007). Chronic nicotine doses down-regulate PDE4 isoforms that are targets of antidepressants in adolescent female rats. *Biological Psychiatry, 61*(1), 56–64.

Ptito, M., & Kupers, R. (2005). Cross-modal plasticity in early blindness. *Journal of Integrative Neuroscience, 4*(4), 479–488.

Rapoport, J. L., Addington, A. M., Frangou, S., & Psych, M. R. C. (2005). The neurodevelopmental model of schizophrenia: Update 2005. *Molecular Psychiatry, 10*(5), 434–449.

Roffman, J. L., Marci, C. D., Glick, D. M., Dougherty, D. D., & Rauch, S. L. (2005). Neuroimaging and the functional neuroanatomy of psychotherapy. *Psychological Medicine, 35*(10), 1385–1398.

Rubia, K., Halari, R., Cubillo, A., Mohammad, A., Brammer, M., & Taylor, E. (2009). Methylphenidate normalises activation and functional connectivity deficits in attention and motivation networks in medication-naïve children with ADHD during a rewarded continuous performance task. *Neuropharmacology, 57*(7–8), 640–652.

Rummel-Kluge, C., Schuster, T., Peters, S., & Kissling, W. (2008). Partial compliance with antipsychotic medication is common in patients with schizophrenia. *Australian and New Zealand Journal of Psychiatry, 42*(5), 382–388.

Sanes, D., Reh, T., & Harris, W. (2006). *Development of the nervous system.* New York: Academic Press.

Schlaggar, B. L., Brown, T. T., Lugar, H. M., Visscher, K. M., Miezin, F. M., & Petersen, S. E. (2002). Functional neuroanatomical differences between adults and school-age children in the processing of single words. *Science (New York), 296*(5572), 1476–1479.

Seeman, P. (1987). Dopamine receptors and the dopamine hypothesis of schizophrenia. *Synapse (New York), 1*(2), 133–152.

Shaw, P., Gogtay, N., & Rapoport, J. (2010). Childhood psychiatric disorders as anomalies in neurodevelopmental trajectories. *Human Brain Mapping, 31*(6), 917–925.

Shaywitz, B. A., Lyon, G. R., & Shaywitz, S. E. (2006). The role of functional magnetic resonance imaging in understanding reading and dyslexia. *Developmental Neuropsychology, 30*(1), 613–632.

Shaywitz, B. A., Shaywitz, S. E., Blachman, B. A., Pugh, K. R., Fulbright, R. K., Skudlarski, P., … Gore, J. C. (2004). Development of left occipitotemporal systems for skilled reading in children after a phonologically- based intervention. *Biological Psychiatry, 55*(9), 926–933.

Shifman, S., Levit, A., Chen, M., Chen, C., Bronstein, M., Weizman, A., … Darvasi, A. (2006). A complete genetic association scan of the 22q11 deletion region and functional evidence reveal an association between DGCR2 and schizophrenia. *Human Genetics, 120*(2), 160–170.

Spear, L. P. (2009). Heightened stress responsivity and emotional reactivity during pubertal maturation: Implications for psychopathology. *Development and Psychopathology, 21*(1), 87–97.

Stansfield, K. H., & Kirstein, C. L. (2006). Effects of novelty on behavior in the adolescent and adult rat. *Developmental Psychobiology, 48* (1), 10–15.

Sulik, K. K., Johnston, M. C., & Webb, M. A. (1981). Fetal alcohol syndrome: embryogenesis in a mouse model. *Science (New York), 214*(4523), 936–938.

Teicher, M. H., Andersen, S. L., & Hostetter, J. C. (1995). Evidence for dopamine receptor pruning between adolescence and adulthood in striatum but not nucleus accumbens. *Developmental Brain Research, 89*(2), 167–172.

Thompson, P. M., Vidal, C., Giedd, J. N., Gochman, P., Blumenthal, J., Nicolson, R., … Rapoport, J. L. (2001). Mapping adolescent brain change reveals dynamic wave of accelerated gray matter loss in very early-onset schizophrenia. *Proceedings of the National Academy of Sciences of the United States of America, 98*(20), 11650–11655.

Torres, O. V., Tejeda, H. A., Natividad, L. A., & O'Dell, L. E. (2008). Enhanced vulnerability to the rewarding effects of nicotine during the adolescent period of development. *Pharmacology, Biochemistry, and Behavior, 90*(4), 658–663.

Turkeltaub, P. E., Gareau, L., Flowers, D. L., Zeffiro, T. A., & Eden, G. F. (2003). Development of neural mechanisms for reading. *Nature Neuroscience, 6*(7), 767–773.

Volkow, N. D., Wang, G., Telang, F., Fowler, J. S., Logan, J., Childress, A., … Wong, C. (2006). Cocaine cues and dopamine in dorsal striatum: mechanism of craving in cocaine addiction. *Journal of Neuroscience: The Official Journal of the Society for Neuroscience, 26*(24), 6583–6588.

Walter, H., Berger, M., & Schnell, K. (2009). Neuropsychotherapy: Conceptual, empirical and neuroethical issues. *European Archives of Psychiatry and Clinical Neuroscience, 259*(Suppl. 2), S173–S182.

Wegiel, J., Kuchna, I., Nowicki, K., Imaki, H., Wegiel, J., Marchi, E., … Wisniewski, T. (2010). The neuropathology of autism: defects of neurogenesis and neuronal migration, and dysplastic changes. *Acta Neuropathologica, 119*(6), 755–770.

Wibrand, K., Panja, D., Tiron, A., Ofte, M. L., Skaftnesmo, K., Lee, C. S., … Bramham, C. R. (2010). Differential regulation of mature and precursor microRNA expression by NMDA and metabotropic glutamate receptor activation during LTP in the adult dentate gyrus in vivo. *European Journal of Neuroscience, 31*(4), 636–645.

Wong, D. F., Wagner, H. N., Tune, L. E., Dannals, R. F., Pearlson, G. D., Links, J. M., … Gjedde, A. (1986). Positron emission tomography reveals elevated D2 dopamine receptors in drug-naive schizophrenics. *Science (New York), 234*(4783), 1558–1563.

Wrona, D. (2006). Neural-immune interactions: an integrative view of the bidirectional relationship between the brain and immune systems. *Journal of Neuroimmunology, 172*(1–2), 38–58.

3
Cultural Dimensions of Psychopathology
The Social World's Impact on Mental Disorders[1]

STEVEN REGESER LÓPEZ

University of Southern California
Los Angeles, California

PETER J. GUARNACCIA

Rutgers, The State University of New Jersey
New Brunswick, New Jersey

Over the past several decades, researchers have increasingly examined cultural influences in psychopathology. However, for much of this period, the study of culture and mental disorders was a marginal field of inquiry. This chapter will illustrate how cultural issues have moved to the fore in the study of psychopathology. A landmark event marking this transition came in 1977 when Kleinman heralded the beginning of a "new cross-cultural psychiatry," an inter-disciplinary research approach integrating anthropological methods and conceptualizations with traditional psychiatric and psychological approaches. Mental health researchers were encouraged to respect indigenous illness categories and to recognize the limitations of bio-medical illness categories, such as depression and schizophrenia. Also, the new cross-cultural psychiatry distinguished between disease, a "malfunctioning or maladaptation of biological or psychological processes," and illness, "the personal, interpersonal, and cultural reaction to dis-ease" (p. 9). The perspective that Kleinman and others (Fabrega, 1975; Kleinman, Eisenberg, & Good, 1978) articulated in the 1970s reflected an important direction for the study of culture and psychopathology—to understand the social world within mental illness (Draguns, 1980; Marsella 1980).

Many advances were made during the first decade of the new cross-cultural psychiatry perspective. One was the establishment of the interdisciplinary journal, *Culture, Medicine, and Psychiatry*. This newly founded journal, in conjunction with *Transcultural Psychiatry* in Canada (formerly *Transcultural Psychiatric Research Review*), provided and continues to pro-vide an important forum for cultural research in psychology and psychiatry. Also, during the 1980s, large-scale epidemiologic studies were carried out. The second multinational World Health Organization (WHO) study of schizophrenia was launched and preliminary findings were reported (Sartorius et al., 1986). The Epidemiological Catchment Area (ECA) studies were also conducted during this time frame (Regier et al., 1984). Some may question how cultur-ally informed these classic studies were (Edgerton & Cohen, 1994; Fabrega, 1990; Guarnaccia, Kleinman, & Good, 1990). However, most reviews of culture, ethnicity, and mental disorders today refer to the findings from the WHO and ECA studies to address how social, ethnic, and cultural factors are related to the distribution of psychopathology. Also during this time, the

---

[1] This chapter is adapted from S. R. López and P. J. Guarnaccia (2000). Cultural psychopathology: Uncovering the social world of mental illness. *Annual Review of Psychology, 51*, 571–598.

National Institute of Mental Health funded research centers with the sole purpose of conducting research on and for specific ethnic minority groups (African Americans, American Indians, Latino Americans, and Asian Americans). Some of the research from these centers contributed to the growing cultural psychopathology database (e.g., Cervantes, Padilla, & Salgado de Snyder, 1991; King, 1978; Manson, Shore, & Bloom, 1985; Neighbors, Jackson, Campbell, & Williams, 1989; Rogler, 1989; Sue et al., 1991).

Dialogue across disciplines was also initiated during this time. For example, Kleinman and Good's (1985) influential volume, *Culture and Depression*, brought together the research of not only anthropologists, but also of psychologists and psychiatrists as well as historians and philosophers. Another significant indicator of the field's development was and continues to be its success in attracting new investigators. In sum, these first 10 years can be characterized as an exciting and fertile time for the study of cultural psychopathology.

Despite many advances, the field's main messages were not reaching larger audiences. Investigators were communicating primarily among themselves in their specialty journals and books. On rare occasions, one would find a special issue on cultural research in a mainstream journal (e.g., Butcher, 1987, *Journal of Consulting and Clinical Psychology*). Those findings that did get published in widely distributed journals were scattered among a broad array of journals. Thus, from the perspective of mainstream investigators, the developments of the new cross-cultural psychiatry went largely unnoticed. A telling example of this occurred at a joint meeting of the *Diagnostic and Statistical Manual of Mental Disorders*, fourth edition (*DSM–IV*) task force and the Culture and Diagnosis Work Group in 1991. After two days of intensive discussion of the potential contributions of cultural psychopathology research to *DSM–IV*, the chair of the *DSM–IV* task force commented that this was really interesting work and that the members of the Culture and Diagnosis Work Group should publish this research—this being three years after Kleinman's (1988) *Rethinking Psychiatry* had appeared! In this book, Kleinman provided a comprehensive review of culture, psychopathology, and related research. Drawing on empirical data and theory, he argued that culture matters for the study and treatment of mental disorders. This volume serves as a significant marker in the development of the new cross-cultural psychiatry, which we refer to here as the study of cultural psychopathology.

Key Developments

Conceptual Contributions

Definition of Culture   Central to the study of cultural psychopathology is the definition of culture. Much of the past and even current research relies on a definition of culture that is outdated. In fact, Betancourt and López (1993) wrote a critical review of cultural and psychological research in which culture was defined as the values, beliefs, and practices that pertain to a given ethnocultural group. The strength of this definition is that it begins to unpack culture. Instead of arguing that a given expression of distress resides within a given ethnocultural group, for example, researchers argue that the expression of distress is related to a specific value or orientation. We see this as a significant advancement. It helps researchers begin to operationalize what about culture matters in the specific context. Further, it recognizes the heterogeneity within specific ethnocultural groups. Knowing that someone belongs to a specific ethnic group provides guidelines to potential cultural issues in psychopathology, but it does not imply that that person adheres to all the cultural values and practices of that group.

At the same time, this definition of culture as values, beliefs, and practices has significant limitations (Lewis-Fernandez & Kleinman, 1995). One is that it depicts culture as residing largely within individuals. The emphasis on values and beliefs points out the psychological nature of culture. We argue that culture is manifested in the interaction between people and is highly social in nature. Situating practices (customs and rituals) with values and beliefs gives the impression that the practices in the social world are a function of values and beliefs. For example, people are thought to rely on their family in times of crisis because they are high in *familialism* or family orientation. Investigators rarely examine what about the social world facilitates or fosters reliance on family members. Perhaps harsh environmental conditions contribute to families coming together to overcome adversity. When applying the values and beliefs definition of culture, the social world is subjugated to the psychological world of the individual. Contrary to this perspective, we argue that it is action in the social and physical world that produces culture as much as people's ideas about the world. In our view, the social world interacts on an equal footing with the psychological world in producing human behavior.

A second important limitation of this frequently used definition of culture is that it depicts culture as a static and bounded phenomenon. We assert that culture involves process and change, and that culture is constantly in flux both in its regions of origin and as people bring their cultures with them as they move around the world (Garro, 2001; Greenfield, 1997; Guarnaccia & Rodriguez, 1996). Attempts to mold culture into a set of generalized value orientations or behaviors will continually misrepresent what culture is. Culture is a dynamic and creative process, some aspects of which are shared by large groups of individuals as a result of particular life circumstances and histories. Given the changing nature of our social world and given the efforts of individuals to adapt to such changes, culture can best be viewed as an ongoing process, a system or set of systems in flux (Hong, Morris, Chiu, & Benet-Martinez, 2000).

A related limitation of the values-based definition of culture is that it depicts people as recipients of culture from a generalized "society" with little recognition of the individual's role in negotiating his or her cultural world (Garro, 2000). More recent approaches to culture in anthropology, while not discarding the importance of a person's cultural inheritance of ideas, values, and ways of relating, have focused equally on the emergence of culture from the life experiences and interactions of individuals and small groups. People can change and either add to or reject cultural elements through social processes such as migration and acculturation. A viable definition of culture acknowledges the agency of individuals in establishing their social worlds.

In sum, current views of culture attend much more to people's social world than past views of culture that emphasized the individual. Of particular interest are people's daily routines and how such activities are tied to families, neighborhoods, villages, and social networks. By examining people's daily routines one can identify what matters most to people (Gallimore, Goldenberg, & Weisner, 1993) or what is most at stake for people (Kleinman, 2006; Ware & Kleinman, 1992). Furthermore, this perspective captures the intersubjective and interactional dimensions of culture as it is both a product of group values, norms, and experiences, as well as individual innovations and life histories. The use of this broader definition of culture should help guide investigators away from flat, unidimensional notions of culture to discover the richness of a cultural analysis for the study of psychopathology. An important component of this perspective is the examination of intracultural diversity. In particular, social class, poverty, and gender continue to affect different levels of mental health both within cultural groups and across cultural groups.

Goals of Cultural Research   Culture is important in a number of domains within psychopathology research. It is important in the expression of disorder and distress; a cultural analysis can point out the variability in the manner in which mental illness is manifested. Social and cultural factors can also affect the etiology and prevalence of disorder by differentially placing some at more risk than others for developing psychopathology. In addition, the course of disorder, as reflected in the degree of disability or in the number of clinical relapses, is also related to important cultural factors. We want to encourage all of these lines of inquiry.

Regardless of the specific domain of research, there are two meta-goals of cultural research. Some writers imply that cultural research should test the generality of given theoretical notions. For example, in a thoughtful analysis of cultural research Clark (1987) noted: "Conceptual progress in psychology requires a unified base for investigating psychological phenomena, with culture-relevant variables included as part of the matrix" (p. 465). From Clark's point of view, cross-cultural work can serve to enhance the generality of given conceptual models by adding, when necessary, cultural variables to an existing theoretical model to explain between group and within group variance. Although Clark acknowledges the possibility that a construct developed in one country may not have a counterpart in another country, at no time does she discuss the value of deriving models of distinct clinical entities found in only one country or ethnocultural group. This suggests that for Clark the main purpose of studying culture is to reinforce the universality of existing psychological models by subsuming cross-cultural variations into the mainstream of research.

In contrast, both Fabrega (1990) and Rogler (1989) criticized researchers for attending insufficiently to the cultural specificity of mental illness and mental health. Fabrega examined researchers' use of mainstream instruments and conceptualizations in studying mental disorders among Latinos and challenged such researchers to be bold in their critiques of "establishment psychiatry." Rogler recommended a framework for mainstream psychiatric researchers that attend more fully to culture. For both Fabrega and Rogler, the risk of overlooking cultural variations is much greater in current psychopathology research than the risk of overlooking cultural similarities. Focusing on culture-specific phenomena at this time is of central importance to the further development of the field.

An important conceptual advancement is the recognition of both positions, that is, studying culture to identify general processes and studying culture to identify culture-specific processes. By focusing only on generalities, we overlook the importance of culture-specific phenomena. On the other hand, by emphasizing culture-specific phenomena we overlook the possibility of generalities. The overall purpose of cultural research, therefore, is to advance our understanding of general processes, culture-specific processes, and the manner in which they interact in specific contexts (Beals et al., 2003; Draguns, 1990). The aim of this chapter is to identify culture's mark amid the ubiquity of human suffering.

Major Advances

We now turn to selected developments over the past 22 years in the study of culture and psychopathology. We begin with a discussion of four of the most important projects that were carried out since 1988: the incorporation of cultural factors in the *DSM–IV* (American Psychiatric Association, 1994), the publication of the *World Mental Health* report (Desjarlais, Eisenberg, Good, & Kleinman, 1996), the release of the U.S. Surgeon General's *Supplemental Report on Mental Health: Culture, Race, and Ethnicity* (U.S. Department of Health and Human Services, 2001), and the completion of the Collaborative Psychiatric Epidemiology surveys.

The National Institute of Mental Health (NIMH) funded the establishment of a culture and diagnosis work group to inform the development of the *DSM–IV*. The work group's efforts resulted in three main contributions to *DSM–IV*: (1) inclusion of some discussion on how cultural factors can influence the expression, assessment, and prevalence of disorders in each of the disorder chapters, (2) an outline of a cultural formulation of clinical diagnosis to complement the multiaxial assessment, and (3) a glossary of relevant cultural-bound syndromes from around the world. A more complete documentation of the work group's findings and contributions is available in a special volume growing out of the group's deliberations (Mezzich et al., 1997), in volume 3 of the *DSM–IV Sourcebook* (Widiger et al., 1997), and in other publications (e.g., Alarcón, 1995; Kirmayer 1998; Mezzich, Kleinman, Fabrega, & Parron, 1996). Another major impact of the culture and diagnosis work group was the integration of a large number of senior and junior investigators that brought new energy to the field of cultural psychopathology. Without a doubt the attention given to culture in *DSM–IV* is a major achievement in the history of the classification of mental disorders. Never before had classification schemas or related diagnostic interviews addressed the role of culture in psychopathology to this degree (López & Núñez 1987; Rogler, 1996). (See Kirmayer, 1998, and Lewis-Fernandez & Kleinman, 1995, for a discussion of the limitations of how *DSM–IV* considered culture.)

The cultural considerations for *DSM–IV* provided a foundation on which to build future editions. It is unclear, however, the degree to which culture will be considered in the development of DSM–5. Early review papers indicate that it will be considered in that edition (e.g., Alarcón et al., 2002; Bernal, Cumba-Aviles, & Sacz-Santiago, 2006), however, there is no central cultural work group for this edition as there was for *DSM–IV*. At least for anxiety disorders, culture is being given very careful scrutiny (Lewis-Fernandez et al., 2010).

A second major development within the past 15 years was the publication of the *World Mental Health* report. Desjarlais et al. (1996) compiled research from across the world to identify the range of mental health and behavioral problems (e.g., mental disorders, violence, suicide) particularly among low-income countries in Africa, Latin America, Asia, and the Pacific. The authors derived several conclusions. Perhaps the most significant was that mental illness and related problems exact a significant toll on the health and well-being of people worldwide and produce a greater burden based on a "disability-adjusted life years" index than that from tuberculosis, cancer, or heart disease (Murray & López, 1996). Among all physical and mental disorders, depressive disorders alone were found to produce the fifth greatest burden for women and seventh greatest burden for men.

Another important observation was that mental disorders and behavioral problems are intricately tied to the social world and occur in clusters of intimately linked social and psychological problems. For example, the authors identified the social roots of the poor mental health of women. Among the many factors are hunger (undernourishment afflicts more than 60% of women in developing countries), work-related problems (women are poorly paid for dangerous, labor intensive jobs), and domestic violence (surveys in some low-income communities worldwide report that up to 50 to 60% of women have been beaten). The research on women's mental health illustrates that psychopathology is as much pathology of the social world as pathology of the mind or body.

Based on their findings, Desjarlais et al. (1996) made specific recommendations to advance both mental health policy and research to help reduce the significant burden of mental illness across the world. Their consideration of the social world leads easily to recommending specific interventions to address not only mental health problems but also the social conditions that surround and greatly influence such problems. In addressing the poor mental health of women, for example, they call for coordinated efforts to empower women economically and through education, as well as to reduce violence against women in all its forms. In addition, women's mental health is identified as one of the top five research priorities worldwide. They call for research to examine the social factors that influence women's health in specific cultural contexts and to identify effective community-based interventions in improving their health status (see Winstead & Sanchez, this volume).

The third development was the Surgeon General's *Supplemental Report on Mental Health* concerning culture, race, and ethnicity (U.S. Department of Health and Human Services, 2001). The Surgeon General first published a landmark report on the status of the nation's mental health (U.S. Department of Health and Human Services, 1999). Some observers were concerned that insufficient attention was given to the mental health of the country's ethnic and racial minority groups (Chavez, 2003; López, 2003). In response to this concern and under the leadership of the

Substance Abuse and Mental Health Services Administration, the Surgeon General published a report on the mental health of the nation's four main minority groups: American Indians/Alaska Natives, African Americans, Asian Americans/Pacific Islanders, and Latino Americans. Although the report's focus was mental health care, considerable attention was given to our current understanding of the types of psychopathology common among these groups, based largely on epidemiological and clinical research. One of the major contributions of this report was the synthesis of literature on the mental health of these diverse groups.

The main message of the Surgeon General's report was that "culture counts." "The cultures from which people hail affect all aspects of mental health and illness, including the types of stresses they confront, whether they seek help, what types of help they seek, what symptoms and concerns they bring to clinical attention, and what types of coping styles and social supports they possess" (U.S. Department of Health and Human Services, 2001, p. ii). The Surgeon General's report compiled the best available research that culture matters in these domains. For example, evidence was reviewed regarding the relationship between racism and mental health (Kessler, Mickelson, & Williams, 1999) and ethnicity and psychopharmacology (Lin, Poland, & Anderson, 1995). In addition, the report outlined future directions to address the mental health needs of these underserved communities, including expanding the science base and training mental health scientists and practitioners. In all, this report served two important functions. It brought together the best available mental health research regarding the main U.S. minority groups. Also, because of the status and visibility of the office of the Surgeon General, the report alerted the nation to the mental health needs of these four main ethnic and racial minority groups.

The Collaborative Psychiatric Epidemiology Surveys (CPES) represent the fourth and final major development that is highlighted. The CPES comprises three nationally representative surveys of both majority and minority groups in the United States. Similar instruments and methods were used to foster cross-survey comparisons. The National Comorbidity Survey-Replication (NCS-R; Kessler et al., 2004) was carried out between 2001 and 2003 and was based on a probability sample (N = 9,282) of the United States (the 48 contiguous states) in which Euro-Americans were primarily represented (73%) with much smaller proportions of minority group members (non-Hispanic Blacks 12%, Hispanics 11%, and others 4%). This sample was comprised of English-speaking individuals 18 years and older. The National Survey of American Life (Jackson et al., 2006) was conducted between 2001 to 2003 and focused on national samples of African-origin adults including African Americans (n = 3,570), and Afro-Caribbeans (n = 1,623). In addition, an adolescent sample of 1,200 13- to 17-year-old African Americans and Afro-Caribbeans was studied. Including samples of African Americans and Afro-Caribbeans enabled the examination of the heterogeneity of African origin persons. The National Latino and Asian American Study (NLAAS; Alegría, Takeuchi et al., 2006) was the first mental health survey of nationally representative samples of Latinos (N = 2,554) and Asian Americans (N = 2,095). These surveys were of persons 18 years and older and were conducted from 2002 to 2003 (Abe-Kim et al., 2007; Alegría et al., 2008). Among the strengths of these surveys were that non-English-speaking persons (Spanish, Tagalog, Chinese, and Vietnamese) were included as well as individuals from several subethnic groups. This enabled the examination of language and differences within ethnic group.

The contributions of the CPES have been most significant. For the first time we have nationally representative samples of three of the major U.S. racial/ethnic minority groups (American Indians are notably missing) and can compare their prevalence rates with that of Euro-Americans with minimal concern for differences in methodologies or representativeness of samples. In addition, we have data for subracial or sub ethnic groups to examine the importance of within-group variability. A recent study of major depression, carried out by Gonzalez, Tarraf, Whitfield, and Vega (2010), reflects both of these important strengths. First, they found that across most of the racial and ethnic groups there is a healthy immigrant effect where immigrants have lower prevalence rates of depression than U.S. born adults of the same ethnic or racial background. Second, as noted previously by other authors (e.g., Alegría et al., 2008), the healthy immigrant effect does not apply to all groups, especially Cubans and Puerto Ricans. A third important finding is that the healthy immigrant effect does not hold for older adults; it appears to "yield to the overwhelming effects of socioeconomic disadvantages in later years" (p. 1050). Although these three findings concern only major depression, they reflect some of the richness of the CPES. Studies based on the CPES will likely continue to contribute to our understanding of the sociocultural context and psychopathology.

Together the *DSM–IV*, the *World Mental Health* report, the Surgeon General's supplemental report on mental health, and the CPES make major contributions to the study of culture and psychopathology and give important visibility and credibility to this important domain of research. At the same time, they illustrate the range of conceptualizations of culture and the importance of the social domain. For *DSM–IV*, culture tends to be depicted as exotic, through its influence on symptom expression and the noted culture-bound syndromes. Culture is thought to reside largely in persons from "culturally different" groups. There is little attention paid to the influence of culture in every clinical encounter, influencing the client, provider, and the broader community context, regardless of the patient's ethnic or racial background.

The *World Mental Health* report, on the other hand, recognizes the dynamic, social processes linked to culture. Hunger, work, and education, for example, are integrally related to how people adapt or fail to adapt. Clinical phenomena are recognized, but so are behavioral problems not traditionally considered in psychiatric classification systems, such as domestic violence and sexual violence. Throughout, the authors recognize cultural variability as a key dimension of culture and mental health, and they highlight the moral and health implications of controversial practices, such as female circumcision.

The Surgeon General's report falls between both perspectives. It recognizes the importance of culture in specific clinical entities (both culture-bound syndromes and mainstream mental disorder categories). It also acknowledges the importance of the broader social world, though the emphasis tends to be more disorder based and less contextually based than the *World Mental Health* report. The CPES also falls between both perspectives. On the one hand, the main findings focus on *DSM–IV*-defined disorders with little attention to the different ways psychopathology is expressed, given specific sociocultural contexts (for exemptions see Lewis-Fernandez et al., 2009; and Guarnaccia et al., 2010). On the other hand, attention has been given to the sociocultural context and how that relates to disorder and distress (e.g., Gavin et al., 2010). Despite the differences in the treatment of culture, these four research developments indicate that culture as a subject matter is no longer the exclusive purview of cultural psychologists, psychiatrists, and anthropologists. It is now the subject matter of all users of *DSM–IV*, worldwide policymakers, national health policymakers, mental health researchers, and those who care for people with mental disorders.

Disorder-Related Research

We now turn to the examination of selected psychopathology research. We chose the study of anxiety, schizophrenia, and childhood psychopathology because within each of these areas there are systematic studies that examine the cultural basis of the expression of these disorders as well as the social and cultural processes that underlie the development and course of illness.

Anxiety   In this area, we chose to focus our attention on one line of research, the study of *ataques de nervios*, though there are important overviews of this broad area of anxiety research (Guarnaccia, 1997; Guarnaccia & Kirmayer, 1997). The study of *ataques de nervios* is an important line of research because it focuses on a culture-specific phenomenon for which the triangulation of ethnography, epidemiology, and clinical research has made important contributions. Thus, we will be able to examine some ways ethnography informs mainstream research and highlight the important ways culture influences psychopathology.

Ataque de nervios is an idiom of distress particularly prominent among Latinos from the Caribbean, but also recognized among other Latino groups. Symptoms commonly associated with *ataques de nervios* include trembling, attacks of crying, screaming uncontrollably, and verbal or physical aggression. Other symptoms that are prominent in some *ataques* but not others are seizure-like or fainting episodes, dissociative experiences, and suicidal gestures. A general feature experienced by most sufferers of *ataques de nervios* is feeling out of control. Most episodes occur as a direct result of a stressful life event related to family or significant others (e.g., death or divorce). After the *ataque*, people oftentimes experience amnesia of what occurred, but then quickly return to their usual level of functioning (American Psychiatric Association, 1994, p. 845).

Guarnaccia and colleagues initiated a program of research by first carrying out open-ended, descriptive interviews in clinical settings with people who had experienced *ataques de nervios* (De La Cancela, Guarnaccia, & Carrilo, 1986; Guarnaccia, De La Cancela, & Carrillo, 1989). Drawing from the rich description of clinical cases and an understanding of the social history of Puerto Ricans living in the United States, these investigators pointed out an association between social disruptions (family and immediate social networks) and the experience of *ataques*. To build on the ethnographic base, Guarnaccia and colleagues turned to epidemiological research to examine its prevalence in Puerto Rico. They examined data from a large epidemiological study in Puerto Rico (Canino et al., 1987) in which respondents were directly queried as to whether they had suffered an *ataque de nervios* and what the experience was like (Guarnaccia, Canino, Rubio-Stipec, & Bravo, 1993). The prevalence rate was found to be high, 16% of the large community sample ($n = 912$), and *ataques de nervios* were found to be associated with a wide range of mental disorders, particularly anxiety and mood disorders. The social context continued to be important in understanding *ataques de nervios*. *Ataques* were found to be more prevalent among women, persons older than 45, people from lower socioeconomic background, and those with disrupted marital relations. Later, Guarnaccia, Rivera, Franco, and Neighbors (1996) returned to the ethnographic mode to explicate the experience of *ataques* among those persons who had reported suffering an *ataque de nervios* in the epidemiological study. Through in-depth interviewing, the full range of symptoms and the specific social contexts were identified. This "experience-near" research approach enabled Guarnaccia and associates to examine carefully how the social world can become part of the physical self as reflected in *ataques de nervios*.

Clinical research has further examined the relationship between *ataques de nervios* and psychiatric diagnoses. Liebowitz and colleagues (1994) carried out clinical diagnostic interviews of 156 Latino patients from an urban psychiatric clinic that specializes in the treatment of anxiety. They explicated the relationship between patients having an *ataque de nervios* and meeting criteria for panic disorder, other anxiety disorders, or an affective disorder. Their fine-grained analysis suggests that the different expressions of *ataque de nervios* interact with different coexisting psychiatric disorders. Persons with an *ataque de nervios* who also suffer from panic disorder present largely anxiety symptoms. However, in those with an affective disorder, *ataques de nervios* are characterized by emotional lability, especially anger (Salmán et al., 1998). Thus, in addition to the social factors previously noted, these findings suggest that the clinical context may also play a role in understanding *ataque de nervios*. A more recent clinical study from the same site, but with different data, more clearly delineates the borderlines between *ataque de nervios* and panic disorder (Lewis-Fernandez et al., 2002). The investigators noted that key distinguishing features of *ataques* as compared to panic attacks are that *ataques* are most often triggered by some stressful event, that people feel relieved after their *ataques*, and that *ataques* do not follow the same rapid crescendo as panic attacks.

Work on *ataques de nervios* has been extended to children (Guarnaccia, Martinez, Ramirez, & Canino, 2005). In a study of the mental health of children in Puerto Rico, the authors included a question on *ataques de nervios*. They found that *ataques* continue to be reported by Puerto Rican children, particularly adolescent girls. As in adults, *ataques* are more common in children who meet criteria for a range of psychiatric disorders in the anxiety and depression spectrum.

The study of *ataque de nervios* is exemplary for many reasons. What is most striking is the systematic ongoing dialogue between ethnographic, epidemiological, and clinical research methods to advance our understanding of *ataques of nervios* and how the social world interacts with psychological and physical processes in the individual. With the multiple approaches, one observes the shifting of the researchers' lenses (Kleinman & Kleinman, 1991). In the early ethnographic work, Guarnaccia and colleagues drew from a small number of clinical cases and interpreted their findings with broad strokes, focusing on the broader social contexts of the individuals, particularly their migration experience and experiences of marginal social status. In the epidemiological research, the investigators used large, representative samples to identify people with *ataques* and the social correlates of that experience. In this research, the social context is reduced to single questions concerning gender, age, education level, and marital status, which provide some basis for interpretation but certainly lack the richness of ethnographic material. The clinical studies provide an in-depth profile of patients' symptomatology and the symptom patterns of those with and without an *ataque*, but they provide less information about the social world of the sufferer. Each approach has its strengths and limitations. What matters though is not a given strength or limitation of a specific study, but the weaving of multiple studies with multiple approaches to understand the given phenomenon in some depth.

In addition to the ongoing dialogue between research approaches, the research is also exemplary by placing *ataque de nervios* and related mental disorders in their social context. In almost all studies, *ataque de nervios* is presented not as a popular illness (i.e., an illness defined by the community) or clinical entity (i.e., a psychologically defined disorder) that resides within individuals, but as a popular illness that reflects the lived experience of women with little power and disrupted social relations. In adopting multiple approaches, the emphasis given to the social domain is likely to shift. Nevertheless, over the several studies Guarnaccia and his colleagues have maintained considerable attention to the social context. In so doing, they have demonstrated how to include the social world in epidemiological (Guarnaccia et al., 1993), clinical (Salmán et al., 1998), as well as ethnographic studies. This integration resulted in a proposal for a parallel categorization of psychopathology for Puerto Ricans using popular categories that bring together both the psychiatric and social dimensions of distress (Guarnaccia, Lewis-Fernandez, & Rivera Marano, 2003). Overall, the study of *ataque de nervios* provides a model for the investigation of culture and psychopathology, particularly for research that begins with a culture-specific form of distress (Guarnaccia & Rogler, 1999).

Schizophrenia The cultural conception of the self can influence the manner in which disorders are expressed and understood by others. This is articulated in Fabrega's (1989) thoughtful overview of how past anthropologically informed research contributed to the study of psychosis and how future studies can advance our understanding of the interrelations of culture and schizophrenia. According to Fabrega, the effect of schizophrenia on individuals and communities depends on whether they conceive of the self as autonomous and separate from others or as connected and bound to others (Markus & Kitayama, 1991; Shweder & Bourne, 1984). The research that most directly addresses this notion is that which examines the role of social factors in the course of schizophrenia. Two prominent lines of inquiry include the WHO cross-national study of schizophrenia and a series of studies examining the relationship of families' emotional climate to the course of illness. (For an examination of culture and symptom expression in schizophrenia see Brekke & Barrio, 1997, and Weisman et al., 2000.)

The WHO's International Pilot Study on Schizophrenia (IPSS) and the follow-up study, Determinants of Outcomes of Severe Mental Disorder (DOSMD), represent the largest multinational study of schizophrenia to date (IPSS: 9 countries and 1,202 patients; DOSMD: 10 countries and 1,379 patients; Jablensky et al., 1992; World Health Organization, 1979). Many contributions have been made by these investigations, including finding evidence of the comparability of schizophrenia's core symptoms across several countries (for a critique see Kleinman, 1988). The finding that has received the most attention by cultural researchers is that schizophrenia in developing countries has a more favorable course than in developed countries (Weisman, 1997). Some investigators have referred to this basic finding as "arguably the single most important finding of cultural differences in cross-cultural research on mental illness" (Lin & Kleinman, 1988, p. 563). Others have been most critical of methods and interpretations (e.g., Cohen, Patel, Thara, & Gureje, 2008; Edgerton & Cohen, 1994; Hopper, 1991). For example, Edgerton and Cohen (1994) pointed out that the distinction between "developed" and "developing" countries is unclear. Moreover, they argued that the cultural explanation for the differences in course is poorly substantiated. They also suggested that such research could be more culturally informed through the direct measure of specific cultural factors in conjunction with observations of people's daily lives (Hopper, 1991). What is clear is that the WHO findings have provided the basis for an important discussion of method and theory regarding how the course of schizophrenia can be shaped by the social world.

Another line of research addressing culture's role in the course of schizophrenia focuses on families' emotional climate. Based on the early work of Brown, Birley, and Wing (1972), research has found that hospitalized patients who return to households marked by high *expressed emotion* (criticism, hostility, and emotional involvement) are more likely to relapse than those who return to households that are not so characterized (Bebbington & Kuipers, 1994; Butzlaff & Hooley, 1998; Leff & Vaughn, 1985). This line of investigation is important to the study of culture because it points out the importance of the social world. More specifically, cross-national and cross-ethnic studies have uncovered interesting differences in the level and nature of expressed emotion (Jenkins & Karno, 1992). These studies show that cultural factors in the definitions and experiences of schizophrenia affect the emotional climate of families where ill individuals live. Furthermore, these cultural differences have important effects on mental health outcomes.

The most systematic cultural analysis of families' role in schizophrenia has been carried out by Jenkins and her colleagues. In using both clinical research methods based on the prototypic contemporary study of expressed emotion (Vaughn & Leff, 1976) and ethnographic methods based on in-depth interviews, Jenkins and associates extended this line of study to Mexican American families in Los Angeles. In the first major report, Karno et al. (1987) replicated the general finding that patients who return to high expressed emotion families are more likely to relapse than patients who return to low expressed emotion families. Jenkins (1988a) then carried out an in-depth examination of Mexican American families' conceptualization of schizophrenia, specifically *nervios*, and how this differed from a comparable sample of Anglo-American families who viewed schizophrenia largely as a mental illness (Guarnaccia, Parra, Deschamps, Milstein, & Argiles, 1992). Based on both quantitative (coded responses to open-ended questions) and qualitative data, Jenkins (1988b) suggested that Mexican Americans' preference for labeling the family member's schizophrenia as *nervios* is tied to the family members efforts to decrease the stigma associated with the illness and also to promote family support for the ill individual. In subsequent papers, Jenkins (1991, 1993) critiqued the cultural basis of the expressed emotion construct in general, as well as its components of criticism and emotional overinvolvement in particular. An important theoretical contribution to the study of the course of schizophrenia is that Jenkins situates families' expressed emotion not only in the family members' attitudes, beliefs, or even feelings (which is the case in most studies), but also in the patient–family social interaction. Overall, Jenkins's work has brought much needed attention to how serious mental illness is embedded in specific social and cultural contexts.

Building on Jenkins work, López and colleagues have further critiqued the notion of expressed emotion with its focus on negative family functioning, particularly criticism (López, Nelson, Snyder, & Mintz, 1999). They pointed out that at an early juncture in the study of families and relapse, investigators (Brown et al., 1972) opted to focus on aspects of family conflict that predict relapse rather than the pro-social aspects of family functioning that buffer relapse. In a reanalysis and extension of the Mexican American sample (Karno et al., 1987) and a comparable Anglo-American sample (Vaughn, Snyder, Jones, Freeman, & Falloon, 1984), López et al. (2004) found that family warmth predicted relapse for Mexican Americans, whereas criticism predicted relapse for Anglo-Americans. In other words, Mexican American patients who returned to families marked by high warmth were less likely to relapse than were those who returned to families characterized by low warmth. For Anglo-Americans, high criticism was positively related to relapse, but warmth was unrelated to relapse. Subsequent analyses of the Mexican American sample (Breitborde, López, Wickens, Jenkins, & Karno, 2007) provided direct evidence that the presence of high warmth and a moderate degree of emotional overinvolvement were associated with less relapse than the usual relapse rate in the study of expressed emotion (Butzlaff & Hooley, 1998). Moreover, a high level of emotional overinvolvement was associated with a greater-than-usual rate of relapse. Aguilera, López, Breitborde, Kopelowicz, and Zarate (2010) replicated the relationship between emotional overinvolvement and relapse with an independent sample of Mexican Americans. Together these findings point out that for largely immigrant Mexican Americans, there is an ongoing tension between maintaining close family ties (high warmth and moderate degrees of involvement) without becoming too involved (Jenkins, 1993). Although close family connections may be valued (and beneficial), too much closeness can be problematic. (See Kopelowicz et al., 2006, for a behavioral observation study of Mexican American families' interactions with their ill relatives that found a similar dynamic.) In addition to identifying this family dynamic, López and colleagues (2009) found that there is a relatively high number of Mexican American caregivers who are identified as emotionally overinvolved. Together these findings suggest that family interventions with this ethnic group should not simply address family negativity, the emphasis of most family-based treatments (Falloon et al., 1982). Attention to caregivers' emotional overinvolvement is likely to be helpful as well.

López et al. (2004) did not attribute the observed ethnic differences in family processes related to relapse to a set of presumed cultural beliefs associated with the "Mexican culture" or a collectivist culture. Instead, they noted that most of the families and patients of Mexican origin were immigrants and that maintaining family ties was crucial to the survival of low-income immigrants living in a foreign and at times hostile environment. Their maintenance of the value of family support was extended to relatives who developed serious mental illnesses. The latter interpretation is consistent with a view of culture as embedded in the social world, rather than as a set of individual values or beliefs.

In conjunction with two other international studies (Italy: Bertrando et al., 1992; Yugoslavia: Ivanović, Vuletić, & Bebbington, 1994), these findings are consistent with the hypothesis that culture plays a role in the manner in which families respond to relatives with schizophrenia, which in turn influences the course of illness. A limitation of most of these findings is that there was no direct measure of cultural processes (for an exception see Aguilera et al., 2010). Nevertheless, the importance of this research is that the exploration of possible cultural variability led to the beginning of a line of inquiry that examines what families do to prevent relapse. Such research has the potential to add a much needed balance to family research by focusing on both positive and negative aspects of families' behaviors (Weisman, Gomes, & López, 2003). The study of care giving (e.g., Guarnaccia, 1998; Lefley 1998; Ramirez Garcia, Chang, Young, López, & Jenkins, 2006) and families' day-to-day interactions with ill family members will likely shed further light on the importance of families' pro-social functioning.

Childhood Disorders   The study of child psychopathology is a rich field of inquiry for those interested in culture. As noted by Weisz, McCarty, Eastman, Chaiyasit, and Suwanlert (1997), child psychopathology requires attention to the behavior of children as well as the views of adults—parents, teachers, and mental health practitioners—for it is the adults who usually decide whether or not a problem exists. The fact that others determine whether children's behavior is problematic underscores the importance of the social world in defining mental illness and disorders of children and adolescents.

John Weisz and his colleagues have carried out the most systematic research on culture and childhood psychopathology (for a review see Weisz et al., 1997). In their first study, conducted in Thailand and the United States, Weisz, Suwanlert, Chaiyasit, Weiss, and Walter (1987) found that Thai children and adolescents who were referred to mental health clinics reported more internalizing problems than U.S. children and adolescents. In contrast, U.S. children and adolescents reported more externalizing problems than Thai children and adolescents. In follow-up community studies, where the mental health referral process was not a factor in the identification of problem behaviors, the cross-national differences were confirmed for internalizing problems but not for externalizing problems (Weisz, Suwanlert, Chaiyasit, Weiss, Achenbach, & Walter, 1987; Weisz, Suwanlert et al., 1993). The prevalence of externalizing problems among U.S. and Thai youth identified in their respective communities did not differ. Weisz and colleagues argued that the findings with regard to internalizing problems are consistent with the idea that culture shapes the manner in which children and adolescents express psychological distress. Because Thai youth come from a largely Buddhist religious and cultural background that values self-control and emotional restraint, they may be more likely than U.S. youth to express psychological distress in a manner that does not violate cultural norms. (For an analysis of the syndromes across the U.S. and Thai samples, see Weisz, Weiss, Suwanlert, & Chaiyasit, 2003).

In addition to these intriguing findings, two other factors stand out in Weisz and colleagues' research: the systematic nature of the research, and the care with which the research has been conducted. Weisz and colleagues began this line of investigation in mental health clinics, and then used a community survey to rule out the possibility of the influence of referral factors (Weisz, Suwanlert, Chaiyasit, Weiss, Achenbach et al., 1987). Based on these findings, Weisz and Weiss (1991) derived a referability index for specific problem behaviors (e.g., vandalism and poor school work) that specifies the likelihood that a given problem will be referred for treatment, taking into account the problem's prevalence in a given community. In this study, they demonstrated how gender and nationality influence whether or not a problem is brought to the attention of mental health professionals. Subsequently, Weisz and colleagues examined teachers' reports of actual children (Weisz et al., 1989) and both parents' and teachers' ratings of hypothetical cases (Weisz, Suwanlert, Chaiyasit, Weiss, & Jackson, 1991). In a study of teachers' report of problem behaviors, Weisz, Chaiyasit, Weiss, Eastman, and Jackson (1995) found that Thai teachers report more internalizing and externalizing problem behaviors among Thai children than U.S. teachers report among U.S. children. Each of Weisz and colleagues' studies systematically builds on their previous work in advancing an understanding of how adults with differing social roles define children's problem behaviors. Multiple cross-cultural studies using different methods with different research participants provide a rich network of findings to advance our understanding of how the social context shapes the identification of youths' mental health problems.

The care with which Weisz and colleagues carry out their research is best illustrated in the study of teachers' ratings of problem behaviors (Weisz et al., 1995). They found that Thai teachers rate more internalizing and externalizing problem behaviors for Thai students than U.S. teachers rate of their own students. Given that this finding runs counter to the previous clinical and community studies that only found differences for internalizing problems, they devised an innovative observational methodology to assess whether it was something about the children or the teachers that contributed to this contradictory finding. Weisz et al. (1995) employed independent observers of children's school behavior and obtained teacher ratings of the same children who were observed in Thailand and in the United States. One of the independent raters was a bilingual Thai psychologist who had received graduate training in the United States. His participation in both teams of independent observers was critical to assessing the reliability of the Thai and U.S. observers. The relationship between his ratings and those of the other U.S. and Thai raters were equally high, suggesting that the ratings were reliable across both national sites. Interestingly, the observers rated Thai children as having less than half as many problem and off-task behaviors as U.S. children, yet Thai teachers rated the observed students as having many more problem behaviors than U.S. teachers rated their students. These data suggest that Thai teachers have a much lower threshold than U.S. teachers for identifying problem behaviors in their students. Findings in cross-cultural research are often open to multiple interpretations. By using careful methodology across multiple studies, Weisz and collaborators have discerned the specific meaning of their complex set of findings. In doing so, they have highlighted the importance of contextual factors in the assessment of child psychopathology and demonstrate that it is untenable to view the assessment of child psychopathology as culture free.

Developmental researchers are examining more closely the influence of culture on the type and degree of problem behaviors of children and adolescents. Weisz and associates have extended their research in Thailand and the United States to Jamaica and Kenya (Lambert, Weisz, & Knight, 1989; Weisz, Sigman, Weiss, & Mosk, 1993). Other investigators have compared rates of internalizing and externalizing problems in other parts of the world (e.g., Denmark: Arnett & Balle-Jensen, 1993; Puerto Rico: Achenbach et al., 1990). Achenbach et al. (2008) have embarked on the most ambitious project thus far, drawing on hundreds of cross-cultural studies using the Achenbach System of Empirically Based Assessment and delineating sociocultural norms based on nationality.

Other researchers have examined specifically internalizing type problem behaviors (Greenberger & Chen, 1996) or externalizing type problem behaviors (Weine, Phillips, & Achenbach, 1995) in cross-national or cross-ethnic samples. An important trend in this research is that epidemiological research that compares groups cross nationally and suggests possible cultural explanations is now being complemented by research that examines the psychosocial processes associated with children's and adolescents' adjustment or psychopathology. For example, Chen, Greenberger, Lester, Dong, and Guo (1998) examined risk factors (parent–adolescent conflict and perceived peer approval of misconduct) and protective factors (parental warmth and parental monitoring) associated with acting-out problems across four groups of adolescents: European Americans, Chinese Americans, Taipei Chinese, and Beijing Chinese. They found both cross-cultural similarities and differences in the way both family and peer factors contributed to misconduct. Generally the predicted risk and protective factors accounted for a significant amount of variance for misconduct in each of the four groups, however, peer influences were less relevant for the Taipei and Beijing Chinese youth. (See also Polo and López, 2009, as they examined the sociocultural mediators that explain differences in internalizing distress among U.S.-born and immigrant Mexican-origin youth.)

The strength of the more recent studies is that they examine processes that may explain potential cross-national differences and similarities, including social (family and peers) and psychological (values) processes. Thus, an important step has been taken to understand why differences and similarities may occur in behavior problems cross nationally. Although the conceptual models used to frame such research are rich, include social processes, and have a strong empirical tradition in psychological research, they are not well informed by cultural-specific processes of the non-U.S. groups under study. Investigators typically apply models developed largely in the United States. Ethnographic research that attempts to identify what about the social and cultural world might play a role in the expression of distress and disorder among children would be especially welcome. This research could then lead to the direct examination of those culture-specific factors that are believed to affect psychopathology within a given conceptual framework, as evidenced in the work of some developmental researchers (Fuligni, 1998) and as advocated by others (Schneider, 1998). The growing interest of researchers in studying internalizing and externalizing problem behaviors cross nationally and cross ethnically attests to the utility of this approach for enhancing our understanding of culture and childhood psychopathology.

Research Areas With Great Potential to Advance Our Understanding of the Social World

Immigration   There has been a longstanding interest in the role of immigration or acculturation as it relates to mental health and mental disorders. Important studies indicate that among Mexican-origin adults, immigrants have lower prevalence rates than those who are born in the United States (Burnam, Hough, Karno, Escobar, & Telles, 1987; Vega et al., 1998). More recently, Grant et al. (2004) reported that the acculturation effect applied not only to Mexican-origin residents but also to non-Latino White immigrants when compared to non-Latino Whites born in the United States. The same effect has also been reported for Caribbean Blacks from the NSAL; immigrant Caribbean Blacks had lower rates of substance abuse disorders (Broman, Neighbors, Delva, Torres, & Jackson, 2008) and major depression (Williams et al., 2007) than U.S.-born Caribbean Blacks. Alegría and colleagues (Alegría, Canino et al., 2006; Alegría et al., 2008) caution that the immigration/acculturation effect does not universally apply to immigrant groups. In particular, they point out that among Latinos the immigrant/acculturation effect pertains largely to Mexican origin adults, not Cuban Americans or Puerto Ricans, though Puerto Ricans are not really immigrants as they are U.S. citizens whether they live on Puerto Rico or the mainland. Also, for Asian Americans, the immigrant effect primarily applies to women (Takeuchi et al., 2007). Thus available literature suggests that there is strong evidence for an immigration effect; however, it does not apply universally to all immigrant groups.

The social and psychological mechanisms that are responsible for the differing prevalence rates for the immigrant groups are poorly understood at this time. Nevertheless, available studies indicate that research on immigration and acculturation can contribute much to our understanding of how the social world and psychopathology interrelate (Rogler, 1994). A particularly wide-open area of study is the examination of immigration and mental health and disorders among children and adolescents (Gil & Vega, 1996; Guarnaccia & López, 1998; Polo & López, 2009). Not only will immigration/acculturation research be able to address important conceptual and methodological issues in the study of culture, it will also have important policy implications for the delivery of mental health services to underserved communities (Salgado de Snyder, Diaz-Perez, & Bautista, 1998).

American Indians   We are encouraged by the growing interest in the study of psychopathology among U.S. ethnic minority groups. To highlight this area, we have chosen to focus on research with American Indians because we have given little attention to this growing body of literature and because researchers in this area have given considerable attention to social factors. A systematic series of studies has examined the mental health problems of American Indian children (e.g., Beiser, Sack, Manson, Redshirt, & Dion, 1998; Dion, Gotowiec, & Beiser, 1998) and adults (Maser & Dinges, 1992–1993). Although many of these studies use mainstream models of disorder and distress (O'Nell, 1989), there are growing efforts to contextualize the mental health problems within these communities. In one study, Duclos et al. (1998) found that nearly half of the American Indian adolescents detained in the juvenile justice system met the criteria for mental disorders, ranging from substance abuse/dependence (38%) to major depression (10%). These rates were much higher than community surveys of American Indian youth and non-Indian youth. These researchers argue that the juvenile justice system has the potential to serve as an important site for treating these high-risk youth, many of whom would go untreated. In another study, O'Nell and Mitchell (1996) found that the line between normal and pathological drinking among adolescent American Indians is contextually based. Their ethnographic findings suggest that a rigid model of alcohol abuse, defined by biology (frequency and amount of alcohol) or psychology (distress), without significant attention to the sociocultural context (e.g., when and with whom one drinks) is limited in distinguishing between normative and pathological drinking (see Klostermann & Kelley, this volume).

The largest study to date of the mental health of Americans Indians is the American Indian Services Utilization, Psychiatric Epidemiology, Risk and Protective Factors Project (Beals et al., 2003). This project is based on representative samples of adult residents within two reservations (Southwest tribe: $n = 1,446$, and Northern Plains tribe: $n = 1,638$). Among the early findings reported from this research is that when controlling for various demographic correlates, the American Indian samples reported greater lifetime prevalence rates of alcohol abuse and post-traumatic stress disorder and lower lifetime rates of major depression than a national sample from the United States across ethnicities (Beals et al., 2005). More recent studies have examined the role of adversity (e.g., disruptions to children's lives such as parental divorce and traumas such as witnessed violence) in the development of mental disorders. Whitesell et al. (2007), for example, found that both proximal and cumulative distal experiences of adversity were associated with an increased risk of the onset of substance dependence symptoms. Given that ethnographic interviews were also carried out in this large-scale project, we expect in the future more nuanced research reports that examine the social world as it relates to trauma and alcohol disorders.

Conclusion

Cultural psychopathology, the study of culture and the definition, experience, distribution, and course of psychological disorders, is now "on the map." Articles are being published in culture-focused journals as well as mainstream journals (e.g., *American Journal of Psychiatry, Archives of General Psychiatry, Journal of Abnormal Psychology, Journal of the American Academy of Child and Adolescent Psychiatry, Journal of Nervous and Mental Disease*). Substantive areas of psychopathology research are being shaped by cultural research. Efforts to integrate idioms of distress with mainstream constructs are well under way. Examples include studies of *ataques de nervios* and anxiety and affective disorders, and *nervios* and families' conceptualization of serious mental illness. Guarnaccia and Rogler (1999) provided a program for moving some of this research forward. Kleinman's important 1988 book got the message out that culture matters. As evidenced in the Surgeon General's report and the CPES, the message has been received;

cultural research is providing an innovative and fresh perspective to our understanding of several important aspects of psychopathology.

For cultural researchers to build on the empirical and conceptual foundation that has been established, they need to continue to be critical of how culture is conceptualized and how such conceptualizations guide their research. It is clear from this review that culture can no longer be treated solely as an independent variable or as a factor to be controlled for. Rather, culture infuses the full social context of mental health research. Culture is important in all aspects of psychopathology research—the design and translation of instruments, the conceptual models that guide the research, the interpersonal interaction between researcher and research participants, the definition and interpretation of symptom and syndromes, and the structure of the social world that surrounds a person's mental health problems. Cultural psychopathology research requires a framework that incorporates culture in multifaceted ways. For this reason, it is crucial that cultural research not obscure the importance of other social forces such as gender, class, poverty, and marginality that work in conjunction with culture to shape people's everyday lives. The examination of both social and cultural processes is one way to help guard against superficial cultural analyses that ignore or minimize the powerful political economic inequalities that coexist with culture.

A corollary of the need for a broad framework for research is the need for approaches that integrate qualitative and quantitative methods. Cultural psychopathology research can serve as an important site for integrating ethnographic, observational, clinical, and epidemiological research approaches. Mental health problems cannot be fully understood through one lens. Ethnographic research provides insights into the meaning of mental health problems and how they are experienced in their sociocultural context. Observational research captures people's functioning in their daily lives. Clinical research can provide detailed descriptions of psychopathological processes and can contribute to developing treatments to alleviate suffering at the individual as well as social levels. Epidemiological research can identify who is most at risk for psychopathology and broaden perspectives to more generalized processes and populations. It is the integration of these perspectives, through new mixes of methodologies and in the composition of research teams, that will make the cultural psychopathology research agenda succeed.

The ultimate goal of cultural psychopathology research is to alleviate suffering and improve people's lives. This requires attention to the multiple levels of individual, family, community, and the broader social system. Our enhanced notion of culture leads to analysis of the expression and sources of psychopathology at all of these levels. Our commitment to making a difference in people's everyday lives argues for the development of treatment and prevention interventions at these multiple levels as well. The increasing cultural diversity of the United States and the massive movements of people around the globe provide both an opportunity and imperative for cultural psychopathology research.

References

Abe-Kim, J., Takeuchi, D. T., Hong, S., Zane, N., Sue, S., Spencer, M. S., … Alegría, M. (2007). Use of mental health-related services among immigrant and US-born Asian Americans: Results from the National Latino and Asian American Study. *American Journal of Public Health, 97*, 91–98.

Achenbach, T. M., Becker, A., Dopfner, M., Heiervang, E., Roessner, V., Steinhausen, H., & Rothenberger, A. (2008). Multicultural assessment of child and adolescent psychopathology with ASEBA and SDQ instruments: Research findings, applications, and future directions. *Journal of Child Psychology and Psychiatry, 49*, 251–275.

Achenbach, T. M., Bird, H. R., Canino, G., Phares, V., Gould, M. S., & Rubio-Stipec, M. (1990). Epidemiological comparisons of Puerto Rican and U.S. mainland children: Parent, teacher and self-reports. *Journal of the American Academy of Child & Adolescent Psychiatry, 29*(1), 84–93.

Aguilera, A., López, S. R., Breitborde, N. J. K., Kopelowicz, A., & Zarate, R. (2010). Expressed emotion and sociocultural moderation in the course of schizophrenia. *Journal of Abnormal Psychology, 119*(4), 875–885.

Alarcón, R. D. (1995). Culture and psychiatric diagnosis: Impact on DSM-IV and ICD-10. *Psychiatric Clinics of North America,18*, 449–465.

Alarcón, R. D., Bell, C. C., Kirmayer, L. J., Lin, K. M., Ustun, B., & Wisner, K. L. (2002). Beyond the funhouse mirrors: Research agenda on culture and psychiatric diagnosis. In D. J. Kupfer, M. B. First, & D. A. Regier (Eds.), *A research agenda for DSM-V* (pp. 219–281). Washington, DC: American Psychiatric Press.

Alegría, M., Canino, G., Shrout, P. E., Woo, M., Duan, N., Vila, D., … Meng, X. L. (2008). Prevalence of mental illness in immigrant and non-immigrant U.S. Latino groups. *American Journal of Psychiatry, 165*, 359–369.

Alegría, M., Canino, G., Stinson, F. S., & Grant, B. F. (2006). Nativity and DSM-IV psychiatric disorders among Puerto Ricans, Cuban Americans, and non-Latino Whites in the United Status: Results from the National Epidemiologic Survey on Alcohol and related conditions. *Journal of Clinical Psychiatry, 67*, 56–65.

Alegría, M., Takeuchi, D., Canino, G., Duan, N., Shrout, P., Meng, X. L., … Gong, F. (2006). Considering context, place and culture: The National Latino and Asian American Study. *International Journal of Methods in Psychiatric Research, 13*, 208–220.

American Psychiatric Association. (1994). *Diagnostic and statistical manual of mental disorder*s (4th ed.). Washington, DC: Author.

Arnett, J., & Balle-Jensen, L. (1993). Cultural bases of risk behavior: Danish adolescents. *Child Development, 64*, 1842–1855.

Beals, J., Manson, S. M., Mitchell, C. M., Spicer P., AI-SUPERPFP Team. (2003). Cultural specificity and comparison in psychiatric epidemiology: Walking the tightrope in American Indian research. *Culture, Medicine and Psychiatry, 27*, 259–289.

Beals, J., Novins, D. K., Whitesell, N. R., Spicer, P., Mitchell, C. M., & Manson, S. M., AI-SUPERPFP Team. (2005). Prevalence of mental disorders and utilization of mental health services in two American Indian reservation populations: Mental health disparities in a national context. *American Journal of Psychiatry, 162*, 1723–1732.

Bebbington, P., & Kuipers, L. (1994). The predictive utility of expressed emotion in schizophrenia: An aggregate analysis. *Psychological Medicine, 24*, 707–718.

Beiser, M., Sack, W., Manson, S., Redshirt, R., & Dion, R. (1998). Mental health and the academic performance of First Nations and majority-culture children. *American Journal of Orthopsychiatry, 68*, 455–467.

Bernal, G., Cumba-Aviles, E., & Saez-Santiago, E. (2006). Cultural and relational processes in depressed Latino adolescents. In S. R. H. Beach, M. Z. Wamboldt, N. J. Kaslow, R. E. Heyman, M. B. First, L. G. Underwood, & D. Reiss (Eds.), *Relational processes and DSM-V: Neuroscience, assessment, prevention and treatment* (pp. 211–224). Washington, DC: American Psychiatric Press.

Bertrando, P., Beltz, J., Bressi, C., Clerici, M., Farma, T., Invernizzi, G., & Cazzullo, C. L. (1992). Expressed emotion and schizophrenia in Italy: A study of an urban population. *British Journal of Psychiatry, 161*, 223–229.

Betancourt, H., & López, S. R. (1993). The study of culture, race and ethnicity in American psychology. *American Psychologist, 48*, 629–637.

Breitborde, N. J. K., López, S. R., Wickens, T. D., Jenkins, J. H., & Karno, M. (2007). Toward specifying the nature of the relationship between expressed emotion and schizophrenic relapse: The utility of curvilinear models. *International Journal of Methods in Psychiatric Research, 16*(1), 1–10.

Brekke, J. S., & Barrio, C. (1997) Cross-ethnic symptom differences in schizophrenia: The influence of culture and minority status. *Schizophrenia Bulletin, 23*, 305–316.

Broman, C. L., Neighbors, H. W., Delva, J., Torres, M., & Jackson, J. S. (2008). Prevalence of substance use disorders among African Americans and Caribbean Blacks in the National Survey of American Life. *American Journal of Public Health, 98*, 1107–1114.

Brown, G. W., Birley, J. L. T., & Wing, J. K. (1972). Influence of family life on the course of schizophrenic disorders: A replication. *British Journal of Psychiatry, 21*, 241–258.

Burnam, A., Hough, R. L., Karno, M., Escobar, J. I., & Telles, C. (1987). Acculturation and lifetime prevalence of psychiatric disorders among Mexican Americans in Los Angeles. *Journal of Health and Social Behavior, 28*, 89–102.

Butcher, J. N. (1987). Introduction to thte special series. *Journal of Consulting and Clinical Psychology, 55*, 459–460.

Butzlaff, R. L., & Hooley, J. M. (1998). Expressed emotion and psychiatric relapse: A meta-analysis. *Archives of General Psychiatry, 55,* 547–552.

Canino, G. J., Bird, H. R., Shrout, P. E., Rubio-Stipec, M., Bravo, M., Martinez, R., … Guevara, L. M. (1987). The prevalence of specific psychiatric disorders in Puerto Rico. *Archives of General Psychiatry, 44,* 727–735.

Cervantes, R. C., Padilla, A. M., & Salgado de Zinder, V. N. (1991). The Hispanic Stress Inventory: A culturally relevant approach to psychological assessment. *Psychological Assessment, 3,* 438–447.

Chavez, N. (2003). Commentary. *Culture, Medicine and Psychiatry, 27,* 391–394.

Chen, C., Greenberger, E., Lester, J., Dong, Q., & Guo, M. (1998). A cross-cultural study of family and peer correlates of adolescent misconduct. *Developmental Psychology, 34,* 770–81.

Clark, L. A. (1987). Mutual relevance of mainstream and cross-cultural psychology. *Journal of Consulting and Clinical Psychology, 55,* 41–70.

Cohen, A., Patel, V., Thara, R., & Gureje, O. (2008). Questioning an axiom: Better prognosis for schizophrenia in the developing world? *Schizophrenia Bulletin, 34,* 229–244.

De La Cancela, V., Guarnaccia, P., & Carrillo, E. (1986). Psychosocial distress among Latinos. *Humanity Society, 10,* 431–447.

Desjarlais, R., Eisenberg, L., Good, B., & Kleinman, A. (1996). *World mental health: Problems and priorities in low-income countries.* Oxford: Oxford University Press.

Dion, R., Gotowiec, A., & Beiser, M. (1998). Depression and conduct disorder in Native and non-Native children. *Journal of the American Academy of Child and Adolescent Psychiatry, 37,* 736–742.

Draguns, J. G. (1980). Disorders of clinical severity. In H. C. Triandis & J. G. Draguns (Eds.), *Handbook of cross-cultural psychology: Psychopathology* (Vol. 6, pp. 99–174). Boston: Allyn and Bacon.

Draguns, J. G. (1990). Culture and psychopathology: Toward specifying the nature of the relationship. In J. Berman (Ed.), Nebraska Symposium on Motivation *1989: Cross-cultural perspectives* (pp. 235–277). Lincoln: University of Nebraska Press.

Duclos, C. W., Beals, J., Novins, D. K., Martin, C., Jewett, C. S., & Manson, S. M. (1998). Prevalence of common psychiatric disorders among American Indian adolescent detainees. *Journal of the American Academy of Child and Adolescent Psychiatry, 37,* 866–873.

Edgerton, R., & Cohen, A. (1994). Culture and schizophrenia: The DOSMD challenge. *British Journal of Psychiatry, 164,* 222–231.

Fabrega, H. (1975). The need for an ethnomedical science. *Science, 189,* 969–975.

Fabrega, H. (1989). On the significance of an anthropological approach to schizophrenia. *Psychiatry, 52,* 45–65.

Fabrega H. (1990). Hispanic mental health research: A case for cultural psychiatry. *Hispanic Journal of Behavioral Science, 12,* 339–365.

Fallon, I. R. H., Boyd, J. L., McGill, C. W., Razani, J., Moos, H. B., & Gilderman, A. M. (1982). Family management in the prevention of exacerbations of schizophrenia. *New England Journal of Medicine, 396,* 1437–1440.

Fuligni, A. (1998). Authority, autonomy, and parent-adolescent conflict and cohesion: A study of adolescents from Mexican, Chinese, Filipino, and European backgrounds. *Developmental Psychology, 34,* 782–792.

Gallimore, R., Goldenberg, C. N., & Weisner, T. S. (1993). The social construction and subjective reality of activity settings: Implications for community psychology. *American Journal of Community Psychology, 21,* 537–559.

Garro, L. C. (2000). Cultural knowledge as resource in illness narratives: Remembering through accounts of illness. In C. Mattingly & L. C. Garro (Eds.), *Narrative and the cultural construction of illness and healing* (pp. 70–87). Berkeley: University of California Press.

Garro, L. C. (2001). The remembered past in a culturally meaningful life: Remembering as cultural, social and cognitive process. In C. Moore & H. Mathews (Eds.), *The psychology of cultural experience* (pp. 105–147). Cambridge: Cambridge University Press.

Gavin, A. R., Walton, E., Chae, D. H., Alegría, M., Jackson, J. S., & Takeuchi, D. (2010). The associations between socio-economic status and major depressive disorder among Blacks, Latinos, Asians and non-Hispanic Whites: Findings from the Collaborative Psychiatric Epidemiology Studies. *Psychological Medicine, 40,* 51–61.

Gil, A., & Vega, W. A. (1996). Two different worlds: Acculturation stress and adaptation among Cuban and Nicaraguan families in Miami. *Journal of Social and Personal Relations, 13,* 437–458.

Gonzalez, H. M., Tarraf, W., Whitfield, K. E., & Vega, W. A. (2010). The epidemiology of major depression and ethnicity in the United States. *Journal of Psychiatric Research, 44,* 1043–1051.

Grant, B. F., Stinson, F. S., Hasin, D. S., Dawson, D. A., Chou, S. P., & Anderson, K. (2004). Immigration and lifetime prevalence of DSM-IV psychiatric disorders among Mexican Americans and non-Hispanic whites in the United States. *Archives of General Psychiatry, 61*, 1226–1233.

Greenberger, E., & Chen, C. (1996). Perceived family relationships and depressed mood in early and late adolescence: A comparison of European and Asian Americans. *Developmental Psychology, 32*, 707–716.

Greenfield, P. M. (1997). Culture as process: Empirical methods for cultural psychology. In J. W. Berry, Y. H. Poortinga, & J. Pandey (Eds.), *Handbook of Cross-Cultural Psychology: Theory and Method* (Vol. 1, pp. 301–346). Needham Heights, MA: Allyn and Bacon.

Guarnaccia, P. J. (1997). A cross-cultural perspective on the anxiety disorders. In S. Friedman (Ed.), *Treating anxiety disorders across cultures* (pp. 3–20). New York: Guilford.

Guarnaccia, P. J. (1998). Multicultural experiences of family caregiving: A study of African American, European American and Hispanic American families. In H. Lefley (Ed.), *Families coping with illness: The cultural context* (pp. 45–61). San Francisco: Jossey-Bass.

Guarnaccia, P. J., Canino, G., Rubio-Stipec, M., & Bravo, M. (1993). The prevalence of *ataques de nervios* in the Puerto Rico study: The role of culture in psychiatric epidemiology. *Journal of Nervous and Mental Disease, 181*, 157–165.

Guarnaccia, P. J., De La Cancela, V., & Carrillo, E. (1989). The multiple meanings of *ataques de nervios* in the Latino community. *Medical Anthropology, 11*, 47–62.

Guarnaccia, P. J., & Kirmayer, L. (1997). Culture and the DSM-IV anxiety disorders. In T. Widiger, A. Frances, H. A. Pincus, M. B. First, R. Ross, & W. Davis (Eds.), *DSM-IV source book* (Vol. 3, pp. 925–932). Washington, DC: American Psychiatric Press.

Guarnaccia, P. J., Kleinman, A., & Good, B. J. (1990). A critical review of epidemiological studies of Puerto Rican mental health. *American Journal of Psychiatry, 147*, 449–456.

Guarnaccia, P. J., Lewis-Fernandez, R., & Rivera Marano, M. (2003). Toward a Puerto Rican popular posology: *Nervios* and *ataques de nervios*. *Culture, Medicine and Psychiatry, 27*, 339–366.

Guarnaccia, P. J., Lewis-Fernandez, R., Martinez, I., Shrout, P., Guo, J., Torres, M.,...Alegría, M. (2010). Ataques de nervios as a marker of social and psychiatric vulnerability: Results from the NLAAS. *International Journal of Social Psychiatry, 56*, 289–309.

Guarnaccia, P. J., & López, S. (1998). The mental health and adjustment of immigrant and refugee children. *Child and Adolescent Psychiatric Clinics of North America, 7*, 537–553.

Guarnaccia, P. J., Martinez, I., Ramirez, R., & Canino, G. (2005). Are *ataques de nervios* in Puerto Rican children associated with psychiatric disorder? *Journal of the American Academy of Child and Adolescent Psychiatry, 44*, 1184–1192.

Guarnaccia, P. J., Parra, P., Deschamps, A., Milstein, G., & Argiles, N. (1992). Si Dios quiere: Hispanic families' experiences of caring for a seriously mentally ill family member. *Culture, Medicine, and Psychiatry, 16*, 187–215.

Guarnaccia, P. J., Rivera, M., Franco, F., & Neighbors, C. (1996). The experiences of ataques de nervios: Towards an anthropology of emotions in Puerto Rico. *Culture, Medicine, and Psychiatry, 20*, 343–367.

Guarnaccia, P. J., & Rodriguez, O. (1996). Concepts of culture and their roles in the development of culturally competent mental health services. *Hispanic Journal of Behavioral Sciences, 18*, 419–443.

Guarnaccia, P. J., & Rogler, L. H. (1999). Research on culture-bound syndromes: New directions. *American Journal of Psychiatry, 156*, 1322–1327.

Hong, Y., Morris, M. W., Chiu, C., & Benet-Martinez, V. (2000). Multicultural minds: Dynamic constructivist approach to culture and cognition. *American Psychologist, 55*, 709–720.

Hopper, K. (1991). Some old questions for the new cross-cultural psychiatry. *Medical Anthropology Quarterly, 5*, 299–330.

Ivanović, M., Vuletić, Z., & Bebbington, P. (1994). Expressed emotion in the families of patients with schizophrenia and its influence on the course of illness. *Social Psychiatry and Psychiatric Epidemiology, 29*, 61–65.

Jablensky, A., Sartorius, N., Ernberg, G., Ankar, M., Korten, A., Cooper, J. E., … Bertelsen, A. (1992). Schizophrenia: Manifestations, incidence and course in different cultures. *Psychological Medicine, 20*(Suppl.), 1–97.

Jackson, J. S., Torres, M., Caldwell, C. H., Neighbors, H. W., Nesse, R. M., Taylor, R. J., … Williams, D. R. (2006). The National Survey of American Life: A study of racial, ethnic and cultural influences on mental disorders and mental health. *International Journal of Methods in Psychiatric Research, 13*, 196–207.

Jenkins, J. H. (1988a). Conceptions of schizophrenia as a problem of nerves: A cross-cultural comparison of Mexican-Americans and Anglo-Americans. *Social Science and Medicine, 26*, 1233–1243.

Jenkins, J. H. (1988b). Ethnopsychiatric interpretations of schizophrenic illness: The problem of *nervios* within Mexican-American families. *Culture, Medicine, and Psychiatry, 12,* 303–331.

Jenkins, J. H. (1991). Anthropology, expressed emotion, and schizophrenia. *Ethos, 19,* 387–431.

Jenkins, J. H. (1993). Too close for comfort: Schizophrenia and emotional overinvolvement among *Mexicano* families. In A. D. Gaines (Ed.), *Ethnopsychiatry* (pp. 203–221). Albany, NY: State University of New York Press.

Jenkins, J., & Karno, M. (1992). The meaning of expressed emotion: Theoretical issues raised by cross-cultural research. *American Journal of Psychiatry, 149,* 9–21.

Karno, M., Jenkins, J. H., de la Selva, A., Santana, F., Telles, C., López, S., & Mintz, J. (1987). Expressed emotion and schizophrenic outcome among Mexican-American families. *Journal of Nervous and Mental Disease, 175,* 143–151.

Kessler, R., Berglund, P., Chiu, W. T., Demler, O., Heeringa, S., Hiripi, E., … Zheng, H. (2004). The US National Comorbidity Survey-Replication (NCS-R): Design and field procedures. *International Journal of Methods in Psychiatric Research, 13,* 69–92.

Kessler, R. C., Mickelson, K. D., & Williams, D. R. (1999). The prevalence, distribution, and mental health correlates of perceived discrimination in the United States. *Journal of Health and Social Behavior, 40,* 208–230.

King, L. M. (1978). Social and cultural influences on psychopathology. *Annual Review of Psychology, 29,* 405–433.

Kirmayer, L. J. (1998). Editorial: The fate of culture in DSM-IV. *Transcultural Psychiatry, 35,* 339–342.

Kleinman, A. (1988). *Rethinking Psychiatry: From cultural category to personal experience.* New York: Free Press.

Kleinman, A. (2006). *What really matters.* New York: Oxford University Press.

Kleinman, A. M. (1977). Depression, somatization and the "New Cross-Cultural Psychiatry." *Social Science and Medicine, 11,* 3–10.

Kleinman, A., Eisenberg, L., & Good, B. (1978). Culture, illness, and care: Clinical lessons from anthropologic and cross-cultural research. *Annals of Internal Medicine, 88,* 251–258.

Kleinman, A., & Good, B. J. (Eds.). (1985). *Culture and depression.* Berkeley: University of California Press.

Kleinman, A., & Kleinman, J. (1991). Suffering and its professional transformations: Toward an ethnography of experience. *Culture, Medicine, and Psychiatry, 15,* 275–301.

Kopelowicz, A., López, S. R., Zarate, R., O'Brien, M., Gordon, J., Chang, C., & Gonzalez-Smith, V. (2006). Expressed emotion and family interactions in Mexican Americans with schizophrenia. *Journal of Nervous and Mental Disease, 19,* 330–334.

Lambert, M. C., Weisz, J. R., & Knight, F. (1989). Over- and undercontrolled clinic referral problems of Jamaican and American children and adolescents: The culture-general and the culture-specific. *Journal of Consulting and Clinical Psychology, 57,* 467–472.

Leff, J. P., & Vaughn, C. E. (1985). *Expressed emotion in families.* New York: Guilford.

Lefley, H. (Ed.). (1998). *Families coping with illness: The cultural context.* San Francisco: Jossey-Bass.

Lewis-Fernandez, R., Guarnaccia, P. J., Martinez, I. E., Salmán, E., Schmidt, A., & Liebowitz, M. (2002). Comparative phenomenology of *ataques de nervios,* panic attacks, and panic disorder. *Culture, Medicine and Psychiatry, 26,* 199–223.

Lewis-Fernandez, R., Hinton, D. E., Laria, A. J., Patterson, E. H., Hofmann, S. G., Craske, M. G., … Liao, B. (2010). Culture and the anxiety disorders: Recommendations for DSM-V. *Depression and Anxiety, 27,* 212–229.

Lewis-Fernandez, R., Horvitz-Lennon, M., Blanco, C., Guarnaccia, P. J., Cao, Z., & Alegría, M. (2009). Significance of endorsement of psychotic symptoms by US Latinos. *Journal of Nervous and Mental Disease, 197,* 337–347.

Lewis-Fernandez, R., & Kleinman, A. (1995). Cultural psychiatry: Theoretical, clinical and research issues. *Psychiatric Clinics of North America, 18,* 433–448.

Liebowitz, M. R., Salmán, E., Jusino, C. M., Garfinkel, R., Street, L., Cardenas, D. L., … Davies, S. (1994). Ataque de nervios and panic disorder. *American Journal of Psychiatry, 151,* 871–875.

Lin, K. M., & Kleinman, A. M. (1988). Psychopathology and clinical course of schizophrenia: A cross-cultural perspective. *Schizophrenia Bulletin, 14,* 555–567.

Lin, K. M., Poland, R. E., & Anderson, D. (1995). Psychopharmacology, ethnicity and culture. *Transcultural Psychiatric Research Review, 32,* 3–40.

López, S. R. (2003). Reflections on the surgeon general's Report on Mental Health: Culture, Race and Ethnicity. *Culture, Medicine and Psychiatry, 27,* 419–434.

López, S. R, Nelson, K., Polo, A., Jenkins, J. H., Karno, M., Vaughn, C., & Snyder, K. (2004). Ethnicity, expressed emotion, attributions and course of schizophrenia: Family warmth matters. *Journal of Abnormal Psychology, 113,* 428–439.

López, S. R., Nelson, K., Snyder, K., & Mintz, J. (1999). Attributions and affective reactions of family members and course of schizophrenia. *Journal of Abnormal Psychology, 108*, 307–314.

López, S., & Núñez, J. A. (1987). The consideration of cultural factors in selected diagnostic criteria and interview schedules. *Journal Abnormal Psychology, 96*, 270–272.

López, S. R., Ramirez Garcia, J. I., Ullman, J. B., Kopelowicz, A., Jenkins, J., Breitborde, N. J. K., & Placencia, P. (2009). Cultural variability in the manifestation of expressed emotion. *Family Process, 48*, 179–194.

Manson, S. M., Shore, J. H., & Bloom, J. D. (1985). The depressive experience in American Indian communities: A challenge for psychiatric theory and diagnosis. In A. Kleinman & B. J. Good (Eds.), *Culture and depression* (pp. 331–368). Berkeley: University of California Press.

Markus, H. R., & Kitayama, S. (1991). Culture and the self: Implications for cognition, emotion, and motivation. *Psychological Review, 98*, 224–253.

Marsella, A. J. (1980). Depressive experience and disorder across cultures. In H. Triandis & J. Draguns (Eds.), *Handbook of cross-cultural psychology: Psychopathology* (Vol. 6, pp. 237–289). Boston: Allyn and Bacon.

Maser, J. D., & Dinges, N. (1992–1993). The co-morbidity of depression, anxiety and substance abuse among American Indians and Alaska Natives. *Culture, Medicine, and Psychiatry, 16*, 409–577.

Mezzich, J. E, Kleinman, A., Fabrega, H., & Parron, D. L. (Eds.). (1996). *Culture and psychiatric diagnosis: A DSM-IV perspective.* Washington, DC: American Psychiatric Association.

Mezzich, J. E., Kleinman, A., Fabrega, H., Parron, D. L., Good, B. J., Lin, K., & Manson, S. M. (1997). Cultural issues for DSM-IV. In T. A. Widiger, A. J. Frances, H. A. Pincus, R. Ross, M. B. First, & W. Davis (Eds.), *DSM-IV sourcebook* (Vol. 3, pp. 861–1016). Washington, DC: American Psychiatric Association.

Murray, C. J. L., & López, A. D. (1996). *The global burden of disease: A comprehensive assessment of mortality and disability from diseases, injuries, and risk factors in 1990 and projected to 2020.* Cambridge: Harvard University Press.

Neighbors, H. W., Jackson, J. S., Campbell, L., & Williams, D. (1989). The influence of racial factors on psychiatric diagnosis: A review and suggestions for research. *Community Mental Health Journal, 25*, 301–310.

O'Nell, T. (1989). Psychiatric investigations among American Indians and Alaska Natives: A critical review. *Culture, Medicine, and Psychiatry, 13*, 51–87.

O'Nell, T., & Mitchell, C. M. (1996). Alcohol use among American Indian adolescents: The role of culture in pathological drinking. *Social Science and Medicine, 42*, 565–578.

Polo, A. J., & López, S. R. (2009). Culture, context, and the internalizing distress of Mexican American youth. *Journal of Clinical Child and Adolescent Psychology, 38*, 273–285.

Ramirez Garcia, J. I., Chang, C. L., Young, J. S., López, S. R., & Jenkins, J. H. (2006). Family support predicts psychiatric medication usage among Mexican American individuals with schizophrenia. *Social Psychiatry and Psychiatric Epidemiology, 41*, 624–631.

Regier, D. A., Myers, J. K., Kramer, M., Robins, L. N., Blazer, D. G., Hough, R. L., … Locke, B. Z. (1984). The NIMH Epidemiologic Catchment Area program. *Archives of General Psychiatry, 41*, 934–941.

Rogler, L. H. (1989). The meaning of culturally sensitive research in mental health. *American Journal of Psychiatry, 146*, 296–303.

Rogler, L. H. (1994). International migrations: A framework for directing research. *American Psychologist, 49*, 701–708.

Rogler, L. H. (1996). Framing research on culture in psychiatric diagnosis: The case of the DSM-IV. *Psychiatry: Interpersonal and Biological Processes, 59*, 145–155.

Rogler, L. H., Malgady, R. G., & Rodríguez, O. (1989). *Hispanics and Mental Health: A Framework for Research.* Malabar, FL: Krieger.

Salgado de Snyder, V. N., Diaz-Perez, M., & Bautista, E. (1998). Pathways to mental health services among inhabitants of a Mexican village with high migratory tradition to the United States. *Health and Social Work, 23*, 249–261.

Salmán E., Liebowitz, M., Guarnaccia, P. J., Jusino, C. M., Garfinkel, R., Street, L., … Klein, D. F. (1998). Subtypes of ataques de nervios: The influence of coexisting psychiatric diagnosis. *Culture, Medicine, and Psychiatry, 22*, 231–244.

Sartorius, N., Jablensky, A., Korten, A., Ernberg, G., Anker, M., Cooper, J. E., & Day, R. (1986). Early manifestations and first-contact incidence of schizophrenia in different cultures. *Psychological Medicine, 16*, 909–928.

Schneider, B. H. (1998). Cross-cultural comparison as doorkeeper in research on social and emotional adjustment of children and adolescents. *Developmental Psychology, 34*, 793–797.

Shweder, R. A., & Bourne, E. J. (1984). Does the concept of the person vary cross-culturally? In R. A. Shweder & R. A. LeVine (Eds.), *Culture theory: Essays on mind, self and emotion* (pp. 158–199). Cambridge: Cambridge University Press.

Sue, S., Fujino, D. C., Hu, L., Takeuhi, D. T., & Zane, N. W. S. (1991). Community mental health services for ethnic minority groups: A test of the cultural responsiveness hypothesis. *Journal of Consulting and Clinical Psychology, 59,* 533–540.

Takeuchi, D. T., Zane, N., Hong, S., Chae, D. H., Gong, F., Gee, G. C., & Alegría, M. (2007). Immigration related factors and mental disorders among Asian Americans. *American Journal of Public Health, 97,* 84–90.

U.S. Department of Health and Human Services. (1999). *Mental health: A report of the surgeon general.* Rockville, MD: Author.

U.S. Department of Health and Human Services. (2001). *Mental health: Culture, race, and ethnicity—A supplement to Mental health: A report of the surgeon general.* Rockville, MD: Author.

Vaughn, C. E., & Leff, J. P. (1976). The influence of family and social factors on the course of psychiatric illness. *British Journal of Psychiatry, 129,* 125–137.

Vaughn, C. E., Snyder, K. S., Jones, S., Freeman, W. B., & Falloon, I. R. (1984). Family factors in schizophrenic relapse: Replication in California of British research on expressed emotion. *Archives of General Psychiatry, 41,* 1169–1177.

Vega, W. A., Kolody, B., Aguilar-Gaxiola, S., Aldrete, E., Catalana, R., & Caraveo-Anduaga, J. (1998). Lifetime prevalence of DSM-III-R psychiatric disorders among urban and rural Mexican Americans in California. *Archives of General Psychiatry, 55,* 771–778.

Ware, N., & Kleinman A. (1992). Culture and somatic experience: The social course of illness in neurasthenia and chronic fatigue syndrome. *Psychosomatic Medicine, 54,* 546–560.

Weine, A. M., Phillips, J. S., & Achenbach, T. M. (1995). Behavioral and emotional problems among Chinese and American children: Parent and teacher reports for ages 6 to 13. *Journal of Abnormal Child Psychology, 23,* 619–639.

Weisman, A. (1997). Understanding cross-cultural prognostic variability for schizophrenia. *Cultural Diversity and Mental Health, 3,* 3–35.

Weisman, A. G., Gomes, L., & López, S. R. (2003). Shifting blame away from ill relatives: Latino families' reactions to schizophrenia. *Journal of Nervous and Mental Disease, 175,* 143–151.

Weisman, A. G., López, S. R., Ventura, J., Nuechterlein, K. H., Goldstein, M. J., & Hwang, S. (2000). A comparison of psychiatric symptoms between Anglo-Americans and Mexican-Americans with schizophrenia. *Schizophrenia Bulletin, 26,* 817–824.

Weisz, J. R., Chaiyasit, W., Weiss, B., Eastman, K. L., & Jackson, E. W. (1995). A multimethod study of problem behavior among Thai and American children in school: Teacher reports versus direct observation. *Child Development, 66,* 402–415.

Weisz, J. R., McCarty, C. A., Eastman, K. L., Chaiyasit, W., & Suwanlert, S. (1997). Developmental psychopathology and culture: Ten lessons from Thailand. In S. S. Luthar, J. A. Burack, D. Cicchetti, & J. R. Weisz (Eds.), *Developmental psychopathology: Perspectives on adjustment, risk, and disorder* (pp. 568–592). Cambridge: Cambridge University Press.

Weisz, J. R., Sigman, M., Weiss, B., & Mosk J. (1993). Parent reports of behavioral and emotional problems among children in Kenya, Thailand, and the United States. *Child Development, 64,* 98–109.

Weisz, J. R., Suwanlert, S., Chaiyasit, W., Weiss, B., Achenbach, T. M., & Eastman, K. L. (1993). Behavioral and emotional problems among Thai and American adolescents: Parent reports for ages 12–16. *Journal of Abnormal Psychology, 102,* 395–403.

Weisz, J. R., Suwanlert, S., Chaiyasit, W., Weiss, B., Achenbach, T. M., & Trevathan D. (1989). Epidemiology behavioral and emotional problems among Thai and American children: Teacher reports for ages 6–11. *Journal of Child Psychology and Psychiatry and Allied Disciplines, 30,* 471–484.

Weisz, J. R., Suwanlert, S., Chaiyasit, W., Weiss, B., Achenbach, T. M., & Walter, B. R. (1987). Epidemiology of behavioral and emotional problems among Thai and American children: Parent reports for ages 6 to 11 *Journal of the American Academy of Child and Adolescent Psychiatry, 26,* 890–897.

Weisz, J. R., Suwanlert, S., Chaiyasit, W., Weiss, B., & Jackson, E. W. (1991). Adult attitudes toward over- and undercontrolled child problems: Urban and rural parents and teachers from Thailand and the United States. *Journal of Child Psychology and Psychiatry and Allied Disciplines, 32,* 645–654.

Weisz, J. R., Suwanlert, S., Chaiyasit, W., Weiss, B., & Walter, B. (1987). Over- and undercontrolled referral problems among children and adolescents from Thailand and the United States: The *wat* and *wai* of cultural differences. *Journal of Consulting and Clinical Psychology, 55,* 719–726.

Weisz, J. R., & Weiss, B. (1991). Studying the "referability" of child clinical problems. *Journal of Consulting and Clinical Psychology, 59,* 266–273.

Weisz, J. R., Weiss, B., Suwanlert, S., & Chaiyasit, W. (2003). Syndromal structure of psychopathology in children of Thailand and the United States. *Journal of Consulting and Clinical Psychology, 71,* 375–385.

Whitesell, N. R., Beals, J., Mitchell, C. M., Keane, E. M., Spicer, P., Turner, R. J., … Al-SUPERPFP Team. (2007). The relationship of cumulative and proximal adversity to onset of substance dependence symptoms in two American Indian communities. *Drug and Alcohol Dependence, 91,* 279–288.

Widiger, T., Frances, A., Pincus, H. A., First, M. B., Ross, R., & Davis, W. (Eds.). (1997). *DSM-IV source book* (Vol. 3). Washington, DC: American Psychiatric Press.

Williams, D. R., Gonzalez, H. M., Neighbors, H., Nesse, R., Abelson, J. M., Sweetman, J., & Jackson, J. S. (2007). Prevalence and distribution of major depressive disorder in African Americans, Carribean Blacks, and Non-Hispanic Whites: Results from the National Survey of American Life. *Archives of General Psychiatry, 64,* 305–315.

World Health Organization. (1979). *Schizophrenia: An international follow-up study.* New York: Wiley.

4

The Role of Gender, Race, and Class in Psychopathology

BARBARA A. WINSTEAD and JANIS SANCHEZ

Old Dominion University
Norfolk, Virginia

When we consider the occurrence of psychopathology, its etiology, and the effectiveness of its treatment, we generally treat clients and clinicians as if they all belong to the same group. We are not unaware of group differences. Most chapters in this textbook intentionally address issues of gender or race as they are related to the psychological disorder being described. And Smith, in this volume, presents a full description of the importance of culture in understanding psychopathology. But the majority of descriptions of disorders and treatments and research speak of clients and clinicians without reference to their social identities and with the assumption that diagnoses, treatments, and research outcomes can be generally applied to one and all.

By discussing the role of gender, race, and class in psychopathology, this chapter focuses on the differences rather than the universalities. It addresses these questions: (a) Do gender, race, and class affect which psychological disorders individuals experience or how they experience them? (b) Are individuals from different groups treated differently by the mental health system? (c) Do recommended treatments work equally well for individuals from these different groups? (d) Should treatments take the demographic characteristics of the client into account? (e) Do the gender or race of the therapist matter? (f) What difference do gender, race, and class make? (g) And, if they make a difference, why? In the end we will discover that these questions raise more questions. Clear-cut answers are scarce, but the questions themselves shed light on the process of psychological diagnosis and treatment of psychological disorders.

First a word about terminology: *Race* may be considered an outdated term; scientists are in agreement that biological variation among humans does not fall neatly into "racial" groups. The assumption, however, that group differences in physical or mental health have biological foundations remains prevalent; even as the argument that these categories are socially constructed and represent social relationships, often between those with more power and privilege and those with less, gains currency (Mullings & Schulz, 2006). The use of the term "race," then, as opposed to "ethnicity" or "culture," is meant to remind us of these historical and current assumptions and of the advantages (increasing understanding across groups) and hazards (distancing and pathologizing of the "other") of using race as an identifier. "Gender" is also a problematic term (Pryzgoda & Chrisler, 2000). A distinction has often been made between "sex," meaning biological differences between girls and boys, women and men, and "gender," referring to psychological and sociological differences. But how does one sort these out? Gender reminds us again that a simple biological explanation will rarely if ever suffice in understanding human mental health or disorder.

Recent Initiatives Focused on Gender, Race, and Class

Concern about the impact of gender, race, and class on mental health and mental health care is expressed in at least three recent and ongoing national efforts. One is the attention currently being paid to racial and ethnic disparities in health and mental health. The second is interest in "cross-cultural issues" as part of the planning process for the fifth edition of the *Diagnostic and Statistical Manual of Mental Disorders*. The third is the focus on the training of clinical psychologists in cultural competence. That inequities exist in health and health care based on ethnicity is hardly news. But the attention paid to these inequities at the national level is a relatively recent phenomenon. Chang (2003) wrote about the politics of making disparities salient in the mental health community. The publication in 1999 by the U.S. Department of Health and Human Services (USDHHS) of *Mental Health: A Report of the Surgeon General* was a first and was intended as "an up-to-date review of scientific advances in the study of mental health and of mental illnesses that affect at least one in five Americans" (USDHHS, 1999, p. 3). In the preface to this report, Surgeon General Dr. David Satcher acknowledged that "Even more than other areas of health and medicine, the mental health field is plagued by disparities in the availability of and access to its services. These disparities are viewed readily through the lenses of racial and cultural diversity, age, and gender" (p. vi).

Although issues of diversity were considered in the report, its main thrust was universalistic, treating diagnosis and treatment of psychological disorders as if current tests and treatments could and should be equally applied to all individuals. Nelba Chavez, the administrator of the Substance Abuse and Mental Health Services Administration, refused to sign the report on the grounds that insufficient attention was paid to cultural diversity and disparities in mental health care (Chavez, 2003). This led to the development of a supplement to the report, *Mental Health: Culture, Race, and Ethnicity* (USDHHS, 2001), a 200-plus page report summarizing available research on the impact of ethnicity on mental health. The report is organized around presentation of information about the four "most recognized" U.S. minority groups: African Americans, American Indians and Alaska Natives, Asian Americans and Pacific Islanders, and Hispanic Americans. Both the initial report and the culture, race, and ethnicity supplement are available online (http://www.surgeongeneral.gov/library/mentalhealth/cre/).

One of two goals of the U.S. health agenda, *Healthy People 2010*, was the elimination of health disparities. The Office of Minority Health (part of Health, and Human Services), the National Center on Minority Health and Health Disparities, the Centers for Disease Control and Prevention, the National Institutes of Health, and other federal agencies all supported research and programs aimed at research to understand health and mental health disparities and programs to eliminate them. In 2003, the President's New Freedom Commission on Mental Health issued a report, *Achieving the Promise: Transforming Mental Health Care in America*, that speaks explicitly to problems for ethnic minorities in accessing quality mental health care and outlines a plan for research and practice that can close the gap (National Institute on Corrections, 2003). Indeed, Safran et al. (2009) note that mental health disparities have received increased attention. Their graph of the number of publication on mental health disparities shows a small increase between 1995 and 2000 and then a linear increase from around 20 publications per year in 2000 to 180 in 2007.

The *DSM* published by the American Psychiatric Association is the standard used by all mental health professionals for diagnosis of psychological disorders. Concerns with gender and ethnic bias in the criteria for various disorders have been longstanding (Caplan & Cosgrove, 2004). As the American Psychiatric Association plans for the fifth edition of *DSM*, it has established six workgroups that have published preplanning white papers in *A Research Agenda for DSM-V*

(2002). One of these papers (Alarcón et al., 2002) deals with the influence of culture on psychiatric diagnosis, including the influences of ethnicity, language, education, gender, and sexual orientation.

In the disciplines of counseling and clinical psychology there has been a persistent, but increasing, focus on the cultural competence of practitioners. Training in cultural diversity was recommended at the 1973 Vail Conference on graduate education in clinical psychology (Korman, 1974); questions regarding training in cultural diversity became a part of the American Psychological Association (APA) Accreditation Domains and Standards in 1986 and continue to be a focus of consideration in accreditation of clinical, counseling, and school psychology programs; the APA published *Guidelines for Providers of Psychological Services to Ethnic, Linguistic, and Culturally Diversity Populations* (1990) and incorporated awareness of "cultural, individual, and role differences, including those related to age, gender, race, ethnicity, national origin" in its ethics code in 1992 (p. 1598). In 2002 APA approved the *Guidelines on Multicultural Education, Training, Research, Practice, and Organizational Change for Psychologists* (APA, 2002). The Council of National Psychological Associations for the Advancement of Ethnic Minority Interests published *Psychological Treatment of Ethnic Minority Populations* (2003) with recommendations for treatment of Asian American/Pacific Islanders, populations of African descent, Hispanic/Latinos, and American Indians. A joint task force of APA Divisions 17 (Society of Counseling Psychology) and 35 (Society for the Psychology of Women) published *Guidelines for Psychological Practice with Girls and Women* in July 2007 (APA, 2007).

These efforts by the federal government, the American Psychiatric Association, and the APA to identify and address the impact of gender, race, and social class on psychological disorders, their diagnosis, and treatment illustrate the importance of the issue and the recognition that mental health practitioners have a clear responsibility to be familiar with the knowledge base concerning gender, ethnicity, and class and to develop skills that allow them to be competent in their interactions with and treatment of individuals different from themselves. It is unclear, however, if practitioners adhere to these standards.

Although we and many others stress the importance of taking gender, race, and social class into account in our interactions with and responses to clients, the research base for understanding *if* these variables make a difference in prevalence of a disorder or in the effectiveness of an intervention or *how* these variables make a difference generally deal with one or two variables at a time. Thus, this chapter will present research on gender differences and differences by race, ethnicity, and class, but research on the interaction of gender with ethnicity or class is scant. Of great significance when considering race will be whether or not social class, as represented by income and education, is included. In the United States, class and ethnicity are highly interrelated. Although 9.4% of Whites live below the poverty level, 25.8% of African Americans, 25.7%, and 25.3% of Hispanics live below the poverty line (DeNavas-Walt, Proctor, & Smith, 2010). Analyses of ethnicity that do not include social class may confound differences among ethnic groups with differences attributable to income. Even more often overlooked is the connection between gender and poverty. The poverty rate for married-couple families is 5.8%, for single male head-of-household (7% of all families), 16.9%, and for single female head-of-household (19% of all families), 29.9% (DeNavas-Walt et al., 2010).

Even in this brief introduction it may be apparent that, although we continually refer to the intersection among gender, race, and social class, many other documents refer to some of these, all of these, or these plus various other demographic characteristics. The critical issue is placing the individual within the sociocultural context that best helps us to understand and effectively intervene. So, although this chapter focuses on gender, race, and social class, it is understood that these interact with age, sexual orientation, ability, and other variables to form unique experiences for individuals and that the intersection of these variables with others represents combinations that are perceived differently by society and by mental health professionals.

The Role of Gender, Race, and Class in Diagnosis

To understand and treat a psychological disorder requires an accurate diagnosis. The process of diagnosis and treatment is less than perfect, but the goal can be clearly stated: We wish to identify the problem, treat it, and thereby allow the client to lead a more productive and rewarding life. But how do we identify the problem? With physical symptoms, physicians are aided by diagnostic tests that identify abnormalities in biochemistry, histology, or anatomy that signal specific disease processes. With psychological problems, there are rarely physical signs such as an abnormal cell count. We may use diagnostic tests, but these are likely to be based on the self-reports of clients, not blood chemistry or cell cultures. Often psychological diagnosis is accomplished through interviews, in which clinicians learn about symptoms directly from the client, through psychological tests, or through observations of symptoms. What the *DSM* (current edition, *DSM–IV–TR*, American Psychiatric Association, 2000) provides is a set of agreed upon criteria that help clinicians make diagnoses based on sets of symptoms. Psychological diagnosis, following the medical model, leads to present/absent decisions, although many have argued that a continuous rather than a categorical model is better for understanding psychological disorders (Maddux, 2002; Maddux, Gosselin, & Winstead, this volume). With either model, we want to be able to make an accurate assessment of the individual, and to this end we assess the reliability and validity of clinical tests, clinical interviews, and systems for identifying mental disorders (see Widiger; Garb, Lilienfeld, & Fowler, this volume). With a perfectly reliable and valid system we could easily discover if gender, ethnicity, and social class are related to different psychological disorders, if the etiologies or disease courses of these illnesses were similar or different, and ultimately if individuals with different characteristics benefit from similar or different treatments. But with less than perfect diagnostic systems our questions about gender, race, and class become more difficult to answer.

An official nomenclature for identifying mental illnesses was first established in part to create a common language for mental health professionals and researchers (see Widiger, this volume). Beginning in 1980, with *DSM–III*, this goal was largely accomplished in the United States, and research on psychological disorders and treatments adopted this system of diagnosis. Efforts to improve the reliability and validity of the *DSM* have led to revised and updated editions, *DSM–III–R* (APA, 1987), the current *DSM–IV–TR* (APA, 2000), and DSM–5, to be published in May 2013. The purpose of a carefully articulated diagnostic system is to provide clinicians and researchers with an objective-as-possible basis for making decisions about the presence or absence of specific psychopathology. But the question of gender bias in the diagnostic categories themselves (Kaplan, 1983) and of failure to appreciate ethnic and racial variations in perspectives on normality and abnormality (Adebimpe, 1981; Gaines, 1992) were raised almost immediately. Furthermore, to the extent that information relies on the interviewing and interpersonal skills of a diagnostician (as opposed to a standardized survey or interview), the gathering of pertinent information to make this determination may also be influenced by the gender, ethnicity, and class of the client and the interviewer. Even items on standardized scales may introduce bias. Finally, although *DSM* guidelines are in black and white, putting all the symptoms together to arrive at a diagnosis may be influenced by clinician expectations and beliefs about the client based on these demographic characteristics.

DSM–IV–TR Information on Gender, Race, and Class

A fundamental issue, for example, is whether or not the prevalence rates of disorders vary by gender or race. *DSM–IV–TR* includes for many disorders a section that presents information regarding the relation of gender, ethnicity, age, and class to that disorder. Social class is referenced as a link to etiological factors for mental retardation, such as lead poisoning and premature birth, and as a context for understanding undesirable behaviors, such as carrying a weapon or joining a gang, that might be considered indicators of conduct or antisocial disorder but could, in an impoverished or high-crime neighborhood, be self-protective. *DSM–IV–TR* also states that undifferentiated somatization disorder is more common in women of lower socioeconomic status (SES), and that conversion disorders are more common among lower SES and rural individuals. Most of the presentation of cultural features simply exhorts the clinician to be sensitive to cultural variations in symptoms and symptom presentation for various disorders. For example, depression might be experienced as "nerves" or headache among Hispanics or those from the Mediterranean region, "imbalance" in Asian, and problems of the "heart" in Middle Eastern clients (APA, 2000, p. 353). Specific ethnic differences are presented for alcohol-related disorders: lower in Japanese, Chinese, and Korean populations, equal in White and African American, higher in male Hispanics, but lower among female Hispanics. Alcohol abuse is also related to lower education, unemployment, and lower SES, although the abuse of alcohol may well have contributed to these rather than being an outcome of them. Inhalant abuse (e.g., glue sniffing) is noted as a particular problem for Alaskan natives, especially children and adolescents. Although somatization disorder is relatively rare in men, it occurs at a higher rate in Greek and Puerto Rican men. Finally *DSM–IV–TR* takes note of the research (see below) revealing that African Americans are more often diagnosed with schizophrenia than other groups, also noting that whether this is a true difference or the result of bias is unclear. Ethnic differences in bipolar disorder have not been found. Bulimia nervosa is described as "primarily white" (APA, 2000, p. 592).

Although there is interesting but not extensive information in *DSM–IV* on race or social class differences, Hartung and Widiger (1998) conclude that "[m]ost of the mental disorders diagnosed with the *DSM-IV* do appear to have significant differential sex prevalence rates" (p. 280). According to their analysis, the *DSM–IV–TR* provides information on differential sex prevalence for 101 of its 125 described psychological disorders. Excluding disorders that are, by definition, specific to one sex or the other (e.g., female orgasmic disorder, male erectile disorder), 84% of the *DSM–IV* disorders, for which information on prevalence by sex is available, are reported to occur at different rates in females and males. A general summary of these differences indicates that boys and men are more likely to be diagnosed with the infancy, childhood, and adolescent disorders and with substance-related, sexual, gender identity, and impulsive disorders. Girls and women are more likely to be diagnosed with depression, anxiety, somatization, dissociative, and eating disorders. Diagnoses of personality disorders tend to parallel expected sex differences in personality traits or even gender stereotypes: Women are reported to have higher rates of borderline, histrionic, and dependent personality disorders; men are reported to have higher rates of paranoid, schizoid, schizotypal, antisocial, and compulsive personality disorders.

Gender, Race, and Class Bias

As with the ethnic difference in diagnosis of schizophrenia, much has been written about whether sex differences in prevalence rates represent true differences or bias. In 1997 Garb summarized the research literature on gender, race, and social class bias in clinical judgment. In terms of diagnosis, he concluded that there was race bias for diagnosis of schizophrenia and psychotic affective disorders such that Black and Hispanic patients were more likely than White patients to be misdiagnosed with schizophrenia when symptoms suggest psychotic affective disorders and gender bias in that a diagnosis of antisocial personality disorder (APD) is more likely to occur for males and histrionic personality disorder (HPD) for females. Social class was not found to affect diagnoses.

In the following year Widiger (1998) delineated six ways in which diagnoses may reflect bias: "(a) biased diagnostic constructs, (b) biased diagnostic thresholds, (c) biased application of the diagnostic criteria, (d) biased sampling of persons with the disorder, (e) biased instruments of assessment, and/or (f) biased diagnostic criteria" (p. 96). Using these categories as a basis for understanding bias in diagnosis, we will discuss biases in diagnostic standards (e.g., constructs, criteria, and thresholds), biased applications of these diagnostic standards, including assessment instruments, and biased sampling.

Biased Diagnostic Standards Critics of *DSM* have argued that any classification system of psychological disorder represents an ethnocentric construction of what an idealized, or nonpathological, self is. Gaines (1992) suggested that the essential feature of *DSM* diagnoses appears to be the absence of self-control, a Western or European ideal that is incongruent with other cultures. Others argued that the diagnostic constructs were sexist and that women are pathologized by *DSM* diagnostic criteria (Brown, 1992; Caplan, 1991, 1995; Kaplan, 1983; Walker, 1994). HPD and dependent personality disorder (DPD) have been cited as the most egregious examples of gendered, in this case feminine, traits being used to establish the presence of psychopathology (Kaplan, 1983). Kaplan (1983) proposed "independent personality disorder" and "restricted personality disorder" and Pantony and Caplan (1991) suggested "delusional dominating personality disorder" as comparable, but masculine stereotyped, disorders. Others, however, argued that *DSM-III* already included personality disorders that captured maladaptive masculine traits, specifically, APD and compulsive personality disorder (Williams & Spitzer, 1983).

Ross, Frances, and Widiger (1995) suggested: "The *DSM-III/DSM-III-R* personality disorder criteria were constructed, for the most part, by males with little input from systematic empirical research. It would not be surprising to find that male clinicians would have a lower threshold for the attribution of maladaptive feminine traits than for the attribution of maladaptive masculine traits" (p. 212). They go on to describe how the *DSM-IV* Personality Disorders Work Group addressed this problem both by extensive reviews of existing empirical research and by creating more gender-neutral criteria. For example, the HPD item "Inappropriately sexually seductive in appearance or behavior" (*DSM-III-R*, APA, 1987, p. 349) was changed to "interaction with others is often characterized by inappropriate sexually seductive or provocative behavior" (APA, 2000, p. 657). Removing the reference to "appearance" was intended to reduce the possibility that the normal female response to social pressure to appear physically attractive might be viewed as "inappropriately sexually seductive."

Other diagnostic categories also represent a challenge for gender neutrality. Somatization disorder is reported to range from "0.2% to 2% among women and less than 0.2% in men" (*DSM-IV*, 1994, p. 447). Although substantial revisions were made to make criteria less sex biased, *DSM-IV* retains criteria that make a diagnosis in men unlikely. Clients must meet all of the four criteria, and the symptoms reported must not be fully explained by a medical condition. Criterion 3 is "one sexual or reproductive symptom other than pain." The examples given include four symptoms that apply exclusively to women ("irregular menses, excessive menstrual bleeding, vomiting throughout pregnancy"), one that applies to men ("erectile or ejaculatory dysfunction"), and one that may apply more often to women ("sexual indifference"; *DSM-IV*, APA, 1994, p. 449). Hartung and Widiger (1998) concluded: "Research on the epidemiology of the disorder therefore continues to use a criteria set that is biased against making the diagnosis in males, complicating any identification of the disorder in males" (p. 269). They further point out that the World Health Organization criteria for this disorder, while still including menstrual symptoms, also lists gastrointestinal symptoms, abnormal skin sensations, and blotchiness as common symptoms, making it easier for males to be diagnosed with somatization.

The question of criterion bias is further complicated by the issue of the diagnostic validity of specific symptoms for different groups. The purpose of gathering information about a client's feelings, thoughts, and behaviors is to identify, understand, and explain a psychological disorder. It may be the case that certain symptoms are predictive of a diagnostic category, future symptoms, or responsiveness to treatment for some groups, but not for others. An example from the arena of physical illness illustrates this problem. Although heart disease is the number one killer of both women and men in the United States (Giardina, 2000), heart disease is still generally regarded as a greater problem for men than for women. It is estimated that 35% of heart attacks in women are unreported. Women having heart attacks are as likely as men to experience chest pain, but they are somewhat more likely to experience other symptoms, such as breathlessness, perspiration, nausea, and a sensation of fluttering in the heart (Giardina, 2000). An unfamiliar constellation of symptoms may prevent women or health professionals from suspecting the presence of heart disease. In the case of heart attacks, although the underlying condition is the same, the presenting symptoms for women and men are somewhat different. A similar process may occur for psychological disorders. In a study assessing physical aggression as an indicator of antisocial behavior in young children, Spilt, Koomen, Thijs, Stoel, and van der Leij (2010) found that although physically aggressive behavior was distinct from nonaggressive antisocial behaviors for girls and boys, physically aggressive girls used more verbal threats, while physically aggressive boys were more likely to engage in fighting, suggesting that different behaviors were indicative of a common problem in need of detection and intervention.

Being able to identify a criterion that is differentially valid for females or males requires a diagnostic system that is independent of this criterion. In the case of heart disease, whatever the presenting symptoms, the presence or absence of a myocardial infarction can be assessed independently. For psychological disorders, there is no similar confirmation. In reference to establishing criteria for personality disorders, Robins and Guze (1970) advocated for validation studies that would "assess the extent to which the criteria select persons who have a history, present, and/or future consistent with the construct of a (particular) personality disorder" (p. 17). One might also suggest a validity test that considers the effectiveness of standard interventions for persons with and without a particular diagnostic criterion.

According to *DSM–IV* (APA, 1994), "[t]he definition of *mental disorder* ... requires that there be clinically significant impairment or distress" (p. 7). Thresholds for diagnoses should represent the point at which the accumulation of symptoms reaches this level of impairment or distress. But where is it? The issue of thresholds is one of the arguments for a dimensional rather than categorical view of psychopathology (Maddux, 2002; Maddux et al., this volume), but it remains the case that clinicians and clinical researchers are regularly faced with the task of a present versus absent decision in regard to the diagnosis of pathology. Prevalence of a disorder for any particular group will be affected by the setting of this threshold. It is important to note that, for the most part, the number of criteria needed to reach the threshold for a *DSM–IV* diagnosis is established by a committee rather than by empirical research that would justify that particular number.

Biased Application of the Diagnostic Criteria   Diagnosis may also involve objective tests or structured or semistructured interviews. Although bias often suggests subjectivity in judgment, standardized tests can also contain bias. Differential item functioning (DIF) is a term for what happens when a test item has different measurement properties for different groups. Woods, Oltmass, and Turkheimer (2008) evaluated five scales from the Schedule for Nonadaptive and

Adaptive Personality (SNAP) that demonstrated potential bias in previous research. They used a sample with women and men from five ethnic groups. They concluded that gender, ethnicity, or both do indeed affect many SNAP items, and that scores on these scales do not mean the same thing for individuals from different groups. Research of this sort reminds us that "objective" test scores are not bias free and, further, that there are accepted statistical tools for evaluating assessment instruments and improving them.

In keeping with the movement toward using research to inform practice, a 2005 special issue of *Psychological Assessment* focused on evidence-based assessment (EBA), including assessment of major psychological disorders. In their introduction, Hunsley and Mash (2005) specified that "EBAs need to be sensitive to gender, ethnicity, and cultural factors. Scientific evidence for the applicability of assessment tools needs to be demonstrated, not simply assumed on the basis of generalizations from nonrepresentative samples" (p. 252). Anthony and Rowa (2005) admit that for many of the instruments used to assess anxiety disorders, utility across different populations remains an unanswered question. Similarly, in their article on assessment of couple distress, Snyder, Heyman, and Haynes (2005) concluded that "Given that nearly all measures of couple distress were developed and tested on White middle-class married couples, their relevance to, and utility for, assessing ethnic couples, gay and lesbian couples, and low-income couples is unknown" (p. 302).

Joiner, Walker, Pettit, Perez, and Cukrowicz (2005) cited several studies that have demonstrated no evidence for gender or ethnic bias in the commonly used assessment measures for depression. On the other hand, Sprock and Yoder (1997) reviewed studies that suggest that circumstances and age may affect the validity of these instruments. When scales were described as measures of depression, items were endorsed less often by men than by women; but there was no sex difference when the instruments were described as a hassles scales (Page & Bennesch, 1993). In a sample of geriatric patients hospitalized for major unipolar depression Allen-Burge, Storandt, Kinscherf, and Rubin (1994) found that the Beck Depression Inventory (BDI) and the Geriatric Depression scale were more likely to detect depression in elderly women than in elderly men. In addition, depressed women report more symptoms of depression than do depressed men, even when clinicians' judgments of severity of depression do not differ, leading Sprock and Yoder (1997) to suggest that the number of criteria for diagnosis of depression should perhaps be greater for women than for men.

Not surprisingly, on the assessment of personality disorders, Widiger and Samuels (2005) presented a more complex picture. Self-report inventories can provide gender-biased assessments. Problems occur when self-report instruments use responses that do not reflect dysfunction but do apply to one sex or gender more than the other (Lindsay & Widiger, 1995; Widiger, 1998; Widiger & Samuels, 2005). A biased item occurs when men or women (sex bias) or masculine or feminine persons (gender bias) are more likely to endorse the item. The item itself is not a "symptom," nor is it related to general psychopathology, but it does contribute to a scale that measures a personality disorder. Using college students, Lindsay and Widiger (1995) determined that 13–31% of the items from three standardized measures of personality disorder showed some evidence of sex or gender bias according to these criteria.

In a follow-up study Lindsay, Sankis, and Widiger (2000) analyzed outpatients from mental health clinics using updated versions of three instruments: Millon Clinical Multiaxial Inventory-III (MCMI-III), Minnesota Multiphasic Personality Inventory-II (MMPI-II), and Personality Diagnostic Questionnaire-Revised (PDQ-R). Four personality disorder scales (histrionic, dependent, antisocial, and narcissistic) from these instruments were analyzed for sex or gender bias. None of the scale scores from any of the inventories was related to biological sex. Only three scale items showed sex bias (women or men were more likely to endorse them, but the item was unrelated to a measure of psychopathology, the Personality Assessment Inventory);

whereas 36 items suggested gender bias (i.e., the item correlated with a measure of femininity or masculinity but not with the measure of psychopathology). An example of an item that demonstrated sex bias and gender bias was "It's very easy for me to make many friends" from the MCMI-III histrionic scale. This item is not indicative of a psychological problem, but it does contribute to a higher score for histrionic personality disorder. It is also endorsed more frequently by women than by men, and it correlates positively with measures of femininity. This item, then, would tend to give women and feminine individuals higher scores for HPD when they endorse an item that does not represent a maladaptive trait or behavior. Although the few items (three) demonstrating sex bias were all from the histrionic scales, more examples of gender bias were from the narcissistic scale, suggesting that masculine individuals may receive a higher score by endorsing items that reflect adaptive, rather than pathological, characteristics.

Widiger and Samuels (2005) also argue that diagnostic criterion sets themselves are in need of examination for gender bias. Assessment tools based on these criteria as well as interview outcomes will inevitably yield biased outcomes if they are established to diagnose according to definitions of disorder that are inherently biased.

Less attention has been paid to the role of ethnicity in assessment of personality disorder, although Widiger and Samuels (2005) noted finding higher scores for African Americans compared to Whites on the paranoid personality disorder scales of the MCMI-III. As they suggested, it is possible, but not empirically established, that experiences of discrimination and prejudice lead to greater endorsement of items, such as "I am sure I get a raw deal in life," which contributes to the paranoid personality score but may be a reasonable reflection on a life lived facing barriers imposed by racism.

Regardless of the care taken to establish reliable and valid diagnostic tools, the clinicians using the tools or other sources of clinical information may be biased in making diagnoses. Lopez (1989) reviewed the effect of patient variables on clinical judgment. He found evidence of overpathologizing for cases with low social class and diagnostic category biases for race and, to some extent, gender. But he also argued that clinicians can both overpathologize and underpathologize in their judgments of patients and that errors in judgment affect both oppressed and nonoppressed groups and result from information processing biases not just prejudice or discrimination. He cites Luebnitz, Randolph, and Gutsch (1982) who found that lower-class African American patients were more likely to receive a diagnosis of chronic alcohol abuse than White lower-class or African American or White higher-class patients. But given the symptoms presented, the error was more in underdiagnosing alcohol abuse in the White and higher-class African American patients. Similarly, he cited a study by Leinhardt, Seewald, and Zigmond (1982) that suggested that White boys are disproportionately identified as learning disabled. Diagnoses of depression may also be affected by clinician bias. Potts, Burnam, and Wells (1991) compared clinicians' judgments to diagnoses made with a standardized interview assessment and found that there were discrepancies between standardized assessment and clinician judgments in that medical practitioners were less likely to diagnose depression in men and mental health practitioners were more likely to diagnose depression in women. Clearly in the real world of persons interacting with health and mental health practitioners, diagnosis of depression, as with other disorders, is not free of sex bias. Overpathologizing can lead to unnecessary interventions and stigma; underpathologizing leads to lack of treatment and failure to intervene where needed.

Lopez (1989) noted the power of experimental (or analogue) studies in uncovering bias. In his review, 45% of experimental studies examining severity judgments and 55% examining diagnostic judgments revealed bias. In analogue studies clinicians are presented with case histories that are identical except for the sex or ethnicity of the patient. Many studies have focused on gender bias. In these studies half of the clinicians in the research diagnose the "female patient" and half diagnose the "male patient." Given the same information, would clinicians come to the same or different conclusions about the presence of psychological disorders? Warner (1978) gave clinicians ambiguous patient profiles, with a mixture of hysterical and antisocial symptoms (e.g., suicide attempts, no close relationships, self-centered, shoplifting with no remorse for crime, flirtatious). Female profiles were more likely than male profiles to be labeled hysterical (76% vs. 49%) and male profiles were more likely than female to be labeled antisocial (41% vs. 22%). It can be argued that with ambiguous information, clinicians rely on base rates (women *are* more likely to be hysterical; men *are* more likely to be antisocial). The base rates themselves, however, may also represent a biased accumulation of data on women and men. If clinicians use stereotyped perceptions of women and men in their diagnoses (as these studies indicate), then the data based on their clinical judgments will be biased.

To circumvent the issue of base rates, subsequent studies presented clinicians with cases that meet the *DSM* criteria for one or more disorders. Ford and Widiger (1989) created cases that met *DSM–III* criteria for HPD or APD or failed to reach diagnostic criteria for either. HPD was more frequently diagnosed in women, even when the case contained more antisocial than histrionic criteria; and APD was less often diagnosed in women. Adler, Drake, and Teague (1990) developed one case history that met the explicit criteria of four diagnoses: histrionic, narcissistic, borderline, and dependent. Men were more likely to receive a diagnosis of narcissistic personality disorder; women, histrionic personality disorder. There were no differences for borderline or dependent (which was rarely used) personality disorder. In research using a case that met the criteria of borderline personality disorder (BPD) and posttraumatic stress disorder, however, women did receive higher ratings for BPD (Becker & Lamb, 1994). Fernbach, Winstead, and Derlega (1989) created separate vignettes describing clients who met diagnostic criteria for antisocial and somatization disorders and found that there were no sex of vignette differences for somatization disorder; but for APD, although most clients were accurately diagnosed, men (73%) were significantly more likely than women (53%) to receive the diagnosis. Nineteen percent of clinicians made an inaccurate diagnosis of BPD, of these 68% were for the female clients and 32% for the male clients. Crosby and Sprock (2004) further explored the influence of patient sex on diagnosing APD. They provided clinical psychologists with two cases, one meeting minimum criteria for APD, the other used as a distracter. Female clients were underdiagnosed for APD and overdiagnosed for BPD.

If the diagnostic criteria for a disorder are built into the case description, then the presence of clinician bias represents a failure to adhere to the *DSM* diagnostic criteria. Clinicians are coming up with the "wrong" answer when they indicate a diagnostic category other than the one intended. Ford and Widiger (1989) demonstrated that at the level of individual criteria, there is no sex bias. Specific behaviors were rated as indicative of HPD and APD with equal frequency for men and women. But they did find sex bias when assigning clients to one of these diagnostic categories. They concluded that histrionic personality disorder was overdiagnosed in women and underdiagnosed in men. Morey and Ochoa (1989) and Blashfield and Herkov (1996) looked at clinicians' ratings of *DSM* criteria for their own patients and compared ratings on individual criteria with actual diagnoses of these patients. They found weak associations between clinicians' ratings of criteria and the clinicians' diagnoses, suggesting that giving a diagnosis does not necessarily involve an objective formula based on the presence or absence or the total number of certain criteria. Morey and Ochoa (1989) found that clinicians overdiagnose APD in men and BPD in women; and Blashfield and Herkov (1996) replicated these findings. The absence of sex bias for specific criteria in contrast to the presence of sex bias in assigning *DSM*-based diagnoses suggests that dimensional approaches to diagnosis may be less prone to bias than categorical labels, as judgments in the dimensional approach remain at the level of behavioral indicators rather than a summary diagnostic decision.

Another effort to understand the influence of gender on diagnoses of personality disorders had clinicians read one sentence at a time in cases with antisocial, histrionic, or mixed criteria (Flanagan & Blashfield, 2005). In general, the findings confirmed previous research showing that clinicians are more likely to apply HPD to women and APD to men, although gender did not affect diagnoses (inaccurate in these cases) of narcissism or BPD. The staged presentation of diagnostic information also demonstrated that clinicians use gender as a context for understanding symptoms. Clinicians appeared to make "gendered" diagnoses more often when criteria of the disorder were present than when these criteria were not presented.

A great deal has been written about the overdiagnosis of schizophrenia in African Americans and the underdiagnosis of affective disorders (Adembimpe, 1981; Baker & Bell, 1999; Simon, Fleiss, Gurland, Stiller, & Sharpe, 1973). Neighbors, Trierweiler, Ford, and Muroff (2003) cite numerous studies that have found higher rates of schizophrenia in African Americans and mood disorders in Whites. In a study of race disparities in emergency rooms, Kunen, Neiderhauser, Smith, Morris, and Marx (2005) found that, although the observed rate of psychiatric diagnoses (5.27%) was substantially lower than the national prevalence rate (20–28%), African American patients were particularly likely to be undiagnosed. Anxiety and depression were more likely to be diagnosed for White than for African American patients and, even though Whites were more likely to be diagnosed as psychotic, African Americans were more likely than Whites to be diagnosed for schizophrenia. Although differences in prevalence do not necessarily indicate bias, Garb (1997) concluded that bias exists. Indeed, no racial differences in prevalence rates for psychotic disorders were reported in a major epidemiological study (Robins & Regier, 1991) where researchers use structured interviews in community samples to establish, as objectively as possible, actual rates of psychological disorders.

Unlike research on gender bias, which has relied on analogue studies, most studies supporting racial bias have compared diagnoses by hospital or clinic staff with diagnoses from research investigators using chart reviews or structured interviews (e.g., Mukherjee, Shukla, Woodle, Rosen, & Olarte, 1983; Pavkov, Lewis, & Lyons, 1989; Simon et al., 1973). In an early study, Simon et al. (1973) compared diagnoses made by hospital staff with diagnoses made by researchers using structured interviews. For clinical diagnoses, African American patients received more schizophrenia diagnoses and fewer affective disorder diagnoses; but with research diagnoses there were no racial differences. Neighbors et al. (1999) found the agreement between hospital and research diagnoses to be low for both African American and White patients, but the higher rates of schizophrenia diagnoses for African Americans and of mood disorders for Whites remained even with research diagnoses. Nevertheless racial discrepancies were smaller in the more structured assessment (using a *DSM–III* checklist) than in the less structured assessment. In a subsequent study using research interviews, Neighbors et al. (2003) found the same race differences in schizophrenia (African Americans higher) and bipolar disorder (Whites higher), but no differences in major depression or schizoaffective disorder. There were no SES differences among patient groups. In this study they also measured ratings of symptoms and relations between symptoms and diagnoses. Similar profiles were used for diagnosing bipolar disorder, although White patients received higher ratings for hypertalkativeness, which may have led to their higher rate of bipolar diagnosis. But for schizophrenia, more individual symptoms were related to the diagnosis for African Americans than for Whites; and of particular interest, inappropriate affect, although equally observed in the two groups, was considered an indicator of schizophrenia for African Americans but not for Whites (Neighbors et al., 2003).

Examining diagnoses of psychotic patients discharged from a state psychiatric hospital, Strakowski, Shelton, and Kolbrener (1993) found more diagnoses of schizophrenia, especially the paranoid subtype, and fewer diagnoses of affective disorders for African American patients than for White patients. Similarly in a psychiatric emergency clinic, Strakowski et al. (1995)

found more diagnoses for schizophrenia, particularly for African American men. In a study using patients recruited for the *DSM–IV* field trials for schizophrenia and other psychotic disorders, Strakowski, et al. (1996) found that African American patients demonstrated more severe psychotic symptoms, especially first-rank symptoms (i.e., hallucinations, delusions, disordered thinking) than White patients. There were no differences in rates or severity of affective symptoms. In a more recent study, differences in the occurrence of first-rank symptoms were confirmed by Arnold et al. (2004), who used transcripts of audiotapes from structured diagnostic interviews with all cues to ethnicity removed to evaluate the presence of first-rank symptoms. In this study they found that the African American men were more likely than other groups (African American women and White men and women) to be rated as having first-rank symptoms and greater psychopathology by both raters with and without information about race. There were not, however, differences based on race in diagnoses of schizophrenia; but men were significantly more likely to be diagnosed with schizophrenia and less likely to be diagnosed with depression. That no race differences occurred for diagnoses of schizophrenia, mania, or depression is perhaps due to the use of structured interviews by clinicians with extensive training. The presence of an interaction between race and gender, similar to the one found by Strakowski et al. (1995), reminds us of the importance of intersectionality in understanding psychological disorder.

In summary, these studies indicate that less-structured assessments of patients tend to result in higher rates of schizophrenia diagnoses in African Americans compared to Whites, whereas more structured diagnoses show fewer differences. These studies suggest that clinicians may have a bias toward labeling African Americans as schizophrenic. On the other hand, structured assessments and transcripts with race removed (Arnold et al., 2004) suggest that African Americans, especially men, may present with different, perhaps more severe, symptoms. The possibility of sociocultural differences in presentation of mental disorder must always be considered.

An exception to the absence of analogue studies to explore racial bias in diagnosis and the exclusive focus on gender in most analogue studies is the work of Kales et al. (2005) and Loring and Powell (1988). Kales et al. used video vignettes of elderly African American and White women and men describing symptoms that met criteria for major depression but also included cognitive problems, alcohol use, and paranoid thoughts. The vignettes were viewed by primary care physicians. In this well-controlled study, neither gender nor race nor the interaction affected diagnosis or treatment recommendations. These physicians were generally accurate in their diagnoses; 70–80% of cases were diagnosed with major depression. They were even more likely to recommend antidepressants as the first-line treatment (82–90%), although interestingly they were unlikely to refer the patient to a psychiatrist or other mental health professional (9–19.5%). The only variables that affected diagnosis were the physician characteristics of being trained at a non-U.S. medical school or being non-White. These two variables were highly related to each other and predicted being significantly less likely to make a diagnosis of depression. It is possible that the cultural distance (being foreign or foreign-born) led to less comfort in making diagnoses or in less accuracy in diagnosis.

Using written vignettes that included both personality disordered (dependent) and psychotic (undifferentiated schizophrenia) symptoms in the cases to be diagnosed, Loring and Powell (1988) manipulated race (African America vs. White) and gender as demographic characteristics. Vignettes of clients with no information about ethnicity or sex were also included. Finally, they examined gender and race of the psychiatrists as influences on the diagnostic process. They found that modal diagnoses were most accurate in cases *without* information on gender and ethnicity. When this information was introduced, complex patterns of interaction between characteristics of the case and characteristics of the diagnosing psychiatrist occurred. Generally, similarity in race and gender between clinician and client produced the most accurate diagnoses; but male clinicians overdiagnosed depression in women and histrionic personality disorder in White women; and all clinicians overdiagnosed paranoid schizophrenia and paranoid personality disorder in African American men. This study reinforces the conclusion that the interaction of race and gender has a powerful influence on diagnosis.

Loring and Powell (1988) suggested that clinicians are more accurate in their diagnoses when the gender and race of the case are the same as those of the clinician. An exception was the diagnosis of White female clients by White female clinicians that suggested favoring of a less severe diagnosis. Although a full exploration of the interaction of clinician characteristics with patient characteristics is beyond the scope of this chapter, Garb (1997) presented further evidence that clinicians may see less pathology in similar others and more pathology in dissimilar others. For example, Li-Repac (1980) found that White clinicians compared to Chinese American clinicians gave more negative ratings on depression and interpersonal variables to Chinese American clients, and Chinese American clinicians rated White clients as having more severe psychopathology. Tseng, McDermott, Ogino, and Ebata (1982) found that American psychiatrists' ratings of Japanese fathers were more negative than Japanese psychiatrists' ratings. Russell, Fujino, Sue, Cheung, and Snowden (1996) found that for African American, Asian, White, and Hispanic clients, when therapist and client were ethnically matched, therapists' ratings of overall client functioning were more positive. A possible source of bias in diagnosis is the actor–observer effect (Jones & Nisbett, 1987) by which we are more likely to explain our own behavior, or the behavior of those with whom we can identify, in terms of situational factors, but the behavior of others in terms of inner causes, such as a psychological disorder (Poland & Caplan, 2004). This may lead clinicians to overpathologize others, perhaps especially those whose sociocultural context is difficult for the clinician to understand; but it can also lead to underdiagnosing similar others.

These studies indicate that clinicians do use sex and race of client as information that affects their judgment about the diagnosis of a case. Some diagnoses are more prone to this bias than others. Although analogue studies allow the researcher to present clinicians with identical information while varying characteristics of the client, the responses of clinicians to paper-and-pencil or even audio or video versions of a patient cannot completely capture the more interactive process that actually occurs during diagnosis, a process that may be even more susceptible to bias. On the other hand, evidence also suggests that the use of structured interviews, compared to unstructured interviews, can diminish the effects of bias.

Bias in the application of criteria is a reality in the practice of mental health care. Furthermore, to the degree that accurate diagnoses lead to more effective treatment of disorders, biases that lead to inaccurate diagnoses are particularly troublesome.

Biased Sampling The most convenient data for analysis of prevalence rates are those obtained in clinical settings. When individuals come into a clinical setting, either by their own volition or through the actions of others (e.g., parent, courts), they generally receive a diagnosis. Assuming diagnoses are accurate, these data would appear to be a good source of information. But do all individuals with a particular disorder show up in a clinical setting? Factors that bring adults into a clinical setting include willingness to acknowledge the symptoms, willingness to seek treatment, or the persuasive or coercive influence of others. Factors that bring children into a clinical setting include parents' and teachers' perceptions of the severity of the problem and the possibilities for treatment. These factors are likely to be influenced by the gender, race, and class of the affected individual. Women may be more likely to recognize and less resistant to acknowledging that symptoms are indicative of an emotional problem that needs treatment (Yoder, Shute, & Tryban, 1990). Non-Whites are less likely to have access to mental health care, in part due to lack of health insurance, and less likely to use specialized care, often seeking help from primary care services (USDHHS, 2001). Arnold et al. (2004) suggested that one reason first rank symptoms of schizophrenia may be more pronounced in African American men is because they tend to delay seeking mental health treatment. To the extent that rates of psychological disorder seen in clinical populations are the result of differences in help seeking, problem recognition, tolerance or intolerance for symptoms by self or others or attitudes toward mental health care, then differences in prevalence rates in clinical settings will reflect these differences and not just "true" differences in the occurrence of the psychological disorder.

The solution to this dilemma is epidemiological studies with community samples. In these studies, interviewers contact individuals in representative samples and acquire information about symptoms. Diagnosis is accomplished independently of the participants' acknowledgment of or concern about the disorder. Whereas differences in clinical populations reflect differences in the psychological disorders plus differences in various nondisordered behaviors such as help seeking, differences in community samples will not reflect this problem. For numerous disorders, *DSM–IV–TR* (APA, 2000) cites discrepancies in community versus clinical samples or suggests that clinical data may over- or underrepresent different groups due to disorder-specific factors that encourage or discourage treatment seeking. For example, Miltenberger, Rapp, and Long (2006) suggested that the gender difference in trichotillomania (compulsive hair pulling), which is seen far more often in women then men in clinical settings, may result in part from women being more inclined than men to seek treatment for such an appearance-altering problem. More men than women seek help for gambling, but female gamblers may feel stigmatized and unwilling to seek treatment (Hartung & Widiger, 1998).

An excellent example of epidemiological studies is the National Institute of Mental Health's Collaborative Psychiatric Epidemiology Surveys (CPES, 2003), which combines three nationally representative data sets: the National Survey of American Life, the National Comorbidity Survey-Replication, and the National Latino and Asian American Study. Data for these studies were collected between February 2001 and November 2003. Trained nonclinician interviewers conducted fact-to-face computer-assisted interviews, including the World Mental Health Composite International Diagnostic interview. The website lists two books and 232 journal articles based on these data, many focusing on gender, race, and class. Ideally, every disorder would have an adequate and current base of epidemiological data from community samples, but often statements about differences in prevalence rates are based on potentially biased clinical samples.

The Role of Gender, Race, and Class in Treatment

While concerns about gender bias have focused on *DSM* criteria as well as bias in application of criteria and sampling, concerns about racial bias have largely focused on questions of how criteria are applied (i.e., Do racial stereotypes affect diagnosis?; Does sampling affect outcomes, for example, are ethnic minorities more disturbed by the time they reach the clinic or hospital?; How does culture or subculture affect the presentation of symptoms in clinical settings?). It is unlikely that bias has been completely removed from the diagnostic process, and it is critical to remember that diagnosis does influence treatment. But independent of diagnosis, is there evidence that gender, race, and class influence the treatment process and treatment outcomes? As with research on diagnosis, most studies of psychotherapeutic process and outcome have treated gender, race, and class as discrete, rather than interacting, variables. Furthermore, to thoroughly examine the impact of gender, race, and class on treatment outcomes, we should consider the characteristics of the therapist, the type of therapy, the therapy setting, the type of problem, and even the question of access to any therapy at all.

The question of access, whether individuals from different groups have equal opportunities to seek and receive psychotherapeutic treatment, has been the focus of much research on ethnic minorities or persons with low incomes. In general, the majority of individuals identified through epidemiological studies as having psychological disorders do not receive care for these disorders. Using data from the CPES, Wang, Lane et al. (2005) found that within a 1-year period only 41% of those identified with a psychological diagnosis received any care; and González, Tarraf, Whitfield, and Vega (2010) found that only 50.6% of respondents who met major depression criteria had received either pharmacotherapy or psychotherapy and many fewer (21.2%) had received therapy consistent with American Psychiatric Association guidelines. Low income and minority status, however, are additional barriers to receiving mental health care (Cooper-Patrick et al., 1999; González et al., 2010; USDHHS, 2001). Wang, Lane et al. (2005) found that unmet need was greatest for those with low incomes and without insurance and for minorities, the elderly, and rural residents. Furthermore, among the poor, lack of access to transportation or inflexible work schedules, can also work against using mental health resources even when they are available through public mental health services (cf. Armistead et al., 2004, who increased retention in a community intervention program by providing child care and transportation). Because publicly funded programs, such as Medicaid, are intended to provide mental health care for the uninsured, the connection between medical insurance and access to care is complicated. For example, racial disparities in use of publicly supported services are generally small, but data from the National Medical Expenditure Survey (NMES) revealed that African Americans with private insurance are less likely than Whites to use mental health care (Snowden & Thomas, 2000).

For individuals with depressive symptoms as their main reason for a medical visit, Pingitore, Snowden, Sansone, and Klinkman (2001) reported that men, African Americans, other persons of color, and those over 65 were more likely to seek care from a primary care physician, whereas women, Whites, and individuals between 45 and 64 years were more likely to visit a psychiatrist. The level of care provided by primary care physicians was significantly less that the care provided by a psychiatrist. González et al. (2010) found that Mexicans and African Americans were significantly less likely than non-Latino Whites to have received a recommended level of care for depression. Alegría et al. (2002) found that Hispanics, compared to Whites, with low SES, and African Americans, compared to Whites, with higher SES were less likely to use specialty care for mental health problems. Other studies confirm that Hispanics (Cabassa, Zayas, & Hansen, 2006) and African Americans (Cooper-Patrick et al., 1999; Snowden & Pingitore, 2003) are more likely to receive mental health care from a general medical setting than from a mental health specialist. Richardson, Anderson, Flaherty, and Ball (2003) examined treatment for African American and Whites who received a primary diagnosis of major depression in outpatient clinics (both medical and mental health). They found that African Americans were more likely than Whites to receive psychotherapy from substance abuse clinics, but Whites were more likely than African Americans to receive psychotherapy from primary care and specialty mental health clinics. In addition, Kung (2003) found that about 15% of Chinese Americans (in Los Angeles) received mental health specialty care, a figure even lower than that reported for other minority groups. Similarly, Wells, Klap, Koike, and Sherbourne (2001) found that among those with perceived need for alcoholism, drug abuse, or mental health disorders, African Americans and Hispanics were more likely to report unmet need and were less likely to be in active treatment. Additionally, Hispanics, compared to Whites, reported significantly more delays in treatment and less satisfaction in all components of health care. Using the National Comorbidity Survey Replication data, Wang, Berglund et al. (2005) concluded that sociodemographic characteristics that predicted delays in treatment included being male, poorly educated, a member of a racial minority, or married.

Wang, Berglund, and Kessler (2000) found no ethnic or racial differences in access to treatment, but they did find that being African American and not having health insurance predicted not receiving evidence-based care. Young, Klap, Sherbourne, and Wells (2001) also found that African Americans and Hispanics suffering from anxiety or depression were less likely than Whites to receive care congruent with established guidelines. Cabassa et al. (2006) reviewed 16 articles based on seven epidemiological studies and concluded that Hispanic adults compared to non-Latino Whites both underutilize mental health services and are less likely to receive guideline congruent care.

Chow, Jaffee, and Snowden (2003) examined clinical characteristics and mental health service use patterns of Whites, African Americans, Hispanics, and Asians in low and high poverty communities and found that socioeconomic status does moderate the relationship between ethnicity and service access and use. In high-poverty areas Hispanics and Asians were more likely than Whites to use emergency services and Whites were more likely to receive a diagnosis of schizophrenia, perhaps reflecting the downward social mobility of poorly functioning Whites. In low poverty areas, African Americans and Hispanics were more likely than Whites to be referred into mental health services by law enforcement, perhaps reflecting the fact that deviant behavior by minorities in low poverty neighborhoods is more likely to be attended to and constrained. Results were complex but clearly indicate that paths to mental health care differ by both ethnicity and the economic status of one's community.

Rather than examining quality of mental health care at the level of the individual client, Kuno and Rothbard (2005) examined quality of care provided by community mental health centers (CMHCs) in neighborhoods with different income and racial profiles. Using quality indicators, such as use of atypical antipsychotic prescriptions and intensive case management, they found that CMHCs in high income, White areas provided a higher quality of care than CMHCs in low income, African American neighborhoods. This suggests that even when mental health care is available, it may not be of similar quality.

These last two studies also illustrate an inherent problem in the ways in which SES is generally used in mental health research. SES is most commonly measured at the individual or family level. Although there are complex and sophisticated ways to create such a participant specific measure, neighborhood level measurement is often superior to these. Corral and Landrine (2010) made a strong argument for area-based measures of SES, including the fact that low-SES neighborhoods contain poorer quality services and more stressors than high-SES neighborhoods. This is an important consideration in research that examines social class and psychopathology.

Several of these studies that explored in some detail the interplay of ethnicity, income, insurance, and need on access to care nevertheless do not include gender in their studies. When gender is analyzed, the results tend to support the general finding that women are more likely to seek mental health care than men. Cabassa et al. (2006), in their review of epidemiological studies of Hispanic adults, found that several studies, but not all, reported that women, after controlling for other factors, were more likely than men to use mental health services, either from mental health professionals or general medical practices. Kung (2003) reported that in this Chinese American sample, women were significantly more likely than men to seek mental health care. In a large sample of mixed ethnicity, Wang, Berglund et al. (2005) found that women were more likely than men to receive mental health care from general medical services but less likely than men to use psychiatry only. Men are more likely than women to delay seeking treatment (Wang, Lane et al., 2005b). These studies support the general consensus that women are more likely than men to seek psychological treatment (Petry, Tennen, & Affleck, 2000).

Beyond issues of access and general quality of care, we also wanted to know if gender, race, and class affected the type of care delivered and perhaps most importantly the outcomes of treatment. The complexity of the question is revealed if we consider some of the other treatment-relevant variables: sociodemographic characteristics of the therapist (e.g., gender, race, and class), type of therapy, length of therapy, type of problem being treated. Many studies do not have the methodological controls that allow for random assignment of clients to therapists and therapists to clients, making therapist or client characteristics nonexperimental variables. In these cases the possibility that unmeasured variables account for the outcomes must always be kept in mind.

Influence of the Client on Therapy Outcomes

In reviewing the impact of client variables on psychotherapy outcomes, Clarkin and Levy (2004) cited studies showing that higher SES is related to staying longer in psychotherapy and that higher levels of education are related to longer treatment for substance abuse programs, although they also found studies in which SES was not related to remaining in treatment. Wierzbicki and Pekarik (1993), in a meta-analysis of psychotherapy drop out, found that race (minority status), low level of education, and low SES all significantly predicted dropping out of therapy. Reis and Brown (1999), in their review of three decades of research on the unilateral terminator (i.e., a "client who terminates treatment before the clinician believes the client is ready," p. 123), concluded that SES is a reliable predictor of unilateral termination and that despite some nonsignificant results, non-White clients are also more likely to terminate unilaterally. In a more recent study of individual therapy in a substance abuse clinic, researchers found that being female and African American were independent predictors of early treatment drop out (King & Canada, 2004).

Although the focus of research on race and class has mostly been on access to therapy, quality of therapy, and use of therapy (e.g., staying in or dropping out), some research has also examined the effect of client characteristics on therapeutic outcomes. Clarkin and Levy (2004) concluded that neither race nor gender has much impact on therapy outcome. On the other hand, a review by Lam and Sue (2001), while finding that "improvement in therapy is independent of client gender" (p. 480), reported equal numbers of studies that find no difference in outcomes for African Americans compared to Whites and studies that find that African Americans gain less in therapy. They also referenced a study that found that American Indian youth did not benefit as much from substance abuse treatment as Whites (Query, 1985). But they concluded that outcomes for Asian Americans and Hispanics may be similar to those of Whites. Rosenheck, Fontana, and Cottroll (1995) found that African American veterans in treatment for posttraumatic stress disorder (PTSD) were more likely to drop out but also less likely to benefit from therapy than White veterans.

Despite the general conclusions of no sex-of-client effects on therapeutic outcomes, some studies suggest otherwise. Recent studies of substance abuse (Galen, Brower, Gillespie, & Zucker, 2000; Kosten, Gawin, Kosten, & Rounsaville, 1993) and substance abuse plus PTSD (Triffleman, 2001) have found greater severity for women than for men at the beginning of treatment, but equal levels of functioning at the end of treatment, suggesting that women made greater gains during therapy than did men. Ogrodniczuk, Piper, and Joyce (2004) looked at outcomes of short-term group therapy for depression and complicated grief. Women were found to benefit more from this therapy, but they were also found to be more committed to the therapy groups and to be perceived by other group members as more compatible. Both a meta-analysis of child and adolescent outcome research (Weisz, Weiss, Han, Granger, & Morton, 1995) and a study of the psychotherapy outcomes for youth treated in public outpatient programs (Ash & Weis, 2009) found that girls were more likely to benefit from treatment than boys, although Suveg et al. (2009) found no effect for gender on outcomes for individual and family-based interventions for anxiety disorders in a randomized clinical trial.

Issues about women's special needs in substance abuse treatment have been discussed (Wilke, 1994). Treatments included in the studies reviewed above were all outpatient programs. Many interventions for substance abuse or addiction rely, however, on inpatient treatment. Some women may be unable to participate in inpatient treatment or need to terminate treatment prematurely because of child care issues. Although the extent of this problem is not known, some women in need of inpatient treatment may be the sole caregiver for their children (Wilke, 1994). Questions have also been raised about differences in the effectiveness of single-sex and mixed-sex treatment groups. Dahlgren and Willander (1989) found that women in a single-sex group reported better social adjustment and lower alcohol consumption at a 2-year follow-up than did women in a mixed-sex group. Similarly, in a randomized controlled trial, a manual-based 12-session Women's Recovery Group was compared with mixed-gender group drug counseling. Although no differences appeared at the end of treatment, women in the single-sex group showed continued gains and greater reduction in drinking at the 6-month follow-up. Client satisfaction was also significantly higher for women in the single-sex group (Greenfield, Trucco, McHugh, Lincoln, & Gallop, 2007).

Client–Therapist Matching

Many studies have examined client–therapist matching in terms of race or gender on the assumption that greater understanding or credibility will occur when therapist and client share these critical social statuses. The review of client variables by Petry, Tenne, and Affleck (2000) reported mixed results from studies of matching for race. Some find that clients stay in treatment longer, others that there is no effect on retention or outcomes. In their review, Lam and Sue (2001) reported evidence that matching for African Americans is related to the number of sessions (Rosenheck et al., 1995) but not to outcomes, and that matching for Asian American and Hispanics is related to less drop out and more therapy (Gamst, Dana, Der-Karabetian, & Kramer, 2001; Sue, Fujino, Hu, Takeuchi, & Zane, 1991). Subsequent studies found no advantage for ethnic matching for African American children and adolescents, but greater client satisfaction and better child outcomes for ethnically matched Asian Americans (Gamst et al., 2003; Gamst, Dana, Der-Karabetian, & Kramer, 2004). Sterling, Gottheil, Weinstein, and Serota (2001) found no effects for either race or sex matching in terms of retention or outcome in a study of substance abuse treatment for African American cocaine-dependent clients. In a general review of the relationship between ethnic match and termination, Maramba and Hall (2002) concluded that while ethnic similarity reduces rates of treatment drop out and increases the length of time in treatment, the effects are small and do not improve clinical outcome.

In a recent study examining the outcomes from an empirically based treatment, multisystemic therapy (MST) for youth with antisocial behavior, Halliday-Boykins, Schoenwald, and Letourneau (2005) found that caregiver ethnic similarity did matter. The very large sample was diverse and the assignment to a therapist was to next available. The analyses revealed that "when caregivers are ethnically matched with therapists, youths demonstrate greater decreases in symptoms, stay in treatment longer, and are more likely to be discharged for meeting treatment goals" (p. 814). This effect was partly mediated by therapists' greater adherence to the MST protocol in ethnically matched cases.

A diverse sample of children and adolescents seen in outpatient services in mental health facilities also found that race and language matching matter (Hall, Guterman, Lee, & Little, 2002). Ethnic match, but not gender match, was related to lower drop-out rates for Asian American, Mexican American, and African American children. Language match predicted only for Mexican Americans. Ethnic match predicted more treatment sessions for Mexican

Americans and Asian Americans; and language and gender match were additional predictors for Mexican Americans.

Sue, Zane, and their colleagues have argued that the advantages of ethnic matching, when they occur, probably accrue from similarities in problem perception, coping orientation, and goals for treatment (Zane et al., 2005). In a sample of Asian American and White outpatients, they assessed client and therapist for these factors independently and prospectively and found that "treatment-goals match was predictive of session effect and comfort. Coping-orientation match was predictive of less dysphoria after four sessions of treatment [and] … similarities … in perceived distress associated with the problem appeared to result in higher psychosocial functioning at the end of the fourth session" (p. 582). This important study suggests mechanisms by which matching may affect outcomes.

Gender matching has also been a focus of research. Jones and Zoppel (1982) obtained self-reports from clients and therapists regarding the results of therapy. They found that female clients paired with female therapists were perceived by both clients and therapists as having experienced the most positive outcomes, suggesting that sex matching made the difference. But other research fails to support benefits from gender matching. Zlotnick, Elkin, and Shea (1998) took advantage of an exceptional opportunity to investigate sex-of-therapist effects in a well-controlled study, the National Institute of Mental Health Treatment of Depression Collaborative Research Program (TDCRP). In this research all clients were experiencing major depression and were assigned randomly to different treatment conditions, but also to either a female or male therapist. Attrition, treatment outcome (based on the Hamilton Rating Scale for Depression), and client-reported therapist empathy were assessed. Analyses revealed that "among depressed patients, a male or female therapist, or same-versus opposite-gender pairing, was not significantly related to level of depression at termination, to attrition rates, or to the patient's perceptions of the therapist's degree of empathy early in treatment and at termination" (Zlotnick et al., 1998, p. 657). Clients' beliefs about whether a female or male therapist would be more helpful were also assessed prior to therapy, but these beliefs had no impact on outcomes, regardless of whether they were assigned to the person they believed would be more helpful or not. Similarly, in a study of clients randomly assigned to one of three cognitive-behavioral treatment conditions for panic disorder, neither gender of the therapist nor gender match had an effect on therapy outcomes (Huppert et al., 2001).

The current emphasis in psychological treatment is on empirically supported treatments. Once a treatment has been found to be effective in clinical research, we may hypothesize that it will be effective universally, in similarly diagnosed but ethnically different populations; but data suggest that this assumption is not being empirically tested. Weisz, Doss, and Hawley (2005) identified 236 studies of randomized trials testing 386 treatments for children and adolescents. They report that "60% of all the articles failed to include any report on the race or ethnicity of their samples, and more than 70% failed to provide any information on family income or socioeconomic status" (p. 348). Numbers that were reported indicated that although African American youth are generally represented in these samples, other minorities are not. Finally, samples of minority youth are generally too small to test adequately the effectiveness for these groups in comparison to Whites. A major review of treatments for depression failed to address the question of effects for gender, race, or class at all, except to acknowledge that since women are prone to depression in the childbearing years, the relative success of psychotherapy without medication is encouraging (Hollon, Thase, & Markowitz, 2002). The research of Halliday-Boykins et al. (2005), however, that showed that ethnic matching in MST therapy improves outcomes is an important antidote to the assumption that gender, race, and class will not matter once we have established empirically supported treatments.

Gender, Race, and Class and Pharmacotherapy

In previous decades, the exclusion of women and minorities from clinical trials led to a lack of information about the differential responses of women and minorities to psychopharmacological treatment. In 1994 the federal government issued the "NIH Guidelines on the Inclusion of Women and Minorities as Subjects in Clinical Research," including both biomedical and behavioral research.

Results concerning the effects of race on pharmacotherapy are inconsistent. In a study of visits to primary care providers, Lasser, Himmelstein, Woolhandler, McCormick, and Bor (2002) found that African Americans were less likely to receive antidepressant, antianxiety, or any drug therapy, and similar results were found for visits to psychiatrists, except there African American clients were also less likely to receive antipsychotic prescriptions. Similarly, Snowden and Pingitore (2003) found that visits to a primary care physician with a mental health concern led to less pharmacotherapy for African Americans than Whites. On the other hand, in a sample of clients with a primary diagnosis of major depression for whom drug treatments were provided only by specialty mental health clinics, African Americans were more likely than Whites to receive pharmacotherapy.

Results have also indicated that African Americans may be less likely to receive the current standard of care. Kuno and Rothbard (2002) found that African Americans treated for schizophrenia were significantly less likely than Whites to be prescribed nontraditional, second-generation antipsychotics, even when controlling for funding and service types. Similarly, Herbeck et al. (2004) found that African American men, adjusting for clinical, SES, and health-system characteristics, were significantly less likely to receive these drugs and more likely to receive medications that have a greater risk of producing tardive dyskinesia and extrapyramidal side effects. Garb (2005), reviewing research regarding clinical treatment decision making, found that adherence with recommended treatment for schizophrenia was poor and that African American clients often received "excessively high dosages of antipsychotic medicine, and [were] less likely to be on atypical psychotics" (p. 82). These results suggest that African Americans are being overmedicated on traditional drugs and are not benefiting from advances in psychopharmacology.

There are also documented racial differences in attitudes toward psychiatric medication. Schnittker (2003) found that African Americans reported less willingness to use psychiatric medications or to give them to children in their care. These attitudes about pharmacotherapy were predicted by beliefs about efficacy and side effects and are not related to SES, knowledge, religiosity, or medical mistrust.

Women are more likely than men to be prescribed psychotropic drugs, even after controlling for other demographics, health status, SES, and diagnosis (Simoni-Wastila, 2000). But this may reflect women's mental health care–seeking behaviors, as Garb's review (1997) of numerous studies using case vignettes did not find gender effects on recommendations for use of psychotropic medications.

Sex and ethnicity may also affect responses to drug treatment. Differences may include absorption, distribution, metabolism, and elimination, all of which affect the bioavailability of the therapeutic substance. Women, for example, tend to have more fat tissue than men, which affects the metabolism and storage of drugs. Women's endogenous (e.g., menstrual cycle, pregnancy, postpartum, menopause) and exogenous (e.g., birth control pills, hormone replacement therapy) hormone levels also affect drug response (Yonkers & Hamilton, 1995). Estrogen, for example, tends to increase the effectiveness of some antipsychotic drugs (Seeman, 1995), meaning that women could be treated with lower doses; but they may also experience more side effects or toxicity from doses that are safe in men (Yonkers & Hamilton, 1995). Estrogen affects metabolic processes and drug response and estrogen has been tried with mixed to positive results, alone and combined with antidepressants, in treatment for women with refractory depression and for postmenopausal women (Casper, 1998; Kornstein, 1997). Research on the effectiveness of antidepressant medication, however, suggests that women respond more poorly than men to tricyclics and better than men to selective serotonin reuptake inhibitors and monoamine oxidase inhibitors (Kornstein, 1997). On the other hand, female schizophrenics respond better and more rapidly to pharmacological treatment and require lower doses than men in both acute episodes (Szymanski, Lieberman, Alvir, & Mayerhoff, 1995) and ongoing treatment (Tamminga, 1997). Women are also more likely than men to be exposed to more than one psychoactive drug due to a greater incidence of comorbidity, and so drug interaction effects must be considered (Casper, 1998).

There is growing interest in the possibility that different groups, defined by ethnicity, have different responses to drug treatments (Baker & Bell, 1999; Lin & Smith, 2000; Snowden, 2001). Baker and Bell (1999) cited studies that suggest that African Americans, compared to Whites, may have reduced responsiveness to beta blockers and are more likely to be nonresponders to fluoxetine, but may respond better and more rapidly to tricyclic antidepressants and to certain benzodiazepines and to need less lithium to control manic symptoms. The presence of sickle cell anemia in some African Americans may also complicate pharmacotherapy. Ethnic differences in therapeutic levels of lithium, clozapine, and antidepressants have been reported as well as differences between Asian Americans and Whites to haloperidol (Lin & Smith, 2000).

Finally, psychological disorders, especially depression, frequently occur in women 20 to 45 years of age, years when women are likely to bear children. The effects of psychopharmacological agents on maternal health, the health of the developing fetus, and lactation must be understood. To date research suggests that benzodiazepines (antianxiety drugs) lead to craniofacial abnormalities in a fetus and, when taken in late pregnancy, "floppy infant" syndrome; lithium (used in treating bipolar disorder) has been associated with cardiovascular, central nervous system, and mental and physical abnormalities; antidepressant medications have shown no adverse effects in some investigations, but small increased risks of miscarriage or deformities in others; and antipsychotics have yielded mixed outcomes (Casper, 1998). Clearly research clarifying the effects of medication during various stages of pregnancy and during lactation is critical.

Possible Exceptions to No Effects for Sex of Client or Therapist

Although most studies have found that the sex of client and the sex of therapist have relatively little impact on the outcome of psychotherapy, there are particular circumstances in which differences may occur. Liddle (1996) examined therapist sex and sexual orientation as predictors of gay and lesbian clients' reports of therapist practices. She found that gay or bisexual male therapists and gay, bisexual, or heterosexual female therapists were rated as equally helpful but as more helpful than heterosexual male therapists. The fact that men generally have less positive attitudes toward homosexuality than women may help explain why heterosexual male therapists were perceived as least helpful (Liddle, 1996). The therapist's attitude toward client sexual orientation may be a better predictor of outcome than sex or sexual orientation per se.

Certain deleterious effects of psychotherapy are also more likely to occur in some sex-of-therapist–sex-of-client combinations. For example, data suggest that sexual relationships occur between therapist and client in 5–6% of therapy relationships, with 85% of these involving a male therapist with a female client (Lamb & Catanzaro, 1998). This particular negative therapeutic experience is clearly more likely to affect women.

Understanding Gender, Race, and Class

Chang (2003) presented two basic research perspectives for understanding racial (and we would add, gender) differences in mental health and mental health care. The first approach seeks to discover and describe the common factors that predict sociodemographic differences, such as discrimination, poverty, and low social status. The second approach assumes that each group is embedded in a complex and unique set of historical, social, and cultural factors, and that even when common factors are identified, each group may respond differently to them. This approach requires a group-specific approach.

Common factors that affect women and minorities are discrimination and poverty. A series of studies by Landrine, Klonoff, and colleagues have found that sexist discrimination accounted for more variance in depressive and somatic symptoms than life events or daily hassles (Landrine, Klonoff, Gibbs, Manning & Lund, 1995), and that recent and lifetime sex discrimination accounted for the difference between women and men in depressive, anxious, and somatic symptoms (Klonoff, Landrine, & Campbell, 2000). Moradi and DeBlaere (2010) provided an extensive review of the research literature on women's experiences of sex discrimination and its links to psychological and physical health. For African Americans, experiences of racial discrimination are related to low self-esteem, depression, anxiety, and stress-related somatic symptoms (Landrine & Klonoff, 1996; Klonoff, Landrine, & Ullman, 1999). Recently the concept of "race-based trauma" has been discussed as an additional diagnostic category (Carter, 2007). Perceived racial discrimination predicted psychological distress in Hispanic women (Salgado de Snyder, 1987). In a study of urban adolescents in mental health treatment, Surko, Ciro, Blackwood, Nembhard, and Peake (2005) found that perceived racism was associated with exposure to risks, such as violence, sexual abuse and assault, drug abuse, and worry about self and others. Recent research on racial microaggressions, "brief, commonplace, and daily verbal, behavioral, and environmental slights and indignities directed toward Black Americans, often automatically and unintentionally" (Sue, Capodilupo, & Holder, 2008, p. 329), is exploring how these subtle but frequent incidents contribute to experiences of powerlessness and invisibility and may also be a barrier to effective psychotherapy when these occur in the psychotherapeutic relationship (Sue et al., 2007). Racial minorities and women are also more likely than nonminorities and men to live in poverty or have fewer economic resources. Poverty and low income are well-established correlates of depression (Belle & Doucet, 2003).

Other research, however, suggests that belief systems, values, and coping strategies will vary by gender, race, and culture (Brown, Abe-Kim, & Barrio, 2003). In making comparisons, even in an effort to advance understanding, we must consider whether the assumptions that accompany our comparisons, generally that the difference can be attributed to something about the variable (gender, race, class) associated with the difference, are correct. Corral and Landrine (2010) warned us that "researchers rarely measure and control the social contextual correlates of membership in ethnic (and other status) groups" and further that "the plethora of potentially relevant, social contextual correlates of ethnic (and other status) group membership cannot be known a priori" (p. 86). In other words, while we focus on race or socioeconomic status as the risk factor for a disorder, it may, in fact, simply be living in a neighborhood where safety is a day-to-day concern. In this example, if all neighborhoods were equally secure, the effects of race and SES would go away. Sue and Chu (2003) suggested that "rather than developing broad theories to explain the mental health of ethnic minority groups, it may be wiser to begin an inductive process in which separate ethnic groups are studied and examined before construction of a more general theory" (p. 461).

In this era of evidence-based practice, an equally important debate concerns the universality versus specificity of treatment effectiveness. Miranda, Nakamura, and Bernal (2003) argued that although evidence-based treatments have generally been developed and tested on White, middle-class samples, they are likely to be effective for minorities as well. They acknowledged that these therapies should continue to be studied to determine what cultural, social, or environmental conditions affect the quality or acceptability of these treatments. Sue and Zane (2006) disagreed with this argument. They criticized the lack of attention paid to ethnic and cultural minorities in the research on evidence-based interventions and called for not only more research that is inclusive but also research aimed at explaining the effects of cultural variables. Assuming that interventions can and should be adapted for diverse populations, Muñoz and Mendelson (2005) described the development and evaluation of prevention and treatment manuals created for low-income minority populations. They used five principles in developing these manuals: (1) including members of the target group in developing the manual; (2) incorporating relevant cultural values; (3) using religion and spirituality when appropriate; (4) dealing with the stress of acculturation (for those adapting to a new culture); and (5) acknowledging the reality of racism, prejudice, and discrimination. Empirical evaluations of the effectiveness of these manuals were positive (Muñoz & Mendelson, 2005).

Cultural Competence

No review of the research literature can completely capture the complexities of gender, race, and class. Indeed to improve diagnosis and treatment of individual clients we might focus less on the client and more on the therapist. Strategies for developing individual and cultural competence in therapists are critical. The APA's *Guidelines on Multicultural Education, Training, Research, Practice, and Organizational Change for Psychologists* presented six guidelines for enhancing cultural competence: (1) being aware of one's own attitudes and beliefs that can be detrimental in interacting with others who are different; (2) recognizing the importance of multicultural sensitivity, knowledge, and understanding; (3) employing the constructs of multiculturalism and diversity in educating others; (4) recognizing the importance of conducting culture-centered and ethical research with diverse participants; (5) applying culturally appropriate skill in clinical and applied settings; and (6) supporting culturally informed policy development and practices. Sanchez-Hucles and Jones (2006) have reviewed each of these guidelines through the lens of gender. Daniel, Roysircar, Abeles, and Boyd (2004) reviewed research on four elements of cultural competence: self-awareness of attitudes, biases, and assumptions; knowledge about diversity; understanding of gender's interaction with other statuses; and the reality of multiple identities for all individuals. They discussed how these can be incorporated into graduate education and training of clinical psychologists.

Conclusions

This chapter reviews the research literature on gender, race, and class as they affect diagnosis and treatment of psychological disorders. Evidence shows that certain diagnoses (schizophrenia in the case of African Americans, histrionic and, perhaps, borderline personality disorders in the case of women, antisocial personality disorder in the case of men) are more likely to be given to some clients based on certain criteria. Increasing interest in access to mental health care has produced complex findings on the effects of gender, race, and class on use of different services for mental health treatment. Whereas a match between gender of therapist and client may matter in certain situations, there is substantial evidence that matching for race and ethnicity can matter. Research on quality and type of treatment and on pharmacotherapy suggests inequities in treatment and a need for better information about the connections between individual characteristics (including gender and race) and effectiveness of and reactions to psychotropic medications. In an era of establishing and promoting empirically supported treatments, we need to be mindful of the population being treated and we need to ask: Do therapies work equally well with different groups and can psychological interventions be improved by culturally based adaptations? Finally, we need to consider how best to seek greater understanding of the role of gender, race, and class on psychopathology and psychotherapy and we need to continue to focus on developing cultural competence in clinicians.

This chapter makes it abundantly clear that there are very few studies that actually meet the challenge of considering gender, race, and class. Even where all of these sociodemographic variables are assessed, they are often analyzed as individual factors or possibly two-way interactions and the possibilities of higher-order interactions are not pursued. Our discipline's attachment to quantitative, linear, main effect approaches to data may account for this. Research that takes context into account, such as the examination by Chow et al. (2003) of mental health service use by diverse populations in low and high poverty communities and Kuno and Rothbard's (2005) study of quality of care at CMHCs in neighborhoods that vary by income and racial composition, demonstrates the value of doing more than collecting individual reports on sociodemographic variables. Snowden and Yamada (2005) acknowledged that we do not yet understand disparities in mental health care. They call for "more studies of treatment—seeking pathways that favor nonspecialty sources of assistance, improve trust and treatment receptiveness, eliminate stigma, and accommodate culturally distinctive beliefs about mental illness and mental health and styles of expressing mental health-related suffering" (pp. 160–161). Mullings and Schulz (2006) suggested that a better understanding of interactions among gender, race, and class may require a more qualitative approach. This view is supported by Lopez (2003) who argued that reporting of quantitative differences among groups may serve to further marginalize minority groups without helping us to understand them. Without qualitative ethnographic research we may be unable to contextualize and interpret these data.

Mullings and Schulz (2006) pointed out that "it is often difficult to pinpoint how the interaction, articulation, and simultaneity of race, class, and gender affect women and men in their daily lives, and the ways in which these forms of inequality interact in specific situation to condition health" (p. 6). They suggested that gender, race, and class should be viewed as social relationships rather than as characteristics of individuals. Building on this theme, Martin (2006) criticized the supplement to the surgeon general's report and its assumption:

> [T]here is something concrete and real in the world (and increasingly in the brain) that corresponds one to one with the major psychiatric diagnosis. Identifying this real thing … is the proper first step in getting [patients] the proper treatment. Identifying observer bias and removing it will clear the way to more frequently correct diagnosis. But there are … troubling aspects of this view. First, what if the categories into which psychiatry divides disorders themselves already have cultural assumptions embedded in them, not fixed for all time? Second, what if our only route to the real is always through linguistic categories that are necessarily saturated with culturally constituted sets of meanings? (p. 85)

These closing remarks remind us that gender, race, and class are more than sociodemographic characteristics. They constitute essential aspects of the lived experience of individuals who may come to clinicians in need of understanding and assistance. We must determine how to treat these individuals in culturally sensitive and appropriate ways.

References

Adebimpe, V. (1981). Overview: White norms and psychiatric diagnosis of Black patients. *American Journal of Psychiatry, 138,* 279–285.

Adler, D., Drake, R., & Teague, G. (1990). Clinicians' practices in personality assessment: Does gender influence the use of DAM-III Axis II? *Comprehensive Psychiatry, 31,* 125–133.

Alarcón, R. D. Alegría, M., Bell, C. C., Boyce, C. Kirmayer, L. J., Lin, K-M., … Wisner, K. L. (2002). Beyond the funhouse mirrors: Research agenda on culture and psychiatric diagnosis. In D. J. Kupfer, M. B. First, D. A. Regier (Eds.), *A research agenda for DSM-V*™ (pp. 219–266). Washington, DC: American Psychiatric Association.

Alegría, M., Canino, G., Ríos, R. Vera, M., Calderón, J., Rusch, D., & Ortega, A. N. (2002). Mental health care for Latinos: Inequalities in use of specialty mental health services among Latinos, African Americans, and non-Latino Whites. *Psychiatric Services, 53*, 1547–1555.

Allen-Burge, R., Storandt, M., Kinscherf, D. A., & Rubin, E. H. (1994). Sex differences in the sensitivity of two self-report depression scales in older depressed inpatients. *Psychology and Aging, 9*, 443–445.

American Psychiatric Association (APA). (1980). *Diagnostic and statistical manual of mental disorders* (3rd ed.). Washington, DC: Author.

American Psychiatric Association (APA). (1987). *Diagnostic and statistical manual of mental disorders* (3rd ed., rev.). Washington, DC: Author.

American Psychiatric Association (APA). (1994). *Diagnostic and statistical manual of mental disorders* (4th ed.). Washington, DC: Author.

American Psychiatric Association (APA). (2000). *Diagnostic and statistical manual of mental disorders* (4th ed., text rev.). Washington, DC: Author.

American Psychological Association (APA). (2002). *Guidelines on multicultural education, training, research, practice, and organizational change for psychologists.* Washington, DC: Author. Retrieved from http://www.apa.org/pi/oema/resources/policy/multicultural-guidelines.aspx

American Psychological Association (APA). (1990). *Guidelines for providers of psychological services to ethnic, linguistic, and culturally diverse populations.* Washington, DC: Author. Retrieved from (http://www.apa.org/pi/oema/resources/policy/provider-guidelines.aspx

American Psychological Association (APA). (2007). *Guidelines for psychological practice with girls and women.* Washington, DC: Author. Retrieved from (http://www.apa.org/practice/guidelines/girls-and-women pdf

Anthony, M. M., & Rowa, K. (2005). Evidence-based assessment of anxiety disorders. *Psychological Assessment, 17*, 256–266.

Armistead, L. P., Clark, J., Barber, C. N., Dorsey, S., Hughley, J., & Favors, M. (2004). Participant retention in the Parents Matter! program: Strategies and outcome. *Journal of Child and Family Studies, 13*, 67–80.

Arnold, L. M., Keck, P. E., Collins, J., Wilson, R., Fleck, D. E., Corey, K. B., … Strakowski, S. M. (2004). Ethnicity and first-rank symptoms in patients with psychosis. *Schizophrenia Bulletin, 67*, 207–212.

Ash, S. E., & Weis, R. (2009). Recovery among youths referred to outpatient psychotherapy: Reliable change, clinical significance, and predictors of outcome. *Child and Adolescent Social Work Journal, 26*, 399–413. 2003 Retrieved from http://www.apa.org/pi/oema/resources/brochures/treatment-minority.pdf

Baker, F. M., & Bell, C. C. (1999). Issues in the psychiatric treatment of African Americans. *Psychiatric Services, 50*, 362–368.

Becker, D., & Lamb, S. (1994). Sex bias in the diagnosis of borderline personality disorder and posttraumatic stress disorder. *Professional Psychology: Research and Practice, 25*, 55–61.

Belle, D., & Doucet, J. (2003). Poverty, inequality, and discrimination as sources of depression among U.S. women. *Psychology of Women Quarterly, 27*, 101–113.

Blashfield, R. K., & Herkov, M. J. (1996). Investigating clinician adherence to diagnosis by criteria: A replication of Morey and Ochoa (1989). *Journal of Personality Disorders, 10*, 219–228.

Brown, C., Abe-Kim, J. S., & Barrio, C. (2003). Depression in ethnically diverse women: Implications for treatment in primary care settings. *Professional Psychology: Research and Practice, 34*, 10–19.

Brown, L. S. (1992). A feminist critique of personality disorders. In L. S. Brown & M. Ballou (Eds.), *Personality and psychopathology. Feminist reappraisals* (pp. 206–228). New York: Guilford.

Cabassa, L. J., Zayas, L. H., & Hansen, M. C. (2006). Latino adults' access to mental health care: A review of epidemiological studies. *Administration and Policy in Mental Health and Mental Health Services Research, 33*, 316–330.

Caplan, P. J. (1991). How do they decide who is normal? The bizarre, but true, tale of the DSM process. *Canadian Psychology, 32*, 162–170.

Caplan, P. J. (1995). *They say you're crazy. How the world's most powerful psychiatrists decide who's normal.* Reading, MA: Addison-Wesley.

Caplan, P. J., & Cosgrove, L. (Eds.). (2004). *Bias in psychiatric diagnosis.* Lanham, MD: Aronson.

Carter, R. T. (2007). Racism and psychological and emotional injury: Recognizing and assessing race-based traumatic stress. *The Counseling Psychologist, 35*, 144–154.

Casper, R. (1998). The psychopharmacology of women. In R. C. Casper (Ed.), *Women's health: Hormones, emotions and behavior* (pp. 192–218). Cambridge, UK: Cambridge University Press.

Chang, D. F. (2003). An introduction to the politics of science: Culture, race, ethnicity, and the supplement to the surgeon general's Report on Mental Health. *Culture, Medicine and Psychiatry, 27,* 373–383.

Chavez, D. F. (2003). Commentary. *Culture, Medicine and Psychiatry, 27,* 391–393.

Chow, J. C., Jaffee, K., & Snowden, L. (2003) Racial/ethnic disparities in the use of mental health services in poverty areas. *American Journal of Public Health, 93,* 792–797.

Clarkin, J. F., & Levy, K. N. (2004). The influence of client variables on psychotherapy. In M. J. Lambert (Ed.), *Bergin and Garfield's handbook of psychotherapy and behavior change* (5th ed., pp. 194–226). New York: Wiley.

Collaborative Psychiatric Edidemiological Survey (CPES), National Institute of Mental Health. (2003). Available from http://www.icpsr.umich.edu/icpsrweb/CPES/index.jsp

Cooper-Patrick, L., Gallo, J. J., Powe, N. R., Steinwachs, D. M., Eaton, W. W., & Ford, D. E. (1999). Mental health service utilization by African Americans and Whites: Baltimore Epidemiologic Catchment Area follow-up. *Medical Care, 37,* 1034–1045.

Corral, I., & Landrine, H. (2010). Methodological and statistical issues in research with diverse samples: The problem of measure equivalence. In H. Landrine & N. Felipe Russo (Eds.), *Handbook of diversity in feminist psychology* (pp. 83–134). New York: Springer.

Council of National Psychological Associations for the Advancement of Ethnic Minority Interests. (2003). *Psychological treatment of ethnic minority populations.* Washington, DC: Association of Black Psychologists. Retrieved from http://www.apa.org/pi/oema/resources/brochures/treatment-minority.pdf

Crosby, J. P., & Sprock, J. (2004). Effect of patient sex, clinician sex, and sex role on the diagnosis of antisocial personality disorder: Models of underpathologizing and overpathologizing biases. *Journal of Clinical Psychology, 60,* 583–604.

Dahlgren, L., & Willander, A. (1989). Are special treatment facilities for female alcoholics needed? A controlled 2-year follow-up study from a specialized female unit (EWA) versus a missed male-female treatment facility. *Alcoholism: Clinical and Experimental Research, 13,* 499–504.

Daniel, J. H., Roysircar, G., Abeles, N., & Boyd, C. (2004). Individual and cultural-diversity competency: Focus on the therapist. *Journal of Clinical Psychology, 60,* 755–770.

DeNavas-Walt, C., Proctor, B. D., & Smith, J. C. (2010). Income, poverty, and health insurance coverage in the United States: 2009. *Current Population Reports.* (US Census P60-238). Retrieved from http://www.census.gov/prod/2010pubs/p60-238.pdf

Fernbach, B. E., Winstead, B. A., & Derlega, V. J. (1989). Sex differences in diagnosis and treatment recommendations for antisocial personality and somatization disorders. *Journal of Social and Clinical Psychology, 8,* 238–255.

Flanagan, E. H., & Blashfield, R. K. (2005).Gender acts as a context for interpreting diagnostic criteria. *Journal of Clinical Psychology, 61,* 1485–1498.

Ford, M., & Widiger, T. A. (1989). Sex bias in the diagnosis of histrionic and antisocial personality disorders. *Journal of Consulting and Clinical Psychology, 57,* 301–305.

Gaines, A. D. (1992). From DSM-I to DSM-III-R: Voices of self, mastery, and the other: A cultural constructivist reading of US psychiatric classification. *Social Science and Medicine, 35,* 3–24.

Galen, L. W., Brower, K. J., Gillespie, B. W., & Zucker, R. A. (2000). Sociopathy, gender, and treatment outcome among outpatient substance abusers. *Drug and Alcohol Dependence, 61,* 23–33.

Gamst, G., Aguilar-Kitibutr, A., Herdina, A., Hibbs, S., Krishtal, E., Lee, R., … Martenson, L. (2003). Effects of racial match on Asian American mental health consumer satisfaction, *Mental Health Services Research, 5,* 197–208.

Gamst, G., Dana, R. H., Der-Karabetian, A., & Kramer, T. (2001). Asian American mental health centers: Effects of ethnic match and age on global assessment and visitation. *Journal of Mental Health Counseling, 23,* 57–71.

Gamst, G., Dana, R. H., Der-Karabetian, A., & Kramer, T. (2004). Ethnic match and treatment outcomes for child and adolescent mental health center clients. *Journal of Counseling and Development, 82,* 457–465.

Garb, H. N. (1997). Race bias, social class bias, and gender bias in clinical judgment. *Clinical Psychology: Science and Practice, 4,* 99–120.

Garb, H. N. (2005). Clinical judgment and decision making. *Annual Review of Clinical Psychology, 1,* 67–89.

Giardina, E. G. (2000). Heart disease in women. *International Journal of Fertility and Women's Medicine, 45,* 350–357.

González, H. M., Tarraf, W., Whitfield, K. E., & Vega, W. A. (2010). The epidemiology of major depression and ethnicity in the United States. *Journal of Psychiatric Research, 44*, 1043–1051.

Greenfield, S. F., Trucco, E. M., McHugh, R. K., Lincoln, M., & Gallop, R. J. (2007). The women's recovery group study: A stage 1 trial of women-focused group therapy for substance use disorders versus mixed-gender group drug counseling. *Drug and Alcohol Dependence, 90*, 39–47.

Hall, J., Guterman, D. K., Lee, H. B., & Little, S. G. (2002). Counselor-client matching on ethnicity, gender, and language: Implications for counseling school-aged children. *North American Journal of Psychology, 4*, 367–380.

Halliday-Boykins, C. A., Schoenwald, S. K., & Letourneau, E. J. (2005). Caregiver-therapist ethnic similarity predicts youth outcomes from an empirically based treatment. *Journal of Consulting and Clinical Psychology, 73*, 808–818.

Hartung, C. A., & Widiger, T. A. (1998). Gender differences in the diagnosis of mental disorders: Conclusions and controversies of the DSM-IV. *Psychological Bulletin, 123*, 260–278.

Herbeck, D. M., West, J. C., Ruditis, I., Farifteh, R. D., Fitek, D. J., Bell, C. C., & Snowden, L. R. (2004). Variations in use of second-generation antipsychotic medication by race among adult psychiatric patients. *Psychiatric Services, 55*, 677–684.

Hollon, S. D., Thase, M. E., & Markowitz, J. C. (2002). Treatment and prevention of depression. *Psychological Science in the Public Interest, 3*, 39–77.

Huppert, J. D., Bufka, L. F., Barlow, D. H., Gorman, J. M., Shear, M. D., & Woods, S. W. (2001). Therapists, therapist variables, and cognitive-behavioral therapy outcome in a multicenter trial for panic disorder. *Journal of Consulting and Clinical Psychology, 69*, 747–755.

Hunsley, J., & Mash, E. J. (2005). Introduction to the special section on developing guidelines for the evidence-based assessment (EBA) of adult disorders. *Psychological Assessment, 17*, 251–255.

Joiner, T. E. Jr., Walker, R. L., Pettit, J. W., Perez, M., & Cukrowicz, K. C. (2005). Evidence-based assessment of depression in adults. *Psychological Assessment, 17*, 267–277.

Jones, E. E., & Nisbett, R. E. (1987). The actor and the observer: Divergent perceptions of the causes of behavior. In E. E. Jones, D. E. Kanouse, H. H. Kelley, R. E. Nisbett, & S. Valins (Eds.), *Attribution: Perceiving the causes of behavior* (pp. 79–94). Hillsdale, NJ: Erlbaum.

Jones, E. E., & Zoppel, C. L. (1982). Impact of client and therapist gender on psychotherapy process and outcome. *Journal of Consulting and Clinical Psychology, 50*, 259–272.

Kales, H. C., Neighbors, H. W., Valenstein, M., Blow, F. C., McCarthy, J. F., Ignacio, R. V., … Mellow, A. M. (2005). Effect of race and sex on primary care physicians' diagnosis and treatment of late-life depression. *Journal of the American Geriatric Society, 53*, 777–784,

Kaplan, M. (1983). A woman's view of DSM-III. *American Psychologist, 38*, 786–792.

King, A. C., & Canada, S. A. (2004). Client-related predictors of early treatment drop-out in a substance abuse clinic exclusively employing individual therapy. *Journal of Substance Abuse Treatment, 26*, 189–195.

Klonoff, E. A., Landrine, H., & Campbell, R. (2000). Sexist discrimination may account for well-known gender differences in psychiatric symptoms. *Psychology of Women Quarterly, 24*, 93–99.

Klonoff, E. A., Landrine, H., & Ulllman, J. M. (1999). Racial discrimination and psychiatric symptoms among Blacks. *Cultural Diversity and Ethnic Minority Psychology, 5*, 329–339.

Korman, M. (1974). National conference on levels and patterns of professional training in psychology: Major themes. *American Psychologist, 29*, 441–449.

Kornstein, S. G. (1997). Gender differences in depression: Implications for treatment. *Journal of Clinical Psychiatry, 58*(Suppl. 15), 12–18.

Kosten, T. A., Gawin, F. H., Kosten, T. R., & Rounsaville, B. J. (1993). Gender differences in cocaine use and treatment response. *Journal of Substance Abuse Treatment, 10*, 63–66.

Kunen, S., Neiderhauser, R., Smith, P. O., Morris, J. A., & Marx, B. D. (2005). Race disparities in psychiatric rates in emergency departments. *Journal of Consulting and Clinical Psychology, 73*, 116–126.

Kung, W. W. (2003). Chinese Americans' help seeking for emotional distress. *Social Service Review, 77*, 110–158.

Kuno, E., & Rothbard, A. B. (2002). Racial disparities in antipsychotic prescription patterns for patients with schizophrenia. *American Journal of Psychiatry, 159*, 567–572.

Kuno, E., & Rothbard, A. B. (2005). The effect of income and race on quality of psychiatric care in community mental health centers. *Community Mental Health Journal, 41*, 613–622.

Lam, A. G., & Sue, S. (2001). Client Diversity. *Psychotherapy, 38*, 479–486.

Lamb, D. H., & Catanzaro, S. J. (1998). Sexual and nonsexual boundary violations involving psychologists, clients, supervisees, and students: Implication for professional practice. *Professional Psychology: Research and Practice, 29*, 498–503.

Landrine, H., & Klonoff, E. A. (1996). The schedule of racist events: A measure of racial discrimination and a study of is negative physical and mental health consequences. *Journal of Black Psychology, 22,* 144–168.

Landrine, H., Klonoff, E. A., Gibbs, J., Manning, V., & Lund, M. (1995). Physical and psychiatric correlates of gender discrimination: An application of the schedule of sexist events. *Psychology of Women Quarterly, 19,* 473–492.

Lasser, K. E., Himmelstein, D. U., Woolhandler, S. J., McCormick, D., & Bor, D. H. (2002). Do minorities in the United States receive fewer mental health services than Whites? *International Journal of Health Services, 32,* 567–578.

Leinhardt, G., Seewald, A. M., & Zigmond, N. (1982). Sex and race difference in learning disabilities classrooms. *Journal of Educational Psychology, 74,* 835–843.

Liddle, B. J. (1996). Therapist sexual orientation, gender, and counseling practices as they related to ratings of helpfulness by gay and lesbian clients. *Journal of Counseling Psychology, 43,* 394–402.

Lin, K. M., & Smith, M. W. (2000). Psychopharmacotherapy in the context of culture and ethnicity. In P. Ruiz (Ed.), *Ethnicity and Psychopharmacology* (pp. 1–36.). Washington, DC: American Psychiatric Association.

Lindsay, K. A., Sankis, L. M., & Widiger, T. A. (2000). Gender bias in self-report personality disorder inventories. *Journal of Personality Disorders, 14,* 218–232.

Lindsay, K. A., & Widiger, T. A. (1995). Sex and gender bias in self-report personality disorder inventories: Items analyses of the MCMI-II, MMPI, and PDQ-R. *Journal of Personality Assessment, 65,* 1–20.

Li-Repac, D. (1980). Cultural influences on clinical perception: A comparison between Caucasian and Chinese-American therapists. *Journal of Cross-Cultural Psychology, 11,* 327–342.

Lopez, S. (1989). Patient variable biases in clinical judgment. *Psychological Bulletin, 106,* 184–203.

Lopez, S. (2003). Reflections on the surgeon general's Report on Mental Health, Culture, Race, and Ethnicity. *Culture, Medicine and Psychiatry, 27,* 419–434.

Loring, M., & Powell, B. (1988). Gender, race and DSM-III: A study of the objectivity of psychiatric diagnostic behavior. *Journal of Health and Social Behavior, 29,* 1–22.

Luebnitz, R. R., Randolph, D. L., & Gutsch, K. W. (1982). Race and socioeconomic status as confounding variables in the accurate diagnosis of alcoholism. *Journal of Clinical Psychology, 38,* 665–669.

Maddux, J. E. (2002). Stopping the "madness": Positive psychology and the deconstruction of the illness ideology and the *DSM*. In C. R. Snyder & S. J. Lopez (Eds.), *Handbook of positive psychology* (pp. 13–25). New York: Oxford University Press.

Maramba, G. G., & Hall, G. C. N. (2002). Meta-analyses of ethnic match as a predictor of dropout, utilization, and level of functioning. *Cultural Diversity and Ethnic Minority Psychology, 8,* 290–297.

Martin, E. (2006). Moods and representations of social inequality. In A. Schulz & L. Mullings (Eds.), *Gender, race, class, and health* (pp. 60–88). San Francisco, CA: Jossey-Bass.

Miltenberger, R. G., Rapp, J. T., & Long, E. S. (2006). Characteristics of trichotillomanis. In D. W. Woods & R. G. Milenberger (Eds.), *Tic disorders, trichotillomania, and other repetitive behavior disorders* (pp. 133–150). New York: Springer.

Miranda, M., Nakamura, R., & Bernal, G. (2003). Including ethnic minorities in mental health intervention research: A practical approach to a long-standing problem. *Culture, Medicine and Psychiatry, 27,* 467–486.

Moradi, B. & DeBlaere, C. (2010) Women's experiences of sexist discrimination: Review of research and directions for centralizing race, ethnicity, and culture. In B. Landrine & N. Felipe Russo (Eds.), *Handbook of diversity in feminist psychology*. New York: Springer Publishing Co., pp. 172–210.

Morey, L. C., & Ochoa, E. (1989). An investigation of adherence to diagnostic criteria: Clinical diagnosis of the DSM-III personality disorders. *Journal of Personality Disorders, 3,* 180–192.

Mullings, L., & Schulz, A. (2006). Intersectionality and health: An introduction. In A. Schulz & L. Mullings (Eds.), *Gender, race, class, and health* (pp. 3–17). San Francisco, CA: Jossey-Bass.

Muñoz, R. F., & Mendelson, T. (2005). Toward evidence-based interventions for diverse populations: The San Francisco General Hospital prevention and treatment manuals. *Journal of Consulting and Clinical Psychology, 73,* 790–799.

Murkherjee, S., Shukla, S., Woodle, J., Rosen, A. M., & Olarte, S. (1983). Misdiagnosis of schizophrenia in bipolar patients: A multiethnic comparison. *American Journal of Psychiatry, 140,* 1571–1574.

National Institute of Corrections. (2003). *Achieving the promise: Transforming mental health care in America. Final report.* Rockville, MD: President's New Freedom Commission on Mental Health. Retrieved from http://nicic.gov/Library/020228.

National Institutes of Health (NIH) Policy and Guidelines on the Inclusion of Women and Minorities as Subjects in Clinical Research - Amended, October, 2011. http://grants.nih.gov/grants/funding/women_min/guidelines_amended_10_2001.htm

Neighbors, H. W., Trierweiler, S. J., Ford, B. C., & Muroff, J. R. (2003). Racial differences in DSM diagnosis using a semi-structured instrument: The importance of clinical judgment in the diagnosis of African Americans. *Journal of Health and Social Behavior, 43,* 237–256.

Neighbors, H. W., Trierweiler, S. J., Munday, C., Thompson, E. E., Jackson, J. S., Binion, V. J., & Gomez, J. (1999). Psychiatric diagnosis of African Americans: Diagnostic divergence in clinician structured and semistructured interviewing conditions. *Journal of the National Medical Association, 91,* 601–612.

Ogrodniczuk, J. S., Piper, W. E., & Joyce, A. S. (2004). Differences in men's and women's responses to short-term group psychotherapy. *Psychotherapy Research, 14,* 231–243.

Page, S., & Bennesch, S. (1993). Gender and reporting differences in measures of depression. *Canadian Journal of Behavioural Science, 25,* 579–589.

Pantony, K. L., & Caplan, P. J. (1991). Delusional dominating personality disorder: A modest proposal for identifying some consequences of rigid masculine socialization. *Canadian Psychology, 32,* 120–133.

Pavkov, T. W., Lewis, D. A., & Lyons, J. S. (1989). Psychiatric diagnosis and ethnic bias: An empirical investigation. *Professional Psychology: Research and Practice, 20,* 364–368.

Petry, N. M., Tenne, H., & Affleck, G. (2000). Stalking the elusive client variable in psychotherapy research. In C. R. Snyder & R. E. Ingram (Eds.), *Handbook of psychological change* (pp. 88–108). New York: Wiley.

Pingitore, D., Snowden, L., Sansone, R. A., & Klinkman, M. (2001). Persons with depressive symptoms and the treatments they receive: A comparison of primary care physicians and psychiatrists. *International Journal of Psychiatry in Medicine, 31,* 41–60.

Poland, J., & Caplan, P. J. (2004). The deep structure of bias in psychiatric diagnosis. In P. J. Caplan & L. Cosgrove (Eds.), *Bias in psychiatric diagnosis* (pp. 9–23). Lanham, MD: Jason Aronson.

Potts, M. K., Burnam, M. A., & Wells, K. B. (1991). Gender differences in depression detection: A comparison of clinician diagnosis and standardized assessment. *Psychological Assessment, 3,* 609–615.

Pryzgoda, J., & Chrisler, J. C. (2000). Definitions of gender and sex: The subtleties of meaning. *Sex Roles, 43,* 553–569.

Query, J. N. (1985). Comparative admission and follow-up study of American Indians and Whites in a youth chemical dependency unit on the North Central Plains. *International Journal of the Addictions, 20,* 489–502.

Reis, B. F., & Brown, L. G. (1999). Reducing psychotherapy dropouts: Maximizing perspective convergence in the psychotherapy dyad. *Psychotherapy, 36,* 123–136.

Richardson, J., Anderson, R., Flaherty, J., & Bell, C. (2003). The quality of mental health care for African Americans. *Culture, Medicine and Psychiatry, 27,* 487–498.

Robins, E., & Guze, S. B. (1970). Establishment of diagnostic validity of psychiatric illness: Its application to schizophrenia. *American Journal of Psychiatry, 126,* 983–986.

Robins, L. N., & Regier, D. A. (1991). *Psychiatric disorders in America: The epidemiologic catchment area study.* New York: Free Press.

Rosenheck, R., Fontana, A., & Cottroll, C. (1995). Effect of clinician-veteran racial pairing in the treatment of post-traumatic stress disorder. *American Journal of Psychiatry, 152,* 555–563.

Ross, R., Frances, A. J., & Widiger, T. A. (1995). Gender issues in DSM-IV. In J. M. Oldham & M. B. Riba (Eds.), *Review of psychiatry* (Vol. 14, pp. 205–226). Washington, DC: American Psychiatric Press.

Russell, G. L., Fujino, D. C., Sue, S., Cheung, M., & Snowden L. R. (1996). The effects of therapist-client ethnic match in the assessment of mental health functioning. *Journal of Cross-Cultural Psychology, 27,* 598–615.

Safran, M. A., Mays, R. A., Huang, L. N., McCuan, R. Pham, P. K., Fisher, S. K., McDuffie, K. Y., & Trachtenberg, A. (2009). Mental health disparities, *American Journal of Public Health, 99,* 1962–1966.

Salgado de Snyder, V. (1987). Factors associated with acculturative stress and depressive symptomatology among married Mexican immigrant women. *Psychology of Women Quarterly, 11,* 475–488.

Sanchez-Hucles, J., & Jones, N. (2006). Gender issues. In M. G. Constantine (Ed.), *Clinical practice with people of color: A guide to becoming culturally competent* (pp. 183–197). New York, NY: Teachers College Press.

Schnittker, J. (2003). Misgivings of medicine: African Americans' skepticism of psychiatric medication. *Journal of Health and Social Behavior, 44,* 506–524.

Seeman, M. V. (1995). Gender differences in treatment response in schizophrenia. In M. V. Seeman (Ed.), *Gender and psychopathology* (pp. 227–252). Washington, DC: American Psychiatric Press.

Simon, R. J., Fleiss, J. L., Gurland, B. J., Stiller, P. R., & Sharpe, L. (1973). Depression and schizophrenia in hospitalized Black and White mental patients. *Archives of General Psychiatry, 28,* 509–512.

Simoni-Wastila, L. (2000). The use of abusable prescription drugs: The role of gender. *Journal of Women's Health and Gender-Based Medicine, 9,* 289–297.

Snowden, L. R. (2001). Barriers to effective mental health services for African Americans. *Mental Health Services Research, 3,* 181–187.

Snowden, L. R., & Pingitore, D. (2003). Frequency and scope of mental health service delivery to African Americans in primary care. *Mental Health Services Research, 4,* 123–130.

Snowden, L. R., & Thomas, K. (2000). Medicaid and African American outpatient mental health treatment. *Mental Health Services Research, 2,* 115–120.

Snowden, L. R., & Yamada, A-M. (2005). Cultural differences in access to care. *Annual Review of Clinical Psychology, 1,* 143–166.

Snyder, D. K., Heyman, R. E., & Haynes, S. N. (2005). Evidence-based approaches to assessing couple distress. *Psychological Assessment, 17,* 288–307.

Spilt, J. L., Koomen, H. M. Y., Thijs, J. T., Stoel, R. D., & van der Leij, A. (2010). Teachers' assessment of antisocial behavior in kindergarten: Physical aggression and measurement bias across gender. *Journal of Psychological Assessment, 28,* 129–138.

Sprock, J., & Yoder, C. Y. (1997). Women and depression: An update on the report of the APA task force. *Sex Roles, 36,* 269–303.

Sterling, R. C., Gottheil, E., Weinstein, S. P., & Serota, R. (2001). The effect of therapist/patient race- and sex-matching in individual treatment. *Addiction, 96,* 1015–1022.

Strakowski, S. M., Flaum, M., Amador, X., Bracha, H. S., Pandurangi, A. K., Robinson, D., & Tohen, M. (1996). Racial differences in the diagnosis of psychosis. *Schizophrenia Bulletin, 21,* 117–124.

Strakowski, S. M., Lonczak, H. S., Sax, K. W., West, S. A., Crist, A., Mehta, R., & Thienhaus, O. J. (1995). The effects of race on diagnosis and disposition from a psychiatric emergency service. *Journal of Clinical Psychiatry, 56,* 101–107.

Strakowski, S. M., Shelton, R. C., & Kolbrener, M. L. (1993). The effects of race and comorbidity on clinical diagnosis in patients with psychosis. *Journal of Clinical Psychiatry, 54,* 96–102.

Sue, D. W., Capodilupo, C. M., & Holder, A. M. B. (2008). Racial microaggressions in the life experience of Black Americans. *Professional Psychology: Research and Practice, 39,* 329–336.

Sue, D. W., Capodilupo, C. M., Torino, G. C., Bucceri, J. M., Holder, A. M. B., Nadal, K., & Esquilin, M. (2007). Racial microaggressions in everyday life. *American Psychologist, 62,* 271–286.

Sue, S., & Chu, J. Y. (2003). The mental health of ethnic minority groups: Challenges posed by the supplement to the surgeon general's Report on Mental Health. *Culture, Medicine and Psychiatry, 27,* 447–465.

Sue, S., Fujino, D. C., Hu, L., Takeuchi, D. T., & Zane, N. W. (1991). Community mental health services for ethnic minorities: A test of the cultural responsiveness hypothesis. *Journal of Consulting and Clinical Psychology, 59,* 533–540.

Sue, S., & Zane, N. (2006). How well do both evidence-based practices and treatment as usual satisfactorily address the various dimensions of diversity? In J. C. Norcorss, L. E. Beutler, & R. F. Levant (Eds.), *Evidence-based practices in mental health* (pp. 329–337). Washington, DC: American Psychological Association.

Surko, M., Ciro, D., Blackwood, C., Nembhard, M., & Peake, K. (2005). Experience of racism as a correlate of developmental and health outcomes among urban adolescent mental health clients. In K. Peake (Ed.), *Clinical and research uses of an adolescent mental health intake questionnaire: What kids need to talk about* (pp. 235–260). Binghamton, NY: Haworth Social Work Practice Press.

Suveg, C., Hudson, J. L., Brewer, G., Flannery-Schroeder, E., Gosch, E., & Kendall, P. C. (2009). Cognitive-behavioral therapy for anxiety-disordered youth: Secondary outcomes from a randomized clinical trail evaluating child and family modalities. *Journal of Anxiety Disorders, 23,* 341–349.

Szymanski, S., Lieberman, J. A., Alvir, J. M., & Mayerhoff, D. (1995). Gender differences in onset of illness, treatment response, course and biologic indexes in first-episode schizophrenic patients. *American Journal of Psychiatry, 152,* 698–703.

Tamminga, C. A. (1997). Gender and schizophrenia. *Journal of Clinical Psychiatry, 58*(Suppl. 15), 33–37.

Triffleman, E. (2001). Gender differences in a controlled pilot study of psychosocial treatments in substance dependent patients with post-traumatic stress disorder: Design considerations and outcomes. *Alcoholism Treatment Quarterly, 18,* 113–126.

Tseng, W., McDermott, J. F., Ogino, D., & Ebata, K. (1982). Cross-cultural differences in parent-child assessment: U.S.A. and Japan. *International Journal of Social Psychiatry, 28,* 305–317.

U.S. Department of Health and Human Service (USDHHS). (1999). *Mental health: A report of the surgeon general.* Rockville, MD: Public Health Service, Office of the Surgeon General.

U.S. Department of Health and Human Service (USDHHS). (2001). *Mental health: Culture, race, and ethnicity—A supplement to mental health: A report of the surgeon general.* Rockville, MD: Public Health Service, Office of the Surgeon General.

Walker, L. E. A. (1994). Are personality disorders gender biased? In S. A. Kirk & S. D. Einbinder (Eds.), *Controversial issues in mental health* (pp. 22–29). New York: Allyn and Bacon.

Wang, P. S., Berglund, P., & Kessler, R. C. (2000). Recent care of common mental disorders in the United States. *Journal of General Internal Medicine, 15*, 284–292.

Wang, P. S., Berglund, P., Olfson, M., Pincus, H. A., Wells, K. B., & Kessler, R. C. (2005). Failure and delay in initial treatment contact after first onset of mental disorders in the National Comorbidity Survey Replication. *Archives of General Psychiatry, 62*, 603–613.

Wang, P. S., Lane, M., Olfson, M., Pincus, H. A., Wells, K. B., & Kessler, R. C. (2005). Twelve-month use of mental health services in the United States: Results from the National Comorbidity Survey Replication. *Archives of General Psychiatry, 62*, 629–640.

Warner, R. (1978). The diagnosis of antisocial and hysterical personality disorders. *Journal of Nervous and Mental Disease, 166*, 839–845.

Weisz, J. R., Doss, A. J., & Hawley, K. M. (2005). Youth psychotherapy outcome research: A review of critique of the evidence base. *Annual Review of Psychology, 56*, 337–363.

Weisz, J. R., Weiss, B., Han, S. S., Granger, D. A., & Morton, T. (1995). Effects of psychotherapy with children and adolescents revisited: A meta-analysis of treatment outcome studies. *Psychological Bulletin, 117*, 450–468.

Wells, K., Klap, R., Koike, A., & Sherbourne, C. (2001). Disparities in unmet need for alcoholism, drug abuse, and mental health care. *American Journal of Psychiatry, 158*, 2027–2032.

Widiger, T. A. (1998). Invited essay: Sex biases in the diagnoses of personality disorders. *Journal of Personality Disorders, 12*, 95–118.

Widiger, T. A., & Samuels, D. B. (2005). Evidence-based assessment of personality disorders. *Psychological Assessment, 17*, 278–287.

Wierzbicki, M., & Pekarik, G. (1993). A meta-analysis of psychotherapy dropout. *Professional Psychology: Research and Practice, 24*, 190–195.

Wilke, D. (1994). Women and alcoholism: How a male-as-norm bias affects research, assessment, and treatment. *Health and Social Work, 19*, 29–35.

Williams, J. B. W., & Spitzer, R. L. (1983). The issue of sex bias in DSM-III. Critique of a "A woman's view of DSM-III" by Marcie Kaplan. *American Psychologist, 38*, 793–798.

Woods, C. M., Oltmanns, T. F., & Turkheimer, E. (2008). Illustration of MIMIC-Model DIF testing with the Schedule for Nonadaptive and Adaptive Personality. *Journal of Psychopathology and Behavioral Assessment, 31*, 320–330.

Yoder, C. Y., Shute, G. E., & Tryban, G. M. (1990). Community recognition of objective and subjective characteristics of depression. *American Journal of Community Psychology, 18*, 547–566.

Yonkers, K. A., & Hamilton, J. A. (1995). Psychotropic medications. In J. M. Oldham & M. B. Riba (Eds.), *Review of psychiatry* (Vol. 14, pp. 307–332). Washington, DC: American Psychiatric Press.

Young, A. S., Klap, R., Sherbourne, C. D., & Wells, K. B. (2001). The quality of care for depressive and anxiety disorders in the United States. *Archives of General Psychiatry, 58*, 55–61.

Zane, N., Sue, S., Chang, J., Huang, L., Huang, J., Lowe, S., … Lee, E. (2005). Beyond ethnic match: Effects of client-therapist cognitive match in problem perception, coping orientation, and therapy goals on treatment outcomes. *Journal of Community Psychology, 33*, 569–585.

Zlotnick, C., Elkin, I., & Shea, M. T. (1998). Does the gender of a patient or the gender of a therapist affect the treatment of patients with major depression? *Journal of Consulting and Clinical Psychology, 66*, 655–659.

5
Classification and Diagnosis
Historical Development and Contemporary Issues

THOMAS A. WIDIGER

University of Kentucky
Lexington, Kentucky

Aberrant, dysfunctional, and maladaptive thinking, feeling, behaving, and relating are of substantial concern to many professions, the members of which will hold an equally diverse array of beliefs regarding etiology, pathology, and intervention. It is imperative that these individuals are able to communicate meaningfully with one another. The primary purpose of an official diagnostic nomenclature is to provide this common language of communication (Kendell, 1975; Sartorius et al., 1993).

Official diagnostic nomenclatures, however, can be exceedingly powerful, impacting significantly many important social, forensic, clinical, and other professional decisions (Schwartz & Wiggins, 2002). As individuals we think in terms of our language, and the predominant sources of "language" for psychopathology are the fourth edition and its text revision of the American Psychiatric Association's (1994, 2000) *Diagnostic and Statistical Manual of Mental Disorders* (*DSM*) and the 10th edition of the World Health Organization's (WHO) *International Classification of Diseases* (*ICD–10*; WHO, 1992). As such, these nomenclatures have a substantial impact on how clinicians, social agencies, and the general public conceptualize aberrant, problematic, and maladaptive behavior.

Interpreting *DSM–IV–TR* or *ICD–10* as conclusively validated nomenclatures, however, exaggerates the extent of their scientific support (Frances, Pincus, Widiger, Davis, & First, 1990). On the other hand, *DSM–IV–TR* and *ICD–10* are not lacking in credible or compelling empirical support. *DSM–IV–TR* and *ICD–10* contain many flaws, but they are also well-reasoned, scientifically researched, and, for the most part, well-documented nomenclatures that describe what is currently understood by most scientists, theorists, researchers, and clinicians to be the predominant forms of psychopathology (Widiger & Trull, 1993). This chapter presents an overview of the *DSM–IV–TR* diagnostic nomenclature, beginning with historical background, followed by a discussion of the major issues facing the forthcoming DSM–5 and future revisions.

Historical Background

The impetus for the development of an official diagnostic nomenclature was the crippling confusion generated by its absence (Widiger, 2001). "For a long time confusion reigned. Every self-respecting alienist [the 19th-century term for a psychiatrist], and certainly every professor, had his own classification" (Kendell, 1975, p. 87). The production of a new system for classifying psychopathology became a rite of passage in the 19th century for the young, aspiring professor.

> To produce a well-ordered classification almost seems to have become the unspoken ambition of every psychiatrist of industry and promise, as it is the ambition of a good tenor to strike a high C. This classificatory ambition was so conspicuous that the composer Berlioz

was prompted to remark that after their studies have been completed a rhetorician writes a tragedy and a psychiatrist a classification. (Zilboorg, 1941, p. 450)

In 1908 the U.S. Bureau of the Census asked the American Medico-Psychological Association (which subsequently altered its name in 1921 to the American Psychiatric Association) to develop a standard nosology to facilitate the obtainment of national statistics:

> The present condition with respect to the classification of mental diseases is chaotic. Some states use no well-defined classification. In others the classifications used are similar in many respects but differ enough to prevent accurate comparisons. Some states have adopted a uniform system, while others leave the matter entirely to the individual hospitals. This condition of affairs discredits the science. (Salmon, Copp, May, Abbot, & Cotton, 1917, pp. 255–256)

The American Medico-Psychological Association, in collaboration with the National Committee for Mental Hygiene, issued a nosology in 1918 titled *Statistical Manual for the Use of Institutions for the Insane* (Menninger, 1963). This nomenclature, however, failed to gain wide acceptance. It included only 22 diagnoses that were confined largely to psychoses with a presumably neurochemical pathology. "In the late twenties, each large teaching center employed a system of its own origination, no one of which met more than the immediate needs of the local institution" (American Psychiatric Association, 1952, p. v). A conference was held at the New York Academy of Medicine in 1928 to develop a more authoritative and uniformly accepted manual. The resulting nomenclature was modeled after the *Statistical Manual*, but it was distributed to hospitals within the American Medical Association's *Standard Classified Nomenclature of Disease*. Many hospitals used this system, but it eventually proved to be inadequate when the attention of the profession expanded well beyond psychotic disorders during World War II.

ICD–6 and DSM–I

The navy, army, and Veterans Administration developed their own, largely independent nomenclatures during World War II due in large part to the inadequacies of the *Standard Classified*. "Military psychiatrists, induction station psychiatrists, and Veterans Administration psychiatrists, found themselves operating within the limits of a nomenclature specifically not designed for 90% of the cases handled" (American Psychiatric Association, 1952, p. vi). The WHO accepted the authority in 1948 to produce the sixth edition of the *International Statistical Classification of Diseases, Injuries, and Causes of Death* (ICD–6). ICD–6 was the first to include a section devoted to mental disorders (Kendell, 1975), perhaps in recognition of the many psychological casualties of World War II, as well as the increasing impact and contribution of mental health professions within the broader society. The U.S. Public Health Service commissioned a committee, chaired by George Raines (with representatives from a variety of professions and public health agencies), to develop a variant of the mental disorders section of ICD–6 for use within the United States. The United States, as a member of the WHO, was obliged to use ICD–6, but adjustments could be made to maximize its acceptance and utility for the United States. The resulting nomenclature resembled closely the Veterans Administration system developed by Brigadier General William Menninger (brother to Karl Menninger; 1963). Responsibility for publishing and distributing this nosology was given to the American Psychiatric Association (1952) under the title *Diagnostic and Statistical Manual: Mental Disorders* (DSM–I).

DSM–I was generally successful in obtaining acceptance, due in large part to its expanded coverage, including somatoform disorders, stress reactions, and personality disorders. However, the New York State Department of Mental Hygiene, which had been influential in the development of the *Standard Nomenclature*, continued for some time to use its own classification.

DSM–I also included narrative descriptions of each disorder to facilitate understanding and more consistent applications. Nevertheless, fundamental criticisms regarding the reliability and validity of psychiatric diagnoses were also being raised (Zigler & Phillips, 1961). For example, a widely cited reliability study by Ward, Beck, Mendelson, Mock, and Erbaugh (1962) concluded that most of the poor agreement among psychiatrists' diagnoses was largely due to inadequacies of *DSM–I*.

ICD–6 was less successful. The "mental disorders section [of *ICD–6*] failed to gain [international] acceptance and eleven years later was found to be in official use only in Finland, New Zealand, Peru, Thailand, and the United Kingdom" (Kendell, 1975, p. 91). The WHO therefore commissioned a review by the English psychiatrist Erwin Stengel (1959), who reiterated the importance of establishing an official nomenclature.

> A … serious obstacle to progress in psychiatry is difficulty of communication. Everybody who has followed the literature and listened to discussions concerning mental illness soon discovers that psychiatrists, even those apparently sharing the same basic orientation, often do not speak the same language. They either use different terms for the same concepts, or the same term for different concepts, usually without being aware of it. It is sometimes argued that this is inevitable in the present state of psychiatric knowledge, but it is doubtful whether this is a valid excuse. (Stengel, 1959, p. 601)

Stengel attributed the failure of clinicians to accept the mental disorders section of *ICD–6* to the presence of theoretical biases, cynicism regarding any psychiatric diagnoses (some theoretical perspectives opposed the use of any diagnostic terms), and the presence of abstract, highly inferential diagnostic criteria that hindered consistent, uniform applications by different clinicians.

ICD–8 and DSM–II

ICD–6 had been revised to *ICD–7* in 1955, but there were no revisions to the mental disorders. Work began on *ICD–8* soon after Stengel's 1959 report. Considerable effort was made to develop a system that would be used by all of the member countries of the WHO. The final edition of *ICD–8* was approved by the WHO in 1966 and became effective in 1968. A companion glossary, in the spirit of Stengel's recommendations, was to be published conjointly, but work did not begin on the glossary until 1967 and it was not completed until 1972. "This delay greatly reduced [its] usefulness, and also [its] authority" (Kendell, 1975, p. 95). In 1965, the American Psychiatric Association appointed a committee, chaired by Ernest M. Gruenberg, to revise *DSM–I* to be compatible with *ICD–8* and yet also be suitable for use within the United States. The final version was approved in 1967, with publication in 1968.

The diagnosis of mental disorders, however, received substantial criticism during this time (Rosenhan, 1973; Szasz, 1961). A fundamental problem continued to be the absence of empirical support for the reliability, let alone the validity, of its diagnoses (Blashfield & Draguns, 1976). Researchers, however, took to heart the recommendations of Stengel (1959) by developing more specific and explicit criterion sets (Blashfield, 1984). The most influential of these efforts was produced by a group of neurobiologically oriented psychiatrists at Washington University in St. Louis. Their criterion sets generated so much interest that they were published separately in what has become one of the most widely cited papers in psychiatry (Feighner et al., 1972). Research has since indicated that mental disorders can be diagnosed reliably and do provide valid information regarding etiology, pathology, course, and treatment (Kendler, Munoz, & Murphy, 2010).

ICD–9 and DSM–III

By the time Feighner et al. (1972) was published, work was nearing completion on the ninth edition of the *ICD*. The authors of *ICD–9* had decided to include a glossary that would provide more precise descriptions of each disorder, but it was apparent that *ICD–9* would not include the more specific and explicit criterion sets used in research (Kendell, 1975). In 1974, the American Psychiatric Association appointed a task force, chaired by Robert Spitzer, to revise *DSM–II* in a manner that would be compatible with *ICD–9* but would also incorporate many of the current innovations in diagnosis. *DSM–III* was published in 1980 and was remarkably innovative, including (a) a multiaxial diagnostic system (most mental disorders were diagnosed on Axis I, personality and specific developmental disorders were diagnosed on Axis II, medical disorders on Axis III, psychosocial stressors on Axis IV, and level of functioning on Axis V), (b) specific and explicit criterion sets for all but one of the disorders (schizoaffective), (c) a substantially expanded text discussion of each disorder to facilitate diagnosis (e.g., age at onset, course, complications, sex ratio, and familial pattern), and (d) removal of terms (e.g., "neurosis") that appeared to favor a particular theoretical model for the disorder's etiology or pathology (Spitzer, Williams, & Skodol, 1980).

DSM–III–R

An ironic advantage of the specificity and explicitness of the *DSM–III* criterion sets was that a number of mistakes quickly became apparent (e.g., panic disorder in *DSM–III* could not be diagnosed in the presence of a major depression). "Criteria were not entirely clear, were inconsistent across categories, or were even contradictory" (American Psychiatric Association, 1987, p. xvii). Many of these errors and problems were due to the fact that there was insufficient research to guide the authors of the criterion sets. The American Psychiatric Association authorized the development of a revision to *DSM–III* to make corrections and refinements. Fundamental revisions were to be tabled until work began on *ICD-10*. However, it might have been unrealistic to expect the authors of *DSM–III–R* to confine their efforts to refinement and clarification, given the impact, success, and importance of *DSM–III*.

> The impact of DSM-III has been remarkable. Soon after its publication, it became widely accepted in the United States as the common language of mental health clinicians and researchers for communicating about the disorders for which they have professional responsibility. Recent major textbooks of psychiatry and other textbooks that discuss psychopathology have either made extensive reference to DSM-III or largely adopted its terminology and concepts. (American Psychiatric Association, 1987, p. xviii)

It was not difficult to find individuals who wanted to be involved in the development of *DSM–III–R*, and most who were (or were not) involved wanted to have a significant impact. More people were involved in making corrections to *DSM–III* than were used in its original construction and, not surprisingly, there were many proposals for major revisions and even new diagnoses. Four of the diagnoses approved for inclusion by the authors of *DSM–III–R* (i.e., sadistic personality disorder, self-defeating personality disorder, late luteal phase dysphoric disorder [the name for which was subsequently changed to premenstrual dysphoric disorder], and paraphiliac rapism) generated so much controversy that a special ad hoc committee was appointed by the board of trustees of the American Psychiatric Association to reconsider their inclusion. A concern common to all four was that their inclusion might result in harm to women. For example, paraphiliac rapism might be used to mitigate criminal responsibility for rape, and self-defeating personality disorder might be used to blame female victims for having been abused. Another concern was the lack of sufficient empirical support to address or offset these concerns. A compromise was eventually reached in which the two personality disorders and late luteal phase dysphoric disorder were included in an appendix (Endicott, 2000; Widiger, 1995); paraphiliac rapism was deleted entirely.

ICD–10 and DSM–IV

By the time work was completed on *DSM–III–R*, work had already begun on *ICD–10*. The decision of the authors of *DSM–III* to develop an alternative to *ICD–9* was instrumental in developing a highly innovative manual (Kendell, 1991; Spitzer et al., 1980). However, its innovations were also at the cost of decreasing compatibility with the *ICD–9* nomenclature that was used throughout the rest of the world, which is problematic to the stated purpose of providing a common language of communication. In 1988 the American Psychiatric Association appointed a *DSM–IV* task force, chaired by Allen Frances (Frances, Widiger, & Pincus, 1989). Mandates for *DSM–IV* included better coordination with *ICD–10* and improved documentation of empirical support.

The *DSM–IV* committee aspired to use a more conservative threshold for the inclusion of new diagnoses and to have decisions that were guided more explicitly by the scientific literature. Proposals for additions, deletions, or revisions were guided by 175 literature reviews that used a specific format that maximized the potential for critical review, containing, for example, a method section that documented explicitly the criteria for including and excluding studies and the process by which the literature had been reviewed (Frances et al., 1989). The reviews were published within a three-volume *DSM–IV Sourcebook* (Widiger et al., 1994). Testable questions that could be addressed with existing data sets were also explored in 36 studies, which emphasized the aggregation of multiple data sets from independent researchers, and 12 field trials were conducted to provide reliability and validity data on proposed revisions. The results of the 36 studies and 12 field trials were published in the fourth volume of the *DSM–IV Sourcebook* (Widiger et al., 1998). Critical reviews of these 223 projects were obtained by sending initial drafts to advisors or consultants to a respective work group, by presenting drafts at relevant conferences, and by submitting drafts to peer-reviewed journals (Widiger, Frances, Pincus, Davis, & First, 1991).

DSM–IV–TR

One of the innovations of *DSM–III* was the inclusion of a relatively detailed text discussion of each disorder, including information on age of onset, gender, course, and familial pattern (Spitzer et al., 1980). This text was expanded in *DSM–IV* to include cultural and ethnic group variation, variation across age, and laboratory and physical examination findings (Frances, First, & Pincus, 1995). Largely excluded from the text was information concerning etiology, pathology, and treatment, as this material was considered to be too theoretically specific and more suitable for academic texts. Nevertheless, it had also become apparent that *DSM–IV* was being used as a textbook, and the material on age, course, prevalence, and family history was quickly becoming outdated as new information was being gathered.

Therefore, in 1997, the American Psychiatric Association appointed a *DSM–IV* Text Revision Work Group, chaired by Michael First (editor of the text and criterion sets for *DSM–IV*) and Harold Pincus (vice-chair for *DSM–IV*) to update the text material. No substantive changes in the criterion sets were to be considered, nor were any new additions, subtypes, deletions, or other changes in the status of any diagnoses to be implemented. In addition, each of the proposed revisions to the text had to be supported by a systematic literature review that was critiqued by a considerable number of advisors. The *DSM–IV Text Revision* (*DSM–IV–TR*) was published by the American Psychiatric Association in 2000.

The outcome, however, was not entirely consistent with the original intentions. Revisions to the criterion sets for tic disorders and the paraphilias that involved a nonconsenting victim were actually implemented (First & Pincus, 2002), albeit no acknowledgment of these revisions were provided within the manual. In addition, no documentation of the scientific support for the text revisions was provided, due to the inconsistency in the quality of the effort. Rather than have inconsistent or inadequate documentation, it was decided to have none at all.

Continuing Issues for ICD-11 and DSM-5

Work is now well under way for DSM-5, chaired by David Kupfer and Darrel Regier, with an anticipated publication date of 2013. DSM-5 is likely to include a number of major revisions (Frances, 2009). The proposals were posted online on February 10, 2010 (see http://www.dsm5 .org.). Five issues for DSM-5 that will be discussed here are: (1) the empirical support for proposed revisions, (2) the definition of mental disorder, (3) the impact of culture and values, (4) the shift to a neurobiological model, and (5) the shift to a dimensional model.

Empirical Support

Frances et al. (1989) suggested that "the major innovation of DSM-IV will not be in its having surprising new content but rather will reside in the systematic and explicit method by which DSM-IV will be constructed and documented" (p. 375). Frances (2009), the chair of *DSM-IV*, has suggested that the authors of DSM-5 may have flipped this priority on its head, with emphasis now being given to surprising new content and inadequate attention to first conducting systematic, thorough, and balanced reviews to ensure that the proposals have adequate justification and empirical support. Concerns with respect to the process with which DSM-5 was being constructed were perhaps first raised by Robert Spitzer, chair of *DSM-III* and *DSM-III-R*, after having been denied access to the minutes of DSM-5 work group meetings (Decker, 2010). Frances and Spitzer eventually submitted a joint letter to the American Psychiatric Association Board of Trustees on July 7, 2009, expressing a variety of concerns with respect to the process with which DSM-5 was being constructed.

The chair and vice-chair of DSM-5 have stated that the development of DSM-5 is following the procedure used for *DSM-IV*, including literature reviews, data reanalyses, and field trials (Regier, Narrow, Kuhl, & Kupfer, 2010). However, the letter by Frances and Spitzer was initiated by the fact that the field trial for DSM-5 was about to begin before the proposals had received any critical review or even been revealed to the public for input and review. Frances followed this joint letter with additional letters of his own and a series of articles, which eventually led to the decision to postpone the field trial until after all of the proposals had been posted on a website, thereby allowing for at least some external review and public awareness (Decker, 2010). Frances, however, has continued to provide critical reviews through a blog affiliated with *Psychology Today* (Frances, 2010). His primary concern has continued to be that DSM-5 is likely to contain quite a few major revisions without adequate review of the empirical research, with little attention being given to potential costs and risks. The field trial, for instance, will not include any of the *DSM-IV-TR* criterion sets or external validators and will therefore be unable to provide information concerning a shift in the reliability or validity of the diagnostic manual resulting from a proposed revision.

Kendler, Kupfer, Narrow, Phillips, and Fawcett (2009) developed guidelines for DSM-5 work group members. These guidelines indicate that any change to the diagnostic manual should be accompanied by "a discussion of possible unintended negative effects of this proposed change, if it is made, and a consideration of arguments against making this change should also be included" (p. 2). Kendler et al. further stated that "the larger and more significant the change, the stronger should be the required level of support" (p. 2). Some of the DSM-5 literature reviews posted on the DSM-5 website do appear to meet the spirit of the Kendler et al. guidelines (e.g., see the review for the new diagnoses of temper dysregulation of childhood and hypersexual disorder; http://www.dsm5.org). However, others do not.

For example, one of the likely changes to the diagnostic manual will be the creation of a new class of addiction disorders that will subsume both the substance use disorders and pathological gambling and will allow for the diagnosis of additional behavioral addictions, such as Internet and shopping addiction. The posted literature review that provides the rationale and empirical support for this major revision consists of just two sentences indicating that pathological gambling has commonalities with substance dependence, followed by a list of references in which various commonalities can be gleaned (see http://www.dsm5.org). Only one of the articles listed actually directly addresses the question of whether pathological gambling is an addiction syndrome, and it is a review paper by Petry (2006) that is in opposition to the proposal. None of the concerns raised by Petry are addressed.

The DSM–5 personality disorders work group proposes to delete half of the 10 diagnoses, including narcissistic and dependent personality disorders. Kendler et al. (2009) indicated that any such decision should be supported by a literature review concerning the construct validity and clinical utility of the disorders to be deleted. However, no such review was actually conducted. The review that is posted on the website cites only a few studies, none of which concern the five diagnoses proposed for deletion (Skodol, 2010). Yet, there is in fact a considerable body of literature supporting the validity and utility of narcissism (Miller, Widiger, & Campbell, 2010; Ronningstam, 2011) and dependency (Bornstein, 2011). None of this literature has apparently been considered.

Definition of Mental Disorder

The boundaries of the diagnostic manual have been increasing with each edition, and there has long been vocal concern that much of this expansion represents an encroachment into normal problems of living (Caplan, 1995; Folette & Houts, 1996; Maddux, Gosselin, & Winstead, this volume). The coverage will increase substantially with DSM–5, with such new diagnoses as paraphilic coercive disorder, hypersexual disorder, temper dysregulation disorder of childhood, olfactory reference syndrome, hoarding disorder, skin picking disorder, premenstrual dysphoric disorder, pedohebephilic disorder, and binge eating disorder. Frances (2010) suggested that many of these additions represent a further encroachment into normal problems of living.

How the authors of a diagnostic manual can know when a behavior is the result of some form of psychopathology and should then be included within the diagnostic manual remains unclear. Box 5.1 provides the definition of mental disorder provided in *DSM–IV–TR*. This definition was the result of an effort by the authors of *DSM–III* to develop specific and explicit criteria for deciding whether a behavior pattern (homosexuality in particular) should be classified as a mental disorder (Spitzer & Williams, 1982). The intense controversy over homosexuality has largely abated, but the issues raised in this historical debate continue to apply.

For example, to be diagnosed with pedophilia, *DSM–III–R* required only that an adult have recurrent intense urges and fantasies involving sexual activity with a prepubescent child over a period of at least 6 months and have acted on them (or be markedly distressed by them). Every adult who engaged in a sexual activity with a child for longer than 6 months would meet these diagnostic criteria. The authors of *DSM–IV* were therefore concerned that *DSM–III–R* was not providing adequate guidance for determining when deviant sexual behavior is the result of a mental disorder. Presumably, some persons can engage in deviant, aberrant, and even heinous activities without being compelled to do so by the presence of psychopathology. The authors of *DSM–IV*, therefore, added the requirement that "the behavior, sexual urges, or fantasies cause clinically significant distress or impairment in social, occupational, or other important areas of functioning" (American Psychiatric Association, 1994, p. 523).

> ## BOX 5.1   AMERICAN PSYCHIATRIC ASSOCIATION (2000) DEFINITION OF MENTAL DISORDER
>
> In *DSM-IV*, each of the mental disorders is conceptualized as a clinically significant behavioral or psychological syndrome or pattern that occurs in an individual and that is associated with present distress (e.g., a painful symptom) or disability (i.e., impairment in one or more important areas of functioning) or with a significantly increased risk of suffering death, pain, disability, or an important loss of freedom. In addition, this syndrome or pattern must not be merely an expectable and culturally sanctioned response to a particular event, for example, the death of a loved one. Whatever its original cause, it must currently be considered a manifestation of a behavioral, psychological, or biological dysfunction in the individual. Neither deviant behavior (e.g., political, religious, or sexual) nor conflicts that are primarily between the individual and society are mental disorders unless the deviance or conflict is a symptom of a dysfunction in the individual, as described above. (American Psychiatric Association, 2000, p. xxxi)

Spitzer and Wakefield (1999), however, argued that the impairment criteria included in *DSM-IV* were inadequate. They concurred with a concern raised by the National Law Center for Children and Families that *DSM-IV* might contribute to a normalization of pedophilic and other paraphilic behavior by allowing the diagnoses not to be applied if those who have engaged in these acts are not themselves distressed by their behavior or do not otherwise experience impairment. In response, Frances et al. (1995) argued that pedophilic sexual "behaviors are inherently problematic because they involve a nonconsenting person (exhibitionism, voyeurism, frotteurism) or a child (pedophilia) and may lead to arrest and incarceration" (p. 319). Therefore, any person who engaged in an illegal sexual act (for longer than 6 months) would be exhibiting a clinically significant social impairment and would therefore meet the *DSM-IV* threshold for diagnosis. However, one should not use the illegality of an act to determine when an illegal act is a disorder. This undermines the rationale for the inclusion of the impairment criterion to distinguish immoral or illegal acts from abnormal or disordered acts, and it is inconsistent with the definition of a mental disorder that states that neither deviance nor conflicts with the law are sufficient to warrant a diagnosis (see Box 5.1).

The diagnostic criteria for pedophilia were revised in *DSM-IV-TR* to return to what was provided in *DSM-III-R* to avoid the misunderstanding that a denial of distress or impairment would mean that the behavior is considered normal (First & Pincus, 2002). However, the *DSM-IV-TR* criteria again state that simply the presence of the behavior for longer than 6 months indicates the presence of the disorder, thereby providing no meaningful distinction between pedophilic behavior that is willful and volitional from pedophilic behavior that is driven by some form of organismic pathology (First & Frances, 2008). The threshold proposed for DSM–5 is the occurrence of the behavior with at least two children (if both are prepubescent) or three or more (if one is pubescent), or a preference for pedophilic pornography over other forms of pornography (see http://www.dsm5.org). The rationale for these specific requirements is not provided, but it is evident that the intention is to increase the threshold for the diagnosis by requiring more than one partner (albeit a preference for pedophilic pornography will not require any actual pedophilic acts for the diagnosis to be made).

Spitzer and Wakefield (1999) suggested that the distinction between disordered and nondisordered abuse of children should require an assessment for the presence of an underlying, internal pathology (e.g., irrational cognitive schema or neurochemical dysregulation). Wakefield and colleagues have provided examples of other criterion sets from *DSM–IV–TR* that are less politically or socially controversial than pedophilia, which they suggest also fail to make a necessary distinction between maladaptive problems in living and true psychopathology due to the reliance within the criterion sets on indicators of distress or impairment rather than references to pathology (Wakefield & First, 2003). For example, the *DSM–IV–TR* criterion set for major depressive disorder currently excludes most instances of depressive reactions to the loss of a loved one (i.e., uncomplicated bereavement). Depression after the loss of a loved one can be considered a mental disorder though if "the symptoms persist for longer than two months" (American Psychiatric Association, 1994, p. 327). Allowing 2 months to grieve before one is diagnosed with a major depressive disorder might be as arbitrary and meaningless as allowing a person to engage in a sexually deviant act only for 6 months before the behavior is diagnosed as a paraphilia (it is being proposed for DSM–5 to allow just 2 weeks to grieve; see http://www .dsm5.org).

The inclusion of pathology within diagnostic criterion sets (e.g., irrational cognitive schemas, unconscious defense mechanisms, or neurochemical dysregulation) would be consistent with the definition of mental disorder provided in *DSM–IV–TR*, which states that the syndrome "must currently be considered a manifestation of a behavioral, psychological, or biological dysfunction in the individual" (American Psychiatric Association, 2000, p. xxxi; see Box 5.1). However, a limitation of this proposal is that there is currently little agreement over the specific pathology that underlies any particular disorder. There is insufficient empirical support to give preference to one particular cognitive, interpersonal, neurochemical, psychodynamic, or other theoretical model of pathology. The precise nature of this pathology could be left undefined or characterized simply as an "internal dysfunction" (Wakefield, Pottick, & Kirk, 2002), but an assessment of an unspecified pathology is unlikely to be reliable. Clinicians will have very different opinions concerning the nature of the internal dysfunction and quite different thresholds for its attribution.

Alternatively, perhaps the assumption that the expansion of the nomenclature is subsuming normal problems in living is itself questionable. Those who are critical of the nomenclature have decried the substantial expansion of the diagnostic manual since the 1960s (e.g., Follette & Houts, 1996; Kirk, 2005). However, it might have been more surprising to find that scientific research and increased knowledge have failed to lead to the recognition of more instances of psychopathology (Wakefield, 1998, 2001). Perhaps the assumption that only a small minority of the population currently has, or will ever have, a mental disorder (Regier & Narrow, 2002) is also questionable. Very few individuals fail to have at least some physical disorders, and all individuals suffer from quite a few physical disorders throughout their lifetimes. It is unclear why it should be different for mental disorders, as if most have been fortunate to have obtained no problematic genetic dispositions or vulnerabilities and have never sustained any psychological injuries or never experienced significant economic, environmental, or interpersonal stress, pressure, or conflict that would tax or strain psychological functioning.

Optimal psychological functioning, as in the case of optimal physical functioning, might represent an ideal that is achieved by only a small minority of the population. The rejection of a high prevalence rate of psychopathology may reflect the best of intentions, such as concerns regarding the stigmatization of mental disorder diagnoses (Kirk, 2005) or the potential impact on funding for treatment (Regier & Narrow, 2002), but these social and political concerns could also hinder a more dispassionate and accurate recognition of the true rate of a broad range of psychopathology within the population (Widiger & Sankis, 2000).

Wakefield (1992) developed an alternative "harmful dysfunction" definition of mental disorder where dysfunction is a failure of an internal mechanism to perform a naturally selected function (e.g., the capacity to experience feelings of guilt in a person with antisocial personality disorder) and harm is a value judgment that the design failure is harmful to the individual (e.g., failure to learn from mistakes results in repeated punishments, arrests, loss of employment, and eventual impoverishment). Wakefield's model has received substantial attention and was being considered for inclusion in DSM–5 (Rounsaville et al., 2002). However, Wakefield's proposal has also received quite a bit of critical review (e.g., Bergner, 1997; Kirmayer & Young, 1999; Lilienfeld & Marino, 1999; Widiger & Sankis, 2000). A fundamental limitation is its reliance on evolutionary theory, thereby limiting its relevance and usefulness to alternative models of etiology and pathology (Bergner, 1997). Wakefield's model might even be inconsistent with some sociobiological models of psychopathology. Cultural evolution may at times outstrip the pace of biological evolution, rendering some designed functions that were originally adaptive within earlier time periods maladaptive in many current environments (Lilienfeld & Marino, 1999; Widiger & Sankis, 2000). For example, "the existence in humans of a preparedness mechanism for developing a fear of snakes may be a relic not well designed to deal with urban living, which currently contains hostile forces far more dangerous to human survival (e.g., cars, electrical outlets) but for which humans lack evolved mechanisms of fear preparedness" (Buss, Haselton, Shackelford, Bleske, & Wakefield, 1998, p. 538).

Missing from Wakefield's (1992) definition of mental disorder and the definition likely to be included in DSM 5 (Stein et al., 2010) is any reference to dyscontrol. Mental disorders are perhaps best understood as dyscontrolled impairments in psychological functioning (Kirmayer & Young, 1999; Klein, 1999; Widiger & Trull, 1991). "Involuntary impairment remains the key inference" (Klein, 1999, p. 424). Dyscontrol is one of the fundamental features of mental disorder emphasized in Bergner's (1997) "significant restriction" and Widiger and Sankis's (2000) "dyscontrolled maladaptivity" definitions of mental disorder. Including the concept of dyscontrol within a definition of mental disorder would provide a fundamental distinction between mental and physical disorder, as dyscontrol is not a meaningful consideration for a physical disorder.

Fundamental to the concept of a mental disorder is the presence of impairments secondary to feelings, thoughts, or behaviors over which a normal (healthy) person has adequate self-control to alter or adjust to avoid these impairments, if he or she wishes to do so. To the extent that a person willfully, intentionally, freely, or voluntarily engages in harmful sexual acts, drug usage, gambling, or child abuse, the person would not be considered to have a mental disorder. Those who seek professional intervention do so in large part to obtain the insights, techniques, skills, or other tools (e.g., medications) that would increase their ability to better control their mood, thoughts, or behavior.

Dyscontrol as a component of a mental disorder does not imply that a normal person has free will, a concept that is, at best, difficult to scientifically or empirically verify (Bargh & Ferguson, 2000; Howard & Conway, 1986). A person with a mental disorder could be comparable to a computer lacking in the necessary software to combat particular viruses or execute effective programs. Pharmacotherapy alters the neural connections of the central nervous system (the hardware), whereas psychotherapy alters the cognitions (the software) in a manner that increases a person's behavioral repertoire, allowing the person to act and respond more effectively. A computer installed with new software has not been provided free will, rather it has been provided with more options to act and respond more effectively.

Culture and Values

It was the intention of the authors of *ICD–10* to provide a universal diagnostic system, but diagnostic criteria and constructs can have quite different implications and meanings across different cultures. *DSM–IV–TR* addresses cultural issues in three ways. First, the text of *DSM–IV–TR* provides a discussion of how each disorder is known to vary in its presentation across different cultures. Second, an appendix of "culture-bound" syndromes describes disorders that are currently thought to be specific to a particular culture. Third, an additional appendix provides a culturally informed diagnostic formulation that considers the cultural identity of the individual and the culture-specific explanations of the person's presenting complaints (Lim, 2006). Because there is no discussion of cross-cultural issues on the DSM–5 website, it is unclear what revisions, if any, will occur in this area.

There is both a strong and a weak cross-cultural critique of current scientific understanding of psychopathology. The weak critique does not question the validity of a concept of mental disorder but does argue that social and cultural processes affect and potentially bias the

> science of psychopathology and diagnosis: a) by determining the selection of persons and behaviors as suitable material for analysis; b) by emphasizing what aspects of this material will be handled as relevant from a [clinical] standpoint; c) by shaping the language of diagnosis, including that of descriptive psychopathology; d) by masking the symptoms of any putative "universal" disorder; e) by biasing the observer and would-be diagnostician; and f) by determining the goals and endpoints of treatment. (Fabrega, 1994, p. 262)

These concerns are not weak in the sense that they are trivial or inconsequential, but they do not dispute the fundamental validity of a concept of mental disorder or the science of psychopathology. The strong critique, in contrast, is that the construct of mental disorder is itself a culture-bound belief that reflects the local biases of Western society, and that the science of psychopathology is valid only in the sense that it is an accepted belief system of a particular culture (Lewis-Fernandez & Kleinman, 1995; López & Guarnaccia, this volume).

The concept of mental disorder does include a value judgment that there should be necessary, adequate, or optimal psychological functioning (Wakefield, 1992). However, this value judgment is also a fundamental component of the construct of physical disorder (Widiger, 2002). In a world in which there were no impairments or threats to physical functioning, the construct of a physical disorder would have no meaning except as an interesting thought experiment. Meaningful and valid scientific research on the etiology, pathology, and treatment of physical disorders occurs because, in the world as it currently exists, there are impairments and threats to physical functioning. It is provocative and intriguing to conceive of a world in which physical health and survival would or should not be valued or preferred over illness, suffering, and death, but this form of existence is unlikely to emerge anytime in the near future. Placing a value on adequate or optimal physical functioning might be a natural result of evolution within a world in which there are threats to functioning and survival. Likewise, in the world as it currently exists, there are impairments and threats to adequate psychological functioning. It is also provocative and intriguing to conceive of a society (or world) in which psychological health would or should not be valued or preferred, but this form of existence is also unlikely to emerge anytime in the near future. Placing a value on adequate, necessary, or optimal psychological functioning might be inherent to and a natural result of existing in our world. Any particular definition of what would constitute adequate, necessary, or optimal psychological functioning would likely be biased to some extent by local cultural values, but this is perhaps best understood as only the failing of one particular conceptualization of mental disorder (i.e., a weak rather than a strong critique). Valuing adequate, necessary, or optimal psychological functioning could itself still be a logical and natural result of existing in a world in which there are threats to psychological functioning, just as placing a value on adequate, necessary, or optimal physical functioning would be a logical and natural result of existing in a world in which there are threats to physical functioning (Widiger, 2002).

Different societies, cultures, and even persons within a particular culture will disagree as to what constitutes optimal or pathological biological and psychological functioning (López & Guarnaccia, 2000; Sadler, 2005). An important and difficult issue is how best to understand the differences between cultures with respect to what constitutes dysfunction and pathology (Alarcon et al., 2002). For example, simply because diagnostic criterion sets are applied reliably across different cultures does not necessarily indicate that the constructs themselves are valid or meaningful within these cultures (Lewis-Fernandez & Kleinman, 1995). A reliably diagnosed criterion set can be developed for an entirely illusory diagnostic construct. Lewis-Fernandez and Kleinman (1995) argued that it is necessary "to produce a comprehensive nosology that is both internationally and locally valid" (p. 435).

Nevertheless, it is unclear why it should be necessary for the establishment of a disorder's construct validity to obtain cross-cultural (i.e., universal) acceptance. A universally accepted diagnostic system will have an international social utility and consensus validity (Kessler, 1999), but it is also apparent that belief systems vary in their veridicality. Recognition of and appreciation for alternative belief systems are important for adequate functioning within an international community, but respect for alternative belief systems does not necessarily imply that all belief systems are equally valid (Widiger, 2002).

Kirmayer, Young, and Hayton (1995) illustrated well many of the complexities of cross-cultural research. For example, a woman's housebound behavior might be diagnosed as agoraphobic within Western cultures but considered normative (or even virtuous) within a Muslim culture; submissive behavior that is diagnosed as pathologic dependency within Western societies might be considered normative within the Japanese culture. However, simply because a behavior pattern is valued, accepted, encouraged, or even statistically normative within a particular culture does not necessarily mean it is conducive to healthy psychological functioning.

> In societies where ritual plays an important role in religious life ... such societies may predispose individuals to obsessive-compulsive symptoms and mask the disorder when present.... The congruence between religious belief and practice and obsessive-compulsive symptoms also probably contributes to relatively low rates of insight into the irrationality of the symptoms. (Kirmayer et al., 1995, pp. 507, 508)

On the other hand, it is equally important not to assume that what is believed to be associated with maladaptive (or adaptive) functioning in one culture should also be considered to be maladaptive (or adaptive) within all other cultures (Alarcon et al., 2002). "This possible tension between cultural styles and health consequences is in urgent need of further research" (Kirmayer et al., 1995, p. 517), and it is important for this research to go beyond simply identifying differences in behaviors, belief systems, and values across different cultures. This research also needs to address the fundamental question of whether differences in beliefs actually question the validity of any universal conceptualization of psychopathology or suggest instead simply different perspectives on a common, universal issue (see Maddux, Gosselin, & Winstead, this volume).

Shifting to a Neurobiological Model

The authors of *DSM–III* removed terms (e.g., neurosis) that appeared to refer explicitly to psychodynamic constructs to have the manual be atheoretical, or at least be reasonably neutral with respect to alternative models of psychopathology (Spitzer et al., 1980). However, it appears that all theoretical perspectives have found the language of *DSM–IV–TR* to be less than optimal for their own particular perspective. Interpersonal and systems theoretical perspectives, which consider dysfunctional behavior to be due to a pathology of a wider social system rather than simply within the individual, consider the organismic diagnoses of *DSM–IV–TR* to be fundamentally antithetical (Reiss & Emde, 2003). Psychodynamically oriented clinicians bemoan the fact that as the succeeding editions of the manual have become increasingly objective, descriptive, and atheoretical, they have inevitably minimized the subjective and inferential aspects of diagnosis on which most psychodynamically oriented clinicians depend, leading to the development of their own diagnostic manual, the *Psychodynamic Diagnostic Manual* (PDM Task Force, 2006). Behaviorists argue that the organismic perspective of *DSM–IV* is inconsistent with the situational context of dysfunctional behavior (Folette & Houts, 1996). Even those in neurobiologically oriented psychiatry are unhappy. "Although there is a large body of research that indicates that a neurobiological basis for most mental disorders, the DSM definitions are virtually devoid of biology" (Charney et al., 2002, pp. 31–32).

DSM–I favored a psychodynamic perspective (American Psychiatric Association, 1952; Spitzer et al., 1980). In striking contrast, the American Psychiatric Association and the National Institute of Mental Health (NIMH) are shifting explicitly toward a neurobiological orientation. For example, a reading of the table of contents of any issue of the two leading journals of psychiatry (i.e., *American Journal of Psychiatry* and *Archives of General Psychiatry*) will evidence a strong neurobiological orientation. *DSM–IV* included a new section of the text devoted to laboratory and physical examination findings (Frances et al., 1989). All of the laboratory tests included therein are concerned with neurobiological findings, with no reference to any laboratory test that would be of particular relevance to a cognitive, psychodynamic, or interpersonal-systems clinician. The definition of mental disorder in DSM–5 will refer to a "psychobiological dysfunction" in recognition that mental disorders ultimately reflect a dysfunction of the brain (Stein et al., 2010). The head of the NIMH has indicated that priority for funding in the future will be given to studies that formally adopt a "clinical neuroscience" perspective that contributes to an understanding of mental disorders as "developmental brain disorders" (Insel, 2009, p. 132). This is being accomplished in part through the development of research domain criteria (RDoC) that will represent a biological alternative to DSM–5, "with a strong focus on biological processes, and emphasis on neural circuits" (Sanislow et al., 2010, p. 633). "The RDoC framework conceptualizes mental illnesses as brain disorders" (Garvey et al., 2010, p. 749). As indicated by Miller (2010), "over the next 2 to 3 years, NIMH will encourage researchers to shift from using DSM criteria in their grant proposals to using the RDoC categories" (p. 1437), such as fear circuitry disorder.

It is unlikely that one could create a diagnostic manual that is entirely neutral or atheoretical. In fact, if a diagnostic manual is to be guided by the existing empirical support (Frances et al., 1989), the manual would inevitably favor the theoretical perspective that has obtained the greatest empirical support. However, the diagnostic manual should probably continue to at least attempt to remain above the competitive fray rather than embrace any particular team, including the one that currently has the most points. The *DSM* is used by clinicians and researchers from a wide variety of theoretical perspectives, including (but not limited to) neurobiological, psychodynamic, interpersonal, cognitive, behavioral, humanistic, systems, and feminist (Widiger & Mullins-Sweatt, 2008). An important function of the manual is to provide a common means for communication among and research concerning these competing theoretical orientations in a language that would not favor one perspective over the other (Frances et al., 1989). A language that purposely favors one particular perspective would not provide an equal playing field and would have an insidiously subtle, cumulative effect on the subsequent scientific research and discourse (Wakefield, 1998). It might be impossible to construct a diagnostic manual that is truly theoretically neutral, but this is not a compelling reason for abandoning the effort, particularly if the manual is to be used for research attempting to determine the validity of alternative theoretical perspectives.

Shifting to a Dimensional Model of Classification

"DSM-IV-TR is a categorical classification that divides mental disorders into types based on criterion sets with defining features" (American Psychiatric Association, 2000, p. xxxi). This categorical classification is consistent with the medical tradition in which it is believed (and often confirmed in other areas of medicine) that individual disorders have specific etiologies, pathologies, and treatments (Zachar & Kendler, 2007). The intention of the diagnostic manual is to help the clinician determine which particular disorder is present, the diagnosis of which would indicate the presence of a specific pathology that would explain the occurrence of the symptoms and suggest a specific treatment that would ameliorate the patient's suffering (Frances et al., 1995; Kendell, 1975).

It is evident, however, that *DSM–IV–TR* routinely fails in guiding a clinician to the identification of one specific disorder. Despite the best efforts of the authors of each revision to the diagnostic manual to revise the criterion sets to increase their specificity, multiple diagnoses are the norm (Widiger & Clark, 2000). As expressed by the vice-chair of DSM–5, "the failure of DSM-III criteria to specifically define individuals with only one disorder served as an alert that the strict neo-Kraepelinian categorical approach to mental disorder diagnoses advocated by Robins and Guze (1970), Spitzer, Endicott, and Robins (1978), and others could have some serious problems" (Regier, 2008, p. xxi). As expressed by Kupfer, First, and Regier (two of whom are the chair and vice-chair of DSM–5):

> In the more than 30 years since the introduction of the Feighner criteria by Robins and Guze, which eventually led to DSM-III, the goal of validating these syndromes and discovering common etiologies has remained elusive. Despite many proposed candidates, not one laboratory marker has been found to be specific in identifying any of the DSM-defined syndromes. Epidemiologic and clinical studies have shown extremely high rates of comorbidities among the disorders, undermining the hypothesis that the syndromes represent distinct etiologies. Furthermore, epidemiologic studies have shown a high degree of short-term diagnostic instability for many disorders. With regard to treatment, lack of treatment specificity is the rule rather than the exception. (Kupfer, First, & Regier, 2002, p. xviii)

Most (if not all) mental disorders appear to be the result of a complex interaction of an array of interacting biological vulnerabilities and dispositions with a number of significant environmental, psychosocial events that often exert their progressive effects over a developing period of time (Rutter, 2003). The symptoms and pathologies of mental disorders appear to be highly responsive to a wide variety of neurobiological, interpersonal, cognitive, and other mediating and moderating variables that develop, shape, and form a particular individual's psychopathology profile. This complex etiological history and individual psychopathology profile are unlikely to be well described by single diagnostic categories that attempt to make distinctions at nonexistent discrete joints along the continuous distributions (Widiger & Samuel, 2005).

The categorical model of classification is failing in many ways, including an absence of a provision of reliably distinct boundaries, an absence of a credible rationale for diagnostic thresholds, inadequate coverage of existing clinical populations, and the absence of specific etiologies and treatments (Kupfer et al., 2002; Widiger & Trull, 2007). In 1999, a DSM–5 Research Planning Conference was held under joint sponsorship of the American Psychiatric Association and the NIMH, the purpose of which was to set research priorities that would optimally inform future classifications. An impetus for this effort was the frustration with the existing nomenclature (Kupfer et al., 2002). At this conference, research planning work groups were formed to develop white papers that would set a research agenda for DSM–5. The nomenclature work group, charged with addressing fundamental assumptions of the diagnostic system, concluded that it is "important that consideration be given to advantages and disadvantages of basing part or all of DSM-V on dimensions rather than categories" (Rounsaville et al., 2002, p. 12).

The white papers developed by the research planning work groups were followed by a series of international conferences whose purpose was to enrich further the empirical database in preparation for the eventual development of DSM–5. (A description of this conference series can be found at http://www.dsm5.org.) The first conference was devoted to shifting personality disorders to a dimensional model of classification (Widiger, Simonsen, Krueger, Livesley, & Verheul, 2005). The chapter by Presnall and Widiger (this volume) discusses the dimensional model of personality disorder proposed for DSM–5. The final conference was devoted to dimensional approaches across the diagnostic manual, including substance use disorders, major depressive disorder, psychoses, anxiety disorders, and developmental psychopathology, as well as the personality disorders (Helzer, Kraemer et al., 2008).

Work on DSM–5 is now well under way, and it is evident that a primary goal is to shift the manual toward a dimensional classification (Helzer, Wittchen, Krueger, & Kraemer, 2008; Regier et al., 2010). Nevertheless, the shifts likely to be taken in DSM–5 will neither be fundamental nor significant. "What is being proposed for DSM–V is not to substitute dimensional scales for categorical diagnoses, but to add a dimensional option to the usual categorical diagnoses for DSM–V" (Kraemer, 2008, p. 9).

As acknowledged by Helzer, Kraemer, and Krueger (2006), "our proposal not only preserves categorical definitions but also does not alter the process by which these definitions would be developed. Those charged with developing criteria for specific mental disorders would operate just as their predecessors have" (p. 1675). Dimensional proposals for DSM–5 are only to develop "supplementary dimensional approaches to the categorical definitions that would also relate back to the categorical definitions" (Helzer, Wittchen et al., 2008, p. 116). These dimensions will only serve as ancillary descriptions that will lack any official representation within a patient's medical record (i.e., they will have no official alphanumerical code and may then not even be communicated to any public health care agency). In sum, "what is being proposed for DSM–V is not to substitute dimensional scales for categorical diagnoses, but to add a dimensional option to the usual categorical diagnoses for DSM–V" (Kraemer, 2008, p. 9). In the end, DSM–5 will remain a categorical diagnostic system.

Conclusions

Nobody is fully satisfied with, or lacks valid criticisms of, *DSM–IV–TR*. This is unlikely to change with DSM–5. Zilboorg's (1941) suggestion that budding 19th-century theorists and researchers cut their first teeth by providing a new classification of mental disorders still applies, although the rite of passage today is to provide a critique of the *DSM*.

Nobody, however, appears to suggest that all official diagnostic nomenclatures be abandoned. The benefits do appear to outweigh the costs (Salmon et al., 1917; Stengel, 1959). Everybody finds fault with this language, but there is at least the ability to communicate disagreement. Communication among researchers, theorists, and clinicians would be much worse in the absence of this common language.

Nevertheless, as an official diagnostic nomenclature *DSM–IV–TR* is an exceedingly powerful document with a considerable impact on how psychopathology is not only diagnosed but also understood and treated. Persons think in terms of their language, and DSM–5 will govern the manner in which clinicians think about psychopathology for many years to come, for better or for worse.

References

Alarcon, R. D., Bell, C. C., Kirmayer, L., Lin, K-H, Ustun, B., & Wisner, K. (2002). Beyond the fun-house mirrors: Research agenda on culture and psychiatric diagnosis. In D. J. Kupfer, M. B. First, & D. A. Regier (Eds.), *A research agenda for DSM-V* (pp. 219–281). Washington, DC: American Psychiatric Association.

American Psychiatric Association. (1952). *Diagnostic and statistical manual: Mental disorders.* Washington, DC: Author.

American Psychiatric Association. (1968). *Diagnostic and statistical manual of mental disorders* (2nd ed.). Washington, DC: Author.

American Psychiatric Association. (1980). *Diagnostic and statistical manual of mental disorders* (3rd ed.). Washington, DC: Author.

American Psychiatric Association. (1987). *Diagnostic and statistical manual of mental disorders* (3rd ed., rev. ed.). Washington, DC: Author.

American Psychiatric Association. (1994). *Diagnostic and statistical manual of mental disorders* (4th ed.). Washington, DC: Author.

American Psychiatric Association. (2000). *Diagnostic and statistical manual of mental disorders* (4th ed., rev. ed.). Washington, DC: Author.

Bargh, J. A., & Ferguson, M. J. (2000). Beyond behaviorism: On the automaticity of higher mental processes. *Psychological Bulletin, 126,* 925–945.

Bergner, R. M. (1997). What is psychopathology? And so what? *Clinical Psychology: Science and Practice, 4,* 235–248.

Blashfield, R. K. (1984). *The classification of psychopathology. Neo-Kraepelinian and quantitative approaches.* New York: Plenum.

Blashfield, R. K., & Draguns, J. G. (1976). Evaluative criteria for psychiatric classification. *Journal of Abnormal Psychology, 85,* 140–150.

Bornstein, R. F. (2011). Reconceptualizing personality pathology in DSM-5: Limitations in evidence for eliminating DSM-IV syndromes. *Journal of Personality Disorders, 25*(2), 235–247.

Buss, D. M., Haselton, M. G., Shackelford, T. K., Bleske, A. L., & Wakefield, J. C. (1998). Adaptations, exaptations, and spandrels. *American Psychologist, 53,* 533–548.

Caplan, P. J. (1995). *They say you're crazy: How the world's most powerful psychiatrists decide who's normal.* Reading, MA: Addison-Wesley.

Charney, D. S., Barlow, D. H., Botteron, K., Cohen, J. D., Goldman, D., Gur, R. E., … Zaleman, S. J. (2002). Neuroscience research agenda to guide development of a pathophysiologically based classification system. In D. J. Kupfer, M. B. First, & D. A. Regier (Eds.), *A research agenda for DSM-V* (pp. 31–84). Washington, DC: American Psychiatric Association.

Decker, H. S. (2010). *A moment of crisis in the history of American psychiatry.* Retrieved from http://historypsychiatry.wordpress.com/2010/04/27/a-moment-of-crisis-in-the-history-of-american-psychiatry

Endicott, J. (2000). History, evolution, and diagnosis of premenstrual dysphoric disorder. *Journal of Clinical Psychiatry, 62*(Suppl. 24), 5–8.

Fabrega, H. (1994). International systems of diagnosis in psychiatry. *Journal of Nervous and Mental Disease, 182,* 256–263.

Feighner, J. P., Robins, E., Guze, S. B., Woodruff, R. A., Winokur, G., & Munoz, R. (1972). Diagnostic criteria for use in psychiatric research. *Archives of General Psychiatry, 26,* 57–63.

First, M. B., & Frances, A. J. (2008). Issues for DSM-V: Unintended consequences of small changes: the case of paraphilias. *American Journal of Psychiatry, 165,* 1240–1241.

First, M. B., & Pincus, H. A. (2002). The DSM-IV Text Revision: Rationale and potential impact on clinical practice. *Psychiatric Services, 53,* 288–292.

Folette, W. C., & Houts, A. C. (1996). Models of scientific progress and the role of theory in taxonomy development: A case study of the DSM. *Journal of Consulting and Clinical Psychology, 64,* 1120–1132.

Frances, A. J. (2009, June 26). A warning sign on the road to DSM-V: Beware of its unintended consequences. *Psychiatric Times, 26*(8), 1–4.

Frances, A. J. (2010, April 13). *The missing risk/benefit analyses for DSM-5.* Retrieved from http://www.psychologytoday.com/blog/dsm5-in-distress/201004/the-missing-riskbenefit-analyses-dsm5

Frances, A. J., First, M. B., & Pincus, H. A. (1995). *DSM-IV guidebook.* Washington, DC: American Psychiatric Press.

Frances, A. J., Pincus, H. A., Widiger, T. A., Davis, W. W., & First, M. B. (1990). DSM-IV: work in progress. *American Journal of Psychiatry, 147,* 1439–1448.

Frances, A. J., Widiger, T. A., & Pincus, H. A. (1989). The development of DSM-IV. *Archives of General Psychiatry, 46,* 373–375.

Garvey, M., Heinssein, R., Pine, D. S., Quinn, K., Sanislow, C., & Wang, P. (2010). Research domain criteria (RDoc); toward a new classification framework for research on mental disorders. *American Journal of Psychiatry, 167,* 748–751.

Helzer, J. E., Kraemer, H. C, & Krueger, R. F. (2006). The feasibility and need for dimensional psychiatric diagnoses. *Psychological Medicine, 36*, 1671–1680.

Helzer, J. E., Kraemer, H. C., Krueger, R. F., Wittchen, H-U., Sirovatka, P. J., & Regier, D. A. (Eds.). (2008). *Dimensional approaches in diagnostic classification*. Washington, DC: American Psychiatric Association.

Helzer, J. E., Wittchen, H-U., Krueger, R. F., & Kraemer, H. C. (2008). Dimensional options for DSM-V: the way forward. In J. E. Helzer, H. C. Kraemer, R. F. Krueger, H-U. Wittchen, P. J. Sirovatka, & D. A. Regier (Eds.), *Dimensional approaches to diagnostic classification. Refining the research agenda for DSM-V* (pp. 115–127). Washington, DC: American Psychiatric Association.

Howard, G. S., & Conway, C. G. (1986). Can there be an empirical science of volitional action? *American Psychologist, 41*, 1241–1251.

Insel, T. R. (2009). Translating scientific opportunity into public health impact. A strategic plan for research on mental illness. *Archives of General Psychiatry, 66*, 128–133.

Kendell, R. E. (1975). *The role of diagnosis in psychiatry*. London: Blackwell Scientific Publications.

Kendell, R. E. (1991). Relationship between the DSM-IV and the ICD-10. *Journal of Abnormal Psychology, 100*, 297–301.

Kendell, R. E., & Jablensky, A. (2003). Distinguishing between the validity and utility of psychiatric diagnosis. *American Journal of Psychiatry, 160*, 4–12.

Kendler, K. S., Kupfer, D., Narrow, W., Phillips, K., & Fawcett, J. (2009). *Guidelines for making changes to DSM-V*. Unpublished manuscript.

Kendler, K. S., Munoz, R. A., & Murphy, G. (2010). The development of the Feighner criteria: a historical perspective. *American Journal of Psychiatry, 167*, 134–142.

Kessler, R. C. (1999). The World Health Organization International Consortium in Psychiatric Epidemiology: initial work and future directions—the NAPE lecture. *Acta Psychiatrica Scandinavica, 99*, 2–9.

Kirk, S. A. (Ed.). (2005). *Mental disorders in the social environment: Critical perspectives*. New York: Columbia University Press.

Kirmayer, L. J., & Young, A. (1999). Culture and context in the evolutionary concept of mental disorder. *Journal of Abnormal Psychology, 108*, 446–452.

Kirmayer, L. J., Young, A., & Hayton, B. C. (1995). The cultural context of anxiety disorders. *Psychiatric Clinics of North America, 18*, 503–521.

Klein, D. F. (1999). Harmful dysfunction, disorder, disease, illness, and evolution. *Journal of Abnormal Psychology, 108*, 421–429.

Kraemer, H. C. (2008). DSM categories and dimensions in clinical and research contexts. In J. E. Helzer, H. C. Kraemer, R. F. Krueger, H-U. Wittchen, P. J. Sirovatka, & D. A. Regier (Eds.), *Dimensional approaches to diagnostic classification. Refining the research agenda for DSM-V* (pp. 5–17). Washington, DC: American Psychiatric Association.

Kupfer, D. J., First, M. B., & Regier, D. A. (Eds.). (2002). Introduction. In D. J. Kupfer, M. B. First, & D. A. Regier (Eds.), *A research agenda for DSM-V* (pp. xv–xxiii). Washington, DC: American Psychiatric Association.

Lewis-Fernandez, R., & Kleinman, A. (1995). Cultural psychiatry. Theoretical, clinical, and research issues. *Psychiatric Clinics of North America, 18*, 433–446.

Lilienfeld, S. O., & Marino, L. (1999). Essentialism revisited: Evolutionary theory and the concept of mental disorder. *Journal of Abnormal Psychology, 108*, 400–411.

Lim, R. F. (Ed.). (2006). *Clinical manual of cultural psychiatry*. Washington, DC: American Psychiatric Press.

López, S. R., & Guarnaccia, J. J. (2000). Cultural psychopathology: Uncovering the social world of mental illness. *Annual Review of Psychology, 51*, 571–598.

Menninger, K. (1963). *The vital balance*. New York: Viking Press.

Miller, G. (2010, March 19). Beyond DSM: Seeking a brain-based classification of mental illness. *Science, 327*, 1437.

Miller, J. D., Widiger, T. A., & Campbell, W. K. (2010). Narcissistic personality disorder and the DSM-V. *Journal of Abnormal Psychology, 119*(4), 640–649.

PDM Task Force. (2006). *Psychodynamic diagnostic manual*. Silver Springs, MD: Alliance of Psychoanalytic Organizations.

Petry, N. M. (2006). Should the scope of addictive behaviors be broadened to include pathological gambling? *Addiction, 101*(Suppl. 1), 152–160.

Regier, D. A. (2008). Forward: dimensional approaches to psychiatric classification. In J. E. Helzer, H. C. Kraemer, R. F. Krueger, H-U. Wittchen, P. J. Sirovatka, & D. A. Regier (Eds.), *Dimensional approaches to diagnostic classification. Refining the research agenda for DSM-V* (pp. xvii–xxiii). Washington, DC: American Psychiatric Association.

Regier, D. A., & Narrow, W. E. (2002). Defining clinically significant psychopathology with epidemiologic data. In J. E. Hulzer & J. J. Hudziak (Eds.), *Defining psychopathology in the 21st century. DSM-V and beyond* (pp. 19–30). Washington, DC: American Psychiatric Publishing.

Regier, D. A., Narrow, W. E., Kuhl, E. A., & Kupfer, D. J. (2010). The conceptual development of DSM-V. *American Journal of Psychiatry, 166*, 645–655.

Reiss, D., & Emde, R. N. (2003). Relationship disorders are psychiatric disorders: Five reasons they were not included in DSM-IV. In K. A. Phillips, M. B. First, & H. A. Pincus (Eds.), *Advancing DSM. Dilemmas in psychiatric diagnosis* (pp. 191–223). Washington, DC: American Psychiatric Association.

Robins, E., & Guze, S. B. (1970). Establishment of diagnostic validity in psychiatric illness: its application to schizophrenia. *American Journal of Psychiatry, 126*, 107–111.

Ronningstam, E. (2011). Narcissistic personality disorder in DSM-V. In support of retaining a significant diagnosis. *Journal of Personality Disorders, 25*(2), 248–259.

Rosenhan, D. L. (1973). On being sane in insane places. *Science, 179*, 250–258.

Rounsaville, B. J., Alarcon, R. D., Andrews, G., Jackson, J. S., Kendell, R. E., Kendler, K. S., & Kirmayer, L. J. (2002). Toward DSM-V: Basic nomenclature issues. In D. J. Kupfer, M. B. First, & D. A. Regier (Eds.), *A research agenda for DSM-V* (pp. 1–30). Washington, DC: American Psychiatric Press.

Rutter, M. (2003, October). *Pathways of genetic influences on psychopathology.* Zubin Award address at the 18th annual meeting of the Society for Research in Psychopathology, Toronto, Ontario.

Sadler, J. Z. (2005). *Values and psychiatric diagnosis.* Oxford, UK: Oxford University Press.

Salmon, T. W., Copp, O., May, J. V., Abbot, E. S., & Cotton, H. A. (1917). Report of the committee on statistics of the American Medico-Psychological Association. *American Journal of Insanity, 74*, 255–260.

Sanislow, C. A., Pine, D. S., Quinn, K. J., Kozak, M. J., Garvey, M. A., Heinssen, R. K., Sung-En Wang, P., & Cuthbert, B. N. (2010). Developing constructs for psychopathology Research: Research domain criteria. *Journal of Abnormal Psychology, 119*(4), 631–639.

Sartorius, N., Kaelber, C. T., Cooper, J. E., Roper, M., Rae, D. S., Gulbinat, W., … Regier, D. A. (1993). Progress toward achieving a common language in psychiatry. *Archives of General Psychiatry, 50*, 115–124.

Schwartz, M. A., & Wiggins, O. P. (2002). The hegemony of the DSMs. In J. Sadler (Ed.), *Descriptions and prescriptions: Values, mental disorders, and the DSM* (pp. 199–209). Baltimore, MD: Johns Hopkins University Press.

Skodol, A. (2010, February 10). *Rationale for proposing five specific personality types.* Retrieved from http://www.dsm5.org/ProposedRevisions/Pages/RationaleforProposingFiveSpecificPersonalityDisorderTypes.aspx

Spitzer, R. L., Endicott, J., & Robins E. (1978). Research diagnostic criteria. Rationale and reliability. *Archives of General Psychiatry, 35*, 773–782.

Spitzer, R. L., & Wakefield, J. C. (1999). DSM-IV diagnostic criterion for clinical significance: Does it help solve the false positives problem? *American Journal of Psychiatry, 156*, 1856–1864.

Spitzer, R. L., & Williams, J. B. W. (1982). The definition and diagnosis of mental disorder. In W. R. Gove (Ed.), *Deviance and mental illness* (pp. 15–32). Beverly Hills, CA: Sage.

Spitzer, R. L., Williams, J. B. W., & Skodol, A. E. (1980). DSM-III: The major achievements and an overview. *American Journal of Psychiatry, 137*, 151–164.

Stein, D. J., Phillips, K. A., Bolton, D., Fulford, K. W. M., Sadler, J. Z., & Kendler, K. S. (2010). What is a mental/psychiatric disorder? From DSM-IV to DSM-V. *Psychological Medicine, 40*(11), 1759–1765.

Stengel, E. (1959). Classification of mental disorders. *Bulletin of the World Health Organization, 21*, 601–663.

Szasz, T. S. (1961). *The myth of mental illness.* New York: Hoeber-Harper.

Wakefield, J. C. (1992). The concept of mental disorder: on the boundary between biological facts and social values. *American Psychologist, 47*, 373–388.

Wakefield, J. C. (1998). The DSM's theory-neutral nosology is scientifically progressive: Response to Follette and Houts (1996). *Journal of Consulting and Clinical Psychology, 66*, 846–852.

Wakefield, J. C. (2001). The myth of DSM's invention of new categories of disorder: Hout's diagnostic discontinuity thesis disconfirmed. *Behaviour Research and Therapy, 39*, 575–624.

Wakefield, J. C., & First, M. B. (2003). Clarifying the distinction between disorder and nondisorder: Confronting the overdiagnosis (false-positives) problem in DSM-V. In K. A. Phillips, M. B. First, & H. A. Pincus (Eds.), *Advancing DSM. Dilemmas in psychiatric diagnosis* (pp. 23–55). Washington, DC: American Psychiatric Association.

Wakefield, J. C., Pottick, K. J., & Kirk, S. A. (2002). Should the DSM-IV diagnostic criteria for conduct disorder consider social context? *American Journal of Psychiatry, 159*, 380–386.

Ward, C. H., Beck, A. T., Mendelson, M., Mock, J. E., & Erbaugh, J. K. (1962). The psychiatric nomenclature. Reasons for diagnostic disagreement. *Archives of General Psychiatry, 7*, 198–205.

Widiger, T. A. (1995). Deletion of the self-defeating and sadistic personality disorder diagnoses. In W. J. Livesley (Ed.), *The DSM-IV personality disorders* (pp. 359–373). New York: Guilford.

Widiger, T. A. (2001). Official classification systems. In W. J. Livesley (Ed.), *Handbook of personality disorders* (pp. 60–83). New York: Guilford.

Widiger, T. A. (2002). Values, politics, and science in the construction of the DSM. In J. Sadler (Ed.), *Descriptions and prescriptions: Values, mental disorders, and the DSM* (pp. 25–41). Baltimore, MD: Johns Hopkins University Press.

Widiger, T. A., & Clark, L. A. (2000). Toward DSM-V and the classification of psychopathology. *Psychological Bulletin, 126*, 946–963.

Widiger, T. A., Frances, A. J., Pincus, H. A., Davis, W. W., & First, M. B. (1991). Toward an empirical classification for DSM-IV. *Journal of Abnormal Psychology, 100*, 280–288.

Widiger, T. A. Frances, A. J., Pincus, H. A., First, M. B., Ross, R. R., & Davis, W. W. (Eds.). (1994). *DSM-IV sourcebook* (Vol. 1). Washington, DC: American Psychiatric Association.

Widiger, T. A., Frances, A. J., Pincus, H. A., Ross, R., First, M. B., Davis, W. W., & Kline, M. (Eds.). (1998). *DSM-IV sourcebook* (Vol. 4). Washington, DC: American Psychiatric Association.

Widiger, T. A., & Mullins-Sweatt, S. (2008). Classification. In M. Hersen & A. M. Gross (Eds.), *Handbook of clinical psychology.* Volume 1. *Adults* (pp. 341–370). New York: Wiley.

Widiger, T. A., & Samuel, D. B. (2005). Diagnostic categories or dimensions: A question for DSM-V. *Journal of Abnormal Psychology, 114*, 494–504.

Widiger, T. A., & Sankis, L. M. (2000). Adult psychopathology: Issues and controversies. *Annual Review of Psychology, 51*, 377–404.

Widiger, T. A., Simonsen, E., Krueger, R., Livesley, J., & Verheul, R. (2005). Personality disorder research agenda for the DSM-V. *Journal of Personality Disorders, 19*, 317–340.

Widiger, T. A., & Trull, T. J. (1991). Diagnosis and clinical assessment. *Annual Review of Psychology, 42*, 109–133.

Widiger, T. A., & Trull, T. J. (1993). The scholarly development of DSM-IV. In J. A. Costa e Silva & C. C. Nadelson (Eds.), *International review of psychiatry* (Vol. 1, pp. 59–78). Washington, DC: American Psychiatric Press.

Widiger, T. A., & Trull, T. J. (2007). Plate tectonics in the classification of personality disorder: shifting to a dimensional model. *American Psychologist, 62*, 71–83.

World Health Organization. (1992). *The ICD-10 classification of mental and behavioural disorders. Clinical descriptions and diagnostic guidelines.* Geneva: Author.

Zachar, P., & Kendler, K. S. (2007). Psychiatric disorders: a conceptual taxonomy. *American Journal of Psychiatry, 164*, 557–565.

Zigler, E., & Phillips, L. (1961). Psychiatric diagnosis: A critique. *Journal of Abnormal and Social Psychology, 63*, 607–618.

Zilboorg, G. (1941). *A history of medical psychology*. New York: Norton.

6

Psychological Assessment and Clinical Judgment

HOWARD N. GARB

Lackland Air Force Base
San Antonio, Texas

SCOTT O. LILIENFELD

Emory University
Atlanta, Georgia

KATHERINE A. FOWLER

National Institutes of Mental Health
Silver Springs, Maryland

What major advances have occurred in the assessment of psychopathology over the past 25 years? Many psychologists would argue that the most important breakthroughs include the development of explicit diagnostic criteria, the growing popularity of structured interviews, and the proliferation of brief measures tailored for use by mental health professionals conducting empirically supported treatments (e.g., Antony & Barlow, 2002). Others would disagree. Even an advance that most mental health professionals have embraced, the use of explicit criteria for making psychiatric diagnoses, has been challenged (Beutler & Malik, 2002). For example, Weiner (2000) referred to the fourth edition of the *Diagnostic and Statistical Manual of Mental Disorders* (*DSM–IV*; American Psychiatric Association, 1994) as "a psychometrically shaky, inferential nosological scheme involving criteria and definitions that change from one revision to the next" (p. 436; see also Widiger, this volume). Controversies abound in the domain of assessment, and most beginning readers of this literature are left with little guidance regarding how to navigate the murky scientific waters.

This chapter will provide such guidance. Specifically, we discuss fundamental conceptual and methodological issues in the assessment of psychopathology, with a particular focus on recent developments and advances. We compare different types of assessment instruments, including structured interviews, brief self-rated and clinician-rated measures, projective techniques, self-report personality inventories, and behavioral assessment and psychophysiological methods. We also review research on the validity of assessment instruments and research on clinical judgment and decision making.

Our principal goal in this chapter is to assist readers with the task of becoming well-informed and discerning consumers of the clinical assessment literature. In particular, we intend to provide readers with the tools necessary to distinguish scientifically supported from unsupported assessment instruments and to make valid judgments on the basis of the former instruments.

Psychometric Principles

Before describing the validity of assessment instruments and research on clinical judgment and decision making, we must first clarify the meaning of three key terms: reliability, validity, and treatment utility (see also the *Standards for Educational and Psychological Testing*, American Educational Research Association, American Psychological Association, & National Council on Measurement in Education [AERA, APA, & NCME], 1999).

Reliability refers to consistency of measurement. It is evaluated in several ways. If all of the items of a test are believed to measure the same trait, we want the test to possess good internal consistency: Test items should be positively intercorrelated. If a test is believed to measure a stable trait, then the test should possess test–retest reliability: on separate administrations of the test, clients should obtain similar scores. Finally, when two or more psychologists make diagnoses or other judgments for the same clients, interrater reliability should be high: Their ratings should tend to agree.

Traditionally, interrater reliability was evaluated by calculating the percentage of cases on which raters agree. For example, two psychologists might agree on diagnoses for 80% of the patients in a unit. However, percentage agreement is unduly affected by base rates. In this context, a *base rate* refers to the prevalence of a disorder. When the base rates of a disorder are high, raters may agree on a large number of cases because of chance. For example, if 80% of the patients in a chronic psychiatric inpatient unit suffer from schizophrenia, then two clinicians who randomly make diagnoses of schizophrenia for 80% of the patients will agree on the diagnosis of schizophrenia for about 64% of the cases ($0.8 \times 0.8 = 0.64$). Thus, a moderately high level of agreement is obtained even though diagnoses are made arbitrarily. By calculating kappa or an intraclass correlation coefficient (ICC), one can calculate the level of agreement beyond the chance level of agreement. This calculation is accomplished by taking into account the base rates of the disorder being rated.

When interpreting kappa and ICC, one generally uses the following criteria: Interrater reliability is poor for values below 0.40, fair for values between 0.40 and 0.59, good for values between 0.60 and 0.74, and excellent for values above 0.75 (Fleiss, 1981, p. 218). However, these criteria are typically used for making judgments (e.g., diagnoses or predictions of behavior), not for scoring test protocols. For scoring protocols, a reliability coefficient of at least 0.90 is desirable (Nunnally, 1978, pp. 245–246). Reliability should be higher for scoring tests than for making clinical judgments because if a test cannot be scored reliably, judgments based on those test scores will necessarily have poor reliability.

According to the *Standards for Educational and Psychological Testing* (AERA et al., 1999), *validity* refers to "the degree to which evidence and theory support the interpretations of test scores" (p. 9). Put another way, validity is good if the use of a test allows us to draw accurate inferences about clients (e.g., if the use of test scores helps us provide correct descriptions of traits, psychopathology, and diagnoses).

Reliability and validity differ in important ways. Reliability refers to the consistency of test scores and judgments; validity refers to the accuracy of interpretations and judgments. When reliability is good, validity can be good or poor. For example, two psychologists can agree on a client's diagnosis, yet both can be wrong. Or a client can obtain the same scores on two administrations of a test, yet inferences made using the test scores may be invalid. In contrast, when reliability is poor, validity is necessarily also poor. For example, if two psychologists cannot agree on a client's diagnosis, at least one of them is not making a valid diagnosis.

Different types of evidence can be obtained to evaluate validity. First, evidence can be based on test content (*content validity*). For example, a measure of a specific anxiety disorder, such as obsessive-compulsive disorder, should include an adequate representation of items to assess the principal features of this disorder, in this case obsessions and compulsions. To ensure content validity, many structured interviews contain questions that inquire comprehensively about the *DSM* criteria for anxiety disorders and other conditions (e.g., *Anxiety Disorders Interview Schedule–IV*, *ADIS–IV*; Brown, Di Nardo, & Barlow, 1994). Second, evidence can be based on the relation between tests. A test should show moderate or high correlations with other tests that measure the same attribute or diagnosis (*convergent validity*) and low correlations with tests that measure other attributes and diagnoses (*discriminant validity*). When test scores are used to forecast future outcomes, psychologists refer to this as *predictive validity*. When these scores are correlated with indices or events measured at approximately the same time, psychologists refer to this as *concurrent validity*.

The validity of an assessment instrument can also be evaluated by examining its internal structure (*structural validity*; see Loevinger, 1957). If a test generates many scores that do not intercorrelate as expected, this result may suggest that inferences based on those test scores are wrong. For example, one problem with the Rorschach Inkblot Test is that scores that are purported to reflect psychopathology are highly correlated with the number of responses produced by clients (Lilienfeld, Wood, & Garb, 2000, p. 34). That is, the more responses a client produces on the Rorschach, the greater the likelihood the client will generate responses that ostensibly indicate the presence of psychopathology. For example, a single Rorschach food response is purportedly indicative of dependent personality traits, but the more overall responses a client produces, the greater the likelihood of the client making a food response.

When we describe the content validity, convergent validity, or structural validity of an assessment instrument, we are also describing its construct validity. A construct is a theoretical variable that cannot be measured perfectly. More specifically, constructs are hypothesized attributes of individuals that cannot be observed directly, such as extraversion or schizophrenia (Cronbach & Meehl, 1955; but see Boorsboom, Mellenbergh, & Van Heerden, 2004, for a critique). Construct validity is a broad concept that subsumes content validity, convergent validity, and structural validity.

A number of statistics can be used to evaluate the validity of assessment instruments. Researchers commonly calculate correlations between a test and other measures, including scores on related tests. Other statistics can yield even more useful information. For example, results on sensitivity and specificity are presented routinely in the literature on medical tests, but only infrequently in the literature on psychological assessment (Antony & Barlow, 2002). *Sensitivity* is the likelihood that one will test positive if one has a specified mental disorder. *Specificity* is the likelihood one will test negative if one does not have the specified disorder. Ideally, one attempts to maximize both sensitivity and specificity, although there may be cases in which one elects to emphasize one statistic over the other. For example, if one were attempting to predict suicidal tendency in a large group of patients, one would probably be more concerned with sensitivity than specificity. Other important statistics are positive and negative predictive power. *Positive predictive power* describes the likelihood of a disorder given the presence of a particular result on an assessment instrument. *Negative predictive power* describes the likelihood of the absence of a disorder given the absence of the particular result on the assessment instrument.

The concepts of sensitivity, specificity, positive predictive power, and negative predictive power are illustrated in Table 6.1. In this scenario, provisional diagnoses of a mood disorder are made when the *T*-score for Scale 2 (Depression) of the Minnesota Multiphasic Personality Inventory–2 (MMPI–2) is ≥ 65 (the standard cutoff for psychopathology on the MMPI–2).[1] In the sample with a base rate of 50% (50% of the clients are depressed), 500 clients are depressed and 500 clients are not depressed. For the 500 clients who are depressed, 425 have a *T*-score of ≥ 65. Thus, sensitivity is equal to 425/500 = 85%. Computations for specificity, positive predictive power, and negative predictive power are also presented in Table 6.1.

---

[1] We use the term *provisional diagnoses* because formal diagnoses of psychiatric disorders should not be made on the basis of the MMPI–2 alone.

Table 6.1 Effect of Base Rate on Positive Predictive Power (PPP), Negative Predictive Power (NPP), Sensitivity, and Specificity

	Base Rate = 50%						
	Depressed						
Scale 2 (D)	**Yes**	**No**	**Total**	**PPP**	=	**425/575**	=	**73.9%**
$T^3 \geq 65$	425	150	575	NPP	=	350/425	=	82.4%
$T < 65$	75	350	425	Sensitivity	=	425/500	=	85.0%
Total	500	500	1,000	Specificity	=	350/500	=	70.0%

	Base Rate = 2%						
	Depressed						
Scale 2 (D)	**Yes**	**No**	**Total**	**PPP**	=	**17/311**	=	**5.0%**
$T^3 \leq 65$	17	294	311	NPP	=	686/689	=	99.6%
$T < 65$	3	686	689	Sensitivity	=	17/20	=	85.0%
Total	20	980	1,000	Specificity	=	686/980	=	70.0%

Depending on the statistic used to evaluate validity, accuracy can vary with the base rate of the behavior being predicted (Meehl & Rosen, 1955; also see Greene, 2000, pp. 365–366). As can be seen from Table 6.1, when percentage correct, positive predictive power, and negative predictive power are used to describe validity, accuracy varies with the base rate. For example, percentage correct is 425 + 350 ÷ 1,000 = 77.5% when the base rate is 50%, and 17 + 686 ÷ 1,000 = 70.3% when the base rate is 2%. In contrast, when sensitivity and specificity are used to describe validity, accuracy does not vary with the base rate. Put another way, when percentage correct, positive predictive power, and negative predictive power are used to describe accuracy, the same test will be described as having varying levels of accuracy depending on the base rates in different samples. In general, positive predictive power tends to decrease when base rates decrease, whereas negative predictive power tends to increase when base rates decrease. Thus, statistically rare events (e.g., suicide) are difficult to predict, whereas common events (e.g., no suicide) are relatively easy to predict.

When reading about positive findings for a test score, psychologists should be aware that the score may not work well in their work setting if the base rate in their work setting differs widely from the base rate in the study. If the base rate for a disorder is 0.5 in a study but 0.01 in a clinic, one can expect results for positive predictive power to be much less favorable in the clinic. Nevertheless, a large body of psychological research indicates that psychologists tend to (a) neglect or greatly underuse base rates when making judgments and predictions, and (b) focus too heavily on whether a client falls above or below a test's cutoff score (Finn & Kamphuis, 1995). As a consequence, clinicians' judgments can sometimes be grossly inaccurate when the base rates of the phenomenon in question are extreme (e.g., very low).

Signal detection theory (SDT) often provides the most useful information regarding the validity of an assessment instrument. SDT is a statistical approach that is used when the task is to detect a signal, such as the presence of major depression in a client. By using SDT, we can describe the validity of an assessment instrument across all base rates and across all cutoff scores (the signal is said to be present when a client's score exceeds the cutoff score). Different clinicians may set different cutoff scores for the same test; it is important that our estimate of the validity of a test not be influenced by the placement of the cutoff score. As observed by McFall and Treat (1999): "There is no longer any excuse for continuing to conduct business as usual, now that SDT-based indices represent a clear and significant advance over traditional accuracy indices such as sensitivity, specificity, and predictive power" (p. 227). Although such indices as sensitivity, specificity, and predictive power are informative, we agree with McFall and Treat that in many cases the use of SDT is more appropriate and comprehensive.

Other important psychometric concepts are norms, incremental validity, and treatment utility. *Norms* are scores that provide a frame of reference for interpreting a client's results. For the assessment of psychopathology, normative data can be collected by administering a test to a representative sample of individuals in the community. If a client's responses are similar to the normative data, psychologists should be very cautious about inferring the presence of psychopathology. When norms for a test do not accurately reflect the population of interest, clinicians may make inaccurate and potentially harmful judgments even if the test is valid. For example, a test may be a good measure of a thought disorder, but a clinician interpreting a client's test results may erroneously conclude that the client has a thought disorder if the norms give a false impression of how people in the community perform on the test. Historically, problems with norms have been as serious as, if not more serious than, problems with validity (Wood, Garb, & Nezworski, 2007).

Incremental validity describes the extent to which an instrument contributes information above and beyond already available information (e.g., other measures). For example, the use of a psychological test may allow clinicians to make judgments at a level better than chance, but judgments made using interview and test information may not be more accurate than judgments based on interview information only. One major criticism of the Rorschach Inkblot Test is that it does not provide useful information beyond that which can be obtained using more easily administered instruments, such as questionnaires (Lilienfeld et al., 2000).

Treatment utility describes the extent to which an assessment instrument contributes to decisions about treatment that lead to better outcomes. An assessment instrument could have good validity and good incremental validity, yet not lead to improved treatment outcomes. Surprisingly, few researchers have examined the treatment utility of assessment instruments (Harkness & Lilienfeld, 1997).

Assessment Instruments

Interviews

Unstructured interviews are used predominantly in clinical practice, whereas structured and semistructured interviews are used predominantly in research. One exception is that structured and semistructured interviews are used for clinical care in a growing number of university-based clinics. When conducting an unstructured interview, a psychologist is responsible for deciding what questions to ask. In contrast, when conducting a structured interview, questions are standardized. As one might surmise, semistructured interviews represent a balance between structured and unstructured interviews, providing guidance for interviewers but affording them some flexibility.

Reliability

The interrater reliability of unstructured interviews is generally good as long as a clinician attends to diagnostic criteria (Garb, 1998, pp. 41–42). For example, acceptable levels of interrater reliability were obtained for many, but not all, diagnostic categories in the *DSM–III* field trials and in the field trials for the 10th revision of the *International Classification of Mental and Behavioural Disorders* (*ICD–10*, World Health Organization, 1992; American Psychiatric Association, 1980, pp. 470–471; Sartorius et al., 1993). However, clinicians who participated in the *DSM–III* and *ICD–10* field trials were familiar with, and presumably adhered to, the diagnostic criteria. Other studies indicate that many mental health professionals do not attend to criteria when making diagnoses, but instead make diagnoses by comparing patients with their concept of the typical person with a given mental disorder (e.g., Blashfield & Herkov, 1996; Garb, 1996; Morey & Ochoa, 1989). When psychologists do not adhere to diagnostic criteria, interrater reliability is often poor.

The use of semistructured and structured interviews tends to lead to both good adherence to diagnostic criteria and good interrater reliability (Antony & Barlow, 2002; Rogers, 1995). For example, the *ADIS–IV* (Brown et al., 1994) requires interviewers to inquire about the *DSM–IV* criteria for anxiety disorders. Favorable reliability results have been found for this instrument: kappa values have ranged from 0.67 to 0.86 for diagnoses of the *DSM–IV* anxiety disorders (Brown, Di Nardo, Lehman, & Campbell, 2001).

Validity

Some psychologists have argued that diagnoses should not be made using the *DSM* criteria. For example, as already noted, Weiner (2000) argued that the *DSM* criteria are questionable, in part because they are inconsistent across editions of the manual. However, virtually all mental disorders are *open concepts* marked by (a) intrinsically fuzzy boundaries, (b) an indicator list that is potentially infinite, and (c) an unclear inner nature (Meehl, 1986). Although diagnostic criteria sometimes change in response to changing social norms and political pressures, they more often change as more is learned about a disorder. For example, we may eventually learn that certain individuals who meet the *DSM–IV* criteria for schizophrenia actually have disorders that have not yet been identified. Still, the construct of schizophrenia can be useful even though we are aware that the meaning of the term is somewhat imprecise and will change as more research is conducted. *DSM* diagnoses can be valid and useful even when we possess an incomplete understanding of the nature, etiology, course, and treatment of the conditions categorized.

As already noted, structured and semistructured interviews are used routinely in research. When important discoveries are made about the nature, etiology, course, or treatment of a disorder, they support the validity of the instruments used in the studies. For example, if a structured interview is used to select participants for a study on treatment outcome and the treatment intervention is found to be effective, one can infer that a client who obtains a specific diagnosis on the structured interview is likely to respond to the treatment. Thus, the bulk of the evidence on validity that supports structured and semistructured interviews derives from studies on psychopathology and treatment outcome. Similarly, evidence that supports the validity of the *DSM* criteria supports the validity of assessment instruments that help to determine if a participant satisfies those criteria. Because there is no gold standard for evaluating the validity of structured interviews (Faraone & Tsuang, 1994) or other assessment measures in psychopathology research, validity is established by evaluating "the degree to which evidence and theory support the interpretations of test scores" (AERA et al., 1999, p. 9).

There are several reasons to believe that structured interviews are more valid than unstructured interviews, at least when clinicians conducting unstructured interviews do not adhere to diagnostic criteria. First, interrater reliability tends to be better for structured and semistructured interviews, so all things being equal they are more likely to be valid. Second, many structured interviews are designed to inquire comprehensively about the *DSM* criteria. To the extent that the *DSM* criteria have been validated, the validity of these structured and semistructured interviews will be supported. Third, when interviews and self-report instruments are used to diagnose personality disorders, clinicians using unstructured interviews typically show the lowest agreement with other assessment instruments. In his review of the literature, Widiger (2002) noted that "the worst median convergent validity coefficient was obtained in the only study to have used unstructured interviews by practicing clinicians" (p. 463).

Additional evidence raises questions about the validity of diagnoses made by many practicing clinicians. Agreement between structured interview diagnoses and diagnoses made in clinical practice is generally poor (e.g., Brockington, Kendell, & Leff, 1978; Molinari, Ames, & Essa, 1994; Steiner, Tebes, Sledge, & Walker, 1995). For example, in one study (Steiner et al., 1995), clinical diagnoses made for 100 patients were compared with diagnoses made by research investigators using a structured interview. An overall weighted kappa coefficient indicated that agreement between the two interview methods was poor (kappa = 0.25). Values for kappa are typically higher when one structured interview is compared with another, although to a surprising degree this issue has not been studied for some widely used interviews (Rogers, 1995). Thus, based on the available evidence, one *cannot* argue that it makes little difference whether one conducts an unstructured or structured interview.

Although structured interviews generally appear to be more valid than unstructured interviews, their limitations need to be recognized. Because these limitations are shared with unstructured interviews, they do not indicate that unstructured interviews possess advantages over structured interviews. First, it is relatively easy for respondents to consciously underreport or overreport psychopathology on structured interviews (Alterman et al., 1996). Moreover, few structured interviews contain validity scales designed to detect dishonest or otherwise aberrant responding. Second, because memory is fallible, reports in interviews are often inaccurate or incomplete, even when clients are not intentionally trying to deceive the interviewer (Henry, Moffitt, Caspi, Langley, & Silva, 1994). Third, when clinicians are instructed to make use of medical records and other information in addition to structured interviews, considerable clinical judgment is required to describe and diagnose the client because information from different sources may conflict. This requirement is a potential limitation because clinical judgment is fallible.

Finally, an important methodological advance in evaluating the validity of interviews is the LEAD standard. LEAD is an acronym for *longitudinal, expert,* and *all data*. When using the LEAD standard (Spitzer, 1983), diagnoses made by using interviews are compared with diagnoses made by collecting longitudinal data. Using this approach, clients are followed over time to provide longitudinal data for making diagnoses, and diagnoses are made by expert clinicians using all relevant data. Although the LEAD standard can help us learn about the validity of diagnoses, it has rarely been used. Using this approach, one can more accurately evaluate the validity of diagnoses based on unstructured, structured, or semistructured interviews.

Brief Self-Rated and Clinician-Rated Measures

Brief measures have been developed for monitoring psychotherapy progress and providing information necessary to deliver standardized evidence-based interventions. To an extent seldom found for other assessment instruments, treatment utility has been established for measures used to monitor psychotherapy progress.

A number of systems have been developed for monitoring psychotherapy progress, and in particular for identifying clients who have made little or no progress during psychotherapy and who are at risk for deteriorating. For example, research suggests that it can be helpful to administer the Outcome Questionnaire-45 (OQ–45; Lambert & Finch, 1999) to clients prior to every session. The OQ–45 takes about 5 to 7 min to complete, and it measures constructs related to level of functioning including: (a) distress and symptoms, (b) interpersonal problems, and (c) problems related to social role performance. Normative data have been collected, making it possible to identify clients who have made less progress than 95% of the clients who obtained the same initial OQ–45 score (Lambert, Harmon, Slade, Whipple, & Hawkins, 2005). Results obtained in Germany and the United States demonstrate that clients tend to have better outcomes when therapists are alerted to poorly progressing clients (e.g., Lambert et al., 2003;

Percevic, Lambert, & Kordy, 2004). For example, for clients identified as being at risk, deterioration rates decreased from 21 to 13% when therapists were provided with feedback information (Lambert et al., 2003).

In addition, brief self-rated and clinician-rated measures have been constructed to provide information necessary to deliver standardized, evidence-based interventions. For example, the Beck Depression Inventory–II, the Beck Anxiety scale, and other scales are frequently used to assess depression and anxiety (Beck & Steer, 1990; Beck, Steer, & Brown, 1996). In addition, psychologists who use cognitive behavioral techniques to treat panic disorder frequently use brief measures to describe (a) the severity and frequency of panic-related symptoms, (b) cognitions or beliefs that are frequently associated with panic disorder, (c) clients' perceptions of their control over threatening internal situations, and (d) panic-related avoidance behaviors (e.g., Baker, Patterson, & Barlow, 2002). Because psychologists who use cognitive behavioral techniques are not usually concerned with measuring broad areas of psychopathology and personality, brief self-rated and clinician-rated measures are typically best suited for their needs.

The reliability and validity of many of these measures appears to be adequate. For example, the Panic Disorder Severity Scale (PDSS; Shear et al., 1997) is a seven-item scale that can be completed by either the clients or clinicians to describe key features of panic disorder with agoraphobia. When completed by a clinician, the ratings are based on information that has been gathered in interview and therapy sessions. Ratings are made for frequency of panic, anxiety about future panic attacks, magnitude of distress during panic, interference in social functioning, interference in work functioning, and avoidance behaviors. The PDSS possesses excellent interrater reliability (kappa = 0.87; Shear et al., 1997). In addition, PDSS ratings are correlated significantly with other measures of features of panic disorder. For example, Shear et al. (1997) obtained a correlation of $r - .55$ for the relation between total scores on the PDSS and severity ratings for panic disorder on the *ADIS–IV*. Equally important is evidence related to the content of the scale items: The PDSS was designed to assess problems that are important for treatment planning. In fact, a reason that brief self-rated and clinician-rated measures are popular is that they evaluate dimensions believed to be important for treatment planning. That is, they are designed to (a) evaluate problems that need to be addressed in treatment, and (b) provide information that is required to implement empirically based treatment interventions (see Stewart & Chambless, this volume). Finally, the PDSS can be used to track a client's progress. This use bears important implications for treatment use. For example, if the measure is administered during the course of treatment and indicates that a client is not improving, the clinician should consider trying a different intervention. In one study (Shear et al., 1997), clients were classified as treatment responders and nonresponders on the basis of ratings made by independent evaluators. A different group of evaluators made PDSS ratings for all clients before and after treatment. In contrast to nonresponders, responders showed statistically significant improvement on the PDSS.

Although reliability and validity appear to be fair for many self-rated and clinician-rated measures, the evaluation of their validity has been limited. Rather than compare the results from one of these measures with the results of a structured interview or with another self-rated or clinician-rated measure, it would be helpful to use behavioral assessment methods to evaluate validity. This approach has rarely been used, but the results from one study are provocative. When behavioral assessment methods were used to evaluate the validity of clients' statements, clients were found to overestimate the frequency and intensity of their panic attacks on a structured interview and on a brief self-rated test (Margraf, Taylor, Ehlers, Roth, & Agras, 1987).

Behavioral Assessment Methods and Psychophysiological Assessment

Behavioral assessment methods and psychophysiological assessment can provide valuable information. For example, by using diary measures, one can ask a client to record and rate the frequency and intensity of panic attacks shortly after symptoms occur. Or one can monitor a client's eating or smoking habits. By making ratings shortly after symptoms or behaviors occur, the results are more likely to be accurate than when based on retrospective reports. The increased accessibility of palmtop computers may eventually render it easier to collect and analyze self-monitoring data (data describing clients' ongoing behavior recorded by the clients themselves).

Behavioral assessment tests and other behavioral observation techniques can also provide valuable information. Behavioral assessment tests (also known as behavioral approach tests and behavioral avoidance tests) involve asking clients to enter situations that typically make them anxious, that they avoid, or both. For example, a client with a phobia can be instructed to approach a feared object (e.g., a spider) and a client with an obsessive-compulsive disorder can be instructed to switch off an electrical appliance and leave the room without checking it. During and after behavioral assessment tests, clients rate their level of anxiety. Other techniques include observing clients in role-play situations and in natural settings (without their being instructed to confront feared situations). For example, observations can be made of children in classrooms or of patients in psychiatric units.

Psychophysiological techniques can also provide valuable information. For example, a polysomnographic evaluation, which is conducted in a sleep lab, can provide valuable information about how well a client is sleeping (Savard & Morin, 2002). Similarly, measures of psychophysiological arousal can provide important information in the assessment of posttraumatic stress disorder, especially with respect to treatment process and outcome (Litz, Miller, Ruef, & McTeague, 2002). One team of investigators found that by playing a tape of combat sounds and measuring participants' heart rates, systolic blood pressure, and muscle tension with a forehead electromyogram, combat veterans with posttraumatic stress disorder could be discriminated from other veterans with 95.5% accuracy (Blanchard, Kolb, Pallmeyer, & Gerardi, 1982). Nevertheless, it will be important to cross-validate these findings in an independent sample. Because the psychophysiological assessment of other disorders has been confined largely to the laboratory, the extent to which these findings generalize to naturalistic settings remains unclear.

Global Measures of Personality and Psychopathology

Projective techniques and *self-report personality* inventories are designed to measure broad aspects of personality and psychopathology. Projective techniques include the Rorschach, Thematic Apperception Test (TAT), and human figure drawings. Self-report personality inventories include the MMPI–2 (Butcher, Dahlstrom, Graham, Tellegen, & Kaemmer, 1989), the Minnesota Multiphasic Personality Inventory-2-Restructured Form (MMPI–2–RF; Ben-Porath & Tellegen, 2008), the Personality Assessment Inventory (PAI; Morey, 1991), and the Millon Clinical Multiaxial Inventory–III (MCMI–III; Millon, 1994). Projective techniques are relatively unstructured: Stimuli are frequently ambiguous (e.g., inkblots, as in the case of the Rorschach) and response formats are typically open-ended (e.g., telling a story in response to a drawing of individuals interacting, as in the case of the TAT). In contrast, self-report personality inventories are relatively structured: Stimuli are fairly clear-cut (e.g., statements with which a client agrees or disagrees) and response formats are constrained (e.g., on the MMPI–2–RF, one can make a response of "true" or "false"). In general, validity findings are more encouraging for self-report personality inventories than for projective techniques, although exceptions have been found (see Lilienfeld et al., 2000; Wood, Nezworski, Lilienfeld, & Garb, 2003).

Projective Techniques

A common argument for using projective techniques is that they can circumvent a client's purported defenses and therefore can be used to evaluate conscious and unconscious processes. For example, some psychologists believe that when clients look at Rorschach inkblots and report what they see, they cannot invent faked responses because they do not know the true meaning of their Rorschach responses. However, research demonstrates that projective techniques are vulnerable to faking. For example, in one study (Albert, Fox, & Kahn, 1980), normal participants were instructed to fake paranoid schizophrenia. Presumed experts in the use of the Rorschach (Fellows of the Society for Personality Assessment) were unable to detect faking of psychosis. Diagnoses of malingering were made for 4% of the psychotic participants, 9% of the informed fakers (they were informed about the nature of disturbed thought processes and paranoid schizophrenia, but not about the Rorschach), 7% of uninformed fakers, and 2% of normal participants who were not instructed to fake. Diagnoses of psychosis were made for 48% of the psychotic participants, 72% of the informed fakers, 46% of the uninformed fakers, and 24% of the normal participants who were not instructed to fake.

A problem with many projective techniques is that they are difficult to score.[2] For example, the Comprehensive System (CS; Exner, 1993) is the most popular system for scoring the Rorschach. Exner (1993, p. 23), the developer of the CS, claimed that interrater reliability is better than 0.85 for all CS scores. However, results from other studies indicate that this result is true for only about half of the CS scores (Acklin, McDowell, Verschell, & Chan, 2000; Nakata, 1999; Shaffer, Erdberg, & Haroian, 1999; but see Meyer et al., 2002). Furthermore, in one study (Guarnaccia, Dill, Sabatino, & Southwick, 2001), the average scoring accuracy was only about 65%. In comparison, scoring is typically excellent for other types of tests (e.g., intelligence tests and personality inventories). For example, interrater reliability coefficients for the scoring of the Wechsler Adult Intelligence Scale, Third Edition (WAIS–III) have a median value of 0.95 and a minimum value of 0.90.

Another problem with projective techniques is that psychologists rarely use normative data when interpreting TAT protocols and human figure drawings, even though the availability of normative data can help to prevent the overperception of psychopathology. Furthermore, serious problems have surfaced regarding the normative data for the Rorschach. First, Exner (2001b) reported that his 1993 CS adult normative sample contained an error of enormous magnitude: The sample was described as being composed of 700 distinct protocols, but it actually contained 479 distinct protocols with 221 protocols counted twice. Subsequently, the CS adult normative sample has been revised (Exner, 2001b), but even this sample has been reported to contain errors (Meyer & Richardson, 2001). Second, Exner (personal communication, December 8, 2000) refused to make the current CS adult normative sample available for examination, even though J. M. Wood, a prominent critic of the CS, offered to pay for any expenses this would incur (J. M. Wood, personal communication, August 5, 2000).[3] Third, three of the strongest advocates for the Rorschach have subsequently discouraged clinicians from using the CS norms for children, even though they have already been used for many years. They also presented data that raise questions about the CS norms for adults (Meyer, Erdberg, & Shaffer, 2007). Finally, and most important, despite scattered claims to the contrary (e.g., Butcher, 2010), the use of the CS norms is likely to lead to the overperception of psychopathology (Hamel, Shaffer, & Erdberg, 2000; Shaffer et al., 1999; Wood, Nezworski, Garb, & Lilienfeld, 2001b; also see Aronow, 2001; Exner, 2001a; Hunsley & Di Giulio, 2001; Meyer, 2001; Widiger, 2001; Wood, Nezworski, Garb, & Lilienfeld, 2001a). For example, in one study (Hamel et al., 2000), the Rorschach was

---

[2] In fact, the TAT is rarely scored in clinical practice (see Lilienfeld et al., 2000).

[3] There has also been a heated argument over the accessibility of studies that have been cited to support the CS. Unpublished studies sponsored by Rorschach workshops are frequently cited as evidence supporting the CS, but attempts to obtain copies of papers describing the studies have frequently been unsuccessful (Nezworski & Wood, 1995; Wood, Nezworski, & Stejskal, 1996a, 1996b; but also see Exner, 1995, 1996). Copies of all correspondence will be provided on request.

administered to a group of 100 relatively normal school children. Children were excluded from the study if they had a history of mental disorder. Even though an independent measure (the Conners Parent Rating Scale–92; Conners, 1989) revealed that the children were healthier than average, the results for the Rorschach indicated that the typical child in the sample suffered from "a distortion of reality and faulty reasoning approaching psychosis" and "an affective disorder that includes many of the markers found in clinical depression" (p. 291).

The evidence for the construct validity of most projective techniques is at best mixed. In several meta-analyses, effect sizes for the Rorschach have ranged from $d = 0.25$ to 0.35, indicating that some positive findings have been reported (e.g., Garb, Florio, & Grove, 1998; Hiller, Rosenthal, Bornstein, Berry, & Brunell-Neuleib, 1999; Meyer & Archer, 2001; Parker, Hanson, & Hunsley, 1988). However, positive validity findings for the Rorschach, TAT, and human figure drawings have rarely been independently replicated (Lilienfeld et al., 2000).

The following criteria for evaluating the construct validity of assessment instruments were proposed by Wood, Nezworski, and Stejskal (1996b): (a) test scores should demonstrate a consistent relation to a particular symptom, trait, or disorder; (b) results must be obtained in methodologically rigorous studies; and (c) results must be replicated by independent investigators. Few scores for the Rorschach, TAT, and human figure drawings satisfy these criteria. For the Rorschach, the criteria have been satisfied for scores intended to detect thought disorder and psychotic conditions marked by thought disorder (e.g., schizophrenia), predict psychotherapy outcome, and assess behaviors related to dependency (e.g., Acklin, 1999; Bornstein, 1999; Jorgensen, Andersen, & Dam, 2000; Meyer & Handler, 1997). For the TAT, the criteria have been satisfied for the assessment of achievement motives, the identification of child sexual abuse history, and the detection of borderline personality disorder (Spangler, 1992; Westen, Lohr, Silk, Gold, & Kerber, 1990; Westen, Ludolph, Block, Wixom, & Wiss, 1990). For human figure drawings, the criteria have been satisfied only for distinguishing global psychopathology from normality (Naglieri & Pfeiffer, 1992). Ironically, over half of the indices that have been empirically supported are rarely used by psychologists in clinical practice. Some of these indices are difficult to score, whereas others were not incorporated into Exner's CS—the Rorschach scoring system that most clinicians use.

Most projective indices, including those used widely in clinical practice, have received relatively little empirical support. In commenting on the CS, Meyer and Archer (2001) offered a related observation:

> Yet many variables given fairly substantial interpretive emphasis have received little or no attention (Weiner, 2001). These include the Coping Deficit Index, Obsessive Style Index, Hypervigilance Index, active-to-passive movement ratio, D-score, food content, anatomy and X-ray content, Intellectualization Index, and Isolation Index. (p. 496)

Moreover, in a comprehensive review of research on the relation between Rorschach scores and psychiatric diagnoses (Wood, Lilienfeld, Garb, & Nezworski, 2000), Rorschach scores did not show a well-demonstrated relationship to major depressive disorder, posttraumatic stress disorder (PTSD), anxiety disorders other than PTSD, dissociative identity disorder, conduct disorder, psychopathy, or personality disorders. Moreover, a recent targeted meta-analysis showed that a variety of commonly used Rorschach indices display negligible validity for detecting psychopathy (Wood et al., 2010). Despite these negative findings, the Rorschach continues to be used by psychologists for the diagnosis of these disorders. Similarly, although the Rorschach and human figure drawings are sometimes used by mental health professionals to help decide whether a child has been sexually abused (Oberlander, 1995), their use for this task has not been consistently supported (e.g., Garb, Wood, & Nezworski, 2000; Trowbridge, 1995).

Personality Inventories

Self-report personality inventories require clients to indicate whether a statement describes them. However, contrary to widespread claims, self-report personality inventories do not require clients to be able to accurately describe their symptoms and personality traits. The "dynamics" of self-report personality inventories were described by Meehl (1945):

> A self-rating constitutes an intrinsically interesting and significant bit of verbal behavior, the non-test correlates of which must be discovered by empirical means. [The approach is free] from the restriction that the subject must be able to describe his own behavior accurately.... The selection of items is done on a thoroughly empirical basis using carefully selected criterion groups. (p. 297)

Thus, whereas the validity of brief self-rated tests rests on the content of items, the validity of self-report personality inventories rests on empirical research that relates test items (and test scales) to client characteristics. This approach has met with some success. For example, results from a meta-analysis indicate that the MMPI can be useful for detecting overreporting and underreporting of psychopathology (Berry, Baer, & Harris, 1991).

Scientific support for personality inventories has been mixed. One positive feature is that psychologists who use self-report personality inventories almost always use norms. Also, the norms of major self-report personality inventories, such as the MMPI–2–RF, are representative of U.S. adults or adolescents in the community. There is no evidence that these norms make relatively normal individuals appear pathological.

In contrast, the validity of the primary scales of some tests (e.g., the MMPI–2, the MMPI–2–RF, the Personality Assessment Inventory) has generally been supported, whereas the validity evidence for the scales of other widely used tests (e.g., the MCMI–III) is weaker and less consistent. For example, Rogers, Salekin, and Sewell (1999) reviewed the research on the MCMI–III and concluded that it should not be used in forensic settings (also see Dyer & McCann, 2000; Rogers, Salekin, & Sewell, 2000). Even for the MMPI–2, half of the supplementary scales have not been consistently supported (e.g., Greene, 2000, pp. 218–269). Despite these negative findings, positive results on validity have been consistently replicated by independent investigators for a large number of MMPI–2 and MMPI–2–RF scores. For example, research has demonstrated that Scale 4 ("Psychopathic Deviate") is correlated positively with criminal behaviors and recidivism risk (see Greene, 2000, p. 148), whereas Scale 9 ("Hypomania") is correlated with such characteristics as impulsiveness, extraversion, and superficiality in social relationships (e.g., Graham, Ben-Porath, & McNulty, 1997). In addition, although the new MMPI–2–RF scales are controversial in some quarters (Butcher, 2010), evidence suggests that they are valid for detecting many psychopathological characteristics and may even possess incremental validity above and beyond the original MMPI–2 scales (e.g., Sellbom, Ben-Porath, Lilienfeld, Patrick, & Graham, 2005). In clinical judgment studies, judgments were more valid when psychologists had been given results from personality inventories than when given results from projective techniques (e.g., Garb, 1989, 1998, 2003). In fact, in several studies, validity actually decreased, at least slightly, when Rorschach results were made available in addition to brief biographical or questionnaire results (e.g., Whitehead, 1985).

On the negative side, evidence for the utility of personality inventories in treatment planning is scarce, and the *very* little evidence that exists has not been supportive (Garb, Lilienfeld, Nezworski, Wood, & O'Donohue, 2009). Specifically, when researchers have used manipulated assessment designs to randomly assign some clinicians to receive specific assessment information (e.g., the MMPI–2), and others do not receive such information, there were no detected significant differences in treatment outcome (Lima et al., 2005). Therapists in this study were 25 doctoral students in clinical psychology who each received about 3 to 5 hr per week of supervision with a licensed clinical psychologist.

Clinical Judgment and Decision Making

Experience, Training, and Clinical Judgment

When confronted with evidence regarding the poor validity of specific assessment instruments, such as projective techniques, some clinicians retort that their extensive clinical experience permits them to extract useful inferences from these instruments. In other words, the argument goes, validation studies fail to capture the rich and subtle information that highly seasoned practitioners can obtain from certain assessment measures. For example, in response to review articles demonstrating that a mere handful of Rorschach variables are empirically supported (Lilienfeld et al., 2000, 2001), several practitioners, in messages to the Rorschach Discussion and Information Group, maintained that the negative research evidence was largely irrelevant because their numerous years of clinical experience with the Rorschach endowed them with special judgmental and predictive powers.

Nevertheless, these arguments do not withstand careful scrutiny because the relation between clinical experience and judgmental accuracy has been weak in most studies of personality and psychopathology assessment (Dawes, 1994). For example, when given MMPI (e.g., Graham, 1967) or Rorschach (e.g., Turner, 1966) protocols, clinicians did not produce more valid ratings of psychopathology or personality than did psychology graduate students (see Garb, 1989, 1998, for reviews). Nor is there evidence that presumed experts on certain personality measures outperform other clinicians. In one striking example, Levenberg (1975) asked clinicians to identify children as either normal or abnormal on the basis of their protocols on the Kinetic Family Drawing test, a commonly used human figure drawing measure. Whereas a group of doctoral-level psychologists was correct for 72% of cases, the author of two books on the Kinetic Family Drawing test was correct for only 47% of cases. Turner (1966) provided similar findings on the Rorschach.

One potential exception to the finding that experience and accuracy are negligibly related was reported in a study by Brammer (2002). To help them make diagnoses, psychologists and psychology graduate students were allowed to ask questions and ask for specific items of information. The number of years of clinician experience was significantly associated with the number of correct diagnoses made ($r = .33$), as well as with the number of diagnostically specific questions asked ($r = .51$). Brammer's findings raise the intriguing possibility that experience is related to validity on tasks that require clinicians to structure complex tasks, such as formulating a psychiatric diagnosis by honing in on potential problem areas and then asking progressively more specific questions (see also Clavelle & Turner, 1980).

Some clinicians could contend that although the overall relation between experience and accuracy tends to be weak, many clinicians in real-world settings know which of their judgments are likely to be accurate. Nevertheless, for the use of projective techniques and some other assessment instruments, the relation between the validity of clinicians' judgments and their confidence in these judgments is generally weak. For example, Albert et al. (1980) found no significant relation between validity and confidence when practitioners were asked to use Rorschach protocols to detect malingering. For the MMPI, there is some evidence that confidence is positively related to the validity of clinicians' judgments, but only when these judgments are reasonably valid (e.g., Goldberg, 1965). That is, when psychologists use the MMPI to assist in making diagnoses, they tend to be able to state correctly which of their diagnostic judgments are most likely to be correct.

In contrast to the dispiriting findings concerning the value of clinical experience for personality assessment judgments, the research literature supports the value of training on certain assessment instruments. For example, in several studies psychologists using MMPI protocols made more valid personality judgments than did lay judges (e.g., Aronson & Akamatsu, 1981; see Garb,

1989, for a review). Nevertheless, research does not support the value of training in the inter-pretation of projective protocols. For example, in one study (Gadol, 1969), clinical psychologists and undergraduates were equally accurate when asked to make personality ratings of psychiatric patients on the basis of Rorschach protocols. Similar findings emerged when psychologists were compared with lay judges in their ability to distinguish psychopathology from normality on the basis of human figure drawings or sentence completion tests (see Garb, 1989, for a review).

Why Clinicians Often Do Not Benefit From Experience

Why are practitioners often unable to benefit from clinical experience? Although the reasons are manifold (see Arkes, 1981; Dawes, Faust, & Meehl, 1989; Garb, 1989), we focus on six here. The first three concern the nature of the feedback available to clinicians, and the remaining three rea-sons concern cognitive processes that influence the selection and interpretation of this feedback.

Nature of Feedback

First, in contrast to physicians in most domains of organic medicine, psychologists rarely receive clear-cut feedback concerning their judgments and predictions (Meehl, 1973). Instead, the feedback psychologists receive is often vague, ambiguous, open to multiple interpretations, and delayed. For example, if a clinician concludes that an adult client was sexually abused in childhood on the basis of an unstructured interview and Rorschach protocol, this judgment is difficult to falsify. If the client were to deny a history of abuse or express uncertainty about it, the clinician could readily maintain that the interpretation may still be correct because the cli-ent may have forgotten or repressed the abuse (although the scientific evidence for repression is controversial; see Holmes, 1990). Moreover, when clinicians receive feedback regarding their predictions (e.g., forecasts of violence), it is often substantially delayed, thereby introducing the potential distorting effects of memory.

Second, clinicians typically have access to only a subset of the data needed for accurate judg-ments, a quandary referred to by Gilovich (1991) as the "missing data problem." For example, clinicians may perceive certain psychological conditions (e.g., nicotine dependence) to be more chronic and unremitting than they are (Schacter, 1982) because they are selectively exposed to individuals who remain in treatment. Cohen and Cohen (1984) referred to this effect as the "clinician's illusion."

Third, some feedback that clinicians receive from clients is misleading. Meehl (1956) referred to an individual's tendency to accept highly generalized but nonobvious personality descriptions as the *P. T. Barnum effect*, after the circus entrepreneur who quipped that "I like to give a little something to everybody" and "A sucker is born every minute." Numerous studies demonstrate that most individuals who present with Barnum descriptions (e.g., "You have a great deal of unused potential," "At times you have difficulty making up your mind") find such descriptions to be highly compelling, particularly when they believe that these descriptions were tailored for them (Logue, Sher, & Frensch, 1992; Snyder & Larson, 1972). The Barnum effect demonstrates that personal validation, the informal method of validating test feedback by relying on respon-dents' acceptance of this feedback, is a highly fallible barometer of actual validity. In addition, because clients are often impressed by Barnum feedback, such feedback can fool clinicians into believing that their interpretations are more valid than they really are. The same process can also explain why astrologers and palm readers are often confident that their interpretations are accurate (see Wood et al., 2003).

Cognitive Processes

Fourth, a substantial body of literature documents that individuals are prone to *confirmatory bias*, the tendency to selectively seek out and recall information consistent with one's hypotheses and to neglect information inconsistent with these hypotheses. Several investigators have found that clinicians fall prey to confirmatory bias when asked to recall information regarding clients. For example, Strohmer, Shivy, and Chiodo (1990) asked counselors to read three versions of a case history of a client, one containing an equal number of descriptors indicating good self-control and poor self-control, one containing more descriptors indicating good control than poor self-control, and one containing more descriptors indicating poor than good self-control. One week after reading this case history, psychotherapists were asked to offer as many factors as they could remember that "would be helpful in determining whether or not [the client] lacked self-control" (p. 467). Therapists offered more information that would be helpful for confirming than disconfirming the hypothesis that the client lacked self-control, even in the condition in which the client was described or characterized primarily by good self-control descriptors.

There also is evidence that clinicians are sometimes prone to premature closure in diagnostic decision making: they may tend to reach conclusions too quickly (Garb, 1998). For example, Gauron and Dickinson (1969) reported that psychiatrists who observed a videotaped interview frequently formed diagnostic impressions within 30 to 60 s. Premature closure may both reflect and produce confirmatory bias. It may reflect confirmatory bias because clinicians may reach rapid conclusions by searching only for data that confirm preexisting hypotheses. It may produce confirmatory bias by effectively halting the search for data that could disconfirm such hypotheses.

Fifth, investigators have shown that clinicians, like all individuals, are prone to illusory correlations, which has generally been defined as the perception of (a) a statistical association that does not actually exist, or (b) a stronger statistical association than is actually present. Illusory correlations are likely to arise when individuals hold powerful a priori expectations regarding the covariation between certain events or stimuli. For example, many individuals are convinced that a strong correlation exists between the full moon and psychiatric hospital admissions, even though studies have demonstrated repeatedly that no such association exists (Rotton & Kelly, 1985).

In a classic study of illusory correlation, Chapman and Chapman (1967) examined why psychologists perceive clinically meaningful associations between signs on the draw-a-person (DAP) test (e.g., the drawing of large eyes) and psychiatric symptoms (e.g., suspiciousness) even though research has demonstrated that these associations do not exist (Kahill, 1984). They presented undergraduate participants with DAP protocols that were purportedly produced by psychiatric patients with certain psychiatric symptoms (e.g., suspiciousness). Each drawing was paired randomly with two of these symptoms, which were listed on the bottom of each drawing. Undergraduates were asked to inspect these drawings and estimate the extent to which certain DAP signs co-occurred with these symptoms. Chapman and Chapman found that participants "discovered" that certain DAP signs tended to consistently co-occur with certain psychiatric symptoms, even though the DAP signs and symptoms had been randomly paired. For example, participants mistakenly perceived large eyes in drawings as co-occurring with suspiciousness and broad shoulders in drawings as co-occurring with doubts about manliness. Interestingly, these are the same associations that tend to be perceived by clinicians who use the DAP (Chapman & Chapman, 1967). Illusory correlation has been demonstrated with other projective techniques, including the Rorschach (Chapman & Chapman, 1969) and sentence completion tests (Starr & Katkin, 1969). Scientifically minded practitioners need to be aware of the phenomenon of illusory correlation, which suggests that clinicians can be convinced of the validity of assessment indicators in the absence of validity.

Finally, it can be difficult to learn from clinical experience unless one thinks in probabilistic terms (Einhorn, 1988). Unfortunately, this skill can be very difficult to learn. For example, individuals tend to overestimate the likelihood that they would have predicted an outcome after they have become aware of the outcome, an effect termed *hindsight bias* (Arkes, Faust, Guilmette, &

Hart, 1988; Fischhoff, 1975). Thus, if a client commits suicide and an investigation is conducted, the investigators may conclude that the suicide could have been predicted, in part because of hindsight bias. Similarly, when asked to rate the likelihood of one event occurring and the same event plus another event occurring, individuals will often give a higher rating for the likelihood of both events occurring, an effect termed *conjunction bias* (Garb, 2006; Tversky & Kahneman, 1983). For example, for a particular client, if one diagnosis seems likely (e.g., major depressive disorder) and another diagnosis seems unlikely (e.g., antisocial personality disorder), then some clinicians may believe the likelihood of a client having both diagnoses is greater than the likelihood of the client have only the less likely disorder. However, according to probability theory, the probability of events A and B, $P(A \cap B)$, cannot be greater than the probability of event A, $P(A)$, or the probability of event B, $P(B)$. Because clinicians do not naturally think probabilistically, they sometimes engage in deterministic reasoning. Every clinician can generate explanations why a client behaves a particular way or has a particular disorder, but these explanations may not be correct. Clinicians do not necessarily have complete information about every client, and some of the information they do have is likely to contain error. For this reason, we should not unquestioningly accept a theory or case formulation simply because it seems compelling and seems to explain all of the available information.

Group Biases in Judgment

A large number of studies have examined biases related to the demographic characteristics of clients (e.g., their race, gender, or socioeconomic status; for a review, see Garb, 1997; Maddux, Gosselin, & Winstead, this volume). Bias occurs when the validity of a clinical judgment or test differs by demographic characteristics of clients (e.g., when the validity of judgments is better for White clients than for Black clients). The most frequent type of bias discussed by psychologists is *slope bias*, which involves differences in validity coefficients across groups. When a test or clinical judgment yields a significantly higher validity coefficient in one group than another (slope bias), the test or judgment exhibits differential validity (Anastasi & Urbina, 1997). Note that the mere presence of group differences on a test is not sufficient to infer bias; bias requires that the clinical judgment or test be less valid for one group than for another. We will briefly describe results for gender bias, race bias, and social class bias.

Sex Bias

Sex role stereotypes are a cause for concern in the diagnosis of psychopathology, especially for the diagnosis of personality disorders. When two groups of clinicians are given one of two case vignettes, and the case vignettes are identical except for the designation of gender, then histrionic personality disorder is more likely to be diagnosed in women and antisocial personality disorder is more likely to be diagnosed in men. Both male and female clinicians exhibit this bias (e.g., Adler, Drake, & Teague, 1990; Ford & Widiger, 1989). Ford and Widiger (1989) found that clinicians were not biased when they made ratings for the individual criteria that comprise these diagnoses. This finding suggests that the bias is linked to clinicians' perceptions of the diagnoses themselves, not to the *DSM* criteria for these disorders.

Race Bias

In a number of studies conducted in clinical settings, race bias has been shown to occur in psychiatric diagnosis, the prescription of psychiatric medications, violence prediction, and child abuse reporting (Garb, 1997, 1998). When the effect of social class was controlled, race still emerged as an important predictor. African American and Hispanic patients were less likely to be diagnosed with a psychotic mood disorder and more likely to be diagnosed with schizophrenia compared with White patients exhibiting similar symptoms (e.g., Mukherjee, Shukla, Woodle, Rosen, &

Olarte, 1983; Simon, Fleiss, Gurland, Stiller, & Sharpe, 1973). This occurred even when a diagnosis of schizophrenia was inappropriate. Additionally, African American patients received a larger number of antipsychotic medications, injections of antipsychotic medications, and psychiatric medications overall. Moreover, clinicians have exhibited race bias when predicting the occurrence of violence in institutional settings, including psychiatric wards and prisons. In these studies, they have overestimated the risk of violence for Black inpatients and inmates. However, for clients residing in the community, race bias was not found for the prediction of violence. Race was a potent predictor of failure to report child abuse: Cases of child abuse were less likely to be reported if the child was White than Black (Hampton & Newberger, 1985).

Social Class Bias

Social class bias has been demonstrated only sparsely in psychiatric diagnosis and treatment (Garb, 1997, 1998). One finding that has emerged is the relation of social class to psychotherapy decisions. Clinicians were more likely to recommend middle-class individuals than lower-class individuals for psychotherapy and expected them to do better in therapy when both groups were recommended. Additionally, middle-class clients were more likely to be recommended for insight-focused therapy, whereas lower-class clients received more recommendations for supportive therapy (see Garb, 1997, for a review).

Methodological Recommendations

Several methodological steps can be taken to improve the quality of psychological assessment and the judgments derived from psychological tests. First, more sophisticated procedures can be used to evaluate validity. For example, to evaluate the validity of diagnoses, one can use the LEAD standard (Spitzer, 1983; also see Garb, 1998, pp. 45–53). Use of the LEAD standard, which was described earlier, allows researchers to ascertain the validity of structured interviews and other assessment instruments. In addition, the criteria proposed by Wood et al. (1996b) should be used to determine if an assessment instrument is valid for its intended purpose. For example, if positive validity findings have been obtained in two studies but not in two others, one would conclude that the assessment instrument does not meet the Wood et al. (1996b) criteria because the results were not consistent.

A second recommendation is that item response theory (IRT) be used to construct and evaluate tests. IRT is an alternative to traditional (classical) test theory. It can be used as a methodological and statistical tool for a number of purposes, including test construction, evaluating a test, and using person-fit indices to assess how well a trait (or construct) describes an individual. For example, using person-fit indices, one may conclude that a trait is not relevant to a person if the person responds in an idiosyncratic manner (e.g., endorses severe but not moderate symptoms of depression). IRT also permits test constructors to determine which items are most discriminating at different levels of the trait in question. For example, IRT analyses could reveal that a measure of depression adequately distinguishes nondepressed from moderately depressed individuals, but not moderately from severely depressed individuals.

Although well established in achievement and aptitude testing, IRT has been applied infrequently to personality assessment. This is partly because cognitive constructs are better understood than personality constructs. Put another way, construct validity issues have been more formidable for personality measurement. Just the same, in a relatively few studies, IRT has been applied successfully to personality assessment. For example, historically, linear factor analyses have been used to describe the structure of the MMPI and MMPI–2. Because MMPI and MMPI–2 items are dichotomous (true–false questions), and because linear factor analysis assumes that ratings are normally distributed and not dichotomous, it is more appropriate to use nonlinear factor analysis or multidimensional IRT methods. Using IRT to uncover the factor structure of the MMPI–2, Waller (1998) found important differences between his results and those of previous factor analyses.

Third, the use of computers for making judgments and decisions is becoming increasingly important in the assessment of psychopathology. Findings from a meta-analysis (Grove, Zald, Lebow, Snitz, & Nelson, 2000) suggest that computer programs can be successfully developed for this purpose. The utility of these programs derives from well-established (although still largely neglected) findings that actuarial (statistical) formulas based on empirically established relations between predictors and criteria are almost always superior to or at least equal to clinical judgment (Dawes et al., 1989; Grove & Meehl, 1996). However, relatively few well-validated computer programs are available for clinical tasks (Garb, 2000). As observed by Wood, Garb, Lilienfeld, and Nezworski (2002):

> Substantial progress has been made in developing computerized algorithms to predict violence, child abuse and neglect, and recidivism among juvenile offenders.... However, there are still no well-validated algorithms for making diagnoses [or case formulations], ... describing personality traits and psychopathology, or making treatment decisions. (p. 534)

Similarly, Snyder (2000) concluded that popular computer programs that have been used for years to interpret test results (e.g., for the MMPI–2 and the Rorschach) are inadequately validated. Research is needed to develop and validate new computer programs that provide valid descriptions of a client's personality and psychopathology.

Conclusions

Assessing psychopathology is an activity fraught with potential error and bias. However, by attending to research findings, psychologists can avoid using test scores that are invalid, and they can become familiar with the strengths and weaknesses of clinical judgment. In this way, errors that are potentially detrimental to clients can be avoided. For example, the use of the CS norms for interpreting Rorschach protocols can lead to false positives in the assessment of psychopathology. By not using the CS norms, or by using them with extreme caution, one can avoid making harmful judgments such as misdiagnosing normal clients as pathological.[4]

Some psychologists argue that although scientific research is important, we should also rely on clinical experience to determine if an assessment instrument is valuable. Indeed, some even argue that when research and clinical experience conflict, we should place a higher premium on the latter. Psychologists are frequently encouraged to use the Rorschach and other projective techniques because they seem to provide rich clinical data (e.g., Karon, 2000). However, clinical experience can be fallible for a host of reasons, including biased feedback, illusory correlation, confirmatory bias, and deterministic reasoning (Dawes et al., 1989; Garb, 1998). The scientific method, not clinical experience, is the best method for minimizing error and resolving controversies. Scientific techniques, such as double-blind designs and control groups, are essential tools that researchers have developed to protect themselves from being misled (Lilienfeld, 2002, 2010). As McFall (1991) noted:

> [There is a] commonly offered rationalization that science doesn't have all the answers yet, and until it does, we must do the best we can to muddle along, relying on our clinical experience, judgment, creativity, and intuition (cf., Matarazzo, 1990). Of course, this argument reflects the mistaken notion that science is a set of answers, rather than a set of processes or methods by which to arrive at answers. Where there are lots of unknowns—and clinical

---

[4] For a case history describing a client who was apparently harmed by interpretations of the Rorschach, see Garb, Wood, Lilienfeld, and Nezworski (2002).

psychology certainly has more than its share—it is all the more imperative to adhere as strictly as possible to the scientific approach. Does anyone seriously believe that a reliance on intuition and other unscientific methods is going to hasten advances in knowledge? (pp. 76–77)

Finally, as noted by McFall (cited in Trull & Phares, 2001, p. 62), one feature that should distinguish clinical and counseling psychologists from most other mental health professionals is their scientific training (see also Baker, McFall, & Shoham, 2009). To ignore research findings because they make us feel uncomfortable is to neglect our most distinctive and positive attribute: our training in, and our willingness to be guided by, science.

References

Acklin, M. W. (1999). Behavioral science foundations of the Rorschach test: Research and clinical applications. *Assessment, 6*, 319–326.

Acklin, M. W., McDowell, C. J., Verschell, M. S., & Chan, D. (2000). Interobserver agreement, intraobserver reliability, and the Rorschach Comprehensive System. *Journal of Personality Assessment, 74*, 15–47.

Adler, D. A., Drake, R. E., & Teague, G. B. (1990). Clinicians' practices in personality assessment: Does gender influence the use of DSM-III Axis II? *Comprehensive Psychiatry, 31*, 125–131.

Albert, S., Fox, H. M., & Kahn, M. W. (1980). Faking psychosis on the Rorschach: Can expert judges detect malingering? *Journal of Personality Assessment, 44*, 115–119.

Alterman, A. I., Snider, E. C., Cacciola, J. S., Brown, L. S. Jr., Zaballero, A., & Siddiqui, N. (1996). Evidence of response set effects in structured research interviews. *Journal of Nervous and Mental Disease, 184*, 403–410.

American Educational Research Association (AERA), American Psychological Association, & National Council on Measurement in Education. (1999). *Standards for educational and psychological testing.* Washington, DC: AERA.

American Psychiatric Association. (1980). *Diagnostic and statistical manual of mental disorders* (3rd ed.). Washington, DC: Author.

American Psychiatric Association. (1994). *Diagnostic and statistical manual of mental disorders* (4th ed.). Washington, DC: Author.

Anastasi, A., & Urbina, S. (1997). *Psychological testing* (7th ed.). New York: Macmillan.

Antony, M. M., & Barlow, D. H. (Eds.). (2002). *Handbook of assessment and treatment planning for psychological disorders.* New York: Guilford.

Arkes, H. R. (1981). Impediments to accurate clinical judgment and possible ways to minimize their impact. *Journal of Consulting and Clinical Psychology, 49*, 323–330.

Arkes, H. R., Faust, D., Guilmette, T. J., & Hart, K. (1988). Eliminating the hindsight bias. *Journal of Applied Psychology, 73*, 305–307.

Aronow, E. (2001). CS norms, psychometrics, and possibilities for the Rorschach technique. *Clinical Psychology: Science and Practice, 8*, 383–385.

Aronson, D. E., & Akamatsu, T. J. (1981). Validation of a Q-sort task to assess MMPI skills. *Journal of Clinical Psychology, 37*, 831–836.

Baker, T. B., McFall, R. M., & Shoham, V. (2009). Current status and future prospects of clinical psychology: Toward a scientifically principled approach to mental and behavioral health care. *Psychological Science in the Public Interest, 9*, 67–103.

Baker, S. L., Patterson, M. D., & Barlow, D. H. (2002). Panic disorder and agoraphobia. In M. M. Antony & D. H. Barlow (Eds.), *Handbook of assessment and treatment planning for psychological disorders* (pp. 67–112). New York: Guilford.

Beck, A. T., & Steer, R. A. (1990). *Manual for the Beck Anxiety Inventory.* San Antonio, TX: Psychological Corporation.

Beck, A. T., Steer, R. A., & Brown, G. K. (1996). *Beck Depression Inventory manual* (2nd ed.). San Antonio, TX: Psychological Corporation.

Ben-Porath, Y. S., & Tellegen, A. (2008). *Minnesota Multiphasic Personality Inventory-2-Restructured Form (MMPI-2-RF): Manual for administration, scoring, and interpretation.* Minneapolis: University of Minnesota Press.

Berry, D. T. R., Baer, R. A., & Harris, M. J. (1991). Detection of malingering on the MMPI: A meta-analysis. *Clinical Psychology Review, 11*, 585–598.

Beutler, L. E., & Malik, M. L. (Eds.). (2002). *Rethinking the DSM: A psychological perspective*. Washington, DC: American Psychological Association.

Blanchard, E. B., Kolb, L. C., Pallmeyer, T. P., & Gerardi, R. J. (1982). A psychophysiological study of post-traumatic stress disorder in Vietnam veterans. *Psychiatric Quarterly, 54*, 220–229.

Blashfield, R. K., & Herkov, M. J. (1996). Investigating clinician adherence to diagnosis by criteria: A replication of Morey and Ochoa (1989). *Journal of Personality Disorders, 10*, 219–228.

Bornstein, R. F. (1999). Criterion validity of objective and projective dependency tests: A meta-analytic assessment of behavioral prediction. *Psychological Assessment, 11*, 48–57.

Borsboom, D., Mellenbergh, G. J., & Van Heerden, J. (2004). The concept of validity. *Psychological Review, 111*, 1061–1071.

Brammer, R. (2002). Effects of experience and training on diagnostic accuracy. *Psychological Assessment, 14*, 110–113.

Brockington, I. F., Kendell, R. E., & Leff, J. P. (1978). Definitions of schizophrenia: Concordance and prediction of outcome. *Psychological Medicine, 8*, 387–398.

Brown, T. A., Di Nardo, P., & Barlow, D. H. (1994). *Anxiety disorders interview schedule for DSM-IV*. San Antonio, TX: Psychological Corporation.

Brown, T. A., Di Nardo, P. A., Lehman, C. L., & Campbell, L. A. (2001). Reliability of DSM-IV anxiety and mood disorders: Implications for the classification of emotional disorders. *Journal of Abnormal Psychology, 110*, 49–58.

Butcher, J. N. (2010). Personality assessment from the nineteenth to the early twentieth century: Past achievements and contemporary challenges. *Annual Review of Clinical Psychology, 6*, 1–20.

Butcher, J. N., Dahlstrom, W. G., Graham, J. R., Tellegen, A., & Kaemmer, B. (1989). *Manual for the administration and scoring of the MMPI-2*. Minneapolis: University of Minnesota Press.

Chapman, L. J., & Chapman, J. P. (1967). Genesis of popular but erroneous psychodiagnostic observations. *Journal of Abnormal Psychology, 72*, 193–204.

Chapman, L. J., & Chapman, J. P. (1969). Illusory correlation as an obstacle to the use of valid psychodiagnostic signs. *Journal of Abnormal Psychology, 74*, 271–280.

Clavelle, P. R., & Turner, A. D. (1980). Clinical decision-making among professionals and paraprofessionals. *Journal of Clinical Psychology, 36*, 833–838.

Cohen, P., & Cohen, J. (1984). The clinician's illusion. *Archives of General Psychiatry, 41*, 1178–1182.

Conners, K. (1989). *Manual for Conners' rating scales*. North Tonawanda, NY: Multi-Health Systems.

Cronbach, L. J., & Meehl, P. E. (1955). Construct validity in psychological tests. *Psychological Bulletin, 52*, 281–302.

Dawes, R. M. (1994). *House of cards: Psychology and psychotherapy built on myth*. New York: Free Press.

Dawes, R. M., Faust, D., & Meehl, P. E. (1989). Clinical versus actuarial judgment. *Science, 243*, 1668–1674.

Dyer, F. J., & McCann, J. T. (2000). The Millon clinical inventories, research critical of their forensic application, and Daubert criteria. *Law and Human Behavior, 24*, 487–497.

Einhorn, H. J. (1988). Diagnosis and causality in clinical and statistical prediction. In D. C. Turk & P. Salovey (Eds.), *Reasoning, inference, and judgment in clinical psychology* (pp. 51–70). New York: Free Press.

Exner, J. E. (1993). *The Rorschach: A Comprehensive System: Vol. 1: Basic Foundations* (3rd ed.). New York: Wiley.

Exner, J. E. (1995). Comment on "Narcissism in the Comprehensive System for the Rorschach." *Clinical Psychology: Science and Practice, 2*, 200–206.

Exner, J. E. (1996). Comment on "The Comprehensive System for the Rorschach: A Critical Examination." *Psychological Science, 7*, 11–13.

Exner, J. E. (2001a). A comment on "The Misperception of Psychopathology: Problems With the Norms of the Comprehensive System for the Rorschach." *Clinical Psychology: Science and Practice, 8*, 386–388.

Exner, J. E. (2001b). *A Rorschach workbook for the Comprehensive System* (5th ed.). Asheville, NC: Rorschach Workshops.

Faraone, S. V., & Tsuang, M. T. (1994). Measuring diagnostic accuracy in the absence of a "gold standard." *American Journal of Psychiatry, 151*, 650–657.

Finn, S. E., & Kamphuis, J. H. (1995). What a clinician needs to know about base rates. In J. Butcher (Ed.), *Clinical personality assessment: Practical approaches* (pp. 224–235). New York: Oxford University Press.

Fischhoff, B. (1975). Hindsight ≠ foresight: The effect of outcome knowledge on judgment under uncertainty. *Journal of Experimental Psychology: Human Perception and Performance, 1*, 288–299.

Fleiss, J. (1981). *Statistical methods for rates and proportions* (2nd ed.). New York: Wiley.

Ford, M., & Widiger, T. (1989). Sex bias in the diagnosis of histrionic and antisocial personality disorders. *Journal of Consulting and Clinical Psychology, 57*, 301–305.

Gadol, I. (1969). The incremental and predictive validity of the Rorschach test in personality assessments of normal, neurotic, and psychotic subjects. (UMI No. 69-4469). *Dissertation Abstracts, 29,* 3482B.

Garb, H. N. (1989). Clinical judgment, clinical training, and professional experience. *Psychological Bulletin, 105,* 387–396.

Garb, H. N. (1996). The representativeness and past-behavior heuristics in clinical judgment. *Professional Psychology: Research and Practice, 27,* 272–277.

Garb, H. N. (1997). Race bias, social class bias, and gender bias in clinical judgment. *Clinical Psychology: Science and Practice, 4,* 99–120.

Garb, H. N. (1998). *Studying the clinician: Judgment research and psychological assessment.* Washington, DC: American Psychological Association.

Garb, H. N. (2000). Computers will become increasingly important for psychological assessment: Not that there's anything wrong with that! *Psychological Assessment, 12,* 31–39.

Garb, H. N. (2003). Incremental validity and the assessment of psychopathology in adults. *Psychological Assessment, 15,* 508–520.

Garb, H. N. (2006). The conjunction effect and clinical judgment. *Journal of Social and Clinical Psychology, 25,* 1048–1056.

Garb, H. N., Florio, C. M., & Grove, W. M. (1998). The validity of the Rorschach and the Minnesota Multiphasic Personality Inventory: Results from meta-analyses. *Psychological Science, 9,* 402–404.

Garb, H. N., Lilienfeld, S. O., Nezworski, M. T., Wood, J. M., & O'Donohue, W. T. (2009). Can quality improvement processes help psychological assessment meet the demands of evidence-based practice? *Scientific Review of Mental Health Practice, 7* (1), 15–22.

Garb, H. N., Wood, J. M., Lilienfeld, S. O., & Nezworski, M. T. (2002). Effective use of projective techniques in clinical practice: Let the data help with selection and interpretation. *Professional Psychology: Research and Practice, 33,* 454–463.

Garb, H. N., Wood, J. M., & Nezworski, M. T. (2000). Projective techniques and the detection of child sexual abuse. *Child Maltreatment, 5,* 161–168.

Gauron, E. F., & Dickinson, J. K. (1969). The influence of seeing the patient first on diagnostic decision-making in psychiatry. *American Journal of Psychiatry, 126,* 199–205.

Gilovich, T. (1991). *How we know what isn't so.* New York: Free Press.

Goldberg, L. R. (1965). Diagnosticians versus diagnostic signs: The diagnosis of psychosis versus neurosis from the MMPI. *Psychological Monographs, 79*(9, Whole No. 602).

Graham, J. R. (1967). A Q-sort study of the accuracy of clinical descriptions based on the MMPI. *Journal of Psychiatric Research, 5,* 297–305.

Graham, J. R., Ben-Porath, Y. S., & McNulty, J. L. (1997). Empirical correlates of low scores on the MMPI-2 scales in an outpatient mental health setting. *Psychological Assessment, 9,* 386–391.

Greene, R. L. (2000). *The MMPI-2: An interpretive manual.* Needham Heights, MA: Allyn and Bacon.

Grove, W. M., & Meehl, P. E. (1996). Comparative efficiency of informal (subjective, impressionistic) and formal (mechanical, algorithmic) prediction procedures: The clinical-statistical controversy. *Psychology: Public Policy and Law, 2,* 293–323.

Grove, W. M., Zald, D. H., Lebow, B. S., Snitz, B. E., & Nelson, C. (2000). Clinical versus mechanical prediction: A meta-analysis. *Psychological Assessment, 12,* 19–30.

Guarnaccia, V., Dill, C. A., Sabatino, S., & Southwick, S. (2001). Scoring accuracy using the Comprehensive System for the Rorschach. *Journal of Personality Assessment, 77,* 464–474.

Hamel, M., Shaffer, T. W., & Erdberg, P. (2000). A study of nonpatient preadolescent Rorschach protocols. *Journal of Personality Assessment, 75,* 280–294.

Hampton, R. L., & Newberger, E. H. (1985). Child abuse incidence and reporting by hospitals: Significance of severity, class and race. *American Journal of Public Health, 75,* 56–60.

Harkness, A. R., & Lilienfeld, S. O. (1997). Individual differences science for treatment planning: Personality traits. *Psychological Assessment, 9,* 349–360.

Henry, B., Moffitt, T. E., Caspi, A., Langley, J., & Silva, P. A. (1994). On the "Remembrance of Things Past": A longitudinal evaluation of the retrospective method. *Psychological Assessment, 6,* 92–101.

Hiller, J. B., Rosenthal, R., Bornstein, R. F., Berry, D. T. R., & Brunell-Neuleib, S. (1999). A comparative meta-analysis of Rorschach and MMPI validity. *Psychological Assessment, 11,* 278–296.

Holmes, D. S. (1990). The evidence for repression: An examination of sixty years of research. In J. L. Singer (Ed.), *Repression and dissociation: Implications for personality theory, psychopathology, and health* (pp. 85–102). Chicago: University of Chicago Press.

Hunsley, J., & Di Giulio, G. (2001). Norms, norming, and clinical assessment. *Clinical Psychology: Science and Practice, 8,* 378–382.

Jorgensen, K., Andersen, T. J., & Dam, H. (2000). The diagnostic efficiency of the Rorschach Depression Index and the Schizophrenia Index: A review. *Assessment, 7,* 259–280.

Kahill, S. (1984). Human figure drawing in adults: An update of the empirical evidence, 1967–1982. *Canadian Psychology, 25,* 269–292.

Karon, B. P. (2000). The clinical interpretation of the thematic apperception test, Rorschach, and other clinical data: A reexamination of statistical versus clinical prediction. *Professional Psychology: Research and Practice, 31,* 230–233.

Lambert, M. J., & Finch, A. E. (1999). The Outcome Questionnaire. In M. E. Maruish (Ed.), *The use of psychological testing for treatment planning and outcomes assessment* (2nd ed., pp. 831–869). Mahwah, NJ: Erlbaum.

Lambert, M. J., Harmon, C., Slade, K., Whipple, J. L., & Hawkins, E. J. (2005). Providing feedback to psychotherapists on their patients' progress: Clinical results and suggestions. *Journal of Clinical Psychology/In Session, 61,* 165–174.

Lambert, M. J., Whipple, J. L., Hawkins, E. J., Vermeersch, D. A., Nielsen, S. L., & Smart, D. W. (2003). Is it time for clinicians to routinely track patient outcome? A meta-analysis. *Clinical Psychology: Science and Practice, 10,* 288–301.

Levenberg, S. B. (1975). Professional training, psychodiagnostic skill, and Kinetic Family Drawings. *Journal of Personality Assessment, 39,* 389–393.

Lilienfeld, S. O. (2002). When worlds collide: Social science, politics, and the Rind et al. (1998) child sexual abuse meta-analysis. *American Psychologist, 57,* 176–188.

Lilienfeld, S. O. (2010). Can psychology become a science? *Personality and Individual Differences, 49,* 281–288.

Lilienfeld, S. O., Wood, J. M., & Garb, H. N. (2000). The scientific status of projective techniques. *Psychological Science in the Public Interest, 1,* 27–66.

Lilienfeld, S. O., Wood, J. M., & Garb, H. N. (2001, May). What's wrong with this picture? *Scientific American, 284,* 80–87.

Lima, E. N., Stanley, S., Kaboski, B., Reitzel, L. R., Richey, J. A., Castro, Y., … Joiner, T. E. Jr. (2005). The incremental validity of the MMPI-2: When does therapist access not enhance treatment outcome? *Psychological Assessment, 17,* 462–468.

Litz, B. T., Miller, M. W., Ruef, A. M., & McTeague, L. M. (2002). Exposure to trauma in adults. In M. M. Antony & D. H. Barlow (Eds.), *Handbook of assessment and treatment planning for psychological disorders* (pp. 215–258). New York: Guilford.

Loevinger, J. (1957). Objective tests as instruments of psychological theory. *Psychological Reports, 3,* 635–694.

Logue, M. B., Sher, K. J., & Frensch, P. A. (1992). Purported characteristics of adult children of alcoholics: A possible "Barnum effect." *Professional Psychology: Research and Practice, 23,* 226–232.

Margraf, J., Taylor, C. B., Ehlers, A., Roth, W. T., & Agras, W. S. (1987). Panic attacks in the natural environment. *Journal of Nervous and Mental Disease, 175,* 558–565.

Matarazzo, J. D. (1990). Psychological assessment versus psychological testing: Validation from Binet to the school, clinic, and courtroom. *American Psychologist, 45,* 999–1017.

McFall, R. M. (1991). Manifesto for a science of clinical psychology. *Clinical Psychologist, 44,* 75–88.

McFall, R. M., & Treat, T. A. (1999). Quantifying the information value of clinical assessments with signal detection theory. *Annual Review of Psychology, 50,* 215–241.

Meehl, P. E. (1945). The dynamics of "structured" personality tests. *Journal of Clinical Psychology, 1,* 296–303.

Meehl, P. E. (1986). Diagnostic taxa as open concepts: Metatheoretical and statistical questions about reliability and construct validity in the grand strategy of nosological revision. In T. Millon & G. Klerman (Eds.), *Contemporary directions in psychopathology* (pp. 215–231). New York: Guilford.

Meehl, P. E., & Rosen, A. (1955). Antecedent probability and the efficiency of psychometric signs, patterns, or cutting scores. *Psychological Bulletin, 52,* 194–216.

Meehl, P. E. (1956). Wanted—A good cookbook. *American Psychologist, 11,* 263–272.

Meehl, P. E. (1973). Why I do not attend case conferences. In P. E. Meehl (Ed.), *Psychodiagnosis: Selected papers* (pp. 225–302). Minneapolis: University of Minnesota Press.

Meyer, G. J. (2001). Evidence to correct misperceptions about Rorschach norms. *Clinical Psychology: Science and Practice, 8,* 389–396.

Meyer, G. J., & Archer, R. P. (2001). The hard science of Rorschach research: What do we know and where do we go? *Psychological Assessment, 13,* 486–502.

Meyer, G. J., Erdberg, P., & Shaffer, T. W. (2007). Toward international normative reference data for the Comprehensive System. *Journal of Personality Assessment, 89,* S201–S216.

Meyer, G. J., & Handler, L. (1997). The ability of the Rorschach to predict subsequent outcome: A meta-analysis of the Rorschach prognostic rating scale. *Journal of Personality Assessment, 69,* 1–38.

Meyer, G. J., Hilsenroth, M. J., Baxter, D., Exner, J. E., Fowler, J. C., Piers, C. C., & Resnick, J. (2002). An examination of interrater reliability for scoring the Rorschach Comprehensive System in eight data sets. *Journal of Personality Assessment, 78*, 219–274.

Meyer, G. J., & Richardson, C. (2001, March). *An examination of changes in form quality codes in the Rorschach Comprehensive System from 1974 to 1995.* Presented at the midwinter meeting of the Society for Personality Assessment, Philadelphia, PA.

Millon, T. (1994). *The Millon Clinical Multiaxial Inventory-III manual.* Minneapolis, MN: National Computer Systems.

Molinari, V., Ames, A., & Essa, M. (1994). Prevalence of personality disorders in two geropsychiatric inpatient units. *Journal of Geriatric Psychiatry and Neurology, 7*, 209–215.

Morey, L. C. (1991). *Personality Assessment Inventory: Professional manual.* Tampa, FL: Psychological Assessment Resources.

Morey, L. C., & Ochoa, E. S. (1989). An investigation of adherence to diagnostic criteria: Clinical diagnosis of the DSM-III personality disorders. *Journal of Personality Disorders, 3*, 180–192.

Mukherjee, S., Shukla, S., Woodle, J., Rosen, A. M., & Olarte, S. (1983). Misdiagnosis of schizophrenia in bipolar patients: A multiethnic comparison. *American Journal of Psychiatry, 140*, 1571–1574.

Naglieri, J. A., & Pfeiffer, S. I. (1992). Performance of disruptive behavior-disordered and normal samples on the Draw-A-Person: Screening procedure for emotional disturbance. *Psychological Assessment, 4*, 156–159.

Nakata, L. M. (1999). Interrater reliability and the Comprehensive System for the Rorschach: Clinical and non-clinical protocols. (Doctoral dissertation, Pacific Graduate School of Psychology, 1999). *Dissertation Abstracts International, 60*, 4296B.

Nezworski, M. T., & Wood, J. M. (1995). Narcissism in the Comprehensive System for the Rorschach. *Clinical Psychology: Science and Practice, 2*, 179–199.

Nunnally, J. (1978). *Psychometric theory* (2nd ed.). New York: McGraw-Hill.

Oberlander, L. B. (1995). Psycholegal issues in child sexual abuse evaluations: A survey of forensic mental health professionals. *Child Abuse and Neglect, 19*, 475–490.

Parker, K. C. H., Hanson, R., & Hunsley, J. (1988). MMPI, Rorschach, and WAIS: A meta-analytic comparison of reliability, stability, and validity. *Psychological Bulletin, 103*, 367–373.

Percevic, R., Lambert, M. J., & Kordy, H. (2004). Computer-supported monitoring of patient treatment response. *Journal of Clinical Psychology, 60*, 285–299.

Rogers, R. (1995). *Diagnostic and structured interviewing: A handbook for psychologists.* Odessa, TX: Psychological Assessment Resources.

Rogers, R., Salekin, R. T., & Sewell, K. W. (1999). Validation of the Millon Clinical Multiaxial Inventory for Axis II disorders: Does it meet the *Daubert* standard? *Law and Human Behavior, 23*, 425–443.

Rogers, R., Salekin, R. T., & Sewell, K. W. (2000). The MCMI-III and the *Daubert* standard: Separating rhetoric from reality. *Law and Human Behavior, 24*, 501–506.

Rotton, J., & Kelly, I. W. (1985). Much ado about the full moon: A meta-analysis of lunar-lunacy research. *Psychological Bulletin, 97*, 286–306.

Sartorius, N., Kaelber, C. T., Cooper, J. E., Roper, M. T., Rae, D. S., Gulbinat, W., … Regier, D. A. (1993). Progress toward achieving a common language in psychiatry: Results from the field trial of the clinical guidelines accompanying the WHO classification of mental and behavioral disorders in *ICD-10*. *Archives of General Psychiatry, 50*, 115–124.

Savard, J., & Morin, C. M. (2002). Insomnia. In M. M. Antony & D. H. Barlow (Eds.), *Handbook of assessment and treatment planning for psychological disorders* (pp. 523–555). New York: Guilford.

Schacter, S. (1982). Recidivism and self-cure of smoking and obesity. *American Psychologist, 37*, 436–444.

Sellbom, M., Ben-Porath, Y. S., Lilienfeld, S. O., Patrick, C. J., & Graham, J. R. (2005). Assessing psychopathic personality traits with the MMPI-2. *Journal of Personality Assessment, 85*, 334–343.

Shaffer, T. W., Erdberg, P., & Haroian, J. (1999). Current nonpatient data for the Rorschach, WAIS-R, and MMPI-2. *Journal of Personality Assessment, 73*, 305–316.

Shear, M. K., Brown, T. A., Barlow, D. H., Money, R., Sholomskas, D. E., Woods, S. W., … Papp, L. A. (1997). Multicenter collaborative panic disorder severity scale. *American Journal of Psychiatry, 154*, 1571–1575.

Simon, R. J., Fleiss, J. L., Gurland, B. J., Stiller, P. R., & Sharpe, L. (1973). Depression and schizophrenia in hospitalized black and white mental patients. *Archives of General Psychiatry, 28*, 509–512.

Snyder, C. R., & Larson, G. R. (1972). A further look at student acceptance of general personality interpretations. *Journal of Consulting and Clinical Psychology, 38*, 384–388.

Snyder, D. K. (2000). Computer-assisted judgment: Defining strengths and liabilities. *Psychological Assessment, 12*, 52–60.

Spangler, W. D. (1992). Validity of questionnaire and TAT measures of need for achievement: Two meta-analyses. *Psychological Bulletin, 112*, 140–154.

Spitzer, R. L. (1983). Psychiatric diagnosis: Are clinicians still necessary? *Comprehensive Psychiatry, 24*, 399–411.

Starr, B. J., & Katkin, E. S. (1969). The clinician as an aberrant actuary: Illusory correlation and the incomplete sentences blank. *Journal of Abnormal Psychology, 74*, 670–675.

Steiner, J. L., Tebes, J. K., Sledge, W. H., & Walker, M. L. (1995). A comparison of the structured clinical interview for DSM-III-R and clinical diagnoses. *Journal of Nervous and Mental Disease, 183*, 365–369.

Strohmer, D. C., Shivy, V. A., & Chiodo, A. L. (1990). Information processing strategies in counselor hypothesis testing: The role of selective memory and expectancy. *Journal of Counseling Psychology, 37*, 465–472.

Trowbridge, M. M. (1995). Graphic indicators of sexual abuse in children's drawings: A review of the literature. *Arts in Psychotherapy, 22*, 485–493.

Trull, T. J., & Phares, E. J. (2001). *Clinical Psychology* (6th ed.). Belmont, CA: Wadsworth.

Turner, D. R. (1966). Predictive efficiency as a function of amount of information and level of professional experience. *Journal of Projective Techniques and Personality Assessment, 30*, 4–11.

Tversky, A., & Kahneman, D. (1983). Extensional vs. intuitive reasoning: The conjunction fallacy in probability judgment. *Psychological Review, 90*, 293–315.

Waller, N. G. (1998). Searching for structure in the MMPI. In S. E. Embretson & S. L. Hershberger (Eds.), *The new rules of measurement* (pp. 185–217). Mahwah, NJ: Erlbaum.

Weiner, I. B. (2000). Using the Rorschach properly in practice and research. *Journal of Clinical Psychology, 56*, 435–438.

Weiner, I. B. (2001). Advancing the science of psychological assessment: The Rorschach Inkblot method as exemplar. *Psychological Assessment, 13*, 423–432.

Westen, D., Lohr, N., Silk, K. R., Gold, L., & Kerber, K. (1990). Object relations and social cognition in borderlines, major depressives, and normals: A thematic apperception test analysis. *Psychological Assessment, 2*, 355–364.

Westen, D., Ludolph, P., Block, M. J., Wixom, J., & Wiss, F. C. (1990). Developmental history and object relations in psychiatrically disturbed adolescent girls. *American Journal of Psychiatry, 147*, 1061–1068.

Whitehead, W. C. (1985). Clinical decision making on the basis of Rorschach, MMPI, and automated MMPI report data. (Doctoral dissertation, University of Texas Southwestern Medical Center at Dallas, 1985). *Dissertation Abstracts International, 46*, 2828.

Widiger, T. A. (2001). The best and the worst of us? *Clinical Psychology: Science and Practice, 8*, 374–377.

Widiger, T. A. (2002). Personality disorders. In M. M. Antony & D. H. Barlow (Eds.), *Handbook of assessment and treatment planning for psychological disorders* (pp. 453–480). New York: Guilford.

Wood, J. M., Garb, H. N., Lilienfeld, S. O., & Nezworski, M. T. (2002). Clinical assessment. *Annual Review of Psychology, 53*, 519–543.

Wood, J. M., Garb, H. N., & Nezworski, M. T. (2007). Psychometrics: Better measurement makes better clinicians. In S. O. Lilienfeld & W. T. O'Donohue (Eds.), *The great ideas of clinical science: The 17 concepts that every mental health practitioner should understand* (pp. 77–92). New York: Brunner-Routledge.

Wood, J. M., Lilienfeld, S. O., Garb, H. N., & Nezworski, M. T. (2000). The Rorschach test in clinical diagnosis: A critical review, with a backward look at Garfield (1947). *Journal of Clinical Psychology, 56*, 395–430.

Wood, J. M., Lilienfeld, S. O., Nezworski, M. T., Garb, H. N., Allen, K. H., & Wildermuth, J. L. (2010). Validity of Rorschach inkblot scores for discriminating psychopaths from nonpsychopaths in forensic populations: A meta-analysis. *Psychological Assessment, 22*, 336–349.

Wood, J. M., Nezworski, M. T., Garb, H. N., & Lilienfeld, S. O. (2001a). Problems with the norms of the Comprehensive System for the Rorschach: Methodological and conceptual considerations. *Clinical Psychology: Science and Practice, 8*, 397–402.

Wood, J. M., Nezworski, M. T., Garb, H. N., & Lilienfeld, S. O. (2001b). The misperception of psychopathology: Problems with the norms of the Comprehensive System for the Rorschach. *Clinical Psychology: Science and Practice, 8*, 350–373.

Wood, J. M., Nezworski, M. T., Lilienfeld, S. O., & Garb, H. N. (2003). *What's wrong with the Rorschach? Science confronts the controversial inkblot test.* San Francisco, CA: Jossey-Bass.

Wood, J. M., Nezworski, M. T., & Stejskal, W. J. (1996a). The Comprehensive System for the Rorschach: A critical examination. *Psychological Science, 7*, 3–10.

Wood, J. M., Nezworski, M. T., & Stejskal, W. J. (1996b). Thinking critically about the Comprehensive System for the Rorschach: A reply to Exner. *Psychological Science, 7*, 14–17.

World Health Organization. (1992). *The ICD-10 classification of mental and behavioural disorders. Clinical descriptions and diagnostic guidelines.* Geneva: Author.

7

Psychotherapy Research

REBECCA E. STEWART and DIANNE L. CHAMBLESS

University of Pennsylvania
Philadelphia, Pennsylvania

The focus of this book is on the study of psychopathology and its assessment and treatment. Understanding psychopathology is an important part of the science of psychology in its own right, but it is more than pure science. Psychopathology research plays an important role in the development of interventions to ameliorate mental disorders and to promote well-being. Almost every chapter in Part II of this text includes material on treatment for the disorders in question, usually based on the outcome of treatment research. Where does this information come from? This chapter will describe the process by which psychotherapy research is conducted and the controversies surrounding the proper nature and role of such research.

Psychotherapy Research

Psychotherapy research is a broad field encompassing a number of streams of research. *Process research*, designed to identify and delineate the important events in therapy, typically addresses what happens in a therapeutic session and investigates such variables as therapist behaviors, client behaviors, and interactions between the therapist and the client. For example, a common theme in psychoanalytic therapy research is the characteristics of transference (Connolly, Crits-Christoph, Barber, & Luborsky, 2000). *Outcome research* focuses on the effects of psychotherapy, both immediate and long-term changes in the problems for which a person seeks or is referred for treatment as well as improvement on broader variables such as quality of life or interpersonal functioning. Not surprisingly, process research is often linked to outcome research so as to identify factors that may be important in treatment outcome. For example, meta-analyses indicate that the better the client–therapist alliance, the better the treatment outcome, with the alliance accounting for about 5% of the variance in improvement (Martin, Garske, & Davis, 2000).

Yet other questions in psychotherapy research include prediction of treatment outcome—what are the characteristics of clients who do well in this treatment—or, to answer a more sophisticated question, who will do well in this treatment but not in that treatment? For example, Barber and Muenz (1996) showed that in treatment of major depression, interpersonal therapy was better for clients with obsessive-compulsive personality traits, whereas cognitive-behavior therapy was better for clients with avoidant personality traits. Such findings demonstrate *moderation* of treatment outcome by a patient characteristic, in this case, specific personality traits. Finally, *mediation* of treatment outcome is an important area of study. Mediation research asks, what are the mechanisms underlying treatment efficacy? For example, in a study comparing several forms of treatment for attention-deficit/hyperactivity disorder Hinshaw et al. (2000) found that the impact of treatment on children's social skills at school was mediated by parents' use of negative or ineffective discipline. In other words, to the degree that treatment reduced parents' use of negative or ineffective discipline, children's social skills at school improved. Although all of these forms of psychotherapy research are important, the focus in this chapter will be mainly be on psychotherapy outcome research.

A Prototypical Psychotherapy Outcome Study

There is no one method of outcome research accepted by all types of psychotherapy researchers. What is described here is the reigning paradigm for major studies such as those funded by the National Institute of Mental Health in which the efficacy of one or more treatments is tested, as well as the paradigm accepted for research on empirically supported treatments, which will be defined in a later section. We will address some of the controversies about this paradigm later in this chapter. To establish *efficacy*, a psychological intervention is tested under well-controlled circumstances. If it proves to be beneficial in multiple studies, then researchers may turn their attention to *effectiveness* research, in which the generalization of the treatment's benefits to less well-controlled, more real world circumstances is examined. Hence, the first efforts have a strong focus on internal validity, whereas later efforts may concentrate on external validity (Moras, 1998). In yet later stages, researchers may focus on issues of cost-effectiveness and the ease of dissemination of a treatment to a wide audience of clinicians, settings, and consumers (Baker, McFall, & Shoham, 2008).

Research Designs

Both single case experiments (Barlow & Hersen, 1973) and randomized controlled trials (RCTs) allow close controls on the internal validity of research. These experimental methods, properly conducted, allow the investigator to draw causal inferences about the efficacy of a treatment. Because RCTs are far more common, We will focus on this approach here. In RCTs, patients are randomly assigned to the treatment of interest or to one or more control groups or alternative treatments. Without random assignment, it would be impossible to know whether any differences observed among treatments were due to the treatments or to systematic preexisting differences among patients. Control groups are used to determine whether any improvement with treatment might be due simply to effects such as the passage of time, the assessment procedures (e.g., talking at length about your problems with the clinical assessor), or to making a decision to do something about the problem. The simplest control group is a *waiting list condition*, where clients receive the treatment under investigation after a prescribed delay during which they participate in assessment. Usually the delay period is for the length of the treatment, but for severely distressed clients, this may be shortened for ethical reasons. Waiting list conditions are similar to the delay many clients undergo when they seek treatment at clinics, but there are drawbacks, including the ethical concern about postponing treatment and the fact that a number of clients will seek treatment elsewhere or lose their resolve to undergo treatment during the waiting period.

Waiting list control conditions allow the researcher to draw an important conclusion that perhaps many consumers want to know: Does the treatment work better than no treatment? However, such control groups are unsatisfactory if the researcher or consumer wants to know whether the treatment adds to the so-called nonspecific effects of psychotherapy. That is, does the treatment work because of placebo effects, the belief in and hope of change that occur when people think they are getting treatment? Does the treatment work simply because the clients get to talk with a sympathetic person about their problems? If so, there is nothing that is specifically helpful about this treatment versus any other, and no justification for having highly trained psychotherapists versus counselors with less training deliver the treatment. *Placebo control conditions* (e.g., a pill placebo combined with regular brief meetings with a supportive psychiatrist) and *alternative therapy conditions* (e.g., supportive counseling) provide for another level of analysis than the waiting list control group. However, these control groups are also not without their problems. For ethical reasons, patients given a placebo receive the real treatment at the end of the treatment period, but many may drop out before that time to seek other treatment if it is available. If patients who received supportive counseling are not satisfied with their improvement in treatment, they may get additional treatment during the follow-up period, which precludes controlled assessment of long-term outcome.

Finally, the researcher may choose to compare the treatment of interest to various medications or to other forms of psychotherapy known or believed to be efficacious for the types of problems being treated. Comparisons of two or more types of psychotherapy are less common at this point than is research designed to develop and test the efficacy of one treatment. For many disorders there are not yet two or more psychological approaches that have each been determined to yield satisfactory treatment benefits relative to waiting list or placebo control groups, making such comparisons premature. However, comparisons of psychotherapy with medication and with the combination of medication and psychotherapy are frequently conducted.

Typically in the development of a particular treatment, the research follows this course: First, an uncontrolled study is initiated in which the effects of the treatment are tested by comparing clients' status before and after treatment; second, comparisons are made with waiting list control groups; third, comparisons are made with placebo or basic counseling; and fourth, comparisons are made with medication or other efficacious psychotherapies. At each stage, the comparisons become more stringent, and the number of participants required for the research increases. Statistically significant effects between a treatment and waiting list control group may be obtained with 25 patients per condition, but comparisons between two efficacious treatments or between psychotherapy and a medication will require 50 or more patients per group to be able to detect differences in efficacy that are clinically important (Kazdin & Bass, 1989). Consider that the typical psychotherapy–medication trial includes the following conditions: psychotherapy plus placebo, medication alone, medication plus psychotherapy, pill placebo plus clinical management (meetings with a supportive, encouraging psychiatrist for medication monitoring), and perhaps psychotherapy without pill placebo (to control for any effects of the patients' thinking they are on medication, which may have a positive or negative impact). For such a trial, then, 250 or more patients are required, often requiring multiple treatment sites to obtain enough participants. As a result, these studies are very expensive to mount and virtually impossible to conduct without major government grants. For this reason, psychotherapy research proceeds more slowly than pharmacotherapy research, which is funded largely by the pharmaceutical industry. There is, of course, no psychotherapy industry to fund research in this area.

Defining the Intervention

For pharmacotherapy researchers, it is fairly easy to define the treatment intervention: Provide the drug (or pill placebo identical in appearance) in the proper therapeutic dosage and monitor its use and side effects. For psychotherapy researchers, the process is more difficult. The researcher must carefully describe the treatment approaches being studied such that the study therapists and the ultimate readers of the study (clinicians and other researchers) know exactly what treatment was tested. This is accomplished by writing a treatment manual that details the principles and procedures used in the treatment. How structured such manuals are tends to vary with the type of therapy tested. For example, cognitive-behavioral treatment manuals are often highly detailed, frequently with session-by-session outlines. In contrast, manuals for psychodynamic psychotherapy may rely on broader brush strokes, describing treatment principles and the types of conditions under which the therapist chooses one possible intervention over another, such as when to interpret the patient's behavior versus when to be supportive.

Manuals often become more and more highly detailed across research trials and end up being book length.

Manuals are critical to treatment research in that they permit dissemination of efficacious treatments (others can read how the treatments were done) and because they provide the operational definition of the treatment. Labels for treatments are often not sufficiently informative. For example, there are many versions of psychodynamic treatment, some of which are radically different from others. Just which dynamic treatment approaches were followed in this study? Using manuals also tightens the internal validity of the study by reducing unwanted experimental variance. When therapists have a treatment manual to follow, there is less variability in the outcomes of the individual therapists employed in the treatment trial (Crits-Christoph et al., 1991).

It is not enough that the study therapists are provided with a treatment manual. They must also be trained in delivering this treatment and then monitored during the study for their adherence to the treatment manual and their competence in carrying out the treatment. Trained raters watch videotapes of treatment sessions and use rating scales to determine whether therapists are following the key procedures of the treatment and are avoiding mixing in other treatments that are not to be included in this study. Expert raters also watch these tapes to code the therapists' skill. Ensuring that the therapists delivered the treatment in at least a minimally competent way is vital to the eventual acceptance of the study and the treatment. Readers can easily reject findings counter to their own beliefs if they can discount the results because therapist competence and adherence were not demonstrated.

Selecting the Treatment Sample and Assessing Outcome

An early step in designing a treatment outcome study is selecting the target population and the sample. Again, an operational definition is required. Earlier in the history of psychotherapy research, the description of the study sample was often quite broad, for example, in the case of neurotic outpatients. The present practice is to define study samples more precisely, usually with a specific diagnosis from the *Diagnostic and Statistical Manual of Mental Disorders* (American Psychiatric Association, 1994), such as borderline personality disorder. However, samples may also be defined on the basis of characteristics other than formal diagnoses. For example, Markman, Renick, Floyd, Stanley, and Clements (1993) developed a program designed to prevent marital dissatisfaction and divorce and targeted unselected engaged couples. Others have created programs to reduce drinking and problems associated with alcohol use in college students who drink heavily but do not meet the diagnostic criteria for an alcohol use disorder (Carey, Carey, Maisto, & Henson, 2006).

The researcher also determines the study's exclusion criteria. Who is omitted? Thus, for example, acutely suicidal patients who require immediate hospitalization are excluded from most outpatient studies for ethical reasons. Alcohol- and substance-dependent patients are usually excluded from trials for treatment of other disorders they may have until their chemical dependencies have been addressed because these problems tend to interfere with progress in other areas. In the intake process, the typical RCT screens out about two thirds of the people who initially contacted the project (Westen & Morrison, 2001). This means that for the 250-patient medication versus psychotherapy RCT described earlier, over 750 potential participants would need to be screened for the study.

To determine who enters the study and who improves in treatment, reliable and valid means of assessing the patients' problems and symptom severity are required. Questionnaire measures are often used to assess change in treatment, but interviews are commonly employed to make initial diagnoses as well as to monitor change over time. Interviewers must be carefully trained to be reliable in their assessments, and their reliability across the course of the study must be monitored by another trained rater who is uninformed as to the initial diagnosis or severity rating.

Empirically Validated Treatments

Several of the chapters in Part II of this volume mention the terms *empirically validated treatments* or *empirically supported treatments* (ESTs). In general these terms are used interchangeably to refer to treatments that have met the standards set by one or more groups who have reviewed the psychotherapy literature to identify treatments that work for particular disorders or presenting problems (see Chambless & Ollendick, 2001, for a review). These efforts were initiated in the United States by Division 12 (Society of Clinical Psychology) of the American Psychological Association (APA). Division 12's task force on the Promotion and Dissemination of Psychological Procedures (later the Committee on Science and Practice) defined ESTs as treatments that were *probably efficacious* or *efficacious*. Probably efficacious treatments are those that have been found to be superior to waiting list control groups in two or more studies, that have been found to be superior to another treatment in at least one study, or that have been found to be superior to another treatment in multiple studies but only tested by one research group. Efficacious treatments were defined as those that have proved more beneficial than placebo conditions or alternative treatments by more than one research group. (These are abbreviated criteria. A complete description can be found in Chambless et al., 1998.) In both cases, when multiple studies were available, the preponderance of the most exacting evidence had to favor the treatment's efficacy. Moreover, treatments had to be tested according to the methods described in this section for rigorous psychotherapy research. DeRubeis and Crits-Christoph (1998) provided examples of the efficacy evidence for a number of treatments of adult disorders.

At the time of their 2001 review, Chambless and Ollendick noted that the various review groups tackling the psychotherapy literature had identified 108 ESTs for adults and 37 for children. Although an updated comprehensive review has not yet been published, APA's Division 12 maintains an updated, online version of the list of empirically supported treatments, listing treatments with "strong," "modest," and "controversial" research support (http://www .psychologicaltreatments.org). With support from the National Institute for Health and Clinical Excellence (in the United Kingdom), an additional website has been developed to help consumers and therapists access information about ESTs (http://www.nice.org.uk). The identification of ESTs may be categorized as a part of the *evidence-based practice* movement. According to the principles of evidence-based practice, clinicians are encouraged to integrate the best research evidence regarding possible treatment of a patient with their clinical expertise and consideration of the patient's characteristics and values (Levant, 2005; Sackett, Straus, Richardson, Rosenberg, & Haynes, 2000). Thus, evidence-based practice includes not only EST research but also any other sort of evidence the practitioner might bring to bear on treatment decisions, for example, knowledge of the importance of building positive expectations for change and of developing a strong working alliance with the client. Compilations of ESTs are intended to serve as quick guides for clinicians, students, and educators who want to learn more about how to effectively treat a variety of disorders but who do not have time or the expertise to conduct extensive literature reviews themselves. Presently the Commission on Accreditation of the American Psychological Association, which reviews and accredits doctoral programs and internships in professional psychology in the United States, requires that at least some of a student's didactic and practical training be devoted to the study of ESTs (Office of Program Consultation and Accreditation, 2009). The newly developed Psychological Clinical Science Accrediting System for clinical psychology programs places even heavier emphasis on training in empirically supported treatments for doctoral students (Baker et al., 2008; http://www.pcsas.org).

A Costly Endeavor

We have covered only a partial list of the requirements for conducting a sound psychotherapy research trial (see Chambless & Hollon, in press, for a more complete description). However, this should be sufficient to understand that the psychotherapy researcher's efforts must be exhaustive and are exhausting! In addition, such research requires a great deal of patience. Psychotherapy trials often take 5 years to complete the evaluation of all patients' progress from the beginning to the end of treatment and another 2 years to complete assessment of treatment response at follow-up. The amount of time required to treat each participant is great, ranging from about 12 sessions of treatment of at least 50 min each to a year or more of treatment for severe psychopathology such as borderline personality disorder. The amount of effort that goes into treating and assessing each patient and the process of treatment and the requirements for highly trained personnel to carry out these activities makes such research a very expensive endeavor. Moreover, one study is not sufficient to demonstrate convincingly that a treatment is efficacious. Multiple replications, especially by other researchers not intimately involved in the development of the treatment, are essential.

Effectiveness Research

Once a treatment's efficacy has been established, it is time to export or disseminate the treatment to the community to test whether it works outside the hot house of the research clinic, that is, to conduct *effectiveness research.* Such tests include determining whether treatments work with the type of patients who may not have participated in university-based research trials (e.g., less-educated patients), in primary care practices, and community mental health centers, when provided by less highly trained personnel, and so forth. Because the focus of such research is on external validity or generalization beyond the research clinic, the designs are often less tightly controlled and may be simple pretest–posttest studies with no control group. In such cases, "benchmarking" may be used. That is, the results of the effectiveness study may be compared to those in published efficacy research. It typically takes many years to move from the initial uncontrolled pilot studies, through efficacy research, to the effectiveness stage of research. However, demonstrating effectiveness of research-proven efficacious in RCTs is now a major thrust of the National Institute of Mental Health, and this has served to move research more quickly to tests of effectiveness (see Baker et al., 2008, for examples of ESTs with established effectiveness).

Given that psychotherapy research is difficult to conduct and very costly, why do it? We turn to this question next.

The Case for Psychotherapy Research

First, Do No Harm

The U.S. Food and Drug Administration requires rigorous testing of medications before they are made available to the public through their physicians. The rationale is that it is important to determine before dissemination whether the drug has harmful effects and whether its beneficial effects outweigh any harmful effects observed. There is no formal equivalent for testing new psychological interventions. Rather, psychologists' ethical code (American Psychological Association, 2002) exhorts them to let clients know whether a treatment is experimental and to avoid the use of treatments that might be harmful. That is, psychologists are largely expected to police themselves, although occasionally a state licensing board may take action against a psychologist using bogus treatments for which he or she has made unsubstantiated claims.

Some would argue that it is unnecessary to test psychological procedures before their widespread use because psychotherapy is undoubtedly beneficial or, at worst, innocuous. We take issue with this claim on two grounds. First, psychotherapy can be harmful. For example, Dishion, McCord, and Poulin (1999) found that peer group interventions for delinquent teens increased adolescent problem behavior and negative life outcomes in adulthood compared with control conditions. This research project, and others like it, was critical in determining that a seemingly logical treatment was actually harmful. Bootzin and Bailey (2005) and Lilienfeld (2007) provide other examples of treatments that may produce more harm than good, such as critical incident stress debriefing, a commonly used method of immediate (1-week posttrauma) crisis counseling designed to combat posttraumatic stress disorder (PTSD). In some studies participants in groups using this intervention approach have had more, rather than fewer, PTSD symptoms postintervention than participants in control groups.

Second, an ineffective treatment is in itself harmful. An example is facilitated communication for autistic children, which ostensibly enabled children with developmental disabilities to communicate using a computer keyboard and to demonstrate that they were far more cognitively capable than was apparent. This intervention generated great excitement until controlled research repeatedly demonstrated that the results either did not occur or were created, in all likelihood unknowingly, by the facilitator (Herbert, Sharp, & Gaudiano, 2002). Without this research, many parents would have continued to have their hopes cruelly and falsely raised, and resources for the treatment of these severely disabled children would have continued to be diverted from programs that might be genuinely helpful and assigned instead to a bogus intervention.

Some disorders worsen without effective treatment. Under these circumstances, providing a patient with an ineffective treatment when effective ones exist is not innocuous. For example, we have seen patients with severe anxiety disorders who had years, even decades, of ineffective treatment while they lost their jobs, their friends, their avocations, and their life savings. When the efficacy of cognitive-behavioral treatments for such disorders has been repeatedly demonstrated (see Williams, this volume), withholding such treatment in the face of patient deterioration is not a neutral act. The ethics code of the American Psychological Association (2002) requires that psychologists refer clients who are not improving in their care for other treatment. Without psychotherapy research, clinicians cannot know what effective treatments are available.

Psychotherapists as Decision Makers

Others claim that psychotherapy research is unnecessary because practicing clinicians know best how to treat their patients based on their clinical training, expertise, and lore (Silver, 2001; Silverman, 1996). There is a surprising dearth of research on psychotherapists' decision making. However, in a recent survey of psychologists in private practice, clinicians reported that they were most likely to rely on their clinical experiences when making treatment decisions (Stewart & Chambless, 2007). How accurate is clinical judgment? There is a large body of research on clinicians' decision making regarding psychological assessments, much of which suggests clinical experience does not increase practitioners' ability to reach valid conclusions if they rely on clinical judgment rather than empirical data in the assessment process (see Garb, Lilienfeld, & Fowler, this volume). Making a decision about how to treat a new client or a client who is not responding to the present treatment plan is the result of an assessment process and is likely subject to the same errors in judgment if clinical experience is the only guide.

Kadden, Cooney, Getter, and Litt (1989) asked therapists of inpatients with alcohol dependence to predict which of two aftercare treatment programs would be better for their patients. The patients were randomly assigned to one of two treatments, and the authors found that patient data (e.g., severity of psychopathology) predicted which treatment would work better for certain patients. In contrast, the inpatient therapists predicted no better than chance which treatments would work for certain patients, despite their extensive contact with these patients; much more contact than merely an outpatient therapist usually has to take place before embarking on a treatment plan. Schulte, Kunzel, Pepping, and Schulte-Bahrenberg (1992) randomly assigned patients with phobias to standardized treatment with exposure or to an individualized program of cognitive-behavior therapy of the therapist's device. The same therapists participated in both conditions. Therapists in this study were significantly more effective in treating patients with phobic disorders when they were constrained to use the EST of choice (exposure) than they were when they were allowed to devise their own treatment plans, which typically included less exposure than the mandated treatment. These therapists, then, although experienced in treating phobic disorders, thought they could do better than the research-supported efficacious treatment by developing a treatment plan for their clients. They were wrong. Much more research is needed to test whether clinicians are more effective when they follow the treatment recommended by the research literature rather than when they follow their clinical intuitions, but so far the evidence indicates they should follow the data. This may be a distasteful thought to many practitioners (Silverman, 1996).

Why might clinical experience be a less accurate guide to treatment decisions than psychotherapists tend to believe? A variety of forces converge to make decisions about psychotherapy based on unsystematic observation vulnerable to error (Dawes, Faust, & Meehl, 1989). The amount of information that must be processed in psychotherapy is enormous and it taxes the cognitive capacity of humans as information processors. This leaves clinicians open to the many cognitive biases that influence the attention, selection, and interpretation of feedback they may receive. It is easy for even the most well meaning of us to deceive ourselves under such circumstances.

A historical example is readily known to many students of abnormal psychology. In the early 1770s, Franz Mesmer developed a technique based on his theory of animal magnetism, which posited the existence of palliative magnetic fluids in nature. With a combination of light, music, and chanting, Mesmer produced *mesmerism*, which allegedly moved the magnetic fluids, curing the body and mind of diseases (Pattie, 1994). Mesmer enjoyed great success and popularity with his procedure in Europe. What may be less likely to be covered in undergraduate texts is the debunking of mesmerism. King Louis XVI commissioned the French Academy of Sciences, including Benjamin Franklin, then resident in Paris, to investigate Mesmer and his therapeutics. Using an early and literal example of the single blind study (wherein patients do not know which treatment they are receiving), the commissioners blindfolded patients so that they would not know whether they were being mesmerized. They discovered that patients' responses depended not on the treatment procedure, but on whether they believed they had been mesmerized, in short, on the placebo effect. Franklin concluded, "Some think it will put an end to Mesmerism, but there is a wonderful deal of credulity in the world, and deceptions as absurd have supported themselves for ages" (cited in Isaacson, 2004, p. 427). The case of mesmerism illustrates the dangers of reliance on uncontrolled observations of practitioners and patients.

Thinking that a treatment works when it does not is one kind of mistake a therapist may make, but what about the other type of mistake, when therapists think a treatment may be harmful when it is actually beneficial? Prolonged exposure to images, thoughts, and other stimuli associated with trauma has by far the greatest evidentiary base for treatment of posttraumatic stress disorder (Foa, Rothbaum, Riggs, & Murdock, 1991). However, despite its strong endorsement by experts, prolonged exposure is underutilized by clinicians in the field, who cite a variety of reasons for their reluctance, none of which are empirically based (Becker, Zayfert, & Anderson, 2004). In particular, clinicians feared that prolonged exposure leads to symptom worsening. In contrast, the available evidence shows that patients who receive exposure therapy experience better outcomes and no reliable worsening of symptoms compared to patients in waiting list conditions and other treatments (Cahill et al., 2010).

Garb et al. (this volume) describe a number of cognitive biases that may affect clinicians' decision making in the assessment process. These also come into play in practitioners' assessments of treatment efficacy. Psychotherapists are in a particularly difficult situation, in that unless they make concerted efforts to systematically collect information on their practice, they rarely receive clear-cut feedback on their outcomes. Patients often leave treatment without explanation—some because they are doing better, and some because they are dissatisfied. Others may leave saying they are feeling better because they are uncomfortable with telling their therapist that they are disgruntled. Moreover, many factors contribute to patients' improvement or deterioration, only one of which is the patient's psychotherapy, making causal attributions difficult even when it is clear that a patient is doing well or not. Such an information vacuum is fertile ground for cognitive errors. We will present a few examples here.

First, many problems for which people seek treatment are subject to so-called *spontaneous remission*. That is to say, clients get better because the disorder has run its course or because other forces in their environment or their own efforts have led to improvement. The waiting list control group is designed to detect such improvement and to prevent researchers from concluding that a treatment is efficacious when change would have occurred without the intervention. Practitioners, however, have no control group and thus are subject to the "illusory correlation," believing that their interventions led to the change when, in fact, there was no causal connection. In addition, once clinicians, like anyone else, begin to believe that an intervention is beneficial for a certain type of client, they may tend to look for evidence that supports their hypothesis and ignore evidence to the contrary. This is called the *myside bias*.

The operation of the *availability heuristic* means that certain types of memory errors are likely. When clinicians search their memory banks for an intervention that was helpful in the past for a particular situation, they may recall a salient example of a time the intervention was associated with dramatic improvement and forget all the times it did not help. The availability heuristic may also account for the "clinician's illusion." Cohen and Cohen (1984) coined this term to describe psychotherapists' beliefs that clinical disorders are more severe and enduring than epidemiological evidence indicates. Vessey, Howard, Lueger, Kächele, and Mergenthaler (1994) demonstrated that most clients stay in psychotherapy for 6 months or less, but that those clients who do remain long term take up an increasing part of the therapist's practice as they accrue. Thus, it is easy for practitioners to conclude erroneously that most patients who enter treatment are long term and that psychopathology is generally unremitting because these are the cases that readily come to mind. Absent systematic records, it appears that practitioners cannot accurately calculate the characteristics of their caseloads (Knesper, Pagnucco, & Wheeler, 1985). Yet how long clients stay in treatment seems relatively simple, discrete information compared to the assessment of clients' response to treatment interventions.

Do psychotherapists really know how well their patients are doing? Perhaps not. Hannan et al. (2005) compared the judgment of clinicians in a college counseling center to a research-derived algorithm for prediction of treatment failure and found that clinicians were quite poor at predicting outcome, whereas the actuarial method worked very well. Hannan and colleagues noted that therapists rarely predicted deterioration, even though it occurred in 42 of 550 patients. In contrast, the empirical method identified all of the patients who would become reliably worse, although it also generated numerous false-positive results, that is, a prediction of deterioration when deterioration did not occur. Nevertheless, the false positives did have poorer outcomes than those not identified as likely treatment failures. These data speak to the importance of collecting data in clinical practice rather than relying on unsystematic observation.

The purpose of this discussion is not to insinuate that clinicians are incompetent or unresponsive to facts, but rather to make the point that clinicians are subject to the same illusions, biases, and memory distortions as anyone else and that they deal with very complex data. Nor is this discussion meant to downplay the importance of clinical lore and intuition. Clinical experience is a rich source of hypotheses about disorders and their treatments that, when submitted to experimental testing, have led to a variety of efficacious treatments. Nonetheless, the reliance of many clinicians on clinical judgment is exceedingly problematic in light of the literature on the superiority of data-based predictions over clinical judgment.

Rejection of Psychotherapy Research

As noted previously, some practitioners reject the importance of psychotherapy research for their practice, believing clinical expertise is all that is required. Others object to specific aspects of EST research, the predominant paradigm at present. We will present a few of those objections here (see also Chambless & Ollendick, 2001; Norcross, Beutler, & Levant, 2006).

Nonspecific Factors Rule

According to some authors (e.g., Ahn & Wampold, 2001; Wampold et al., 1997), the only important factors in psychotherapy outcome are so-called nonspecific factors that are common to all treatments. These include hope, expectation of change, and a good relationship with the therapist. A great deal of research bears witness to the importance of such factors in treatment outcomes (Orlinsky, Grawe, & Parks, 1994), and it is a rare psychologist who would argue that better treatment results are obtained by having an uncaring attitude toward one's clients and communicating to them that therapy is unlikely to work. The controversy, therefore, is not over the importance of the nonspecific factors but rather concerns whether different treatment interventions have an impact above and beyond these factors. In our view, this will depend on whether particular treatments rely on specific and effective treatment interventions attuned to the psychopathology of a disorder. For example, in a recent meta-analysis, Siev and Chambless (2007) demonstrated that cognitive-behavior therapy is significantly more effective for panic disorder than are relaxation-based therapies, whereas this is not the case for generalized anxiety disorder. This difference may arise because the psychopathology of panic disorder is now well understood, and effective treatment interventions have been carefully designed to address it. Treatment of generalized anxiety disorder leads to significant change, but the degree to which patients improve remains unsatisfactory in that fewer than half change to a clinically significant degree. Accordingly, researchers in that area are reconsidering the best approach based on having taken another look at core features of the disorder. For example, Dugas, Schwartz, and Francis (2004) highlighted the importance of focusing on these patients' intolerance of uncertainty and reported very promising preliminary results of treatment that includes such a focus (Dugas & Koerner, 2005).

Adherents to the nonspecific factors model of therapy efficacy might assert that when cognitive-behavior therapy is found to be more effective than another treatment, such as relaxation training, as in the Siev and Chambless (2007) meta-analysis, it must be because the nonspecific components of cognitive-behavior therapy were stronger than those in the comparison treatment. Unfortunately, researchers in cognitive-behavior therapy have not always included measures of nonspecific factors such as the therapeutic relationship. When they have, the superiority of cognitive-behavior therapy to applied relaxation training is evident despite their equivalence on expectations of improvement and the quality of the therapeutic relationship (Clark et al., 2006).

Treatment Manuals Are Rigid and Rob Therapists of Creativity

Psychotherapists differ as to whether they consider psychotherapy to be an art, a science, or a mixture of those things. Those who believe therapy is an art have expressed contempt for the constraint implied in treatment that is guided by a manual, a necessary component of EST research (Silverman, 1996). Such practitioners often indicate that they approach each client as an individual and avoid being guided by nomothetic treatment research as channeled through treatment manuals. There seem to be two misconceptions at play here. One is that the practitioner really can approach each client de novo, without any ideas about what might be helpful for him or her. After all, if there is nothing a therapist can be taught about how to treat particular clients, then there is no point in training for psychotherapy. Few are likely to agree this is the case. Rather, therapists likely draw on informal observations they learned from their supervisors or conclude from their own clinical experience to be helpful with a particular kind of case. As soon as a psychotherapist says "In my experience this sort of client is best approached in this way," she or he is making a probabilistic statement. We would argue that there is great value in clearly articulating these clinical observations and testing their validity. This is precisely what is done when a treatment manual is constructed and an RCT is conducted.

The second misconception is the idea that psychotherapists who use ESTs must follow treatment manuals in a robotic fashion such that they are robbed of their therapeutic creativity and not allowed to use their skills. Certainly some manuals are structured more than others, but it is impossible for the thousands of decisions that each therapist must make to be codified. Although manuals provide extensive descriptions of specific procedures within a treatment, flexibility is inherently necessary so that the therapist can respond to the patient and maintain a good therapeutic relationship (Kendall, Chu, Gifford, Hayes, & Nauta, 1998). Nonetheless, the goal is to detail as many of the treatment decisions as possible so that therapists who are not highly expert in the treatment of a particular disorder are able to learn from the experience of experts to carry out the treatment competently.

ESTs' Efficacy Does Not Generalize to Clinical Practice

Characteristics of Research Participants

The claim is often made that ESTs will not work in clinical practice settings, usually because the clients in practice settings are purported to be more severe or to have more comorbid conditions than clients treated in research studies (Persons & Silberschatz, 1998). Westen and Morrison (2001) estimated that the average inclusion rate for studies of depression, panic disorder, and generalized anxiety disorder ranged from 32 to 36%. They inferred from these data that the more difficult cases were being excluded from research trials, and thus the efficacy of ESTs for these disorders was likely overblown. Stirman and colleagues have conducted several studies challenging this conclusion.

In the first of these studies, Stirman, DeRubeis, Crits-Christoph, and Brody (2003) developed the concept of the virtual clinic. That is, they hypothesized that many patients might be excluded from one RCT because they did not have the disorder in question, whereas they would fit inclusion criteria for another RCT being run down the virtual hallway by another researcher. For example, the patient may have applied for treatment of panic disorder and was excluded because she had a primary diagnosis of social phobia. However, she would be eligible for a different RCT in the virtual clinic, the study for social phobia. To test this idea, these authors mapped information from charts of patients seeking treatment through a managed care program to the inclusion and exclusion criteria of nearly 100 RCTs for individual therapies. Of those patients who had diagnoses represented in the RCT literature, 80% of these patients would have been eligible for at least one study. Patients who failed to match to studies in the existing literature mostly would have been excluded, not because their problems were too complex but because they failed to meet minimum severity criteria.

Another charge is that patients with comorbid conditions are excluded from RCTs. Because people with comorbid conditions are more likely to receive treatment than those with a single disorder (Kessler et al., 1994), it would be difficult indeed to conduct RCT research if this were the case. Nonetheless, the psychotherapy researcher must make a hierarchy of disorders so that the problem most in need of treatment is addressed. In a second study, using records of patients who had been screened out of RCTs, Stirman, DeRubeis, Crits-Christoph, and Rothman (2005) found that all patients who had a primary diagnosis of a disorder represented in the RCT literature would have been included in at least one RCT, regardless of their Axis I or II comorbidity.

Transportability of EST to Clinical Settings

A second claim regarding generalization is that ESTs will not work once taken from their ivory tower settings into the real world of clinical practice. This is the domain of effectiveness research, and there is a burgeoning literature on the effectiveness of ESTs. Examples include research demonstrating the benefits of ESTs with ethnic minority clients (e.g., Carter, Sbrocco, Gore, Marin, & Lewis, 2003), ESTs administered by clinic personnel instead of highly trained research therapists (e.g., Foa et al., 2005), ESTs in community mental health and primary care settings (e.g., Bedi et al., 2000; Merrill, Tolbert, & Wade, 2003), and ESTs with patients who either have not been asked to agree to random assignment to treatment (e.g., Juster, Heimberg, & Engelberg, 1995) or have refused to be randomized (e.g., Stiles et al., 2006). In a recent meta-analysis, Stewart and Chambless (2009) synthesized 56 effectiveness studies of cognitive-behavioral therapy for adult anxiety disorders tested in less-controlled, real-world circumstances. They found that this approach is effective in clinically representative conditions and that the results from effectiveness studies are in the range of those obtained in major efficacy trials. Although more research on effectiveness is clearly needed and meta-analyses of effectiveness studies for other disorders have yet to be completed, based on the available data, the arguments that ESTs do not generalize to clinical settings and the clients seen therein do not hold up.

EST Lists Are Unfair

Psychologists of some theoretical orientations believe that the EST approach is unfair to their preferred psychotherapy method and argue that, because not all treatments have been tested, the playing field is not level (Stiles et al., 2006). This represents some confusion about what the designation of a treatment as an EST means. That a treatment is termed empirically supported does not constitute a claim that it has been shown to be superior to other treatments. Rather, it has been shown to be efficacious in comparison with control conditions, which might or might not include another type of psychotherapy. Moreover, an untested treatment may be effective, but its benefits are simply unknown. If one prefers a treatment with efficacy evidence (and admittedly we do), then ESTs are superior to treatments without such evidence, but this is a different type of superiority.

Cognitive-behavioral researchers have been at the forefront of developing treatment manuals and protocols, and the preponderance of EST research has been in cognitive-behavioral treatments. This is not surprising given the traditional emphasis of cognitive-behavioral treatments on specifying procedures and identifying symptoms and treatment goals. Although researchers of other orientations, for example, psychodynamic psychotherapy, have also produced manuals (e.g., Milrod, Busch, Cooper, & Shapiro, 1997), the research on these interventions is limited compared to research on cognitive-behavioral therapy. In part this might account for Stewart and Chambless's (2007) findings that private practitioners with a psychodynamic orientation have less positive attitudes about the utility of EST-type treatment research for their practice than cognitive-behavioral and eclectic therapists. In the decades since the publication of the first Division 12 EST task force report (Task Force, 1995), research has provided some support for the efficacy of short-term psychodynamic therapy. The Division 12 Committee on Science and Practice currently lists two forms of short-term psychodynamic therapy as possibly efficacious: short-term psychodynamic psychotherapy for depression and short-term psychoanalytic therapy for panic disorder (http://www.psychologicaltreatments.org). More short-term dynamic treatments will undoubtedly appear on lists of ESTs in the future. This may make the EST concept more acceptable to psychologists of this orientation.

The prospect for rigorously controlled outcome research on long-term psychodynamic psychotherapy is less hopeful. Certainly patients cannot ethically be kept in control conditions for years. Accordingly, the remaining approach to controlled research (see section on "Research Designs") would require very large studies in which long-term dynamic psychotherapy is compared to another active treatment. Such research would be extremely expensive, and few patients or public health systems would be able to afford access to this treatment even if it proved effective, making the public health significance low. In addition, dropout rates in long-term treatment research are very high, threatening the internal validity of the research. Perhaps for these reasons, funding agencies are reluctant to support research on long-term therapy. As a result, psychodynamic therapists who focus on long-term treatment may rely on case reports and conceptualizations based on clinical experience and on uncontrolled research (e.g., Leichsenring & Rabung, 2008) to inform the theory and practice of this form of therapy.

Conclusions

We began this chapter with a statement that psychopathology research serves psychotherapy research. We end with the observation that psychotherapy research serves psychopathology research. That is, there is a reciprocal feedback loop between these two forms of research that is mutually beneficial. For example, cognitive theory of panic disorder stresses the importance of frightening misinterpretations of bodily sensations to the development and maintenance of this problem (Clark, 1986). Treatment aimed at changing these cognitions has proved to be highly effective (see Siev & Chambless, 2007, for a meta-analytic review), and, closing the feedback loop, Teachman, Marker, and Clerkin (2010) have determined that changing beliefs about bodily sensations is critical to the efficacy of cognitive therapy for panic disorder. Thus, psychopathology research informs treatment, and treatment research informs the understanding of the psychopathology of this disorder.

The reciprocal feedback loop can also identify when something is wrong with either the theory or the treatment. For example, it was originally postulated that the "sine qua non of marriage was the quid pro quo" (Gottman, 1998, p. 181). In other words, in happy couples there was an equitable exchange of positive behaviors. This theory led to the use of contingency contracting in marital behavioral therapy, wherein spouses were trained to contract for a desired behavior on the part of their partners by agreeing to reciprocate by doing something that their partners wanted. However, systematic research on couples' interactions revealed that this was precisely the wrong thing to do. In fact, insistence on the equitable exchange of behaviors actually characterized unhappy marriages. Thus, the increased knowledge about marital satisfaction led to improvements in marital therapy, namely the removal of contingency contracting as a basic intervention.

On the basis of these and many other such examples, We argue that progress in applied clinical psychology occurs when treatments are based on a solid understanding of the psychopathology of a given disorder and when those treatments are rigorously evaluated not only for their efficacy and effectiveness but also for the causal factors underlying their benefits. In this fashion, treatments may be honed more precisely to concentrate on the critical elements in outcome, making psychotherapeutic interventions more efficient and more effective.

References

Ahn, H., & Wampold, B. E. (2001). Where oh where are the specific ingredients? A meta analysis of component studies in counseling and psychotherapy. *Journal of Counseling Psychology, 48*(3), 251–257.

American Psychiatric Association. (1994). *Diagnostic and statistical manual of mental disorders* (4th ed.). Washington, DC: Author.

American Psychological Association. (2002). *Ethical principles of psychologists and code of conduct*. Retrieved from http://www.apa.org/ethics/

Baker, T. B., McFall, R. M., & Shoham, V. (2008). Current status and future prospects of clinical psychology: Toward a scientifically principled approach to mental and behavioral health care. *Psychological Science in the Public Interest, 9*(2), 67–103.

Barber, J. P., & Muenz, L. R. (1996). The role of avoidance and obsessiveness in matching patients to cognitive and interpersonal psychotherapy: Empirical findings from the Treatment for Depression Collaborative Research Program. *Journal of Consulting and Clinical Psychology, 64*(5), 951–958.

Barlow, D. H., & Hersen, M. (1973). Single-case experimental designs: Uses in applied clinical research. *Archives of General Psychiatry, 29*(3), 319–325.

Becker, C. B., Zayfert, C., & Anderson, E. (2004). A survey of psychologists' attitudes towards and utilization of exposure therapy for PTSD. *Behaviour Research and Therapy, 42*(3), 277–292.

Bedi, N., Chilvers, C., Churchill, R., Dewey, M., Duggan, C., Fielding, K., … Williams, I. (2000). Assessing effectiveness of treatment of depression in primary care: Partially randomised preference trial. *British Journal of Psychiatry, 177*, 312–318.

Bootzin, R. R., & Bailey, E. T. (2005). Understanding placebo, nocebo, and Iatrogenic treatment effects. *Journal of Clinical Psychology, 61*(7), 871–880.

Cahill, S. P., Foa, E. B., Jayawickreme, N., Rauch, S. A. M., Resick, P. A., Riggs, D. S., & Rothbaum, B. O. (2010). *Primum non nocere (first do no harm): Symptom worsening and improvement after prolonged exposure for PTSD*. Manuscript submitted for publication.

Carey, K. B., Carey, M. P., Maisto, S. A., & Henson, J. M. (2006). Brief motivational interviewing for heavy college drinkers: A randomized controlled trial. *Journal of Consulting and Clinical Psychology, 74*, 943–954.

Carter, M. M., Sbrocco, T., Gore, K. L., Marin, N. W., & Lewis, E. L. (2003). Cognitive-behavioral group therapy versus a wait-list control in the treatment of African American women with panic disorder. *Cognitive Therapy and Research, 27*(5), 505–518.

Chambless, D. L., Baker, M. J., Baucom, D. M., Beutler, L. E., Calhoun, K. S., Crits-Christoph, P., … Woody, S. R. (1998). Update on empirically validated therapies, II. *Clinical Psychologist, 51*(1), 3–16.

Chambless, D. L., & Hollon, S. D. (in press). Treatment validity for intervention studies. In H. Cooper (Ed.), *APA handbook of research methods in psychology*. Washington, DC: American Psychological Association.

Chambless, D. L., & Ollendick, T. H. (2001). Empirically supported psychological interventions: Controversies and evidence. *Annual Review of Psychology, 52*, 685–716.

Clark, D. M. (1986). A cognitive approach to panic. *Behaviour Research and Therapy, 24*(4), 461–470.

Clark, D. M., Ehlers, A., Hackmann, A., McManus, F., Fennell, M., Grey, N., … Wild, J. (2006). Cognitive therapy versus exposure and applied relaxation in social phobia: A randomized controlled trial. *Journal of Consulting and Clinical Psychology, 74*(3), 568–578.

Cohen, P., & Cohen, J. (1984). The clinician's illusion. *Archives of General Psychiatry, 41*(12), 1178–1182.

Connolly, M. B., Crits-Christoph, P., Barber, J. P., & Luborsky, L. (2000). Transference patterns in the therapeutic relationship in supportive-expressive psychotherapy for depression. *Psychotherapy Research, 10*(3), 356–372.

Crits-Christoph, P., Baranackie, K., Kurcias, J. S., Beck, A. T., Carroll, K, … Zitrin, C. (1991). Meta-analysis of therapist effects in psychotherapy outcome studies. *Psychotherapy Research, 1*(2), 81–91.

Dawes, R. M., Faust, D., & Meehl, P. E. (1989). Clinical versus actuarial judgment. *Science, 243*(4899), 1668–1674.

DeRubeis, R. J., & Crits-Christoph, P. (1998). Empirically supported individual and group treatments for adult mental disorders. *Journal of Consulting and Clinical Psychology, 66*, 37–52.

Dishion, T. J., McCord, J., & Poulin, F. (1999). When interventions harm: Peer groups and problem behavior. *American Psychologist, 54*(9), 755–764.

Dugas, M. J., & Koerner, N. (2005). Cognitive-behavioral treatment for generalized anxiety disorder: Current status and future directions. *Journal of Cognitive Psychotherapy. Special Issue: Cognitive Approaches to Insomnia, 19*(1), 61–81.

Dugas, M. J., Schwartz, A., & Francis, K. (2004). Intolerance of uncertainty, worry, and depression. *Cognitive Therapy and Research, 28*(6), 835–842.

Foa, E. B., Hembree, E. A., Cahill, S. P., Rauch, S. A. M., Riggs, D. S., Feeny, N. C., & Yadin, E. (2005). Randomized trial of prolonged exposure for posttraumatic stress disorder with and without cognitive restructuring: Outcome at academic and community clinics. *Journal of Consulting and Clinical Psychology, 73*(5), 953–964.

Foa, E. B., Rothbaum, B. O., Riggs, D. S., & Murdock, T. B. (1991). Treatment of posttraumatic stress disorder in rape victims: A comparison between cognitive-behavioral procedures and counseling. *Journal of Consulting and Clinical Psychology, 59*(5), 715–723.

Gottman, J. M. (1998). Psychology and the study of the marital processes. *Annual Review of Psychology, 49*, 169–197.

Hannan, C., Lambert, M. J., Harmon, C., Nielsen, S. L., Smart, D. W., Shimokawa, K., & Sutton, S. W. (2005). A lab test and algorithms for identifying clients at risk for treatment failure. *Journal of Clinical Psychology, 61*(2), 155–163.

Herbert, J. D., Sharp, I. R., & Gaudiano, B. A. (2002). Separating fact from fiction in the etiology and treatment of autism: A scientific review of the evidence. *Scientific Review of Mental Health Practice: Objective Investigations of Controversial and Unorthodox Claims in Clinical Psychology, 1*, 23–43.

Hinshaw, S. P., Owens, E. B., Wells, K. C., Kraemer, H. C., Abikoff, H. B., Arnold, L. E., … Wigal, T. (2000). Family processes and treatment outcome in the MTA: Negative/ineffective parenting practices in relation to multimodal treatment. [Special issue.] *Journal of Abnormal Child Psychology, 28*(6), 555–568.

Isaacson, W. (2004). *Benjamin Franklin: An American life.* New York: Simon and Schuster.

Juster, H. R., Heimberg, R. G., & Engelberg, B. (1995). Self selection and sample selection in a treatment study of social phobia. *Behaviour Research and Therapy, 33*(3), 321–324.

Kadden, R. M., Cooney, N. L., Getter, H., & Litt, M. D. (1989). Matching alcoholics to coping skills or interactional therapies: Posttreatment results. *Journal of Consulting and Clinical Psychology, 57*(6), 698–704.

Kazdin, A. E., & Bass, D. (1989). Power to detect differences between alternative treatments in comparative psychotherapy outcome research. *Journal of Consulting and Clinical Psychology, 57*, 138–147.

Kendall, P. C., Chu, B., Gifford, A., Hayes, C., & Nauta, M. (1998). Breathing life into a manual: Flexibility and creativity with manual-based treatments. *Cognitive and Behavioral Practice, 5*(2), 177–198.

Kessler, R. C., McGonagle, K. A., Zhao, S., Nelson, C. B., Hughes, M., Eshleman, S., … Kendler, K. S. (1994). Lifetime and 12-month prevalence of DSM-III-R psychiatric disorders in the United States: Results from the National Comorbidity Study. *Archives of General Psychiatry, 51*(1), 8–19.

Knesper, D. J., Pagnucco, D. J., & Wheeler, J. R. (1985). Similarities and differences across mental health services providers and practice settings in the United States. *American Psychologist, 40*(12), 1352–1369.

Leichsenring, F., & Rabung, S. (2008). Effectiveness of long-term psychodynamic psychotherapy: A meta-analysis. *Journal of the American Medical Association, 300*(13), 1551–1565.

Levant, R. F. (2005). *Report of the 2005 presidential task force on evidence-based practice.* Retrieved from http://www.apa.org/practice/resources/evidence/evidence based-report.pdf

Lilienfeld, S. O. (2007). Psychological treatments that cause harm. *Perspectives on Psychological Science, 2*(1), 53–70.

Markman, H. J., Renick, M. J., Floyd, F. J., Stanley, S. M., & Clements, M. (1993). Preventing marital distress through communication and conflict management training: A 4- and 5-year follow-up. *Journal of Consulting and Clinical Psychology, 61*(1), 70–77.

Martin, D. J., Garske, J. P., & Davis, M. K. (2000). Relation of the therapeutic alliance with outcome and other variables: A meta-analytic review. *Journal of Consulting and Clinical Psychology, 68*(3), 438–450.

Merrill, K. A., Tolbert, V. E., & Wade, W. A. (2003). Effectiveness of cognitive therapy for depression in a community mental health center: A benchmarking study. *Journal of Consulting and Clinical Psychology, 71*(2), 404–409.

Milrod, B. L., Busch, F. N., Cooper, A. M., & Shapiro, T. (1997). *Manual of panic-focused psychodynamic psychotherapy.* Arlington, VA: American Psychiatric Publishing.

Moras, K. (1998). Internal and external validity of intervention studies. In A. S. Bellack & M. Hersen (Eds.), *Comprehensive clinical psychology* (Vol. 3, pp. 201–224). Oxford, UK: Elsevier.

Norcross, J. C., Beutler, L. E., & Levant, R. F. (2006). *Evidence-based practices in mental health: Debate and dialogue on the fundamental questions.* Washington, DC: American Psychological Association.

Office of Program Consultation and Accreditation. (2009). *Guidelines and principles for accreditation of programs in professional psychology.* Washington, DC: American Psychological Association.

Orlinsky, D. E., Grawe, K., & Parks, B. K. (1994). Process and outcome in psychotherapy: Noch einmal. In E. A. Bergin, & S. L. Garfield (Eds.), *Handbook of psychotherapy and behavior change* (4th ed., pp. 270–376). Oxford, UK: Wiley.

Pattie, F. A. (1994). *Mesmer and animal magnetism: A chapter in the history of medicine.* Hamilton, NY: Edmonston.

Persons, J. B., & Silberschatz, G. (1998). Are results of randomized controlled trials useful to psychotherapists? *Journal of Consulting and Clinical Psychology, 66*(1), 126–135.

Sackett, D. L., Straus, S. E., Richardson, W. S., Rosenberg, W., & Haynes, R. B. (2000). *Evidence-based medicine: How to practice and teach EBM* (Vol. 2). London: Churchill Livingstone.

Schulte, D., Kunzel, R., Pepping, G., & Schulte-Bahrenberg, T. (1992). Tailor-made versus standardized therapy of phobic patients. *Advances in Behavior Research and Therapy, 14*(2), 67–92.

Siev, J., & Chambless, D. L. (2007). Specificity of treatment effects: Cognitive therapy and relaxation for generalized anxiety and panic disorders. *Journal of Consulting and Clinical Psychology, 75*(4), 513–522.

Silver, R. J. (2001). Practicing professional psychology. *American Psychologist, 56*(11), 1008–1014.

Silverman, W. H. (1996). Cookbooks, manuals, and paint-by-numbers: Psychotherapy in the 90's. *Psychotherapy: Theory, Research, Practice, Training, 33*(2), 207–215.

Stewart, R. E., & Chambless, D. L. (2007). Does psychotherapy research inform treatment decisions in private practice? *Journal of Clinical Psychology, 63*(3), 267–281.

Stewart, R. E., & Chambless, D. L. (2009). Cognitive–behavioral therapy for adult anxiety disorders in clinical practice: A meta-analysis of effectiveness studies. *Journal of Consulting and Clinical Psychology, 77*(4), 595–606.

Stiles, W. B., Hurst, R. M., Nelson-Gray, R., Hill, C. E., Greenberg, L. S., Watson, J. C., … Castonguay, L. G. (2006). What qualifies as research on which to judge effective practice? In J. C. Norcross, L. E. Beutler, & R. F. Levant (Eds.), *Evidence-based practices in mental health: Debate and dialogue on the fundamental questions* (pp. 57–131). Washington, DC: American Psychological Association.

Stirman, S. W., DeRubeis, R. J., Crits-Christoph, P., & Brody, P. E. (2003). Are samples in randomized controlled trials of psychotherapy representative of community outpatients? A new methodology and initial findings. *Journal of Consulting and Clinical Psychology, 71*(6), 963–972.

Stirman, S. W., DeRubeis, R. J., Crits-Christoph, P., & Rothman, A. (2005). Can the randomized controlled trial literature generalize to nonrandomized patients? *Journal of Consulting and Clinical Psychology, 73*(1), 127–135.

Task Force on Promotion and Dissemination of Psychological Procedures. (1995). Training in and dissemination of empirically-validated psychological treatments: Report and recommendations. *Clinical Psychologist, 48*, 3–23.

Teachman, B. A., Marker, C. D., & Clerkin, E. M. (2010). Catastrophic misinterpretations as a predictor of symptom change during treatment for panic disorder. *Journal of Consulting and Clinical Psychology, 78*(6), 964–973.

Vessey, J. T., Howard, K. I., Lueger, R. J., Kächele, H., & Mergenthaler, E. (1994). The clinician's illusion and the psychotherapy practice: An application of stochastic modeling. *Journal of Consulting and Clinical Psychology, 62*(4), 679–685.

Wampold, B. E., Mondin, G. W., Moody, M., Stich, F., Benson, K., & Ahn, H. (1997). A meta-analysis of outcome studies comparing bona fide psychotherapies: Empirically, "all must have prizes." *Psychological Bulletin, 122*(3), 203–215.

Westen, D., & Morrison, K. (2001). A multidimensional meta-analysis of treatments for depression, panic, and generalized anxiety disorder: an empirical examination of the status of empirically supported therapies. *Journal of Consulting and Clinical Psychology, 69*(6), 875–899.

Part II
Common Problems of Adulthood

8
Anxiety Disorders

S. LLOYD WILLIAMS

Ruhr-Universität Bochum
Bochum, Germany

To understand anxiety disorder means to understand both anxiety and disorder as scientific ideas. People are anxious about many different things to many different degrees. But nearly everyone knows anxiety from firsthand experience. We speak of ourselves as feeling anxious, tense, nervous, afraid, worried, scared, and the like. We use these terms not only to describe feelings but also to explain behaviors. We say things like, "She left because she was afraid" or "He couldn't speak because he was too nervous." Scientists too hold that fear and anxiety, terms this chapter will use as synonyms, cause many behaviors, normal and abnormal, adaptive and maladaptive. This anxiety theory of behavior is widely believed. But the meaning of anxiety and its power to strongly influence behavior are far from clear.

Anxiety: Mental Disorder or Psychosocial Problem?

Among its other meanings, the term *anxiety* designates sets of proposed mental disorders called anxiety disorders. The concept of anxiety disorder is even more difficult to understand than the concept of anxiety. The psychological responses that define anxiety are subject to controversy, as discussed below. But whatever anxiety exactly is, it certainly exists. There can be no doubt that people feel afraid; sometimes very much so. But whether anxiety *disorder* exists is open to dispute. Many books on abnormal psychology and psychopathology have a chapter whose title seems to proclaim anxiety disorder theory true. The present chapter bears the same title, but it rejects anxiety disorder theory without reservation.

This chapter will first contrast anxiety disorders with the principal psychosocial problems that define anxiety disorders. The contrast will point to the advantages we gain when we shift our attention from illusory anxiety disorders to the all-too-real psychosocial problems that define them (cf. Persons, 1986). Then we will consider the nature, origin, and treatment of those psychosocial problems.

Mental Disorder Theory

To understand the idea of anxiety disorder and its conceptual and empirical difficulties, we must first understand the mental disorder theory on which it is based. Mental disorder theory holds that some problems in behavior and consciousness are mental disorders (or mental illnesses, symptoms, psychopathology, syndromes, or similar disease-like states), as defined in diagnostic manuals of mental disorders, such as the American Psychiatric Association's various editions of the *Diagnostic and Statistical Manual of Mental Disorders—DSM–II* (1962), *DSM–III* (1980), *DSM–III-R* (1987), *DSM–IV* (1994), and the current *DSM–IV–TR* (2000)—or the World Health Organization's *International Classification of Diseases* (*ICD–10*; 1992). The individual mental disorders listed in these manuals are grouped into classes such as anxiety disorders, mood disorders, somatoform disorders, and so on, based on the idea that the disorders within each class share some, but not other, critical features. Each disorder is defined mainly by a key problem or a few key problems, such as panic attacks in panic disorder, depressed mood in dysthymic disorder, or bodily fears or complaints in somatoform disorder. But many other kinds of information are also considered in diagnosing each of these mental disorders. Mental disorder theory holds that if we know that someone has a given mental disorder, we thereby should know the major outlines of the person's problems and those problems' likely associated features and outcomes (Regier, Narrow, Kuhl, & Kupfer, 2009). Mental disorder theory dominates practice in, and research on, helping people change (see Widiger, this volume). This has broad negative implications because mental disorders do not correspond closely to psychological reality.

"The Boundary Between Normality and Pathology"?   The formal principles and statistical standards that define mental disorder are neither well specified nor widely accepted (see Maddux, Gosselin, & Winstead, this volume; Widiger, this volume). The *DSM* offers a narrative definition, but it adds, "it must be admitted that no definition specifies precise boundaries for the concept of 'mental disorder'" (American Psychiatric Association, 2000, p. xxxi). *DSM* defines mental disorders mainly by listing them, each with an accompanying operational definition, which together reveal "the boundary between normality and pathology" (American Psychiatric Association, 2000, p. xxxi). Mental disorder theory thus assumes that the human psychological being consists of two dissimilar domains: the normal and the pathological. Mental disorder is *pathological*, that is, it is fundamentally *different* from all other mental things. And *DSM* and *ICD* hold that we must measure mental disorder quite differently from the way we measure other mental things.

Anxiety Disorder Theory

The 12 anxiety disorders proposed by *DSM–IV–TR* are listed in Table 8.1, separately as the 9 specific anxiety disorders and the 3 nonspecific anxiety disorders, each with the principal broad psychosocial problem(s) that defines it. In mental disorder theory the 9 specific anxiety disorders are particularly important as being, in principle, the most informative. But if a person has prominent anxiety, panic, phobic avoidance, obsessions, or compulsions that do not fit the pattern of a specific anxiety disorder, he or she might nonetheless have a nonspecific anxiety disorder. Disorder 12, the last listed in Table 8.1, "Anxiety disorder not otherwise specified," is the most nonspecific anxiety disorder, and it is the most commonly diagnosed of *all* mental disorders (Maser et al., 2009).

Discussion is lively about these proposed anxiety disorders and about possible difficulties in *DSM*'s conception of them (e.g., Craske et al., 2010; Wittchen, Gloster, Beesdo-Baum, Fava, & Craske, 2010). But few question whether anxiety disorder exists. Anxiety disorder theory, like its parent mental disorder theory, has never borne its burden of proof, that is, the burden of showing itself to be valid. We have rarely asked—and never demanded—that it do so. The failings of mental disorder theory are clear in the light of the simpler more accurate *psychosocial problem theory*.

Psychosocial Problem Theory

In psychosocial problem theory (Williams, 2008; Williams & Margraf, 2011), inspired by social cognitive theory (Williams & Cervone, 1998; cf. Bandura, 1986; Mischel, 1968), people's mental and behavioral difficulties, including their anxieties, are *psychosocial problems*, not mental disorders. Psychosocial problems differ from mental disorders in fundamental and far-reaching ways.

Anxiety Disorder–Defining Psychosocial Problems   The major broad psychosocial problems most important in defining the *DSM* anxiety disorders are shown in the right column of Table 8.1.

Table 8.1 The Anxiety Disorders in *DSM–IV–TR* and Their Major Defining Psychosocial Problems

DSM–IV–TR Anxiety Disorder	Major Defining Psychosocial Problem(s)
Specific Anxiety Disorders	
1. Panic disorder without agoraphobia	Panic attacks
2. Panic disorder with agoraphobia	Panic attacks, agoraphobic avoidance, anxiety
3. Agoraphobia without a history of panic disorder	Agoraphobic avoidance, anxiety
4. Specific phobia	Specific phobic avoidance, anxiety
5. Social phobia (social anxiety disorder)	Social phobic avoidance, anxiety
6. Obsessive-compulsive disorder	Obsessions, compulsions
7. Posttraumatic stress disorder	Reexperiencing trauma, numbing, trauma-related phobic avoidance, anxiety, arousal
8. Acute stress disorder	Reexperiencing trauma, dissociation, trauma-related phobic avoidance, anxiety, arousal
9. Generalized anxiety disorder	Worry, anxiety
Nonspecific anxiety disorders	
10. Anxiety disorder due to a general medical condition	Panic attacks, anxiety, obsessions, compulsions
11. Substance-induced anxiety disorder	Panic attacks, anxiety, obsessions, compulsions
12. Anxiety disorder not otherwise specified	Phobic avoidance, anxiety

We will consider some of these in detail below. Briefly and simply, a panic attack is a sudden surge of intense fear. Compulsion is a senseless repetitive behavior one feels compelled to do. Obsession is, similarly, a compelled troubling repetitive pattern of thought. Anxiety is feeling afraid, and it is not strictly necessary for diagnosing some anxiety disorders, as discussed below. Phobic avoidance is persistent avoidance of a harmless object or activity, which can be perceived as threatening, aversive, or unmanageable. *DSM* phobic disorders include agoraphobic, specific, and social phobic avoidance and anxiety, and avoidance of trauma-related stimuli in the stress disorders. The troubling thoughts emphasized among the anxiety disorders include obsession, worry, and the distressing reexperiencing of traumatic events. Dissociative reactions of several types are emphasized in acute stress disorder.

For this chapter I have selected five of these psychosocial problems for scrutiny: (1) phobic avoidance, (2) compulsive behavior, (3) anxiety, (4) panic, and (5) troubling thoughts. These psychosocial problems are compelling realities, problems in their own right, whereas anxiety disorders are abstractions created by committees. Psychosocial problem theory holds that the *DSM* disorder abstractions divert us from, rather than inform us about, people's concrete problems. Psychosocial problem theory proposes that once we know that a person has panic attacks, then we learn little more from knowing whether or not the person has panic disorder. Once the extent of a person's social fears is known, then whether or not the person has social anxiety disorder adds essentially no information (Williams, 2008; Williams & Margraf, 2011).

Psychosocial Problem Assessment   The nature of psychosocial problems is evident in the principles of psychosocial problem assessment (Williams & Margraf, 2011):

1. Psychosocial problems are commensurable and continuous with the psychological person as a whole; the same psychobiological dimensions apply to problems and non-problems alike (Williams & Cervone, 1998; Maddux et al., this volume); and both are measured in accordance with the same psychometric principles.

2. Every kind of psychosocial problem can vary widely in its severity and in finely graduated increments.

3. A psychosocial problem is measured as a *potential* problem whose measurement scale includes zero (no problem), then increases in increments of severity to as extreme, intense, disabling, frequent, distressing, or otherwise bad as the problem can be.

4. A psychosocial problem's defining subproblems (if any) intercorrelate substantially.

5. A psychosocial problem is measured additively in that its defining subproblems are summed to yield a single dimensional problem severity score.

6. Psychosocial problems are defined inclusively, without exclusion criteria.

7. Psychosocial problems are measured flexibly, with freedom (within psychometrically permissible limits) to define problem dimensions, to set single or multiple cut points, and to dichotomize, truncate, rescale, combine, or subdivide basic problem dimensions as fits the assessment context.

A psychosocial problem can be a single behavior or a single rating, an example being an anxiety rating given during a behavioral task. Often a psychosocial problem is indexed as the sum of multiple responses. For example, any self-report anxiety inventory (e.g., the Beck Anxiety Inventory; Beck, Epstein, Brown, & Steer, 1988) and any behavioral test of phobic avoidance (e.g., Williams, Kinney, & Falbo, 1989) is a dimensional psychosocial problem measurement. Psychosocial problem measurement principles yield powerful tools for describing human problems. And they leave no place for mental disorder in the measurement or explanation of behavior.

Anxiety Disorders Distort Psychological Reality

The grouping of some kinds of problems into a class of anxiety disorders and the disorder concept itself distort psychological reality and degrade information about people in varied ways. I will consider a few distorting features of anxiety disorders here before I describe their defining psychosocial problems in subsequent sections.

Disorders Distort by Dichotomization   A mental disorder is a false dichotomy because it inherently divides a person into two unlike parts, one normal but the other pathological. Neither part actually exists. What exists is a person whose mental and behavioral problems can come in many sizes, and which problems are woven inseparably into the fabric of her or his life as a whole. That every kind of problem is fundamentally graduated is growing hard to deny (Smith & Oltmanns, 2009). Phobic avoidance, compulsive rituals, disturbing intrusive thinking, and feelings of anxiety and panic are plainly graduated problems (e.g., Brown & Barlow, 2009; Ruscio, 2010; Slade & Grisham, 2009), so they can be fully measured only with a graduated yardstick.

Wide agreement exists that human mental and behavioral problems can, and do, come in many different sizes (e.g., Kupfer, 2005; Maddux et al., this volume). *DSM* implicitly accepts graduated measurement when it tells us we need to know the number of panicky sensations a person has, the amount of time he or she spends in compulsive ritualizing, and the like. But then *DSM* tells us to trade that graduated problem information for a dichotomous illness judgment: disordered or not disordered. This is a very bad trade. To transform a graduated dimension into a dichotomy is "willful discarding of information. It has been shown that when you so mutilate a variable, you typically reduce its squared correlation with behavior about 36% (Cohen, 1983). Don't do it" (Cohen, 1990, p. 1307). The inherently dichotomous nature of any mental disorder and the inherently graduated nature of any psychosocial problem suggest that the widely anticipated merging of the two concepts in the forthcoming DSM–5 (e.g., Regier et al., 2009; Smith & Oltmanns, 2009) is likely to lead to trouble. This joining in the *DSM* could well be the death of *DSM* and of the mental disorder concept behind it.

Disorders Distort by Heterogeneity and "Comorbidity"   People with a given anxiety disorder tend to be highly heterogeneous with respect to their actual individual problems (Barlow, 2002). Having almost any problem markedly increases the likelihood of having almost any other problem (Boyd et al., 1987). The phobic behaviors, compulsive rituals, anxious and panicky feelings, and troubling thoughts that define anxiety disorders occur frequently in people diagnosed with any anxiety disorder, with no disorder, and with nonanxiety disorders (de Waal, Arnold, Eekhof, & van Hemert, 2004; Kessler et al., 2006; Michail & Birchwood, 2009). These facts call into question the *DSM*'s assumption that particular problematic responses cluster neatly into certain disorders, and these in turn cluster neatly into such superordinate classes as mood disorders and anxiety disorders. That people often must be diagnosed with multiple mental disorders (Davis, Barlow, & Smith, 2010) also defeats the idea that a mental disorder is a single shorthand label to efficiently characterize a person's problems as a whole (Regier et al., 2009). The reality is that far from a succinct accurate label, an anxiety disorder diagnosis diverts us from the psychosocial problems it wants to explain.

Disorders Distort by Disconnecting Themselves from Their Own Symptoms   Mental disorders are disconnected from the very psychological responses they consist of. One reason is that a disorder often conjoins little-correlated problems, and the conjoining alone introduces discord between disorders and their defining problems. The *DSM* diagnosis panic disorder with agoraphobia, for example, weds two largely uncorrelated problems—agoraphobic behavior and panic attacks (Craske & Barlow, 1988; Wittchen et al., 2010)—discussed further below, into a joint predictor with fixed relative weights. Each of these two problems would be more accurately and more usefully measured on its own separate dimension (Williams, 1985; cf. Wittchen et al., 2010).

People often have the types of problems that define a particular disorder, yet they do not have the disorder. Nearly the opposite can also occur, that a person has few of the problems that define a disorder, but she or he has the disorder! These points are illustrated by the large discrepancies between panic attack (the psychosocial problem) and panic disorder (the mental illness) and between agoraphobic avoidance (the problem) and agoraphobic disorder (the mental illness). A panic attack is a sudden surge of intense fear, and agoraphobic avoidance is behavioral avoidance of certain activities or settings in the community (we will consider some nuances in defining panic and agoraphobia in later sections).

Striking is that "A DSM-IV diagnosis of panic disorder with agoraphobia conveys no information about frequency and intensity of panic attacks and the severity of agoraphobic avoidance" (Brown & Barlow, 2002, p. 325). A person with this alleged mental disorder can suffer from any level of panic attacks, including none, any level of agoraphobic avoidance, including none, and indeed can have none of either. In *DSM–IV*, people who either avoid or fear agoraphobia-relevant activities, such as riding busses, shopping, or crossing bridges, have panic disorder whether they have panic attacks or not, as long as they were at least briefly bothered by panic at any past time, however remote. Agoraphobic disorder (*DSM–IV* diagnosis panic disorder with agoraphobia or agoraphobia without history of panic disorder) requires only that the person needs companionship in agoraphobic settings or becomes anxious in such settings, not that he or she must avoid them (*ICD–10* agoraphobia requires avoidance). A person not panicky, anxious, or phobically avoidant (beyond requiring companionship at times) can be validly diagnosed as having current *DSM–IV* panic disorder with agoraphobia.

Disorders Distort by Stringent Thresholds and Nonspecificity   More common than having a disorder without having its symptoms is having its symptoms without having the disorder. Many psychosocial problems, including avoidance, compulsive behavior, troubling thoughts, and anxiety, mild or severe, are excluded from the scope of mental disorders either outright or by placement in a nonspecific disorder category (Widiger, this volume), in either case denying people the full putative benefits of the disorder-based system. Arbitrarily stringent but immutably fixed diagnostic thresholds spawn an abundance of neither-fish-nor-fowl "subthreshold disorders" (Kessler, Chiu, Demler, Merikangas, & Walters, 2005), an almost nonsensical term that seems to mean disorders that are not disorders. Subthreshold whatever-they-ares arise, for example, from the *DSM* rule that to count an anxiety attack as a panic attack for diagnosing panic disorder, it must be accompanied by at least four responses from a longer list, although an attack with only two or three such responses (e.g., a smothering sensation and a feeling of imminent death) can be intense and have serious psychological sequelae (Margraf, Taylor, Ehlers, Roth, & Agras, 1987). If a person's panic attacks reach full intensity only after 10 minutes, she or he definitely does not have *DSM* panic disorder. Other official *DSM* anxiety disorder symptoms get excluded from the disorder measurement system, such as those left unmeasured by diagnostic interviews when people say no to diagnostic stem questions (Dalrymple & Zimmerman, 2008). Countless additional problems fall into disorder limbo because they are not on the list of official disorder symptoms and therefore receive relatively little attention (Maj, 2005).

Disorders Distort by Exclusion   Perhaps the largest source of discordance between psychosocial problems and the mental disorders they define is the exclusion criteria (i.e., rules that the symptoms must be "not due to" another particular disorder or condition). Panic attacks in both *DSM* and *ICD* often have nothing to do with panic disorder. If panicky people also have obsessions, compulsions, delusions, stress, or any one of diverse phobias, medical conditions, or substance use histories, as panicky people often do (Barlow, 2002), they might well not have *DSM–IV* panic disorder. If panickers are depressed, phobic of just about anything including agoraphobic, or highly anxious between panic attacks, as panicky people often are, they definitely do not have *ICD–10* panic disorder. These exclusion criteria multiply all the dimensional problem information by zero, that is, basically they erase it. The result is that the person's panic attacks become diagnostic nonentities. They simply fall off the mental disorder radar screen.

The preceding failings, among others, have brought mental disorder theory to a crisis. Psychosocial problem theory recommends that we discard the concept of anxiety disorder, but take some of its major defining psychosocial problems, namely (a) phobic avoidance, (b) compulsion, (c) anxiety, (d) panic, and (e) troubling thoughts, as starting points for a new dimension-based model of human problems. These broad psychosocial problems are discussed in the sections that follow.

Psychosocial Problems Described

Psychosocial problem theory and social cognitive theory conceive personality as reflecting the reciprocal interaction between persons, their behaviors, and their environments (Williams & Cervone, 1998). The psychological person consists of the individual's consciousness, physiological states, social roles, and identifying attributes. Behavior refers mainly to a person's potentially publicly observable outward actions. The environment is the person's physical, social, and cultural circumstances. The environmental context is part of personality and of psychosocial problems because people are highly sensitive, and idiosyncratically so, to variations in situations (Mischel, 1990), a phenomenon illustrated vividly by the problems under consideration here (Williams, 1985).

Phobic Avoidance

Overt behavior is a critically important personality domain because people's paths through life, and their inward fulfillments and sufferings along the way, have much to do with what they do, and fail to do, outwardly (Williams & Cervone, 1998). To suffer anxiety in grocery stores or social gatherings is bad, but to be unable to go into them is worse, as it undermines people's very ability to look after their own needs, and it forecloses any hope for a near-normal life. Phobic avoidance and compulsive rituals torture people by robbing them of social and recreational possibilities and even of their livelihoods, by humiliating and depressing them, and by lowering their self-esteem and quality of life. Inner emotional distress can entail terrible suffering. But our most pressing special responsibility is to help people regain outer behavioral functioning, as it is also a key to relieving their inner suffering in many cases (Bandura, 1997; Williams, 1996a). Avoidance behavior significantly hampers people with many kinds of problems, and so it is an important "transdiagnostic" human problem (Wilamowska et al., 2010).

Needless avoidance in at least mild and transitory forms is widespread in psychological life, but when avoidance is marked and persistent, one speaks of *phobia*. Phobia illustrates the "neurotic paradox" of self-defeating behavior in which a person is unable to do an ordinary activity although he or she is otherwise capable, wishes to function normally, and is well aware that the limitation is senseless. Phobias can involve gross disability, for example, outright inability to cross a street or speak to a stranger or be in a room with a small spider. People with phobias also refrain from doing things they could do but would rather not. In *DSM*, but not *ICD*, unwarranted fear towards an activity or object is a phobia even if the person does not avoid it. This chapter loosely refers to either excessive fear or avoidance of something as phobia, but the classical meaning of phobia is senseless behavioral avoidance.

Avoidance in phobia usually is accompanied by some degree of anxiety towards the avoided activity. But it need not be in *DSM* or *ICD*. One of the most important and well-established findings in phobia research is that anxious feelings and avoidant behavior are not highly correlated (Carr, 1979; Lang, 1985; Rachman, 1976), just as panic attacks and agoraphobic behavior are not highly correlated (Craske & Barlow, 1988; Wittchen et al., 2010). This lack of anxiety-behavior (or panic-behavior) correlation is discussed in more detail below. The section emphasizes phobic behavior, while later sections address the anxious and panicky feelings and the troublesome thoughts that can variably accompany phobic behavior and that are problems in their own right.

Phobias vary widely in object, severity, and generality. Some phobias are of highly specific objects or activities (e.g., riding elevators or encountering cats or loud people), whereas generalized phobic patterns can encompass a wide range of seemingly dissimilar activities. Any specific phobia can be a generalized problem when it is severe enough or when the feared object or activity is found in diverse places (e.g., spiders or strangers). Specific phobias tend to occur with other phobias (LeBeau et al., 2010; Lipsitz, Barlow, Mannuzza, Hoffman, & Fyer, 2002), so the distinction between specific and generalized phobias can be difficult to make in any case.

Phobias can occur in constellations, such as agoraphobia, in which a person is simultaneously phobic of at least a few and possibly many or all of about 15 or so distinct community activities such as being away from home, using public transportation, shopping, ascending heights, crossing bridges, riding elevators or escalators, driving a car, and being in an audience. These activities are typically more difficult for the person when unaccompanied. A person need only display a few phobias to earn the agoraphobia label (two in *ICD*), and people said to have agoraphobia also tend to have other large problems (Barlow, 2002; Wittchen et al., 2010), so as Doctor (1982) put it succinctly, "heterogeneity abounds" (p. 210).

Phobias of social scrutiny or of being embarrassed or of causing embarrassment to others are common in agoraphobia and apart from it, and can vary endlessly in form, generality, and severity, between individuals and across different cultural contexts (Bögels et al., 2010). Great variation exists in the number, kinds, and patterning of individuals' phobias and in the diverse other problems that can accompany them, such as sad mood, panic attacks, hypochondriacal concerns, and many others (Barlow, 2002). Even a particular kind of specific phobia can be heterogeneous: A dental-phobic person might dread the confinement, the needle, the drilling, the scents, allergic reactions, panic attacks, or various scary social possibilities (Oosterink, de Jongh, & Aartman, 2009), so the term dental phobia conveys only a modest amount of information regarding a person's problem.

Phobic avoidance or fearful feelings about particular things are common far beyond the problems that diagnostic manuals deem official phobic disorders. Dysfunctional avoidance is a major defining problem of 7 of the 12 anxiety disorders as shown in Table 8.1 and is common among people diagnosed with any anxiety disorder. Moreover, some sexual phobias are called sexual dysfunctions; some phobias of having a bodily deformity, body dysmorphic disorder; some disease phobias, hypochondriasis; some phobias of gaining weight, anorexia nervosa; and so on (Fergus & Valentiner, 2010). The various kinds of avoidance and fear have particular themes and concerns not shared among all phobias, but they are still phobias.

Although the term *phobic avoidance* is restricted to overt behavior, one can maladaptively avoid in the emotional and cognitive sphere too. Such "covert" avoidance, embodied in the criteria for diagnosing posttraumatic stress disorder, has a negative impact psychologically (Solomon & Mikulincer, 2007).

Compulsive Behavior

An important variation on phobic behavior is compulsive behavior. A person with a compulsion carries out one or more actions far beyond reason under a sense of being compelled to do so. Common compulsions include excessive cleaning, repeating, checking, counting, arranging, hoarding, or doubting. Compulsions can involve elaborate rituals that can seem to have more of a symbolic function (e.g., magically decontaminating an object) than any practical effect. One cannot easily overstate the heartbreaking extent of impairment and strangeness of behavior that can be observed in people with severe compulsions (Steketee & Barlow, 2002). Less debilitating but still troubling compulsions appear to be quite common (Fullana et al., 2009). And diverse problem behaviors other than those defined by *DSM* or *ICD* as obsessive-compulsive disorder, such as tics, rituals connected with self-starvation, and dysmorphophobia, can be compulsive in nature (Frost & Steketee, 2002).

Compulsive behaviors tend to be accompanied by obsessions, by a feeling of fear or discomfort that declines with the compulsive behavior, by a sense that the compulsions prevent harm or danger, and by recognition that the behavior is excessive or unreasonable. But, importantly, none of these several features is invariably present or necessary (Steketee & Barlow, 2002). Like phobic disorders, obsessive-compulsive disorder can be diagnosed even when negative emotions such as anxiety are entirely absent; compulsions alone, defined by actions, are sufficient for the diagnosis.

Phobia and compulsion are related and can be viewed for some purposes as passive and active variants, respectively, of avoidance, with phobia avoiding by not doing and compulsion avoiding by doing. Phobic and compulsive behaviors often overlap (Rachman & Shafran, 1998). For example, a woman who dreaded burglars remained fully dressed in bed every night atop the bedcovers (phobia) and spent much time before bed checking and rechecking her window and door locks (compulsion). But not all compulsions serve perceived avoidant ends.

Although most people with phobias do not have marked compulsions, they often engage in defensive rituals when they do the things they would rather avoid (Williams, 1985). Most people with marked compulsions are phobic about compulsion-provoking circumstances, such as compulsive handwashers who phobically avoid contact with potential contaminating objects like door handles (Rachman & Shafran, 1998). Cognitive (or "covert") compulsions also exist, in which people perform rituals in thought, such as checking, counting, reciting, or arranging, perhaps in order to neutralize, undo, or counteract a previous unacceptable thought or action (Steketee & Barlow, 2002).

People can engage in compulsive behavior in response to external circumstances or in response to internal events such as obsessions, which are intrusive unwanted thoughts, images, or impulses that can be experienced as aversive, alien, or frightening. At times external situations and obsessive thoughts operate in concert to provoke rituals. For example, when one man who was obsessed with thoughts about offending God stepped off a curb, he had to *not* think "Damn God!" or he thought he would be eternally damned; usually unsure if he had done it right, he had to step back and repeat it over and over.

Cognitive compulsions can be difficult to distinguish from obsessions (Steketee & Barlow, 2002), as both are maladaptive repetitive thoughts. Obsessive thoughts and compulsive thoughts and behaviors demonstrate complex patterns of interplay, and factor analyses of obsessive-compulsive inventories often find factors other than obsessions and compulsions (e.g., Anholt et al., 2009). Obsession scales correlate highly with compulsion scales (Clark, Antony, Beck, Swinson, & Steer, 2005). Among people with either obsessions or compulsions, perhaps 80% have a mixture of both, but some have only obsessions and others have only compulsions. Either can predominate, and theories and treatments concerning each differ (Frost & Steketee, 2002; Rachman, 1998).

Troubling Thoughts

Obsessive thinking, discussed in the preceding section, is but one of many possible distinctive conscious thought patterns that can often be observed in people with marked fears or phobic avoidance. Some characteristic cognitive activities are also proposed as cognitive mechanisms of fear and avoidance (Bandura, 1997; Beck, 1976; Mathews & MacLeod, 2005), considered later in the section on causes. Here I consider troubling thoughts such as obsessions and worries, which are problems in their own right.

Aversive intrusive thoughts, difficult to control or dismiss, can come not only as obsessive preoccupations and excessive worries, but also as scary images, mad impulses, catastrophic expectations, or horrifying recollections, among others (Borkovec, Shadick, & Hopkins, 1991; Frost & Steketee, 2002; Rapee & Barlow, 1991). Some troubling thoughts are neither fear-provoking nor resisted but simply consume too much time and thereby interfere with the person's life, whereas others can be alien repugnant ideas that the person tries to avoid by phobic maneuvers or to undo by neutralizing compulsive rituals or thoughts (Steketee & Barlow, 2002). Problematic thoughts can occur in people who prominently fear and avoid, regardless of their particular dreaded activities. People with phobias, for example, often perceive the phobic object or activity as dangerous, and they worry, obsess, intrusively remember, fearfully anticipate, and have nightmares about it too (Bandura, 1978).

Indeed, bothersome thoughts such as obsessions, worries, and even hallucinations and delusions are common in psychological life generally (Michail & Birchwood, 2009; Morrison & Wells, 2007). Obsessions and worry are also experienced by people who have no serious problems. "Normal" worries and obsessions are similar to problematic worries and obsessions, although the latter are more frequent and intense and occasion greater anxiety, avoidance, and compulsive rituals (Borkovec et al., 1991; Rachman & de Silva, 1978). Whether intrusive thoughts become problems depends partly on their perceived controllability (Borkovec et al., 1991; Grisham & Williams, 2009; Stapinski, Abbott, & Rapee, 2010) and one's self-perceived efficacy to manage worrisome future possibilities (Cieslak, Benight, & Lehman, 2008). Noteworthy is the pronounced situational specificity of thinking, that it can vary markedly as a function of circumstances, with most individuals finding that particular settings or activities evoke more obsessions, worries, catastrophic thoughts, or the like, than do others (Salkovskis, 1996).

Worries and obsessions can be hard to tell apart; they are similar in being excessive, repetitive, time consuming, having recurrent themes, and often being experienced as uncontrollable and bothersome. Many patterns of troubled thinking show elements of prototypical worries and prototypical obsessions (Fergus & Wu, 2010). Maladaptive worry is not always distinct from constructive preparatory problem solving because in both one thinks of possible dangers and how to prevent or manage them (Craske, 1999).

Nor are the boundaries between the excessive, the unreasonable, and the delusional entirely sharp. People with phobic avoidance, compulsions, panic, or obsessive worrying thoughts often recognize that these are out of proportion to objective reality, but such "insight" is highly variable between individuals and even within individuals across different circumstances (Rachman & Shafran, 1998; Williams & Watson, 1985; Zimmerman, Dalyrmple, Chelminski, Young, & Galione, 2010). Some obsessions are plainly delusional (Frost & Steketee, 2002; O'Dwyer & Marks, 2000). People with psychotic problems frequently display obsessions, compulsions, phobias, panic, anxiety, and posttraumatic stress reactions (Michail & Birchwood, 2009; Morrison & Wells, 2007; Foster, Startup, Potts, & Freeman, 2010). Psychosocial problems combine idiosyncratically and with little respect for official disorder boundaries.

Anxiety

Anxiety has long been a principal proposed cause in theories of avoidance behavior, but anxiety is potentially a serious problem in its own right. What is anxiety? Current usage of the term is anything but clear.

Unimodal, Multimodal, and Polymodal Anxiety　Scientists have conceived anxiety in diverse ways (Hersen, 1973; Lang, 1985). It can be defined *unimodally* by a single kind of response such as subjective fear intensity (Walk, 1956) or physiological arousal (Mowrer, 1960). More commonly anxiety is defined *multimodally* by subjective fear and physiological responses and sometimes by certain ideas. The most multimodal definition I call *polymodal* anxiety because its expansive contents include not only all the usual anxiety responses but also behavior and other responses (Lang, 1985). Because putative anxiety responses in one mode tend to be notably disassociated from putative anxiety responses in a different mode (Lang, 1985), psychosocial problem theory holds that the dissimilar responses are better kept separate terminologically rather than being lumped into an all-purpose but not very meaningful "anxiety" category (Williams, 1987).

Subjective Anxiety　Being afraid means above all feeling afraid, consciously, without which anxiety has no meaning. Fear in consciousness is difficult to describe, but people can indicate how intensely afraid they feel by rating it on a simple scale, for example, from 0 (not anxious or afraid) to 10 (extremely anxious and afraid) in one-point increments. Simple unidimensional fear intensity scales from 0 to 8, 0 to 10, or 0 to 100, with simple instructions to rate one's current fear, are in wide use. This sort of definition has the large advantage that it does not impose meanings on anxiety other than what people themselves mean by simple anchor terms like "afraid" or "anxious." Subjective anxiety has meaning in relation to the psychological context in which people experience it. An anxiety intensity rating indicates straightforwardly how much a particular activity frightens someone (Williams, 1987). Multiple-item anxiety scales are widely used (e.g., the Beck Anxiety Inventory; Beck et al., 1988). Both single-rating and multi-item anxiety scales are psychosocial problem scales that measure *potential* anxiety along a single graduated dimension that ranges from no anxiety to high anxiety.

Panic Anxiety　Panic attacks are sudden rushes of intense anxiety (or discomfort in *DSM*) that can be disturbing and can leave a lasting residue of dread and disability (Batelaan et al., 2010).

Yet people can have panic attacks but not develop serious problems in connection with them (Craske, 1999). Panic attacks vary widely in intensity, duration, and frequency, in the number and kinds of thoughts and sensations that accompany them, and along other graduated dimensions (Barlow, 2002).

Panic attacks also vary in their apparent relation to circumstances. Some panic attacks seem to come spontaneously, as if uncued. But people sometimes find panic attacks to be more likely in certain settings. Early theories considered uncued panic to be a biological event (Barlow, 2002). Apart from people's perception of a cue, cued and uncued panic attacks are similar (Craske, 1991; Kessler et al., 2006). The social cognitive view is that even unexpected anxiety and panic occur in relation to discrete events, but these can be cognitive events such as catastrophic interpretations of perceived bodily states (Clark, 1986; Craske,.1991) or loss of self-efficacy for maintaining cognitive control (Williams & LaBerge, 1994). Panic can be highly responsive to situational and psychological manipulations and interventions (Barlow, 2002; Craske, 1999; Mitte, 2005).

Although panic, like ordinary anxiety, is conventionally defined and conceived in part as bodily arousal, the actual relationship between bodily arousal and panic, like that between bodily arousal and anxiety, is not very strong. Many reported panic attacks come without autonomic arousal, and rapid high autonomic arousal often is not experienced as scary or panicky by an individual (Barlow, 2002; Ehlers, 1993; Margraf et al., 1987). As the essence of anxiety is the subjective feeling of anxiety, the essence of panic is the subjective feeling of panic. The anxiety disorder theory approach to panic is discussed later in this chapter.

Trait Anxiety   Subjective anxiety can be viewed not only as a transitory feeling state but also as an enduring personality trait, a disposition to see circumstances as threatening and to react with fear (e.g., Cattell & Scheier, 1961). Trait anxiety is usually measured by asking people to indicate the self-descriptiveness of various brief statements (Hersen, 1973). Trait conceptions and trait-like inventories abound that measure anxiety in general, without respect to context. Considerable attention has been paid recently to broad generalized traits such as "internalizing" (Markon, 2010) and "neuroticism" or "negative affectivity" (Griffith et al., 2010). The personality trait of anxiety sensitivity (i.e., being generally afraid of feeling anxious sensations) and its measure on the Anxiety Sensitivity Index have become quite popular in research (Naragon-Gainey, 2010).

Trait scores have some predictive ability, but they rarely explain even 15% of the variance in behavior and often far less (Bandura, 1986; Mischel, 1990; Williams & Cervone, 1998). People certainly differ from one another in the amount they are, on the average, distressed (or phobically disabled, or bedeviled by intrusive thoughts, or frightened of being afraid, etc.), but in every case they are troubled by certain definite things and not by others (Chambless, Beck, Gracely, & Grisham, 2000). Small changes in context, like the approach of a cat to a severe cat phobic or a chance reminder of childhood diseases to a worrying mother, can produce marked shifts in behavior, thoughts, and feelings (Beck, 1976; Williams & Cervone, 1998). Idiosyncratic strong variation in an individual's mental states and actions across situations pervades the psychosocial problems we are considering, but is simply ignored by generalized traits (Salkovskis, 1996), as is the idiosyncratic configuration of anxiety-related problems from one person to another.

Psychological treatments involve the person coming into mental and physical contact with the specific things he or she fears, avoids, ritualizes over, or intrusively thinks about, and not with most other things (Barlow, 2002; Craske, 1999). Someone's average tendency to be anxious in general (or anxiety sensitive in general or any other trait in general) tells us little for helping the person change. Trait-like measures continue to inspire much research, which has yielded a clearer understanding of the dimensional structure underlying trait anxiety ratings. But the pervasive situational specificities of behavior (Mischel, 1990) mean that no amount of psychometric insight will ever give us a generalized personality trait that will tell us the specifics of someone's problems. Psychosocial problem theory advocates measuring problematic responses per se when feasible, doing so directly in problematic circumstances when feasible, and otherwise assessing them in a psychologically circumscribed context rather than as generalized context-free traits (Williams & Cervone, 1998). As discussed below, nontrait, context-sensitive cognitions predict and explain people's context-sensitive problem behaviors.

Physiological "Anxiety" Anxiety is widely conceived partly as a physiological response, mainly autonomic arousal and its associated neurochemical mechanisms. Because autonomic arousal per se can be measured physically, without reference to people's consciousness, it is a favored index of fear among investigators who judge subjective feelings to be private events inaccessible to both science and therapy (Lang, 1985). Defining anxiety as physiological arousal gets people's unscientific inner feelings out of the way, but at a high price. Although people commonly describe fear in part by describing how their heart raced or they began to sweat, their bodily perceptions often do not match their bodily expressions (Hoehn-Saric, McLeod, Funderburk, & Kowalski, 2004; Andor, Gerlach, & Rist, 2008). Strong emotions of all kinds tend to come with bodily arousal, but that arousal does not distinguish between fears and other strong emotions, especially negative ones (Hoehn-Saric, 1998). Frightened and panicky people show many patterns of physiological arousal, including no arousal at all (Barlow, 2002; Ehlers, 1993; Margraf et al., 1987; Morrow & Labrum, 1978).

Physiological arousal without subjective fear is common, as when people exercise, feel sexual interest, or merely hear a familiar voice (Lang, 1985). To call some instances of autonomic arousal "anxiety" creates confusion because different autonomic indices can correlate little with one another and can even change in opposite directions within an individual during treatment (Bandura, 1969; Rachman & Hodgson, 1974). The large gap between autonomic physiology and subjective feelings means that autonomic or other bodily responses alone cannot be anxiety. Bodily responses and subjective fear are not two "systems of anxiety." Rather, each must be considered on its own terms (Williams, 1987).

Anxiety as Perception of Physiological Arousal Social cognitive theory holds that physiological arousal per se has less impact on behavior than does the person's perception and interpretation of physiological arousal (Andor et al., 2008; Salkovskis & Warwick, 1986). Bodily perceptions can become a focus of obsessive worrying and can give rise to defensive actions, such as seeking medical help for a racing heart or ritually carrying a bottle of water to wet a dry mouth. Bodily perceptions are implicated in generalized anxiety, panic attacks, and illness phobias (Clark, 1986; Salkovskis & Warwick, 1986; Wells, 2004). The perception of arousal can override the actual arousal (Andor et al., 2008).

Anxiety in Mental Disorder Theory Manuals of mental disorders rely on anxiety as a description, a cause, and an effect of diverse mental illnesses, but are unclear and inconsistent in the way they formally define anxiety and use the concept. In disorder theory, anxiety is multimodal and comes in three different forms: the phenomenon of anxiety, the proposed symptoms of anxiety disorder, and panic attacks. Each of these three forms of anxiety is viewed differently in *ICD–10* and *DSM–IV*.

Anxiety as a Disorder-Related Phenomenon In *DSM–IV–TR*'s glossary, anxiety is "the apprehensive anticipation of future danger or misfortune accompanied by a feeling of dysphoria or somatic symptoms of tension" (American Psychiatric Association, 2000, p. 820). *ICD–10*'s definition of anxiety is looser (note the term "usually" in what follows) yet more elaborate: "Primary symptoms of anxiety … usually involve elements of (a) apprehension (worries about future misfortunes, feeling 'on edge,' difficulty in concentrating, etc.); (b) motor tension (restless fidgeting, tension headaches, trembling, inability to relax); and (c) autonomic overactivity (lightheadedness, sweating, tachycardia … dizziness, dry mouth, etc.)" (World Health Organization, 1992, p. 140). Note that neither definition incorporates avoidance behavior.

The requirement for danger thoughts in *DSM–IV* anxiety and their optional inclusion in *ICD–10* anxiety transform danger thoughts from anxiety's cause into its very definition, and thereby transform Beck's (1976; Beck, Emery, & Greenberg, 1985) perceived danger theory of anxiety into the meaningless claim that anxiety causes itself. It would be better to keep danger thoughts out of the definition of feeling afraid so one can explore the possible role of danger thoughts in making people feel afraid.

Anxiety as a Symptom of Anxiety Disorder   *DSM–IV* and *ICD–10* both propose that dozens of different cognitive, emotional, behavioral, physiological, and perceptual responses (somewhat different between the two manuals) are anxiety disorder symptoms. So according to each manual's definition of anxiety (see the preceding paragraph), some proposed anxiety disorder symptoms are anxiety, whereas other anxiety disorder symptoms are not anxiety. Examples of the former are fearful subjective feelings and physiological overarousal, and of the latter, avoidant behavior and obsessive thoughts. Because the terms *anxiety* and *anxiety symptoms* are used widely as synonyms, mental disorder manuals seem to have further beclouded anxiety's already foggy meaning.

Anxiety as Panic Attack   Disorder manuals also emphasize panic attacks, a variant form of anxiety discussed earlier. *DSM–IV* defines a panic attack as a discrete period of rapidly mounting intense anxiety or discomfort accompanied by certain thoughts, feelings, perceptions, and physiological or other sensations numbering about two dozen, grouped into 13 categories, with responses from at least four categories needed to call a fear attack a panic attack. Notably, avoidance behavior is not part of this definition, but the motivation to avoid panic or to avoid nonpanic but "panic-like" fear attacks, weighs in *DSM*'s definition of agoraphobia. Nearly every one of the two dozen *DSM* panic responses is commonly included in definitions of plain old anxiety. For example, of the 21 items in the Beck Anxiety Inventory (Beck et al., 1988), 15 are *DSM–IV* panic responses. *DSM* distinguishes cued and uncued panic attacks, and it focuses the definition of panic and agoraphobic disorders on uncued panic, although the distinction between the two is not hard and fast (Craske et al., 2010).

Multimodal and Polymodal Anxiety: Three Systems and Beyond   The preceding types of anxiety define it by various nonbehavioral responses. The three-systems analysis (Lang, 1985) went further and threw in maladaptive behavior itself, the very phenomenon anxiety was supposed to explain. Lang (1985) proposed that "the data of anxiety" consist of "verbal reports of distress, fear related behavioral acts," and "patterns of visceral and somatic activation" (pp. 133–134). People no doubt think, feel, act, and respond physiologically, all at once, in nearly everything they do. But as a theory of avoidant behavior the three systems are stillborn. The emotion of anxiety was supposed to be the cause of problematic behavior. Asserting that the emotion and the behavior are one and the same, namely "anxiety," robs both of meaning.

The three systems' verbal report category is sometimes called the cognitive system, but that is ironic because it consists not of actual cognitions but rather of "verbal reports of distress, i.e., reports of anxiety, fear, dread, panic, and associated complaints of worry, obsessions, inability to concentrate, insecurity, and the like" (Lang, 1985, p. 133). Lang also states that these verbal distress reports are of little scientific or therapeutic value: "Feeling states are completely private and represent a poor data resource for the clinician preparing to undertake treatment," and "their unavailability to … observers appears to deny any possibility of scientific investigation" (p. 131). But fortunately, "peculiarities of behavior" and "a variety of [physiological] symptoms … are more yielding to objective analysis" (Lang, 1985, p. 131).

This behavioristic rejection of private experience is jarringly out of tune with psychology's cognitive revolution, which allowed us to start to take people's inner experience seriously on its own terms. The three-systems analysis expanded anxiety to include avoidance, but it did not explain avoidance. To explain avoidance, bioinformational theory elaborated the alleged three systems into a vast polymodal fear network (Lang, 1985; Craske et al., 2008), which is discussed under causes, next.

Causes of Phobic Avoidance and of Related Psychosocial Problems

This review focuses on current psychological causes of problems, although developmental, historical, and biological causes certainly have a role and have been studied extensively (Barlow, 2002; Rachman, 1977; Rapee & Spence, 2004).

Causes of Phobic Avoidance

Recent scientific thinking has emphasized the "transdiagnostic" importance of avoidance behavior, namely that avoidance behavior is often an element of maladaptive psychosocial functioning, irrespective of diagnoses (Wilamowska et al., 2010). The discussion of avoidance in this chapter will focus on phobia as prototypical. Some phobias develop straightforwardly, for example, instated by brief social modeling experiences in monkeys (Mineka, Davidson, Cook, & Keir, 1984) or springing full blown from a single brief traumatic experience (Ehring, Ehlers, & Glucksman, 2008). Scary verbal information alone can engender enduring fear (Field & Lawson, 2003; Rachman, 1977). But most phobias lack discrete precipitating circumstances. And precipitating events produce a phobia in some people but not in others. Phobias appear to be rooted in multiple biological, social, psychological, and environmental circumstances (Rachman, 1977). In the social cognitive approach, historical and biological influences operate mainly via conscious cognitive processes, and especially through perceptions of self-inefficacy, that sustain avoidance behavior in the here and now.

Behavioral avoidance patterns such as phobias and compulsive rituals are correlated to some degree with countless specific inner states, including feelings, cognitions, sensations, and perceptions, any of which in principle could cause avoidance behavior. To isolate inner causes of avoidance behavior one must identify inner states that correlate strongly with that behavior, as only these are likely to emerge as independent causes of behavior. It took scientists a long time to find strong inner predictors of avoidance behavior because for decades their research agenda was dominated by causes like anxious feelings, autonomic arousal, and anxiety-provoking stimuli, to the neglect of conscious cognitions.

Anxiety Theory of Avoidance   Maladaptive avoidance behavior was a principal psychological phenomenon that the concept of anxiety was originally intended to explain. Anxiety was the hypothesized cause and avoidance behavior the explained effect. The psychoanalytic conception that an anxiety drive arising from unconscious threats found symbolic expression in particular phobic or other neurotic behaviors was reformulated in learning terms by two-factor theory (Mowrer, 1960), which proposed that anxiety comes to control avoidant behavior in a two-part process consisting of classical conditioning plus operant conditioning. First, the person learns by classical conditioning to be afraid of a previously neutral stimulus, after having experienced it paired with an aversive stimulus. Then the anxiety provoked by the now-conditioned former neutral stimulus motivates the person to avoid that stimulus, which avoidance is rewarded (operant conditioning) by the decline in anxiety it leads to (Mowrer, 1960; Wolpe, 1958). Important to note is that an actual decline in "hot" fear is required to reinforce the avoidance. The requirement for hot fear is two-factor theory's fatal flaw.

Two-factor theory dominated the study of avoidance for decades and continues to have loyal adherents (e.g., Foa & McNally, 1996; cf. Craske et al., 2008), although a series of important reviews in the late 1960s and 1970s (e.g., Bandura, 1969; Carr, 1979; Rachman, 1976; Seligman & Johnston, 1973) pointed to fundamental problems that two-factor theory never solved. Because it relies on hot anxiety as both the instigator and the motivator of avoidance, two-factor theory inherently cannot explain why maladaptive avoidance behavior so often takes place for prolonged periods with little or no fear, both in research animals (Schwarz, 1989; Seligman & Johnston, 1973) and in severely disabled phobic or compulsive people (Carr, 1979; Spitzer & Williams, 1985; Wittchen et al., 2010).

The point is explicit in *ICD–10*: "It must be remembered that some agoraphobics experience little anxiety because they are consistently able to avoid their phobic situations" (World Health Organization, 1992, p. 136). Most human avoidance behavior is fearless (Carr, 1979). People fill fuel tanks and lock doors in perfect equanimity. Height phobic people walk nonchalantly past tall buildings. Easily executed avoidance behaviors, even highly maladaptive ones, can leave nothing to be afraid of. But sustained phobic avoidance without hot fear is bluntly incompatible with two-factor theory. Also incompatible with two-factor theory is the sustained high fear without phobic avoidance seen, for example, in panic-stricken frequent business fliers. In the social cognitive analysis, discussed below, dysfunctional thinking provokes anxiety, panic, and avoidance. It is the dysfunctional thinking, not the anxiety or the panic, that causes the avoidance behavior.

Mowrer (1960) defined anxiety operationally as autonomic arousal to avoid the then devastating charge of "mentalism" leveled at measures of subjective experience. But autonomic physiology is little related to phobic or compulsive behaviors (or to subjective anxiety; Bandura, 1969; Lang, 1985; Seligman & Johnston, 1973; Williams, 1987). Subjective anxiety is somewhat better correlated with avoidant behavior than is physiology (Williams, Dooseman, & Kleifield, 1984; Williams, Turner, & Peer, 1985), but subjective anxiety also usually accounts for only modest variance in avoidance (Lang, 1985).

Anxiety researchers widely cite Lang's (1985) correct observation that indices of subjective anxiety and of physiological arousal are only modestly correlated with avoidance behavior, but they, like Lang (1985) himself, do not point to the inescapable corollary that anxiety could be at most only a weak cause of avoidance behavior. Causes come in different strengths, and a cause cannot be stronger that its correlation with an effect. Weak correlation means at best weak causation. Anxiety, whether defined as a subjective state or a physiological state, is inherently a weak explanation of avoidance behavior.

As discussed below, cool thoughts about possible future anxiety have considerably stronger a relationship with avoidant behavior than do hot feelings of current anxiety. But such cool thoughts are not part of two-factor theory. Two-factor and other conditioning-based theories (Craske et al., 2010) seek to explain anxious feelings and avoidant behaviors with external conditioning stimuli alone, avoiding mentalism to the greatest extent possible. Subjective anxiety is already mentalistic enough, never mind the "c" word. Cognition in consciousness functions better scientifically than do the mechanistic stimuli, responses, and anxiety drives of two-factor theory (Bandura, 1997; Seligman & Johnston, 1973). Attempts to resurrect two-factor theory cannot ignore the expectations and other cognitions that social cognitive theorists discovered and advanced. But they can reanalyze these cognitions into mechanical stimulus-driven conditioning processes after all (e.g., Davey, 1992; Foa & McNally, 1996). To rehabilitate out-moded theories by retrospectively reframing new cognitive discoveries as mechanical conditioning processes is "post-hoc parsimony" (Wilson, 1978, p. 227). The wisdom of putting new cognitive wine into old conditioning bottles is questionable (Williams, 1996b).

Panic Theory of Avoidance   A variation on the anxiety theory of avoidance, embodied in *DSM–IV* but not in *ICD–10*, holds that agoraphobic avoidance is caused by panic attacks or by non-panic but panic-like attacks. As panic and panic-like are similar to anxiety, so panic theory founders on the same rock that sank two-factor anxiety theory, namely, that panic does not correlate much with agoraphobic behavior (Craske & Barlow, 1988). Panic can be accompanied by extensive phobias, but often it is not, and agoraphobia is common without current panic and without any history of panic attacks (Wittchen et al., 2010). Panic is also common with a host of problems other than agoraphobia (Barlow, 2002; Craske et al., 2010) and occurs in people who have no particular problems at all. Here I review findings that indicate that the anticipation of possible future panic, unlike panic per se, has a strong relationship to avoidance behavior. But anticipation of panic is a conscious cognition, and it is not any part of two-factor theory. As discussed below, another conscious cognitive factor, people's sense of self-efficacy, is yet a better predictor of their phobic avoidance behavior (Williams, 1996a).

Bioinformational Theory of Avoidance   The three-systems idea was mainly a listing of proposed anxiety responses. But bioinformational theory (Lang, 1985; cf. Craske et al., 2008) proposed that the three-system responses reflect a fear structure (also called a fear program or emotion prototype) that underlies avoidance. The fear structure is a largely unconscious associative network of memory nodes containing dozens of interacting language and meaning elements linked to diverse neurophysiological substrates. In this theory "emotions … are fundamentally to be understood as behavioral acts" (Lang, 1985, p. 140) insofar as the deep emotional prototype initially produces a fear reaction unified across the three proposed anxiety systems (i.e., overt behavior, language behavior, and physiology), but inhibitory neural pathways selectively abort some fear responses before they are expressed (Lang, 1985).

Transmuting fearful feelings into avoidant behaviors would be quite a feat of psychic alchemy, given their well-established empirical disassociation. Why the fear prototype would abort its own efferent signals and why evolution would construct special neural pathways to achieve this self-canceling objective are hard to fathom. Barlow (2002) wrote that accepting bioinformational theory's deep unity of fear and avoidance "demands a leap of faith" (p. 57). Bioinformational theory incorporates the latest terminology from neuroscience, cognitive science, and computer science, but it is a big step backwards. Its polyform phenomena governed by countless unconscious and neurobiological mechanisms can tell us little about people's problems. In contrast, social cognitive theories are readily testable and of proven value.

Social Cognitive Theory of Avoidance   Social cognitive theory and a family of related cognitive theories explain phobic and compulsive behavior, anxiety, panic, and bothersome thoughts in terms of people's conscious appraisals of themselves and their circumstances (Bandura, 1997; Beck et al., 1985; Clark, 1999; Rachman, 1998; Salkovskis, 1996; Williams & Cervone, 1998). I call these collectively social cognitive theories because they explain psychosocial problems by people's beliefs, expectations, and judgments about particular things, as represented to themselves in conscious awareness, and about which they potentially can communicate openly. Social cognitions are not generalized trait-like cognitive styles, such as anxiety sensitivity, nor are they generalized information-processing biases, but context-specific thoughts. That context specificity enables them to predict the idiosyncratic patterning of avoidance and fear across situations and time.

Although social cognitive theories are in disagreement about many details, they all view conscious cognition as underlying both anxiety and avoidance. Different social cognitive theories emphasize different kinds of thought, of which outcome expectations and self-efficacy judgments are especially important (Bandura, 1997; Beck et al., 1985; Salkovskis, 1996; Williams & Cervone, 1998). Outcome expectations refer to people's beliefs about the future outcomes of their own actions. Possible negative outcomes can be of several types. People can imagine future dangers (such as possible physical, psychic, or social harms), and they can imagine becoming distressed (anxious or panicky).

Perceived danger is measured as the perceived likelihood, from 0% to 100%, of a harmful outcome; for example, I can be nearly certain that if I walked past that dog it would bite me (Williams & Watson, 1985). Such perceptions of danger have a central causal role in theories derived from the work of Beck (1976), which holds them mainly responsible for the avoidance, fear, and other problems seen in phobia, panic, obsession, compulsion, and stress (Clark, 1999; Salkovskis, 1996). *Anticipated anxiety* is measured as the level of anxiety people think they would reach if they did a certain task; *anticipated panic* is measured as the likelihood, from 0% to 100%, that doing a task would result in a panic attack (Williams, 1996a). Such anticipated distress has been proposed to underlie dysfunctional avoidance (Smits, Powers, Cho, & Telch, 2004). For example, people can anticipate that walking by a dog would be frightening or would provoke panic. Important to note once again is the fundamental difference between a theory that avoidance is prompted by relatively cool cognitive appraisals of hypothetical future fear, and two-factor theory that avoidance is driven along by current hot fear.

A different type of social cognition that is not an outcome expectation, *perceived self-efficacy*, is one's perceived ability to execute an action, for example, seeing oneself as unable to walk past that dog. Self-efficacy scales incorporate no mention of outcomes; the sole question is the extent the person thinks she or he can perform particular actions overtly in behavior, or in the case of thought control self-efficacy, covertly in consciousness. Self-efficacy theory (Bandura, 1997; Maddux, 1995b; Williams, 1996a) holds that avoidance, fear, and scary thoughts arise toward an activity largely because people have a diminished sense that they can act effectively and remain in control. Perceived control is intimately related to perceived self-efficacy because to feel in control a person must judge him- or herself able to enact controlling responses. A sense of control mitigates anxiety and panic (Barlow, 2002; Borkovec et al., 1991; Hofmann, 2005; Stapinski et al., 2010).

The power of the various social cognitions to predict phobic behavior has been compared in diverse studies (summarized in Williams, 1996a; see also Öst, Ferebee, & Furmark, 1997). Both before and after phobia treatment, and in relation to the tasks of an upcoming behavioral avoidance test, people rated their perceived self-efficacy, anticipated anxiety, anticipated panic, and perceived danger. Self-efficacy was consistently the most accurate predictor of behavioral avoidance in the test, and it usually accounted for more than half the variance in behavior. Anticipated anxiety and anticipated panic also proved to be strong predictors of avoidance that each accounted for nearly half the variance in behavior. But importantly, they were consistently less accurate in predicting behavior than was self-efficacy (Williams, 1996a). Perceived danger, rated as the percentage likelihood of a particular harmful outcome occurring, was a weak predictor of behavior.

Self-efficacy consistently remained strongly predictive of phobic behavior when any other cognitive factor (i.e., anticipated anxiety, anticipated panic, or perceived danger) was held constant, whereas each other factor consistently failed to significantly predict behavior when self-efficacy was held constant (Öst et al., 1997; Williams, 1996a). Self-efficacy remains an accurate predictor of future behavior even when relevant past behavior is controlled statistically or does not exist and when noncausal interpretations of the efficacy-behavior link can be ruled out (Williams et al., 1989). These data make clear that people's self-perceptions of their abilities strongly affect their avoidance behavior. Curiously, with a few exceptions (e.g., Benight, Cieslak, Molton, & Johnson, 2008; Cieslak et al., 2008), in recent years the field of anxiety-related research has shunned the measurement of self-efficacy, despite its never-equaled empirical success in predicting future avoidance behavior.

Causes of Anxiety

The preceding section compared several types of social cognition as causes of behavior. But the same social cognitions can be compared as possible causes of subjective anxiety.

Social Cognitive Causes of Anxiety   In much of the phobia research described in the preceding paragraphs, the different social cognitions were assessed in conjunction with measures of subjective anxiety gathered during a behavioral approach test. This enables us to look at the comparative ability of the various social cognitions to predict performance-related subjective anxiety. Analyses showed that anticipated anxiety and anticipated panic were strong predictors of people's subjective anxiety rated during the subsequent behavioral test. Anticipated anxiety and anticipated panic each accounted, separately, for just over half of the variance in performance-related subjective anxiety, whereas self-efficacy accounted for only about one quarter of the variance in performance-related subjective anxiety. The two "anticipated fear" measures (i.e., anticipated anxiety and anticipated panic) each continued to strongly predict performance-related subjective anxiety when either self-efficacy or perceived danger was held constant, whereas the latter two lost all significant predictiveness when either anticipated anxiety or anticipated panic held constant.

Important to note is that people can express high self-efficacy for doing a task but high anticipated anxiety for it as well, in which case they are likely to do the task without great difficulty but with high anxiety (Williams, 1986a). This result suggests that seeing oneself as vulnerable to anxiety (or to panic) causes one (makes one vulnerable) to actually experience anxiety, although how this connection comes about is far from clear (cf. Maddux, 1995a).

Research in the tradition of Beck's (1976) perceived danger theory has continued to examine how perceptions of danger can give rise to anxiety and avoidance (e.g., Stapinski et al., 2010). But danger perceptions are generally weak predictors of the level of anxiety people experience during phobia-related behavioral tests (Williams, 1996a). And when phobic people confront what they dread, danger thoughts are less prominent than Beck (1976) predicted. In one study agoraphobic people were asked to drive a car alone or sit in a small confined space alone while "thinking aloud" on cue (Williams, Kinney, Harap, & Liebmann, 1997). Participants often stated how frightened they felt, and to a lesser extent they expressed uncertainty about performing the task. But they essentially *never* expressed a thought of danger or a thought of a possible harm of any kind. It is puzzling that danger thoughts are only dimly related to agoraphobic behavior and are absent altogether when agoraphobic people confront the worst. Nevertheless, it is clear that maladaptive cognitive appraisals, including danger thoughts, are involved in the development of anxiety and stress reactions (e.g., Meiser-Stedman, Dalgleish, Glucksman, Yule, & Smith, 2009).

Cognitive Processing Bias Causes of Anxiety   Information-processing approaches attribute anxiety partly to cognitive biases, both conscious and unconscious, in anxious people's attention to, perception of, interpretation of, and memory for fear-related information, as well as to biases in cognitive contents in intrusive thoughts and ruminations, compared with nonanxious people (Mathews & MacLeod, 2005; McNally, 1999; Mitte, 2008). In one typical kind of information-processing experiment, people selected for having or not having anxiety, such as a high trait anxiety score or a certain anxiety disorder diagnosis, view briefly presented words related to danger themes or not, and their reaction times on subtasks ostensibly unrelated to the word meanings reveal how they deployed attention as a function of the meanings. Typically, anxious individuals are more attentive to negative items related to their anxiety than are nonanxious individuals for the same items (McNally, 1999). Not all kinds of cognitive operations are equivalently biased in anxious individuals. For example, memory biases in anxiety are more likely for recall than for recognition (Mitte, 2008).

Social cognitive theories concur that people process information differently in relation to their problems than do people without those problems, and that such cognitive biases can contribute to the development of problems and can operate with restricted conscious awareness. At the same time, potential limitations exist in research on information-processing factors. These include the complexity and indefiniteness of the states often being tested (e.g., disorder diagnosis, trait anxiety status), the lack of ecological verisimilitude in the pallid threat stimuli being viewed in a safe laboratory context, and in the behaviors being studied, such as the latency to detect a probe or to name a color appearing on a computer screen, rather than real-world problematic behaviors as such. Moreover, trait-like biases for seeing broad classes of information as threatening, like personality traits of all kinds, have little ability to explain the idiosyncratic patterning of people's problems across situations. Bias effects can be complex, subject to divergent interpretations, and less than robust. For example, sometimes they can be eliminated or even reversed in direction by minor variations in experimental stimuli, participants, or responses (Lim & Kim, 2005; McNally, 1999). And no evidence exists that any information-processing bias, unconscious or otherwise, predicts phobic avoidance or subjective fear reactions remotely as accurately as do conscious social cognitions.

Nevertheless, recent research on training people's information-processing biases suggests that these biases might well play a role in the development and maintenance of anxiety in natural contexts (Mathews, 2006). Induced information-processing biases can lead to anxiety directly, and training that reduces such biases can have a beneficial effect on anxiety (See, McLeod, & Bridle, 2009). The social cognitive view posits that fear and avoidance result from cognitive biases not only in processing information about possible threat, but also about personal self-efficacy, personal vulnerability to anxiety and panic, and other self-reflective cognitive concerns.

Causes of Panic Attacks

Most early research on panic focused on physiological causes (Barlow, 2002). Diverse physical influences, including sodium lactate, carbon dioxide, caffeine, vigorous exercise, and rapid breathing, can induce panic in vulnerable individuals. The sheer variety of bodily influences on panic suggests the possibility of a common psychological mechanism (Clark, 1986).

Social Cognitive Causes of Panic   Psychological models of panic generally conceive it as resulting from perception of threat (Beck et al., 1985), in particular, a vicious cycle of perceiving bodily sensations, interpreting them catastrophically, therefore feeling afraid and apprehensive, which provokes more bodily sensations to be interpreted catastrophically, and so on (Clark, 1986; Rapee, 1993). A self-efficacy analysis places emphasis not only on thoughts of calamity per se, but also on the sense of control or coping, the belief that one can prevent panic by controlling the thoughts that give rise to it, and if need be, can function despite panic, and otherwise can prevent or limit calamitous outcomes (Williams & LaBerge, 1994). Evidence supports a role for cognition in panic, including a sense of control (Barlow, 2002; Casey, Oei, & Newcombe, 2004; Williams & Falbo, 1996). Cognitive processes seem to mediate the effects of psychological and environmental manipulations on biological panic induction and the beneficial effects of panic treatments (Clark, 1993; Hoffman et al., 2007).

Causes of Troubling Thoughts

Social cognitive theories hold that bothersome thoughts such as obsessions and worries occur in the normal stream of consciousness but become problematic as people interpret and respond to them maladaptively. General cognitive deficit theories of obsession fail because, like traits, they are unable to account for the pronounced situational specificity of obsessions (Salkovskis, 1996). Recent theorizing has emphasized an excessive sense of responsibility for preventing potential harmful effects and a corresponding impulse to take neutralizing actions. When people try to avoid or suppress a bothersome intrusion, their neutralizing rituals can increase the thought's frequency and undermine the sense of control, increasing anxiety and spurring greater efforts to exert control, continuing in a vicious cycle (Rachman, 1998; Salkovskis, 1996). Checking itself can undermine confidence in memory, causing more checking (Boschen & Vuksanovic, 2007). Lack of self-efficacy for remembering actions, for distinguishing imagined from real past actions, for maintaining control over thinking, and the like have been called "cognitive confidence" or "thought control confidence," and this kind of self-efficacy has been implicated in obsessions and compulsions (Grisham & Williams, 2009; Hermans et al., 2008).

Theories of worry view it as reinforced by anxiety reduction, by a sense of control, or by perceived risk reduction (Borkovec et al., 1991; Craske, 1999; Stapinski et al., 2010). To the extent that a sense of control over scary thoughts is important, self-efficacy for exercising such control should be important as well (Kent & Gibbons, 1987). Lack of self-efficacy for solving problems appears to have a role in generalized anxiety and worry (Aikins & Craske, 2001).

Treatment of Phobic Avoidance and of Related Psychosocial Problems

Psychological approaches to helping people overcome avoidance and rituals, subjective fear and panic attacks, and worries, obsessions, and intrusive bothersome thoughts have achieved notable successes in recent decades, although much room for improvement remains (Stewart & Chambless, 2009). Behavioral, social, and cognitive interventions can be beneficial in many cases.

Treatment of Phobia and Compulsion

Helping people overcome behavioral disabilities and limitations is important in its own right. It gains additional importance because reducing such avoidance behavior robustly reduces the subjective fear, panic, obsessions, intrusive thoughts, and depressed mood that often go with it.

Performance-based "Exposure" Treatments　　Historically pivotal to phobia treatment was systematic desensitization (Wolpe, 1958) and similar methods derived from it, which guide people to imagine performing their avoided activities. Also influential were modeling methods in which people watched others doing the phobia-related activities. The next major advance was performance-based treatment (sometimes called *in vivo exposure*), in which people directly perform their avoided activities (Agras, Leitenberg, & Barlow, 1968; Bandura, Blanchard, & Ritter, 1969). In performance-based treatment of compulsive rituals, the person engages in ritual-provoking activities (e.g., touches the contaminated door handle or thinks, "Damn God!") but then refrains from the rituals. This method is also called *exposure and response prevention*. Such performance-based methods are reliably more effective than methods based only on imagining or viewing the activities (Bandura et al., 1969; Steketee & Barlow, 2002).

Treatment focused entirely on guiding the person to engage in the phobic activity, with no explicit attention to thinking or feeling, can enduringly eliminate specific phobias and their negative cognitive and emotional accompaniments, within a few hours in many cases, and with widely generalized benefits (Bandura et al., 1969; Ollendick et al., 2009). Even nonbehavioral problems, such as worrying and catastrophizing, appear to be sustained at least partly by subtle or gross avoidance behaviors that insulate people from corrective learning experiences (Rachman, Radomsky, & Shafran, 2008). Because avoidance behavior is a common element of otherwise disparate problems, and because changes in avoidance behavior can powerfully change the subjective anxiety, panic and stress, and intrusive thoughts that often go with it (e.g., Salcioglu, Basoglu, & Livanou, 2007; Vögele et al., 2010; Williams & Falbo, 1996), therapies for diverse problems increasingly place emphasis on identifying and eliminating avoidance behavior. One recent trend is "transdiagnostic" treatments (Wilamowska et al., 2010), which treat dysfunctional avoidance patterns irrespective of diagnosis, using methods developed to treat phobias.

Exposure Concept of Treatment   Treatments based on imagining, watching, or actually doing phobia-related activities are sometimes collectively called *exposure treatment*. The exposure concept likens treatment to Pavlovian extinction, in which unreinforced exposure to the conditioned fear stimulus classically deconditions the person's fear and avoidance (Foa & McNally, 1996). Contact with relevant stimuli is required to learn just about anything. But identical durations of contact with phobic stimuli routinely produce highly disparate degrees of change in phobic behavior, between treatment groups and between individuals within groups (Williams et al., 1984, 1989). The exposure idea cannot explain such variability in benefit because it casts treatment in passive mechanistic terms and points to fixed outer stimuli instead of to flexible inner mental processes.

Guided Mastery Treatment   Treatment based on self-efficacy theory, guided mastery treatment (Williams, 1990), seeks to build a strong sense of self-efficacy by fostering people's performance accomplishments. Although belief that one can do an activity is a cognition, the best way to acquire such a cognition is from firsthand success at doing the activity (Bandura, 1997). Therefore, the guided mastery therapist assists people to succeed at tasks that otherwise would be too difficult, while guiding them to do the tasks proficiently, free of embedded defensive maneuvers and self-restrictions that limit their perceptions of success and hence limit the growth in self-efficacy and in capabilities and the reduction in anxiety that people gain from successes (Williams, 1990; Williams et al., 1989). Assisting people to do what they fear usually produces better results than does simply encouraging them to expose themselves to scary stimuli (Abramowitz, 1996; Feske & Chambless, 1995; Öst, Salkovskis, & Hellstrom, 1991; Williams & Zane, 1989).

Increasing attention in recent years has been given to a method called "one-session treatment" (Ollendick et al., 2009; Öst et al., 1991), which, like guided mastery treatment, traces its roots largely to participant modeling treatment (Bandura et al., 1969). Each of these three methods is undoubtedly potent in helping people with phobias. That the "one-session" name (and implicitly, claim) is an exaggeration is unfortunate. Of course the method is really limited to one session, and that one session eliminates phobias in many people. But a recent careful test of the 3-hours-at-most one session in phobic youth found that about half of the participants continued to be diagnosed with a *DSM*-specific phobia after treatment, and the diagnosis-free other half were not necessarily fear free (Ollendick et al, 2009). In the author's experience with guided mastery treatment (Williams, 1990), some people with a specific phobia can be refractory to performance-based treatment by any name. Even after an experienced therapist has brought to bear carefully devised methods of helping phobic people incrementally perform the phobia-related tasks, and in people who are highly motivated, cooperative, resourceful, and lacking other serious problems, some people make painfully slow progress or none at all. The results of the Ollendick et al. (2009) study thus do not reflect negatively on the treatment method, but suggest that the method's name and its brief application are inapt. They show too that, contrary to myth, specific phobia can be very difficult to treat.

Cognitive Therapies   Given the imperfect results obtained by performance-based treatments to date, investigators have sought to boost treatment power by engaging people's mediating cognitive processes by verbal means. Cognitive therapies designed to help people change their overestimations of danger and to adopt alternative, less self-undermining ways of construing events are widely used in combination with performance-based exposure methods to treat phobic avoidance and rituals (Beck et al., 1985). It has not always been easy to show that cognitive therapies add to the benefits of performance-based exposure treatments (Feske & Chambless, 1995; Fisher & Wells, 2005; Öst, Thulin, & Ramnero, 2005; Williams & Falbo, 1996). Nevertheless, it appears that verbal–cognitive interventions can contribute benefits beyond the benefits from performance-based treatment alone (Clark, 1999).

Treatment of Anxiety

Treatment of Subjective Anxiety   People usually feel anxious about something in particular and often avoid it as well. Mastering the avoidance behavior alone often eliminates any accompanying subjective anxiety as a by-product (Bandura et al., 1969; Öst et al., 1991). When people's anxiety fails to come to an end, despite preforming the activity for sufficient time, social cognitive theory suggests that the therapist needs to guide these people to abandon subtle avoidance maneuvers, defensive activities, and self-protective rituals that circumscribe their sense of mastery and thereby prolong their fear (Williams, 1985; Williams & Zane, 1989).

That phobic people engage in such defensive behaviors, even as they are doing a phobia-related task (i.e., in behaviors now widely called "safety behaviors"), and the significance of such behaviors for the treatment of anxiety, were first described by Williams (1985, pp. 173–174). These avoidance behaviors were called "embedded defensive activities" and they include not only rituals (e.g., carrying a bottle of water in case one's mouth dries out during a fear attack), but also subtle self-restrictions on performance, such as driving the freeway but staying only in the slow lane. It was concluded:

> Embedded defensive activities may in part explain why some people perform feared activities for extended periods with little or no decline in subjective distress…. It is especially important to identify embedded performance restrictions when formulating treatment plans because such maneuvers can provide a basis for direct behavioral intervention to help clients learn to function more effectively and with less discomfort. (Williams, 1985, p. 124)

Williams and Zane (1989) showed the impact these defensive safety behaviors have on anxiety reduction during in vivo exposure in a randomized controlled experiment with agoraphobic people. One group received therapist-supervised in vivo exposure in which the therapist paid attention to their safety behaviors (the "safety-behavior" treatment), while a second group had the identical duration and kind of exposure to the same exposure settings, but the therapist did not pay attention to their safety behaviors (the exposure-only treatment). The safety-behavior treatment produced significantly greater anxiety reductions than did the exposure-only treatment on a posttreatment behavioral test, and the advantage of safety-behavior treatment increased significantly more during the follow-up period.

Although embedded defensive activities were renamed and reinterpreted by Salkovskis (1991) as "safety behaviors," both the label and the interpretation of the behaviors as primarily danger related are open to challenge. The safety behavior label has become standard. But embedded avoidant behaviors and their therapeutic importance were discovered in the light of self-efficacy theory, which sees them not as safety behaviors but as self-efficacy behaviors (i.e., behaviors that can increase and decrease self-efficacy). To illustrate, when an agoraphobic woman first attempts to enter a market, an embedded defensive activity might increase her self-efficacy for performing the task, and thus enable her to do it. For example, she might be more sure she can go into the market if she carries a bottle of water than otherwise. The therapist can strategically recommend and use such self-efficacy modulating behaviors accordingly. But if the woman keeps taking the water bottle after her initial forays into the market, then it will undermine her self-efficacy because she will attribute her success in entering the market, not to her own growing mastery, but to the defensive behavior—she will think, "I could do it only because I had the water with me." The defensive behavior thus quickly evolves from an efficacy- and performance-increasing aid into an efficacy- and performance-undermining dependency. Hence the guided mastery therapist uses such efficacy-enhancing aids only temporarily and quickly withdraws them to foster unaided success, as I have described in detail (Williams, 1990).

Of course subjective anxiety has long been successfully treated by guiding people to imagine themselves encountering stressors and coping effectively with them and by a variety of relaxation and cognitive reappraisal treatment methods (Barlow, 2002; Clark, 1999; Craske, 1999). Some recent studies have explored the combination of conventional cognitive-behavioral methods with techniques based on acceptance and commitment therapy and mindfulness therapy, with promising results (e.g., Roemer & Orsillo, 2007).

Treatment of Panic Attacks   Most people with panic attacks display some avoidance, gross or subtle (Williams, 1985; Williams & Falbo, 1996), so performance-based therapies for avoidance can have a notable impact on panic attacks (Barlow, 2002). Several treatment methods that focused specifically on panic include cognitive therapies designed to increase rational appraisal and decrease catastrophic thoughts, somatic interventions to induce autonomic arousal or other bodily responses in panic (sometimes called interoceptive exposure), and breathing and relaxation techniques designed to normalize and calm physiological arousal (Craske, 1999).

A meta-analysis of 13 studies of panic treatment with cognitive-behavioral therapies, with diverse selection criteria, found rates of panic-free participants after treatment ranging from 53 to 85%, with a weighted mean of 71% (Chambless & Peterman, 2004). In a search for "pure" panic disorder, panic researchers have routinely excluded depressed, agoraphobic, socially phobic, and obsessive panickers from treatment studies. Panickers with few phobias and few other problems are easier to treat than those with more phobias and other problems (Sanchez-Meca, Rosa-Alcazar, Martin-Martinez, & Gomez-Conesa, 2010; Williams & Falbo, 1996). The high level of panic improvement shown by nondepressed, phobia-free panickers likely overestimates the average benefits of panic therapies for panicky people.

Treatment of Troubling Thoughts

Helping people with troubling thoughts often involves a combination of elements administered together. Worries and obsessions are directed toward specific activities or stimuli and are often accompanied by mental or behavioral avoidance reactions or neutralizing rituals, reassurance seeking, and other actions that paradoxically maintain and increase intrusions (Craske, 1999; Rachman, 1998; Salkovskis, 1996). Thus the most widely used technique, regardless of whether the thoughts are worries, obsessions, flashbacks, or visualized future calamities, is with enactive or imaginal performance of avoided activities, with response prevention as appropriate for compulsions (de Silva, Menzies, & Shafran, 2003; Taylor et al., 2003). Thus, a person can deliberately think an intrusive thought then mentally practice not reacting to it. Cognitive treatments (Clark, 1999; Craske, 1999; Rachman & Shafran, 1998) contain a variety of verbal elements, including dialogue aimed at conveying that obsessions are normal, challenging excessive responsibility beliefs and catastrophic meanings, increasing tolerance of uncertainty, as well as methods to try to alter problem imagery, but without trying to decrease the number of intrusive thoughts directly (Salkovskis, 1996).

Prevalence of Disorder or Distribution of Problem Severity Scores?

The extent to which psychological problems occur in the community has been measured by prevalence rates of mental disorders rather than as frequency distributions of dimensional scores. Probably just about everybody has experienced needless avoidance, fears, and unpleasant thoughts now and again, so their prevalence as mental disorders is largely in the eye of the beholder, dependent on which responses and cutoffs one chooses to define disorder and on how assessors actually operationalize them. For example, in one analysis the prevalence of *DSM–III* generalized anxiety disorder dropped from 45% to 9% of the population when the required duration of anxiety increased from 1 month to 6 months and the number of defining responses increased from three to six (Breslau & Davis, 1985).

Prevalence of social phobic disorder ranges from about 2% to 19% of the population, depending on cutoff scores and on how interviewers pose their questions (Stein, Walker, & Forde, 1994). Markedly varying prevalence rates are found for posttraumatic stress disorder mainly because of *DSM*'s imprecise nonoperational definitions (Kessler, Sonnega, Bromet, Hughes, & Nelson, 1995). The prevalence of obsessive-compulsive disorder using *DSM–IV*'s definition is about half of that using *DSM–III*'s definition (Crino, Slade, & Andrews, 2005). The impact of ambiguous psychodiagnostic decision rules is evident in a reanalysis of epidemiological findings applying the *DSM–IV* clinical significance criterion, which lowered the U.S. national prevalence of mental illnesses by 19.2 million people at a single stroke (Narrow, Rae, Robins, & Regier, 2002).

Plainly, the extent of problems in the population would be characterized far better by distributions of problem dimension scores than by frequency counts of mental disorders. But however one might interpret epidemiological findings, they show beyond doubt that serious psychological problems of the kinds described in this chapter are common (Kessler et al., 2005).

Conclusion

I encourage readers to approach anxiety disorder by questioning the meanings of both "anxiety" and "disorder." Calling psychological phenomena by their own proper names without a pseudo-unifying anxiety label removes a comforting illusion of understanding, but it helps us to see problems more clearly on their own terms. Although we say glibly that phobic people avoid because they are anxious, the evidence favors the far different conclusion that phobic people avoid, and are anxious, because they think maladaptive thoughts.

Perhaps more important is to question disorder theory. Most critics of mental disorder oddly conclude with a wish to use psychological dimensions to develop better measures of mental disorder. I disagree fundamentally. Here and now psychosocial dimensions do everything good that disorders do, only better, and without all the distortions. The study of phobia, compulsion, anxiety, panic, and troublesome thoughts is only undermined by working these problems into complexly dichotomous mental disorders. Far from heeding the call to subordinate behavioral science to the mental disorder model, which would be like the victorious General Grant surrendering his army to the defeated General Lee in Mark Twain's tall tale, behavioral scientists can celebrate the ascendance of dimension-based psychosocial problems, and the retiring of dichotomous mental disorders, and never look back.

References

Abramowitz, J. S. (1996). Variants of exposure and response prevention in the treatment of obsessive-compulsive disorder: A meta-analysis. *Behavior Therapy, 27*, 583–600.

Agras, W. S., Leitenberg, H., & Barlow, D. H. (1968). Social reinforcement in the modification of agoraphobia. *Archives of General Psychiatry, 19*, 423–427.

Aikins, D. E., & Craske, M. G. (2001). Cognitive theories of generalized anxiety disorder. *Psychiatric Clinics of North America, 24*, 57–74.

American Psychiatric Association. (1980). *Diagnostic and statistical manual of mental disorders* (3rd. ed.). Washington, DC: Author.

American Psychiatric Association. (1987). *Diagnostic and statistical manual of mental disorders* (3rd rev. ed.). Washington, DC: Author.

American Psychiatric Association. (1994). *Diagnostic and statistical manual of mental disorders* (4th ed.). Washington, DC: Author.

American Psychiatric Association. (2000). *Diagnostic and statistical manual of mental disorders* (4th rev. ed.). Washington, DC: Author.

Andor, T., Gerlach, A. L., & Rist, F. (2008). Superior perception of phasic physiological arousal and the detrimental consequences of the conviction to be aroused on worrying and metacognitions in GAD. *Journal of Abnormal Psychology, 117*, 193–205.

Anholt, G. E., van Oppen, P., Emmelkamp, P. M. G., Cath, D. C., Smit, J. H., van Dyck, R., & van Balkom, A. J. L. M. (2009). Measuring obsessive-compulsive symptoms: Padua Inventory-Revised vs. Yale-Brown Obsessive Compulsive Scale. *Journal of Anxiety Disorders, 23*, 830–835.

Bandura, A. (1969). *Principles of behavior modification*. New York: Holt, Rinehart, and Winston.

Bandura, A. (1978). On paradigms and recycled ideologies. *Cognitive Research and Therapy, 2*(1), 79–103.

Bandura, A. (1986). *Social foundations of thought and action: A social cognitive theory*. Englewood Cliffs, NJ: Prentice-Hall.

Bandura, A. (1997). *Self-efficacy: The exercise of control*. New York: Freeman.

Bandura, A., Blanchard, E. B., & Ritter, B. (1969). Relative efficacy of desensitization and modeling approaches for inducing behavioral, affective, and attitudinal changes. *Journal of Personality and Social Psychology, 13*, 173–199.

Barlow, D. H. (2002). *Anxiety and its disorders*. New York: Guilford.

Batelaan, N. M., de Graaf, R., Penninx, B. W. J. H., van Balkom, A. J. L. M., Vollebergh, W. A. M., & Beekman, A. T. F. (2010). The 2-year prognosis of panic episodes in the general population. *Psychological Medicine, 40*, 147–157.

Beck, A. T. (1976). *Cognitive therapy and the emotional disorders*. New York: International Universities Press.

Beck, A. T., Epstein, N., Brown, G., & Steer, R. A. (1988). An inventory for measuring clinical anxiety: Psychometric properties. *Journal of Consulting and Clinical Psychology, 56*, 893–897.

Beck, A. T., Emery, G., & Greenberg, R. L. (1985). *Anxiety disorders and phobias: A cognitive perspective*. New York: Basic Books.

Benight, C. C., Cieslak, R., Molton, I. R., & Johnson, L. E. (2008). Self-evaluative appraisals of coping capability and posttraumatic distress following motor vehicle accidents. *Journal of Consulting and Clinical Psychology, 76*, 677–685.

Bögels, S. M., Alden, L., Beidel, D. C., Clark, L. A., Pine, D. S., Stein, M. B., & Voncken, M. (2010). Social anxiety disorder: Questions and answers for the DSM-V. *Depression and Anxiety, 27*, 168–189.

Borkovec, T. D., Shadick, R. N., & Hopkins, M. (1991). The nature of normal and pathological worry. In R. M. Rapee & D. H. Barlow (Eds.), *Chronic anxiety: Generalized anxiety disorder and mixed anxiety-depression* (pp. 29–51). New York: Guilford.

Boschen, M. J., & Vuksanovic, D. (2007). Deteriorating memory confidence, responsibility perceptions and repeated checking: Comparisons in OCD and control samples. *Behaviour Research and Therapy, 45*, 2098–2109.

Boyd, J. H., Burke, J. D., Gruenberg, E., Holzer, C. E., Rae, D. S., George, L. K., … Nestadt, G. (1987). The exclusion criteria of DSM-III. In G. L. Tischler (Ed.), *Diagnosis and classification in psychiatry* (pp. 403–424). Cambridge: Cambridge University Press.

Breslau, N., & Davis, G. C. (1985). Further evidence on the doubtful validity of generalized anxiety disorder. *Psychiatry Research, 16*, 177–179.

Brown, T. A., & Barlow, D. H. (2002). Classification of anxiety and mood disorders. In D. Barlow (Ed.), *Anxiety and its disorders* (pp. 292–327). New York: Guilford.

Brown, T. A., & Barlow, D. H. (2009). A proposal for a dimensional classification system based on the shared features of the DSM-IV anxiety and mood disorders: Implications for assessment and treatment. *Psychological Assessment, 21*, 256–271.

Carr, A. T. (1979). The psychopathology of fear. In W. Sluckin (Ed.), *Fear in animals and man* (pp. 199–235). New York: Van Nostrand Reinhold.

Casey, L. M., Oei, T. P. S., & Newcombe, P. A. (2004). An integrated cognitive model of panic disorder: The role of positive and negative cognitions. *Clinical Psychology Review, 24*, 529–555.

Cattell, R. B., & Scheier, I. H. (1961). *The meaning and measurement of neuroticism and anxiety*. New York: Ronald Press.

Chambless, D. L., Beck, A. T., Gracely, E. J., & Grisham, J. R. (2000). Relationships of cognitions to fear of somatic symptoms: A test of the cognitive theory of panic. *Depression and Anxiety, 11*, 1–9.

Chambless, D. L., & Peterman, M. (2004). Cognitive behavior therapy for generalized anxiety disorder and panic disorder: The second decade. In R. L. Leahy (Ed.), *New frontiers of cognitive therapy* (pp. 86–115). New York: Guilford.

Cieslak, R., Benight, C. C., & Lehman, V. C. (2008). Coping self-efficacy mediates the effects of negative cognitions on posttraumatic stress. *Behaviour Research and Therapy, 46*, 788–798.

Clark, D. M. (1986). A cognitive approach to panic. *Behaviour Research and Therapy, 24*, 461–470.

Clark, D. M. (1993). Cognitive mediation of panic attacks induced by biological challenge tests. *Advances in Behaviour Research and Therapy, 15*, 75–84.

Clark, D. M. (1999). Anxiety disorders: Why they persist and how to treat them. *Behaviour Research and Therapy, 37*(Suppl.), S5–S27.

Clark, D. A., Antony, M. M., Beck, A. T., Swinson, R. P., & Steer, R. A. (2005). Screening for obsessive and compulsive symptoms: Validation of the Clark-Beck Obsessive Compulsive Inventory. *Psychological Assessment, 17*, 132–143.

Cohen, J. (1983). The cost of dichotomization. *Applied Psychological Measurement, 7*, 249–253.

Cohen, J. (1990). Things I have learned (so far). *American Psychologist, 45*, 1304–1312.

Craske, M. G. (1991). Phobic fear and panic attacks: The same emotional states triggered by different cues? *Clinical Psychology Review, 11*, 599–620.

Craske, M. G. (1999). Anxiety disorders: *Psychological approaches to theory and treatment*. Boulder, CO: Westview.

Craske, M. G., & Barlow, D. H. (1988). A review of the relationship between panic and avoidance. *Clinical Psychology Review, 8*, 667–685.

Craske, M. G., Kircanski, K., Epstein, A., Wittchen, H.-U., Pine, D. S., Lewis-Fernandez, R., … DSM V Anxiety Disorder Work Group. (2010). Panic disorder: A review of DSM-IV panic disorder and proposals for DSM-V. *Depression and Anxiety, 27*, 93–112.

Craske, M. G., Kircanski, K., Zelikowsky, M., Mystkowski, J., Chowdhury, N., & Baker, A. (2008). Optimizing inhibitory learning during exposure therapy. *Behaviour Research and Therapy, 46*(1), 5–27.

Crino, R. C., Slade, T., & Andrews, G. (2005). The changing prevalence and severity of obsessive-compulsive disorder criteria from DSM-III to DSM-IV. *American Journal of Psychiatry, 162*, 876–882.

Dalrymple, K. L., & Zimmerman, M. (2008). Screening for social fears and social anxiety disorder in psychiatric outpatients. *Comprehensive Psychiatry, 49*, 399–406.

Davey, G. C. L. (1992). Classical conditioning and the acquisition of human fears and phobias: A review and synthesis of the literature. *Advances in Behaviour Research and Therapy, 14*, 29–66.

Davis, L., Barlow, D. H., & Smith, L. (2010). Comorbidity and the treatment of principal anxiety disorders in a naturalistic sample. *Behaviour Therapy, 41*, 396–305.

de Silva, P., Menzies, R. G., & Shafran, R. (2003). Spontaneous decay of compulsive urges: the case of covert compulsions. *Behaviour Research and Therapy, 41*, 129–137.

de Waal, M. W. M., Arnold, I. A., Eekhof, J. A. H., & van Hemert, A. M. (2004). Somatoform disorders in general practice. *British Journal of Psychiatry, 184*, 470–476.

Doctor, R. (1982). Major results of a large-scale survey of agoraphobics. In R. L. DuPont (Ed.), *Phobia: A comprehensive summary of modern treatments* (pp. 203–214). New York: Brunner-Mazel.

Ehlers, A. (1993). Interoception and panic disorder. *Advances in Behaviour Research and Therapy, 15*, 3–21.

Ehring, T., Ehlers, A., & Glucksman, E. (2008). Do cognitive models help in predicting the severity of post-traumatic stress disorder, phobia, and depression after motor vehicle accidents? A prospective longitudinal study. *Journal of Consulting and Clinical Psychology, 76*, 219–230.

Fergus, T. A., & Valentiner, D. P. (2010). Disease phobia and disease conviction are separate dimensions underlying hypochondriasis. *Journal of Behavior Therapy and Experimental Psychiatry, 41*, 438–444.

Fergus, T. A., & Wu, K. D. (2010). Do symptoms of generalized anxiety and obsessive-compulsive disorder share cognitive processes? *Cognitive Therapy and Research, 34*, 168–176.

Feske, U., & Chambless, D. L. (1995). Cognitive behavioral versus exposure only treatment for social phobia: A meta-analysis. *Behavior Therapy, 26*, 695–720.

Field, A. P., & Lawson, J. (2003). Fear information and the development of fears during childhood: effects on implicit fear responses and behavioural avoidance. *Behaviour Research and Therapy, 41*, 1277–1293.

Fisher, P. L., & Wells, A. (2005). How effective are cognitive and behavioral treatments for obsessive-compulsive disorder? A clinical significance analysis. *Behaviour Research and Therapy, 43*, 1543–1558.

Foa, E. B., & McNally, R. J. (1996). Mechanisms of change in exposure therapy. In R. Rapee (Ed.), *Current controversies in the anxiety disorders* (pp. 329–343). New York: Guilford.

Foster, C., Startup, H., Potts, L., & Freeman, D. (2010). A randomised controlled trial of a worry intervention for individuals with persistent persecutory delusions. *Journal of Behavior Therapy and Experimental Psychiatry, 41*, 45–51.

Frost, R. O., & Steketee, G. (2002). *Cognitive approaches to obsessions and compulsions: Theory, assessment, and treatment.* Elsevier: Oxford.

Fullana, M. A., Mataix-Cols, D., Caspi, A., Harrington, H., Grisham, J. R., Moffitt, T. E., & Poulton, R. (2009). Obsessions and compulsions in the community: Prevalence, interfering, help-seeking, developmental stability, and co-occurring psychiatric conditions. *American Journal of Psychiatry, 166*, 329–336.

Griffith, J. W., Zinbarg, R. E., Craske, M. G., Mineka, S., Rose, R. D., Waters, A. M., & Sutton, J. M. (2010). Neuroticism as a common dimension in the internalizing disorders. *Psychological Medicine, 40*, 1125–1136.

Grisham, J. R., & Williams, A. D. (2009). Cognitive control of obsessional thoughts. *Behaviour Research and Therapy, 47*, 395–402.

Hermans, D., Engelen, U., Grouwels, L., Joos, E., Lemmens, J., & Pieters, G. (2008). Cognitive confidence in obsessive-compulsive disorder: Distrusting perception, attention, and memory. *Behaviour Research and Therapy, 46*, 98–113.

Hersen, M. (1973). Self-assessment of fear. *Behavior Therapy, 4*, 241–257.

Hoehn-Saric, R. (1998). Psychic and somatic anxiety: Worries, somatic symptoms, and physiological changes. *Acta Psychiatrica Scandinavica, 98*(Suppl. 393), 32–38.

Hoehn-Saric, R., McLeod, D. R., Funderburk, F., & Kowalski, P. (2004). Somatic symptoms and physiologic responses in generalized anxiety disorder and panic disorder. *Archives of General Psychiatry, 61*, 913 921.

Hofmann, S. G. (2005). Perception of control over anxiety mediates the relation between catastrophic thinking and social anxiety in social phobia. *Behaviour Research and Therapy, 43*, 885–895.

Hofmann, S. G., Meuret, A. E., Rosenfield, D., Suvak, M. K., Barlow, D. H., Gorman, J. M., … Woods, S. W. (2007). Preliminary evidence for cognitive mediation during cognitive-behavioral therapy for panic disorder. *Journal of Consulting and Clinical Psychology, 75*, 374–379.

Kent, G., & Gibbons, R. (1987). Self-efficacy and the control of anxious cognitions. *Journal of Behavior Therapy and Experimental Psychiatry, 18*, 33–40.

Kessler, R. C., Chiu, W. T., Demler, O., Merikangas, K. R., & Walters, E. E. (2005). Prevalence, severity, and comorbidity of 12-month DSM-IV disorders in the National Comorbidity Survey Replication. *Archives of General Psychiatry, 62*, 617–627.

Kessler, R. C., Chiu, W. T., Jin, R., Ruscio, A. M., Shear, K., & Walters, E. E. (2006). The epidemiology of panic attacks, panic disorder, and agoraphobia in the National Comorbidity Survey Replication. *Archives of General Psychiatry, 63*, 415–424.

Kessler, R. C., Sonnega, A., Bromet, E., Hughes, M., & Nelson, C. B. (1995). Posttraumatic stress disorder in the National Comorbidity Survey. *Archives of General Psychiatry, 52*, 1048–1060.

Kupfer, D. (2005). Dimensional models for research and diagnosis: A current dilemma. *Journal of Abnormal Psychology, 114*, 557–559.

Lang, P. J. (1985). The cognitive psychophysiology of emotion: Fear and anxiety. In A. H. Tuma & J. D. Maser (Eds.), *Anxiety and the anxiety disorders* (pp. 131–170). Hillsdale, NJ: Erlbaum.

LeBeau, R. T., Glenn, D., Liao, B., Wittchen, H.-U., Beesdo-Baum, K., Ollendick, T., & Craske, M. G. (2010). Specific phobia: A review of DSM-IV specific phobia and preliminary recommendations for DSM-V. *Depression and Anxiety, 27*, 148–167.

Lim, S.-L., & Kim, J.-H. (2005). Cognitive processing of emotional information in depression, panic, and somatoform disorder. *Journal of Abnormal Psychology, 114*, 50–61.

Lipsitz, J. D., Barlow, D. H., Mannuzza, S., Hoffman, S. G., & Fyer, A. J. (2002). Clinical features of four DSM-IV specific phobia subtypes. *Journal of Nervous and Mental Disease, 190*, 471–478.

Maddux, J. E. (1995a). Looking for common ground: A comment on Kirsch and Bandura. In J. Maddux (Ed.), *Self-efficacy, adaptation, and adjustment: Theory, research, application* (pp. 377–385). New York: Plenum.

Maddux, J. E. (Ed.). (1995b). *Self-efficacy, adaptation, and adjustment: theory, research, application.* New York: Plenum.

Maj, M. (2005). "Psychiatric comorbidity": An artefact of current diagnostic systems? *British Journal of Psychiatry, 186,* 182–184.

Margraf, J., Taylor, C. B., Ehlers, A., Roth, W. T., & Agras, W. S. (1987). Panic attacks in the natural environment. *Journal of Nervous and Mental Disease, 175,* 558–565.

Markon, K. E. (2010). How things fall apart: Understanding the nature of internalizing through its relationship with impairment. *Journal of Abnormal Psychology, 119,* 447–458.

Maser, J. D., Norman, S. B., Zisook, S., Everall, I. P., Stein, M. B., Schettler, P. J., & Judd, L. L. (2009). Psychiatric nosology is ready for a paradigm shift in DSM-V. *Clinical Psychology and Practice, 16,* 24–40.

Mathews, A. M. (2006). Toward an experimental cognitive science of CBT. *Behavior Therapy, 37,* 314–318.

Mathews, A. M., & MacLeod, C. (2005). Cognitive vulnerability to emotional disorders. *Annual Review of Clinical Psychology, 1,* 167–195.

McNally, R. J. (1999). Panic and phobias. In T. Dalgleish & M. J. Power (Eds.), *Handbook of cognition and emotion* (pp. 479–496). New York: Wiley.

Meiser-Stedman, R., Dalgleish, T., Glucksman, E., Yule, W., & Smith, P. (2009). Maladaptive cognitive appraisals mediate the evolution of posttraumatic stress reactions: A 6-month follow-up of child and adolescent assault and motor vehicle accident survivors. *Journal of Abnormal Psychology, 118,* 778–787.

Michail, M., & Birchwood, M. (2009). Social anxiety disorder in first-episode psychosis: Incidence, phenomenology and relationship with paranoia. *British Journal of Psychiatry, 295,* 234–241.

Mineka, S., Davidson, M., Cook, M., & Keir, R. (1984). Observational conditioning of snake fear in rhesus monkeys. *Journal of Abnormal Psychology, 93,* 344–372.

Mischel, W. (1968). *Personality and assessment.* New York: Wiley.

Mischel, W. (1990). Personality dispositions revisited and revised: A view after three decades. In L. A. Pervin (Ed.), *Handbook of personality: Theory and research* (pp. 111–164). New York: Guilford.

Mitte, K. (2005). Meta-analysis of cognitive-behavioral treatments for generalized anxiety disorder: A comparison with pharmacotherapy. *Psychological Bulletin, 131,* 785–795.

Mitte, K. (2008). Memory bias for threatening information in anxiety and anxiety disorders: A meta-analytic review. *Psychological Bulletin, 134,* 886–911.

Morrison, A. P., & Wells, A. (2007). Relationships between worry, psychotic experiences and emotional distress in patients with schizophrenia spectrum diagnoses and comparisons with anxious and non-patient groups. *Behaviour Research and Therapy, 45,* 1593–1600.

Morrow, G. R., & Labrum, A. H. (1978). The relationship between psychological and physiological measures of anxiety. *Psychological Medicine, 8,* 95–101.

Mowrer, O. H. (1960). *Learning theory and behavior.* New York: Wiley.

Naragon-Gainey, K. (2010). Meta-analysis of the relations of anxiety sensitivity to the depressive and anxiety disorders. *Psychological Bulletin, 136,* 128–150.

Narrow, W. E., Rae, D. S., Robins, L. N., & Regier, D. A. (2002). Revised prevalence estimates of mental disorders in the United States. *Archives of General Psychiatry, 59,* 115–123.

O'Dwyer, A., & Marks, I. M. (2000). Obsessive-compulsive disorder and delusions revisited. *British Journal of Psychiatry, 176,* 281–284.

Ollendick, T. H., Öst, L.-G., Reuterskiöld, L., Costa, N., Ciederlund, R., Sirbu, C., … Jarrett, M. A. (2009). One-session treatment of specific phobias in youth: A randomized controlled trial in the United States and Sweden. *Journal of Consulting and Clinical Psychology, 77,* 504–516.

Oosterink, F. M. D., de Jongh, A., & Aartman, I. H. A. (2009). Negative events and their potential risk of precipitating pathological forms of dental anxiety. *Journal of Anxiety Disorders, 23,* 451–457.

Öst, L.-G., Ferebee, I., & Furmark T. (1997). One-session group therapy of spider phobia: Direct versus indirect treatments. *Behaviour Research and Therapy, 35,* 721–732.

Öst, L.-G., Salkovskis, P., & Hellstrom, K. (1991). One-session therapist-directed exposure vs. self-exposure in the treatment of spider phobia. *Behavior Therapy, 22,* 407–422.

Öst, L.-G., Thulin, U., Ramnero, J. (2004). Cognitive behavior therapy vs. exposure in vivo in the treatment of panic disorder with agoraphobia. *Behaviour Research and Therapy, 42,* 1105–1127.

Persons, J. (1986). The advantages of studying psychological phenomena rather than psychiatric diagnoses. *American Psychologist, 11,* 1252–1260.

Rachman, S. (1976). The passing of the two-stage theory of fear and avoidance: Fresh possibilities. *Behaviour Research and Therapy, 14,* 125–131.

Rachman, S. (1977). The conditioning theory of fear acquisition: A critical examination. *Behaviour Research and Therapy, 15,* 375–387.

Rachman, S. (1998). A cognitive theory of obsessions: Elaborations. *Behaviour Research and Therapy, 36,* 385–401.

Rachman, S., & de Silva, P. (1978). Abnormal and normal obsessions. *Behavior Research and Therapy, 16,* 233–248.

Rachman, S., & Hodgson, R. (1974). I. Synchrony and desynchrony in fear and avoidance. *Behaviour Research and Therapy, 12,* 311–318.

Rachman, S., Radomsky, A. S., & Shafran, R. (2008). Safety behavior: A reconsideration. *Behaviour Research and Therapy, 46,* 163–173.

Rachman, S., & Shafran, R. (1998). Cognitive and behavioral features of obsessive-compulsive disorder. In R. P. Swinson, M. M. Anthony, S. Rachman, & M. A. Richter (Eds.), *Obsessive-compulsive disorder* (pp. 51–78). New York: Guilford.

Rapee, R. M. (1993). Psychological factors in panic disorder. *Advances in Behavior Research and Therapy, 15,* 85–102.

Rapee, R. M., & Barlow, D. H. (Eds.). (1991). *Chronic anxiety.* New York: Guilford.

Rapee, R. M., & Spence, S. (2004). The etiology of social phobia. Empirical evidence and an initial model. *Clinical Psychology Review, 24,* 737–767.

Regier, D. A., Narrow, W. E., Kuhl, E. A., & Kupfer, D. J. (2009). The conceptual development of DSM-V. *American Journal of Psychiatry, 166,* 645–650.

Roemer, L., & Orsillo, S. M. (2007). An open trial of an acceptance-based behavior therapy for generalized anxiety disorder. *Behavior Therapy, 38,* 72–85.

Ruscio, A. M. (2010). The latent structure of social anxiety disorder: Consequences of shifting to a dimensional diagnosis. *Journal of Abnormal Psychology, 119,* 662–671.

Salcioglu, E., Basoglu, M., & Livanou, M. (2007). Effects of live exposure on symptoms of posttraumatic stress disorder: The role of reduced behavioral avoidance in improvement. *Behaviour Research and Therapy, 45,* 2268–2279.

Salkovskis, P. M. (1991). The importance of behaviour in the maintenance of anxiety and panic: A cognitive account. *Behavioural Psychotherapy, 19,* 6–19.

Salkovskis, P. M. (1996). Cognitive behavioral approaches to the understanding of obsessional problems. In R. M. Rapee (Ed.), *Current controversies in the anxiety disorders* (pp. 103–133). New York: Guilford.

Salkovskis, P. M., & Warwick, H. M. C. (1986). Morbid preoccupations, health anxiety and reassurance: A cognitive behavioural approach to hypochondriasis. *Behaviour Research and Therapy, 24,* 597–602.

Sanchez-Meca, J., Rosa-Alcanzar, A. I., Martin-Martinez, F., & Gomez-Conesa, A. (2010). Psychological treatment of panic disorder with or without agoraphobia: A meta-analysis. *Clinical Psychology Review, 30,* 37–50.

Schwartz, B. (1989). *Psychology of learning and behavior* (3rd ed.). New York: Norton.

See, J., MacLeod, C., & Bridle, R. (2009). The reduction of anxiety vulnerability through the modification of attentional bias: A real-world study using a home-based cognitive bias modification procedure. *Journal of Abnormal Psychology, 118,* 65–75.

Seligman, M. E. P., & Johnston, J. C. (1973). A cognitive theory of avoidance learning. In F. J. McGuigan & D. B. Lumsden (Eds.), *Contemporary approaches to conditioning and learning* (pp. 69–110). Washington, DC: Winston.

Slade, T., & Grisham, J. R. (2009). A taxometric investigation of agoraphobia in a clinical and a community sample. *Journal of Anxiety Disorders, 23,* 799–805.

Smith, G. T., & Oltmanns, T. F. (2009). Scientific advances in the diagnosis of psychopathology: Introduction to the special section. *Psychological Assessment, 21,* 241–242.

Smits, J. A. J., Powers, M. B., Cho, Y., & Telch, M. J. (2004). Mechanism of change in cognitive-behavioral treatment of panic disorder: Evidence for the fear of fear mediational hypothesis. *Journal of Consulting and Clinical Psychology, 72,* 646–652.

Solomon, Z., & Mikulincer, M. (2007). Posttraumatic intrusion, avoidance, and social functioning: A 20-year longitudinal study. *Journal of Consulting and Clinical Psychology, 75,* 316–324.

Spitzer, R. L., & Williams, J. B. W. (1985). Proposed revisions in the DSM-III classification of anxiety disorders based on research and clinical experience. In A. H. Tuma & J. D. Maser (Eds.), *Anxiety and the anxiety disorders* (pp. 759–773). Hillsdale, NJ: Erlbaum.

Stapinski, L. A., Abbott, M., & Rapee, R. M. (2010). Fear and perceived uncontrollability of emotion: evaluating the unique contribution of emotion appraisal variables to prediction of worry and generalised anxiety disorder. *Behaviour Research and Therapy, 48,* 1097–1104.

Stein, M. B., Walker, J. R., & Forde, D. R. (1994). Setting diagnostic thresholds for social phobia: Considerations from a community study of social anxiety. *American Journal of Psychiatry, 152,* 408–412.

Steketee, G., & Barlow, D. H. (2002). Obsessive-compulsive disorder. In D. H. Barlow (Ed.), *Anxiety and its disorders* (pp. 516–550). New York: Guilford.

Stewart. R. E., & Chambless, D. L. (2009). Cognitive-behavioral therapy for adult anxiety disorders in clinical practice: A meta-analysis of effectiveness studies. *Journal of Consulting and Clinical Psychology, 77,* 595–606.

Taylor, S., Thordson, D. S., Maxfield, L., Fedeoroff, I. C., Lovell, K., & Ogrodniczuk, J. (2003). Comparative efficacy, speed, and adverse effects of three PTSD treatments. *Journal of Consulting and Clinical Psychology, 71,* 330–338.

Vögele, C., Ehlers, A., Meyer, A. H., Frank, M., Hahlweg, K., & Margraf, J. (2010). Cognitive mediation of clinical improvement after intensive exposure therapy of agoraphobia and social phobia. *Depression and Anxiety, 27,* 294–301.

Walk, R. D. (1956). Self ratings of fear in a fear-invoking situation. *Journal of Abnormal and Social Psychology, 52,* 171–178.

Wells, A. (2004). A cognitive model of GAD. In R. G. Heimberg, C. L. Turk, & D. S. Mennen (Eds.), *Generalized anxiety disorder: Advances in research and practice* (pp. 164–186), London: Guilford.

Wilamowska, Z. A., Thompson-Hollands, J., Fairholme, C. P., Ellard, K. K., Farchione, T. J., & Barlow, D. H. (2010). Conceptual background, development, and preliminary data from the unified protocol for transdiagnostic treatment of emotional disorders. *Depression and Anxiety, 27,* 882–890.

Williams, S. L. (1985). On the nature and measurement of agoraphobia. *Progress in Behavior Modification, 19,* 109–144.

Williams, S. L. (1987). On anxiety and phobia. *Journal of Anxiety Disorders, 1,* 161–180.

Williams, S. L. (1990). Guided mastery treatment of agoraphobia: Beyond stimulus exposure. *Progress in Behavior Modification, 26,* 89–121.

Williams, S. L. (1996a). Therapeutic changes in phobic behavior are mediated by changes in perceived self-efficacy. In R. Rapee (Ed.), *Current controversies in the anxiety disorders* (pp. 344–368). New York: Guilford.

Williams, S. L. (1996b). Overcoming phobia: Unconscious bioinformational deconditioning or conscious cognitive reappraisal? In R. Rapee (Ed.), *Current controversies in the anxiety disorders* (pp. 373–376). New York: Guilford.

Williams, S. L. (2008). Anxiety disorders. In J. E. Maddux & B. A. Winstead (Eds.). *Psychopathology: Foundations for a contemporary understanding.* (2nd ed., pp. 141–169). New York: Routledge.

Williams, S. L., & Cervone, D. (1998). Social cognitive theories of personality. In D. F. Barone, M. Hersen, & V. B. Van Hasselt (Eds.), *Advanced personality* (pp. 173–207). New York: Plenum.

Williams, S. L., Dooseman, G., & Kleifield, E. (1984). Comparative effectiveness of guided mastery and exposure treatments for intractable phobias. *Journal of Consulting and Clinical Psychology, 52,* 505–518.

Williams, S. L., & Falbo, J. (1996). Cognitive and performance-based treatments for panic attacks in people with varying degrees of agoraphobic disability. *Behaviour Research and Therapy, 34,* 253–264.

Williams, S. L., Kinney, P. J., & Falbo, J. (1989). Generalization of therapeutic changes in agoraphobia: The role of perceived self-efficacy. *Journal of Consulting and Clinical Psychology, 57,* 436–442.

Williams, S. L., Kinney, P. J., Harap, S., & Liebmann, M. (1997). Thoughts of agoraphobic people during scary tasks. *Journal of Abnormal Psychology, 106,* 511–520.

Williams, S. L., & LaBerge, B. (1994). Panic disorder with agoraphobia. In C. G. Last & M. Hersen (Eds.), *Adult behavior therapy casebook* (pp. 107–123). New York: Plenum.

Williams, S. L., & Margraf, J. (2011). *A mental disorder is less than the psychosocial problems that define it.* Unpublished manuscript. Ruhr-University Bochum, Germany.

Williams, S. L., Turner, S. M., & Peer, D. F. (1985). Guided mastery and performance desensitization treatments for severe acrophobia. *Journal of Consulting and Clinical Psychology, 53,* 237–247.

Williams, S. L., & Watson, N. (1985). Perceived danger and perceived self-efficacy as cognitive determinants of acrophobic behavior. *Behavior Therapy, 16,* 237–247.

Williams, S. L., & Zane, G. (1989). Guided mastery and stimulus exposure treatments for severe performance anxiety in agoraphobics. *Behaviour Research and Therapy, 27,* 237–247.

Wilson, G. T. (1978). The importance of being theoretical: A commentary on Bandura's "Self-efficacy: Toward a unifying theory of behavioral change." *Advances in Behaviour Research and Therapy, 1,* 217–230.

Wittchen, H.-U., Gloster, A. T., Beesdo-Baum, K., Fava, G. A., & Craske, M. (2010). Agoraphobia: A review of the diagnostic classificatory position and criteria. *Depression and Anxiety, 27*, 113–133.

Wolpe, J. (1958). *Psychotherapy by reciprocal inhibition*. Stanford, CA: Stanford University Press.

World Health Organization. (1992). *The ICD-10 classification of mental and behavioural disorders: Clinical description and diagnostic guidelines*. Geneva: Author.

Zimmerman, M., Dalrymple, K., Chelminski, I., Young, D., & Galione, J. N. (2010). Recognition of irrationality of fear and the diagnosis of social anxiety disorder and specific phobia in adults: Implications for criteria revision in DSM-5. *Depression and Anxiety, 27*(11), 1044–1049.

9

Mood Disorders

LAUREN B. ALLOY, DENISE LABELLE, ELAINE BOLAND,
KIM GOLDSTEIN, ABIGAIL JENKINS, BENJAMIN SHAPERO,
SHIMRIT K. BLACK, and OLGA OBRAZTSOVA

Temple University
Philadelphia, Pennsylvania

Consider the case of David, a 24-year-old who sought neuropsychological testing to assess for attention-deficit/hyperactivity disorder (ADHD). David had been taking classes at a local university for the past 4 years to complete his degree. He wanted to be assessed for ADHD because he was experiencing significant difficulties sustaining and paying attention in his classes, and his grades began to suffer. He failed his classes one semester and was placed on academic probation.

Additionally, David was running his own Internet advertising business while attending school. He reported that he was able to keep the business running, but he felt it was suffering due to his current state of disorganization. He was unable to arrive at meetings on time, took poor notes, and had considerable difficulty keeping the business organized. As a result, he was in debt and could not properly manage his finances.

Although many elements of David's story are common in individuals with ADHD, they are also familiar to many people who suffer from severe depression. During David's assessment, he was given a diagnostic interview as well as the Beck Depression Inventory (BDI), a 21-item self-report of depressive symptoms. David reported depressed mood, feelings of hopelessness about his future, irritability, guilt about his failing business and poor academic performance, marked fatigue and sluggishness, anhedonia, and severe sleep disturbance (marked insomnia, sleep continuity disturbance, and early morning awakenings). His symptoms were persistent and severe enough to meet the *Diagnostic and Statistical Manual of Mental Disorders* (*DSM*) criteria for a major depressive episode, and his high score on the BDI—43—indicated this episode was particularly severe. Moreover, David also reported substantial symptoms of anxiety and worry, such as feelings of dread, numbness, hot and cold sweats, shortness of breath, and heart palpitations. Anxiety symptoms are often comorbid in an episode of major depressive disorder and can contribute to the overall impairment of the episode.

Although David had been aware that his mood was lower than he would like it to be, it was not his mood, but rather his inability to keep himself organized, make everyday decisions, or focus on his work that was driving him to seek an assessment for ADHD, which he suspected was the root of his day-to-day difficulties. David was given a battery of neuropsychological tests in addition to diagnostic interviews. Although the results of these assessments were indicative of impairments in attention and concentration, the severity of David's depression and anxiety made it nearly impossible to assign an unequivocal diagnosis of ADHD. Instead, the evaluator recommended that David first seek treatment for his depression and anxiety, as she hypothesized that his attention and concentration symptoms would improve as a result.

David's story is not an uncommon one in clinical settings. Many individuals with moderate to severe depression experience marked impairments in their ability to do their jobs, perform well in school, and stay on top of household chores. However, major depressive disorder is often responsive to treatment either with psychotherapy, pharmacotherapy, or their combination and many see a restoration of their general functioning following a targeted treatment regimen.

We are all familiar, at least casually, with what depression is like. We have all experienced occasional periods of sadness, where nothing seems worth doing, we become tired and slowed down, and our lives are no longer fun. Some have also experienced the opposite state, when we feel on top of the world, excited and reckless, and we become hyperactive and think that we can accomplish anything. In other words, *depression* and *mania*, in mild and temporary forms, are part of everyday existence. For some people, however, these mood swings become so prolonged and extreme that the person's life is seriously disrupted. These conditions are known as *mood disorders* or *affective disorders*.

Mood disorders have been recognized as clinical entities for over 2,000 years. Indeed, Hippocrates described both depression and mania in detail in the fourth century BCE. As early as the first century CE, the Greek physician Aretaeus observed that manic and depressive behaviors sometimes occurred in the same person and seemed to stem from a single disorder. Although they have been studied for centuries, as yet there are no completely satisfactory explanations for the puzzling features of mood disorders. This chapter will first describe the mood disorders as well as their diagnosis, symptoms, dimensions, and risk factors. Then, it will review what is known about the causes and treatment of mood disorders from various theoretical perspectives.

Depressive and Manic Episodes

Typically, mood disorders are episodic. Within days, weeks, or months, a person who has been functioning normally is plunged into despair or becomes euphoric. Once the episode runs its course, the person may return to normal or near-normal functioning, though he or she is likely to have recurrences of mood disturbance. The severity, duration, and nature of the episode (whether depressive or manic) determine the diagnosis. The sections below describe the typical features of depressive and manic episodes.

Major Depressive Episode

Onset of a *major depressive* (MD) *episode* is usually gradual, occurring over a period of several weeks or months, and the episode typically lasts several months and then ends, as it began, gradually (Coryell et al., 1994). Major depressive episodes affect mood, motivation, thinking, somatic, and motor functioning. The characteristic features of a major depressive episode are (see Table 9.1 for the *DSM–IV–TR* diagnostic criteria):

1. *Depressed mood.* Almost all depressed adults report some sadness, ranging from mild melancholy to total hopelessness. Mildly or moderately depressed people may have crying spells; severely depressed individuals often say they feel like crying but cannot. Deeply depressed people see no way that they or anyone else can help them—the *helplessness-hopelessness syndrome.*
2. *Loss of pleasure or interest in usual activities. Anhedonia*, the loss of pleasure or interest in one's usual activities, is the other most common characteristic of a major depressive episode. Even emotional responses to pleasant stimuli are diminished during a major depressive episode (Sloan, Strauss, & Wisner, 2001).
3. *Disturbance of appetite.* Most depressed people have poor appetite and lose weight; however, a minority react by eating more and putting on weight. Whichever type of weight change, the same change tends to occur with each depressive episode (Kendler et al., 1996).

Table 9.1 *DSM–IV–TR* Diagnostic Criteria of Mood Episodes

Manic Episode		
	A.	A discrete period lasting at least 1 week during which the individual feels abnormally euphoric, irritable, or expansive in a way that is clearly different from his or her normal self. If hospitalization is required, duration criteria are not necessary.
	B.	At least three, sometimes more, of the following symptoms must be present during manic episodes:
		1. Feeling unusually self-confident or having significantly increased self-esteem
		2. Needing fewer hours of sleep at night, but feeling completely rested
		3. Feeling unusually talkative or a pressure to keep talking
		4. Experiencing racing (rapid) thoughts
		5. Being unusually and easily distracted by normally irrelevant environmental stimuli
		6. Feeling the desire to accomplish more goals, complete tasks, or start new projects
		7. Getting involved in activities that may reflect poor judgment and may have serious consequences
	C.	The symptoms would not be better explained as a mixed episode
	D.	The symptoms of the manic episode cause problems in the working environment, within the family, or in interpersonal relationships and social activities. Symptoms may be severe enough to necessitate hospitalization or psychotic symptoms may be present.
	E.	The symptoms above are not better explained by substance abuse or the effects of drugs or antidepressant medications or by general medical conditions such as hyperthyroidism.
Hypomanic Episode		
	A.	A discrete period lasting at least 4 days during which the individual feels abnormally euphoric, irritable, or expansive in a way that is clearly different from his or her normal self.
	B.	At least three, sometimes more, of the following symptoms must be present during hypomanic episodes:
		1. Feeling unusually self confident or having significantly increased self-esteem
		2. Needing fewer hours of sleep at night, but feeling completely rested
		3. Feeling unusually talkative or a pressure to keep talking
		4. Experiencing racing (rapid) thoughts
		5. Being unusually and easily distracted by normally irrelevant environmental stimuli
		6. Feeling the desire to accomplish more goals, complete tasks, or start new projects
		7. Getting involved in activities that may reflect poor judgment and may have serious consequences
	C.	There are notable changes and decreases in functioning that are not present when the person is asymptomatic.
	D.	Other people can observe the changes in mood or functioning
	E.	Symptoms are not severe enough to warrant hospitalization. Additionally, there are no psychotic symptoms present.
	F.	The symptoms above are not better explained by substance abuse or the effects of drugs or antidepressant medications or by general medical conditions such as hyperthyroidism.

continued

Table 9.1 *DSM–IV–TR* Diagnostic Criteria of Mood Episodes (Continued)

Major Depressive Episode	A.	A discrete period lasting at least 2 weeks during which an individual experiences a notable change in functioning and at least 5 of the following symptoms (at least one symptom must be depressed mood or loss of interest):
		1. Depressed mood that is experienced almost all day nearly every day
		2. Marked decrease in or loss of interest in pleasurable activities nearly all day, every day
		3. Losing weight without dieting, gaining weight, or noticing a marked decrease or increase in appetite
		4. Difficulty falling asleep or sleeping too much
		5. Feeling restless or unable to sit still, or feeling physically slowed down
		6. Marked fatigue and loss of energy
		7. Feeling guilty for things one has or has not done, as well as inappropriate and excessive guilt or feeling worthless about oneself
		8. Difficulty concentrating
		9. Thoughts of death recurrently or wanting to hurt/kill oneself, though no specific plan or intent is present, or making a suicide attempt
	B.	The symptoms would not be better explained as a mixed episode
	C.	As a result of these symptoms, the individual experiences significant distress or impairments in relationships or the ability to do work.
	D.	The symptoms above are not better explained by substance abuse or the effects of drugs or by general medical conditions such as hypothyroidism.
	E.	The symptoms are not better explained by grief over loss of a loved one.
Mixed Episode	A.	A distinct 1-week period during which criteria for a manic episode and a major depressive episode are simultaneously met every day.
	B.	Mood symptoms during this 1-week period cause impairment in any of the following domains: occupational functioning, social functioning, interpersonal relationships. Psychotic features may be present, and hospitalization may be necessary if severe enough.
	C.	The symptoms above are not better explained by substance abuse, the effects of drugs or antidepressant medications, or a general medical condition.

From American Psychiatric Association. (2000). *Diagnostic and statistical manual of mental health* (4th text rev. ed.) Washington, DC: Author, pp. 356, 362, 365, 368.

4. *Sleep disturbances.* Insomnia is an extremely common feature of depression and can take one or more of three forms. Depressed people may have trouble falling asleep initially, or may awaken repeatedly throughout the night, or may wake up too early in the morning and be unable to fall back to sleep. However, like eating, sleep may increase rather than decrease, with the depressed person sleeping 15 hr a day or more. Depressed individuals who exhibit excessive sleeping are usually the same ones who eat excessively (Kendler et al., 1996).

5. *Psychomotor retardation or agitation.* In *retarded depression*, the most common psychomotor pattern, the depressed person is fatigued, movement is slow and deliberate, posture is stooped, and speech is low and halting, with long pauses before answering. In severe cases, individuals may fall into a mute stupor. Some evidence suggests that the symptom of psychomotor retardation is related to low presynaptic dopamine levels (Paillere Martinot et al., 2001; Smith, this volume). Less frequently, in *agitated depression*, the person shows incessant activity and restlessness—hand wringing and pacing.

6. *Loss of energy.* The depressed person usually exhibits a sharply reduced energy level and may feel exhausted all the time.

7. *Feelings of worthlessness and guilt.* Depressed people see themselves as deficient in whatever attributes they value most: intelligence, beauty, popularity. These feelings of worthlessness are often accompanied by a profound sense of guilt. Depressed individuals believe that any problem is their fault.

8. *Difficulties in thinking.* As in David's case (presented at the start of the chapter), depressed people have trouble concentrating, remembering, and making decisions, even about everyday matters (what to wear, etc.). The harder a mental task, the more difficulty they have (Hartlage, Alloy, Vasquez, & Dykman, 1993).

9. *Recurring thoughts of death or suicide.* Many depressed people have recurrent thoughts of death and suicide. Often, they say they (and everyone else) would be better off if they were dead.

Manic Episode

A typical *manic episode* begins relatively suddenly, over a few days, and is usually shorter than a depressive episode, lasting from several days to several months. The features of a manic episode are as follows (see Table 9.1 for the *DSM–IV–TR* diagnostic criteria):

1. *Elevated, expansive, or irritable mood.* Typically, people in a manic episode feel "high" and on top of the world and have limitless enthusiasm for whatever they are doing. This expansiveness is often mixed with irritability when someone tries to interfere with their behavior. In some cases, irritability is the manic person's dominant mood, with euphoria either intermittent or simply absent.

2. *Inflated self-esteem.* People with mania believe they have highly important plans and special talents and abilities. They tend to see themselves as extremely attractive, powerful, and capable of great achievements, even if they have no such aptitude. They may begin composing symphonies, designing nuclear weapons, or calling the White House with ideas on how to run the country.

3. *Sleeplessness.* Manic episodes are almost always marked by a decreased need for sleep. Manic individuals may sleep only 2 or 3 hr a night, but have twice as much energy as those around them.

4. *Talkativeness.* People with mania tend to talk loudly, rapidly, and constantly. Their speech is often full of puns and jokes that they alone find funny.

5. *Flight of ideas.* Manic individuals' speech often shifts rapidly from topic to topic. They often have racing thoughts; this may be why they speak so rapidly—to keep up with the flow of their ideas.

6. *Distractibility.* Manic individuals are easily distracted. Their attention is frequently pulled by irrelevant and unimportant aspects of the environment.

7. *Hyperactivity.* The expansive mood is usually accompanied by restlessness and increased goal-directed activity—physical, social, occupational, and often sexual.

8. *Reckless behavior.* The euphoria and grandiose self-image of manic people often lead them to impulsive, reckless actions: shopping sprees, reckless driving, careless business investments, sexual indiscretions, and so on. They may impulsively call friends in the middle of the night or spend the family savings on a new sports car.

A *hypomanic episode* is briefer and less severe than a manic episode and does not require impairment, but it has similar symptoms as a manic episode. When a person meets the criteria for major depression and manic episodes simultaneously (e.g., exhibits manic hyperactivity and grandiosity, but also cries and is suicidal), it is called a *mixed episode*. Mixed episodes are not uncommon (Dilsaver, Chen, Shoah, & Swann, 1999) and are proposed as a specifier of mood disorders in the upcoming DSM–5 (see Table 9.1 for the *DSM–IV–TR* criteria for hypomanic and mixed episodes).

Mood Disorder Syndromes

Major Depressive Disorder

People who experience one or more major depressive episodes, with no mania, hypomania, or mixed episodes, have, according to the *DSM, major depressive disorder* (MDD). The prevalence of this disorder during any given month is close to 4% of men and 6% of women. The lifetime risk is about 17% (Ustin, 2001). Major depression is now the fourth leading cause of disability and premature death worldwide (Murray & Lopez, 1996). Depression leads to more office visits than any other medical problem except hypertension and greater impairment—more workdays lost, more time in bed—than chronic medical conditions, such as diabetes or heart disease (Druss, Rosenheck, & Sledge, 2000; Wells & Sherbourne, 1999). Further, although there are effective treatments for depression, most people with major depression do not receive adequate treatment (Young, Klap, Sherbourne, & Wells, 2001). Moreover, each successive generation born since World War II has shown higher rates of depression (Burke, Burke, Rae, & Regier, 1991; Compton, Conway, Stinson, & Grant, 2006; Klerman, 1988). According to some experts, we are in an age of depression.

Course   Major depression is a highly recurrent disorder, with about 80% of all people, with first onset of major depression experiencing at least one recurrence (Judd, 1997). The more previous episodes, the younger the person was at first onset, female gender, family history of depression, the more stressful life events endured recently, the less social support the person received, and the more negative cognitions the individual has the greater the likelihood of recurrence (Belsher & Costello, 1988; Burcusa & Iacono, 2007). Over a lifetime, the median number of episodes per patient is four, with a median duration of 4.5 months per episode (Judd, 1997; Solomon et al., 1997).

The course of recurrent depression varies considerably. Following a depressive episode, some people return to their level of functioning prior to the onset of the disorder, whereas others still show serious impairment in job status, income, marital adjustment, social relationships, and recreational activities 10 years after the episode (Judd et al., 2000). Depression also affects the immune system, leaving people more susceptible to illness and death

(Schleifer, Keller, Bartlett, Eckholdt, & Delaney, 1996; Penninx et al., 2001). Thus, it is difficult for people recovering from a depressive episode to resume their former lives. Indeed, research on "stress generation" indicates that the symptoms and behaviors characteristic of a depressive episode actually generate stressful life events, which in turn can maintain the depression and produce a cycle of chronic stress and impairment (Daley et al., 1997; Liu & Alloy, 2010).

The early course or *prodrome* of depression (early symptoms or signs of an impending episode) has also garnered attention (Iacoviello, Alloy, Abramson, & Choi, 2010; Jackson, Cavanaugh, & Scott, 2003). Certain symptoms, such as sad mood, anhedonia, hopelessness, difficulty concentrating, worrying or brooding, decreased self-esteem, and irritability, are more likely to be present among individuals entering a depressive episode than among demographically similar individuals who did not develop an episode. In addition, the durations of prodromal and residual (symptoms still present as an episode is remitting) phases are correlated, the prodromal and residual symptom profiles are quite similar, and the order of symptom onset during the prodrome is negatively correlated with the order of symptom remission (Iacoviello et al., 2010).

Groups at Risk for Depression   Although depression can strike anyone at any time, some groups are especially vulnerable to experiencing an episode of depression. Research has shown that Hispanic youth, and especially Hispanic girls, tend to have higher rates of depressive symptoms than White or African American youth (McLaughlin, Hilt, & Nolen-Hoeksema, 2007; Twenge & Nolen-Hoeksema, 2002). Some of these differences, however, can be accounted for by controlling for parental education level as well as differences in poverty and perceived support at home and at school (Kennard, Stewart Hughes, Patel, & Emslie, 2006; Mikolajczyk, Bredehorst, Khelaifat, Maier, & Maxwell, 2007). Never-married and formerly married individuals have higher depressive symptoms than those who are married (Mirowsky & Ross, 2003; Turner & Lloyd, 1999). In addition, later-born cohorts have a higher lifetime prevalence of depression (Kessler et al., 2003), which has led to the popular belief that there is currently a depression "epidemic" among today's youth. A large meta-analysis has shown, however, that when concurrent assessment, rather than retrospective recall, is used, there is no evidence for an increased prevalence of child or adolescent depression over the past 30 years (Costello, Erkanli, & Angold, 2006). On the other end of the age spectrum, comorbid conditions associated with aging rather than aging itself may be responsible for the increase in depressive symptoms seen with age (Snowdon, 2001). According to Nguyen and Zonderman (2006), rates of depression remain relatively stable across most of the adult lifespan (ages 25 to 70) and increase thereafter.

One of the most consistent findings in depression research is the gender difference in rates of depression. Epidemiological studies conducted in the United States and European countries have shown that women are twice as likely to develop depression as men (Angst et al., 2002; Kuehner, 2003). In addition, the dramatic gender difference in depression rates in women first emerges during adolescence (Hankin & Abramson, 2001; Nolen-Hoeksema, 2001) and lasts through adulthood. Prior to adolescence, boys and girls tend to have similar rates of depression, and some research has shown that boys might be at an even higher risk for developing depression (Twenge & Nolen-Hoeksema, 2002). These differences in prevalence rates of depression are due to women having a higher risk of first onset, not a difference in the persistence or recurrence of the depressive episodes (Kessler, 2003). There are some cultural groups such as the Old Order Amish and Orthodox Jews that serve as intriguing exceptions to these widespread findings (Angst et al., 2002; Piccinelli & Wilkinson, 2000). Depression rates for women in these groups may be lower because these groups' cultural norms reduce the sexual objectification of girls in adolescence (Hyde, Mezulis, & Abramson, 2008).

A multitude of factors have been implicated in the gender difference in depression rates across the lifespan. Adolescent girls might not welcome the physical changes that accompany puberty as much as boys do, and research has shown that this "body dissatisfaction" is often associated with depressive symptoms (Hankin & Abramson, 2001; Siegel, Yancey, Aneshensel, & Schuler, 1999). Researchers have also identified several psychological factors that contribute to women's vulnerability to developing depression. One is women's interpersonal orientation. It has been suggested that women tend to derive more of their self-worth from their relationships than men (Cyranowski, Frank, Young, & Shear, 2000). Adolescent girls generally score higher than boys on measures of need for social approval and reassurance seeking, which puts them at higher risk for developing depressive symptoms (Rudolph & Conley, 2005). Women's greater interpersonal orientation makes them more susceptible to experiencing more interpersonal stressors, which have been associated with depression (Hammen, 2003).

Although individuals can respond to sad mood in a variety of ways, rumination is especially harmful. *Rumination* involves responding to one's sad mood in a passive manner by repeatedly dwelling on the causes and symptoms of one's depressive mood rather than taking active steps to change one's mood (Nolen-Hoeksema, 1991). Women tend to ruminate more than men in response to sad mood, and controlling for the gender difference in rumination makes the gender difference in depression disappear (Nolen-Hoeksema & Jackson, 2001; Nolen-Hoeksema, Larson, & Grayson, 1999).

Along with biological and psychological factors, social factors also play a role in explaining the higher rates of depression in women. Women experience higher levels of sexual and physical abuse than men, which puts them at a higher risk for developing depression across their lifetimes (Kendler, Gardner, & Prescott, 2002; Weiss, Longhurst, & Mazure, 1999). Childhood sexual abuse has been found to be an especially strong predictor of development of future psychopathology, including depression (Kendler, Kuhn, & Prescott, 2004).

No single factor is implicated in the disparity in rates of depression among men and women. Nolen-Hoeksema and Girgus (1994) proposed a model that suggests that women have a variety of vulnerability factors that interact with new stressors that emerge in adolescence to produce the gender gap in depression.

Bipolar Disorder

Whereas major depression is confined to depressive episodes, *bipolar disorder* typically involves both manic or hypomanic and depressive episodes. Some individuals have a manic or mixed episode—or a series of such episodes—with no depressive episodes. Such cases, though they involve only one "pole," are still classified as bipolar disorder because, aside from the absence of depressive episodes, they resemble the classic bipolar disorder. Some researchers suspect that they are simply cases of insufficient follow-up for depressive episodes. Alternatively, some individuals have both depressive and hypomanic, rather than fully manic, episodes. Thus, *DSM–IV–TR* has divided bipolar disorder into two types. In *bipolar I disorder*, the person has had at least one manic (or mixed) episode and usually, but not necessarily, at least one major depressive episode as well. In *bipolar II disorder*, the person has had at least one major depressive episode and at least one hypomanic episode, but has never met the diagnostic criteria for manic or mixed episode. In a less common pattern, called the *rapid-cycling type*, the person (usually a woman) switches back and forth between depressive and manic or mixed episodes (with at least four mood episodes per year), with little or no "normal" functioning between (Leibenluft, 2000). This pattern, which tends to have a poor prognosis (Leibenluft, 2000), occurs in about 25% of bipolar patients in response to antidepressant medication (Suppes, Dennehy, & Gibbons, 2000).

Table 9.2 Differences Between Bipolar Disorder and Major Depression

	Bipolar Disorder	Major Depression
Gender Ratio	Equal	2:1 (women:men)
Course	More frequent, brief episodes	Less frequent, longer episodes
Prognosis	Greater impairment; but some outcomes of high accomplishment	Less impairment
Prevalence	0.5–3.5% of the U.S. population	17% of the U.S. population
Marital Status	No difference n rates for married vs. unmarried people	Lower rates in married people
Depressive Episodes	Psychomotor retardation common	Psychomotor retardation less common
Genetics	Strong heritability	Weaker heritability
Personality Features	Hyperactivity, ADHD, impulsivity	Dependency, low self-esteem, and obsessional thinking

Adapted from L. B. Alloy, J. H. Riskind, & M. Manos. *Abnormal psychology: Current perspectives* (9th ed.). New York, NY: McGraw-Hill.

The occurrence of manic, hypomanic, or mixed episodes is not all that differentiates bipolar disorder from major depression (see Table 9.2; Rehm, Wagner, & Ivens-Tyndal, 2001). First, bipolar disorder is much less common than major depression, affecting an estimated 0.5 to 3.5% of the world population (Miklowitz & Johnson, 2006). Second, unlike major depression, bipolar disorder occurs in both genders with approximately equal frequency, and bipolar disorder is more prevalent among higher socioeconomic groups. Third, whereas people who are married or have intimate relationships are less prone to major depression, they are not at decreased risk for bipolar disorder. Fourth, people with major depression tend to have histories of low self-esteem, dependency, and obsessional thinking, whereas people with bipolar disorder are more likely to have a history of hyperactivity or ADHD (Sachs, Baldassano, Truman, & Guillo, 2000; Walshaw, Alloy, & Sabb, 2010). Fifth, the depressive episodes in bipolar disorder are more likely to involve psychomotor retardation, excess sleep, and weight or appetite increase than those in major depression (Benazzi, 2000, 2001). Sixth, bipolar disorder mood episodes are generally briefer and more frequent than are those in major depression (Cusin, Serretti, Lattuada, Mandelli, & Smeraldi, 2000). Seventh, bipolar disorder is associated with greater impairment in marital and work functioning, substance use, as well as heightened risk of suicide, and has a worse long-term outcome than major depression (Goodwin & Jamison, 2007; Judd et al., 2005; Kessler et al., 2006; Miklowitz & Johnson, 2006). Finally, bipolar disorder has a stronger genetic predisposition and therefore is more likely to run in families than major depression (Goodwin & Jamison, 2007). Although it previously was believed that major depression had an earlier age of onset than bipolar disorder, it is now common to see bipolar disorder diagnosed in children and adolescents as well, most likely because of greater awareness of the disorder in youth (Youngstrom, Birmaher, & Findling, 2008).

Depression and Bipolar Disorder Spectra

Many people are chronically depressed or experience depressed and expansive mood periods that are not severe enough to merit a major depressive or manic episode diagnosis. Due to the variation in mood disorders, from more mild and chronic to more severe and episodic, many researchers support the notion that both depression and bipolar disorder should be considered as continua or spectra as opposed to discrete disorders (Hankin, Fralye, Lahey, & Waldman, 2005; Merikangas et al., 2007). The DSM–5 is expected to address the dimensional nature of mood disorders and is likely to build on research to date on the spectra of these disorders.

Unipolar Depression Spectrum   Depression can manifest in many different ways and differ in severity and duration. According to the *DSM–IV–TR*, *dysthymic disorder* involves a mild, persistent depression that may occur for 2 or more years. Dysthymic individuals are typically morose, pessimistic, introverted, overconscientious, and incapable of fun (Akiskal & Casano, 1997). In addition, these individuals often have lower energy, low self-esteem, and disturbances of eating, sleeping, and thinking that are associated with MDD, but their functioning is worse (Klein, Schwartz, Rose, & Leader, 2000). Whereas dysthymic disorder is chronic, MDD is usually episodic, although MD episodes can last months or longer. Dysthymic disorder, like MDD, is 1.5 to 3 times more common in women than men, and it has the same neurophysiological abnormalities and responses to antidepressant medication as MDD (Akiskal, Judd, Lemmi, & Gillin, 1997). Researchers have termed it *double depression* when an MD episode is superimposed on dysthymic disorder. *Double depression* (DD) is considered to be on the more severe end of the unipolar depression spectrum. In essence, an individual with dysthymic disorder may sink into a major depressive episode (about 77% of dysthymic individuals develop MDD; Klein et al., 2000) and then recover from the major depression but continue their mild, persistent dysthymia. Kessing (2007) examined the subtypes of depression in a large-scale epidemiological study and found no clear demarcation between mild, moderate, and severe depression, supporting a continuum. In addition, depressive symptoms may change over time, so individuals change diagnosis from meeting criteria for MDD, to minor depression (a subthreshold episode), to dysthymic disorder, DD, and subsyndromal states (Kessing, 2007). Although all three disorders have high rates of recovery, people with DD and dysthymia have more impaired social and physical functioning than those with MDD (Rhebergen et al., 2009). In addition, the more chronic dysthymic disorder is characterized by a worse quality of life, inadequate social support, and slower rates of improvement compared to MDD (Klein, Shankman, & Rose, 2006; Subodh, Avasthi, & Chakrabarti, 2008).

Bipolar Spectrum   Similar to the unipolar spectrum, bipolar disorder can manifest itself in many different ways. Like dysthymic disorder, *cyclothymic disorder* is a chronic condition that may last for years and may never go a few months without a hypomanic or depressive phase. Cyclothymic disorder is mild and persistent and becomes a way of life. For instance, individuals with cyclothymic disorder come to depend on their hypomanic phase to work long hours and catch up on previously delayed tasks before slipping back into a normal or depressed state. Family members often describe cyclothymic individuals as "moody," "high-strung," "hyperactive," and "explosive" (Akiskal, Djenderedjian, Rosenthal, & Khani, 1977). Bipolar disorders appear to form a spectrum of severity from the milder, subsyndromal cyclothymic disorder, to bipolar II disorder, to full-blown bipolar I disorder at the most severe end (Cassano et al., 1999; Goodwin & Jamison, 2007). Three lines of evidence support this spectrum model. First, equivalent rates of bipolar disorder have been reported in the first- and second-degree relatives of cyclothymic disorder and bipolar I individuals (Akiskal et al., 1977; Depue et al., 1981), and increased rates of cyclothymic disorder are found in the first-degree relatives of bipolar patients (Chiaroni, Hantouche, Gouvernet, Azorin, & Akiskal, 2005). In addition, among monozygotic twins, when one twin had bipolar disorder, the co-twin had elevated rates of both bipolar and cyclothymic disorders (Edvardsen et al., 2008). These findings suggest that cyclothymic disorder shares a common genetic diathesis with bipolar disorder. Second, cyclothymic individuals, like bipolar I patients, often experience an induction of hypomanic episodes when treated with tricyclic antidepressants (Akiskal et al., 1977). Finally, individuals with cyclothymic disorder are at increased risk for developing bipolar I or II disorder when followed over time (Akiskal et al., 1977; Birmaher et al., 2009; Kochman et al., 2005; Shen, Alloy, Abramson, & Sylvia, 2008).

Dimensions of Mood Disorder

In addition to the important distinctions between bipolar and depressive disorders, there are certain dimensions that researchers and clinicians have found useful in classifying mood disorders. We discuss three dimensions: psychotic versus nonpsychotic, early versus late onset, and endogenous versus reactive. In addition, we discuss the importance of life events in the onset of mood disorders because this was the original basis of the endogenous–reactive distinction.

Psychotic Versus Nonpsychotic   Some individuals who have episodes of MD or mania may also experience associated symptoms of psychosis. In fact, the diagnosis of MDD or bipolar disorder in the *DSM–IV–TR* can have the additional distinction of "severe with or without psychotic features" (American Psychiatric Association, 2000, pp. 411–417). To get this qualifier for either an MD episode or a manic episode, the psychotic symptoms must occur only during mood episodes, which differentiate psychotic mood disorders from the diagnosis of schizoaffective disorder. Historically, the psychotic characterization was used to describe the severity of the episode, but more recent research suggests that there may be other factors at work (Bora, Yucel, Fornito, Berk, & Pantelis, 2008; Forty et al., 2009).

Major depressive disorder with psychotic features is not uncommon. Roughly 14% of individuals with MDD had a history of episodes with psychotic features (Johnson, Howarth, & Weissman, 1991). Crebbin, Mitford, Paxton, and Turkington (2008) found that the diagnosis of psychotic depression was more prevalent than schizophrenia in first episodes of psychosis. In psychotic depression, hallucinations, delusions, and extreme withdrawal are usually congruent with the depressed mood. For instance, the content of these delusions or hallucinations is generally themed around personal inadequacy, guilt, or deserved punishment. Individuals with psychotic features have generally more severe depressive episodes and greater hormonal disturbances (Contreras et al., 2007). In addition, psychotic features during a depressive episode increase the likelihood of having a future diagnosis of bipolar disorder (Goest et al., 2007).

Episodes of mania with psychotic features are more prevalent than depressive episodes with such features. Estimates of lifetime prevalence of psychotic features occurring during at least one manic episode range from 50 to 75% of those diagnosed with bipolar disorder (Canuso, Bossie, Zhu, Youssef, & Dunner, 2008; Ozyildrim, Cakir, & Yaziki, 2010). Although present to a lesser degree in many manic episodes, thoughts of grandiosity, lack of judgment or insight, and suspiciousness or persecution were at more delusional levels in those with psychotic features.

Researchers continue to debate whether mood disorders with psychotic features are distinct disorders or simply on the more severe end of a spectrum. Kraepelin (1921), in his original classification system, listed all incapacitating mood disorders under the heading "manic-depressive psychosis," which he considered distinct from those episodes at the nonpsychotic level. Some researchers still hold this position. For instance, Bora et al. (2008) suggested that a mood episode with psychotic features may be associated with different genetic and neurobiological markers compared to those without psychotic features. In addition, Forty et al. (2009) suggested that severity is not the only defining characteristic of psychotic depression, but there are predispositions that may lead to psychotic features instead. Other researchers argue that psychotic features are present only at the severe levels of a disorder. For instance, Ozyldirim et al. (2010) described psychotic episodes of mania as more severe, more likely to lead to hospitalization, and less responsive to some medications.

Early Versus Late Onset   Evidence over the past few decades suggests that age at onset is an important factor in the trajectory of mood disorders. In general, people who develop a mood disorder earlier have poorer outcomes. For instance, individuals with recurrent MDD before

15 years old had more clinical features, poorer social outcomes and psychosocial adjustment, and greater anxiety comorbidity than those without recurrent episodes (Hammen, Brennan, Keenan-Miller, & Herr, 2008). In addition, an earlier age of onset of depression is associated with a higher risk of suicide intent (Thompson, 2008). Further, those who developed an earlier onset of dysthymic disorder were more likely to develop MDD than were those with later onset (Klein, Taylor, Dickstein, & Harding, 1988). Heritability may play a role, as the earlier the onset of a depressive disorder, the more likely it is the person has relatives with a mood disorder (Klein et al., 1999).

In recent years, research has also shown similar trajectories in cases of early onset bipolar disorder. Oedegaard, Syrstad, Morken, Askiskal, and Fasmer (2009) found that about 60% of bipolar disorder cases had an early onset (before the age of 20 years) and 13% occurred in childhood (before 13 years of age). Childhood onset has been shown to be associated with a more chronic, severe, and recurrent course of disorder, with poorer functioning and quality of life than adult onset (Birmaher et al., 2009; Perlis et al., 2009). In addition, early onset was associated with a higher percentage of first-degree relatives with a history of mental illness (Rende et al., 2007).

Investigators have begun to examine the early onset of bipolar disorder in children, and many researchers still question the validity of this diagnosis. Bipolar disorder was recognized only recently in children and a lack of consensus on its features remains (Luby & Navsaria, 2010). Even though this issue remains controversial, research has shown that the prevalence of new cases of bipolar disorder in children is increasing (Danner et al., 2009). Some suggest that the increased prevalence may be due to an increase in awareness of childhood onset (e.g., Moreno, Laje, Blanco, Huiping, Schmidt, & Olfson, 2007), whereas others argue that there is an increase in misdiagnosis (e.g., Danner et al., 2009).

Endogenous Versus Reactive   Originally, the terms *endogenous* and *reactive* were used to identify whether or not a depressive episode was preceded by a precipitating event. Those linked to these stressful events were considered to be reactive, whereas those that were not linked to an event were called endogenous (literally, "born from within") and considered to have a more biological basis. Proponents of Kraepelin's tradition make a distinction between nonpsychotic depressions as generally reactive, whereas psychotic depressions are endogenous (Rehm et al., 2001).

Research has subsequently shown that most depressive episodes, including those in bipolar disorder, are preceded by stressful life events (Alloy, Abramson, Urosevic, Bender, & Wagner, 2009; Johnson & Kizer, 2002), and stressful events are a major cause of depressive episodes (Kendler, Karkowski, & Prescott, 1999). In some cases, there is a precipitating event for the first episode, but life events become progressively less important for subsequent recurrences, an effect known as *kindling* (Monroe & Harkness, 2005; Morris, Ciesla, & Garber, 2010). Generally speaking, despite the definition of endogenous and reactive, these terms are no longer used to indicate whether there was a precipitating event, but rather to describe different patterns of symptoms (Rehm et al., 2001). Individuals who show marked anhedonia with associated physical symptoms, such as early morning awakening, weight loss, and psychomotor changes, are described as having a depression that is qualitatively different from those that occur after a death or loss of a loved one, and are thus characterized as endogenous. In the *DSM–IV–TR*, this endogenous characteristic is referred to as melancholic features. Of these symptoms, psychomotor disturbances are the best discriminator of those with melancholic depression compared to those without melancholic features (Parker et al., 2000).

The distinction between endogenous and reactive depression based on symptoms seems to have greater validity. Individuals with endogenous depression differ from those with reactive depression in their sleep patterns. Individuals who prefer evening activities have reported more severe depressive symptoms compared to others based on this biological characteristic (Hidalgo et al., 2009). People with endogenous depression also are more likely to show neurobiological abnormalities and respond to biological treatments, such as electroconvulsive therapy (Rush & Weissenburger, 1994). Accordingly, some researchers still suspect that endogenous depression is more biological, although there is some research to the contrary. For instance, if endogenous depression were more biologically based, research would show that individuals with these features have greater family histories of depression, but numerous studies have shown that they do not (Rush & Weissenburger, 1994). In sum, the distinction between reactive and endogenous depression is generally based on symptom presentation because most mood episodes, whether mania or depression, are preceded by life events.

Life Events in Depression and Bipolar Disorders

Depression is usually precipitated by events that involve failures or uncontrollable interpersonal loss such as death, divorce, or separation (Cronkite & Moos, 1995, Kendler et al., 1999; Monroe, Rohde, Seeley, & Lewinsohn, 1999). By the same token, if a person has social support in the form of close personal relationships, he or she is less likely to succumb to depression in the face of stressful life events (Panzarella, Alloy, & Whitehouse, 2006). Further, stressors that are in part dependent on the individual's behavior (such as a fight) are more likely to lead to depression than events that are independent of their behavior (such as a death in the family; Hammen, 2006; Liu & Alloy, 2010; Rudolph et al., 2000). In addition, some researchers postulate that if an individual holds a specific personality predisposition, events that are specifically congruent with that style tend to predict mood symptoms (e.g., Francis-Raniere, Alloy, & Abramson, 2006). For instance, Francis-Raniere et al. (2006) showed that for personalities characterized by self-criticism and concern about performance evaluation, congruent negative and positive events predicted depressive and hypomanic symptoms, respectively.

The association between stressful life events and depressive episodes differs for first onset of depression and future recurrences. The kindling hypothesis, first postulated by Post (1992), suggests that stressful life events are important for the first onset, but that the association between events and episodes becomes weaker as the number of episodes increases (Kendler, Thornton, & Gardner, 2000; Lewinsohn, Allen, Seeley, & Gotlib, 1999; Monroe & Harkness, 2005). Monroe and Harkness (2005) suggested two interpretations of these findings. The first interpretation is that subsequent episodes are less reliant on stressful events and eventually become autonomous; therefore, depressive episodes may occur without a precipitating event. Their other interpretation is that an event may still be required to precipitate subsequent depressive episodes, but events can be of decreasing severity as individuals experience more episodes, wherein eventually minor events, daily hassles, or expectation of a stressful event could trigger an episode.

Similar to depressive disorders, stressful life events also have been shown to predict symptoms and episodes of mania and depression in bipolar disorder. In depression, negative life events generally precede an episode, whereas both negative and positive life events can precede a hypomanic or manic episode (Alloy, Abramson, Urosevic, Bender, & Wagner, 2009; Johnson, 2005). However, particular types of negative and positive events have been found to trigger bipolar mood episodes. For example, events that disrupt daily social routines (e.g., sleep/wake times, meal times), predict both depressive and hypomanic or manic symptoms and episodes (Malkoff-Schwartz et al., 1998, 2000; Sylvia et al., 2009). In addition, life events involving attainment of or striving toward a desired goal predict increases in manic symptoms or onsets of hypomanic episodes among individuals with bipolar spectrum disorders (Johnson et al., 2008; Nusslock, Abramson, Harmon-Jones, Alloy, & Hogan, 2007). The psychological and neurobiological mechanisms by which life events trigger mood episodes are of considerable importance in ultimately understanding the causes of mood disorders.

Suicide

Of the many reasons why people take their own lives, depression and bipolar disorder are among the most common. Major depressive disorder is the psychiatric diagnosis most commonly associated with suicide, with the risk of suicide among depressed individuals approximately 20 times greater than in the general population (Centers for Disease Control, 2007). Individuals who also have had a manic episode, however, are at even greater risk, with the rates of completed suicide among individuals with a bipolar disorder nearly 60 times greater than the general population (Fountoulakis, Gonda, Siamouli, & Rihmer, 2009).

Prevalence of Suicide

Despite these high rates, suicide may still be underreported for a variety of reasons. For example, the deaths of many people who commit suicide may actually appear accidental. It has been estimated that approximately 15% of fatal automobile accidents are actually suicides (Finch, Smith, & Pokorny, 1970). Another obstacle to obtaining accurate statistics on the prevalence of suicide is the variability in the definition of suicide (Sainsbury & Jenkins, 1982). Although completed suicide is the most severe end of the suicidal spectrum, many other thoughts and behaviors may be considered suicidal. For example, individuals may experience suicidal thoughts, develop plans to commit suicide, or engage in nonfatal suicidal behaviors such as cutting or burning themselves without ever actually attempting or committing suicide. Because many behaviors characterize suicide, a consistent definition of suicide is needed to monitor most effectively the incidence of suicide and examine trends over time and across studies (Goldsmith, Pellmar, Kleinman, & Bunney, 2002).

Along these same lines, research suggests that an individual's intent to die must be taken into account when determining whether behaviors are suicide attempts or not (O'Carroll, Berman, Maris, & Moscicki, 1996). Research suggests that only 39% of people who attempt suicide are truly determined to die, and that another 13% are ambivalent about dying (Kessler, Borges, & Walters, 1999). Furthermore, research since the early 2000s highlights the importance of differentiating suicidal behavior from nonsuicidal self-injury, which is characterized by the direct destruction of bodily tissue without the intent to die (Nock, Joiner, Gordon, Lloyd-Richardson, & Prinstein, 2006).

In 2007, the last year for which statistics are available, more than 34,000 people died by suicide in the United States, making suicide the 11th leading cause of death. At this rate, approximately 91 suicides occur each day and one suicide occurs every 16 minutes in the United States (Centers for Disease Control, 2007). In the general U.S. population, it is estimated that approximately 4.6% of people attempt suicide and around 13.5% think about committing suicide in their lifetimes (Kessler et al., 1999). Many statisticians and public health experts, however, consider these estimates to be far too low, particularly because they are based solely on retrospective self-report measures of suicidal ideation and behaviors, and because they exclude individuals who have actually completed suicide (Madge & Harvey, 1999).

Suicide is also a leading cause of death worldwide. According to the World Health Organization (WHO; 2003), 877,000 people died by suicide in 2002. Although the suicide rates across countries vary greatly, ranging from 0 per 100,000 for men and women in the Dominican Republic to 75.6 men and 16.1 women per 100,000 in Lithuania (WHO, 2003).

Risk Factors for Suicide

A risk factor is a quality or characteristic that places an individual at increased, but not necessarily imminent, risk of suicidal behavior. Risk factors may be stable or transitory, characteristic of the individual or of the environment, and they may have occurred in the past (distal) or be occurring in the present (proximal). Suicide is a complex phenomenon with many causes and is typically a culmination of a variety of biological, psychiatric, and environmental factors (Rihmer, 2007; for a review of risk factors, see the U.S. Department of Health and Human Services' *National Strategy for Suicide Prevention*, 2001, and Table 9.3).

Gender   Although women *attempt* suicide 2 to 3 times as often as men, particularly during adolescence (Centers for Disease Control, 2007; Lewinsohn, Rohde, Seeley, & Baldwin, 2001), men *commit* suicide at nearly 4 times the rate of women and represent approximately 79% of all completed suicides in the United States. A common explanation for this difference in completed suicide is that men tend to choose more lethal methods. Firearms are the most commonly used method of completed suicide among men, whereas poisoning is the most common method of completed suicide among women (Centers for Disease Control, 2007).

Race/Ethnicity   According to the latest statistics from the Centers for Disease Control and Prevention (2007), the highest rates of suicide are found among American Indians and Alaska Natives (14.3 suicide deaths per 100,000) and among non-Hispanic European Americans (13.5 suicide deaths per 100,000). The lowest rates of suicide are seen among Hispanics (6 suicide deaths per 100,000) and non-Hispanic African Americans (5.1 suicide deaths per 100,000). These lower rates among African Americans and Hispanics, however, may be indicative of underreporting and misclassification rather than actual differences due to race or ethnicity (Rockett, Samora, & Cohen, 2006).

Age   In general, the risk of committing suicide increases as a function of age, particularly among men. Older individuals are disproportionately likely to die by suicide, with 14.3 of every 100,000 individuals over 65 years of age dying by suicide. This figure is higher than the national

Table 9.3 Summary of Other Risk Factors for Suicide

Environmental Factors	Biopsychosocial Factors	Sociocultural Factors
Access to lethal means	Previous suicide attempts	Isolation/low social support
Exposure to another's suicide (friend/acquaintance or via the media)	Family history of suicide	Barriers to accessing mental health services
Job loss/financial hardship/ legal problems	Psychopathology, particularly mood disorders, anxiety disorders, certain personality disorders, and schizophrenia	Cultural norms or religious beliefs
Loss of close interpersonal relationships/difficulties in interpersonal problem solving	Alcohol and substance use disorders, particularly when co-occurring with psychopathology	Stigma associated with seeking help
	History of trauma, maltreatment/ abuse, intimate partner violence	Low socioeconomic status
	Hopelessness	
	High levels of impulsivity/aggression	
	Major physical illness	
	Stress	
	Low self-esteem/high self-loathing	

Adapted from U.S. Department of Health and Human Services. (2001). *National strategy for suicide prevention*. Rockville, MD: Author.

average of 11.3 per 100,000 in the general population. Further, this rate increases substantially among white men over 85, with 47 suicides per 100,000 (Centers for Disease Control, 2007).

Suicide rates for adolescents and young adults between ages 15 and 24 have quadrupled among males and doubled among females over the past 60 years. Although suicide rates in this age group have declined almost 30% since 1994, suicide remains the third leading cause of death among 15- to 24-year-olds (Centers for Disease Control, 2007). Approximately 17% of high school students seriously consider suicide each year, and 16.5% make plans for an attempt (Grunebaum et al., 2002). For every youth suicide, it is estimated that 100 to 200 attempts are made (Centers for Disease Control, 2007).

Biology/Genetics   Twin and adoption studies show that the predisposition to engage in suicidal behavior may be at least partly inherited. Relatives of individuals who have died by suicide are 2 to 6 times as likely to commit suicide themselves (Mann et al., 2009). Although the specific genes responsible for increased suicide risk are unknown, genes related to the neurotransmitter serotonin may be potential candidates for suicidal behavior, as altered brain serotonin functioning has been associated with attempted and completed suicide among individuals with depression (Galfalvy, Huang, Oquendo, Currier, & Mann, 2009). In addition, hyperactivity of the hypothalamic-pituitary-adrenal (HPA) axis has been implicated as a risk factor for suicide in major depression (Coryell, Young, & Carroll, 2006).

Mental Disorders   Attempted and completed suicides are very rare in the absence of a major mental disorder (Beautrais, Joyce, Mulder, & Fergusson, 1996), and psychiatric risk factors are often the most powerful and clinically useful predictors of suicide. Approximately 90% of people who attempt or commit suicide have at least one (usually untreated) major mental disorder. The most common disorders associated with suicide are major depression (56–87% of suicide attempts and completions), substance use disorders (26–55%), and schizophrenia (6–13%). In addition, individuals with depression or bipolar disorder who commit or attempt suicide most often do so during a major depressive episode and very rarely during mania (Rihmer, 2007). Specific risk factors within major depressive episodes, in order of significance, include: (1) current suicidal ideation, plan, or wish to die; (2) prior suicide attempt; (3) severe depression characterized by hopelessness and/or guilt; (4) current or recently released psychiatric inpatient status; (5) diagnosis of bipolar II, followed by bipolar I, followed by unipolar depression; (6) depressive mixed states; (7) cyclothymia; (8) psychotic symptoms; and (9) concurrent anxiety disorders, substance use, and serious medical illness (Coryell & Young, 2005; Fiedorowicz et al., 2009; Oquendo et al., 2004; Rihmer, 2007).

Protective Factors   Certain factors may actually *decrease* the risk for suicide. These protective factors include effective treatment for mental disorders and substance abuse, easy access to treatment and support for help seeking, family and adult/teacher/community support, cultural and religious beliefs that discourage suicide, and skills in problem solving and active coping (Centers for Disease Control, 2007; Eisenberg, Ackard, & Resnick, 2007; Meadows, Kaslow, Thompson, & Jurkovic, 2005).

Predicting and Preventing Suicide

The friends and family members of individuals who commit suicide are often shocked, indicating that they were oblivious to the signs. Despite this fact, most suicidal people clearly communicate their intent prior to their death, often to their close relatives. Also, most individuals who commit suicide have visited a psychiatrist or general practitioner within weeks or months of their fatal attempts (Isometsä, Henriksson, Aro, & Heikkinen, 1994). Research suggests, however, that upon these visits to professionals, suicidal individuals were either prescribed vitamins or improper psychotropic medications (Rutz, 1996). Clearly, the recognition and management of presuicidal individuals are poor (Oquendo, Malone, Ellis, Sackeim, & Mann, 1999). Solutions to this problem include better recognition of the signs of suicide, greater awareness of treatment possibilities, and improved training for nonpsychiatric health care professionals and other key personnel who are in positions to recognize the signs of suicide (Gonda, Fountoulakis, Kaprinis, & Rihmer, 2007).

If suicide can be predicted, then perhaps it can be prevented. Researchers have identified several key areas of suicide prevention, including (1) providing education and awareness about the signs of and effective treatments for suicide directed both to the general public and to healthcare providers and school personnel, (2) implementing screening tools for identifying individuals most at risk of suicide so that these individuals might be directed to appropriate treatment, (3) increasing access to mental health services and effective treatments for psychiatric disorders, as individuals who receive appropriate treatment for an underlying psychiatric disorder have the highest likelihood of recovery (Rudd & Joiner, 1998), (4) implementing effective suicide prevention programs, (5) restricting access to lethal means such as firearms, as this may delay a suicide attempt and allow time for the individual to seek help, and (6) managing how suicide is portrayed and reported in the media, as research supports a connection between media portrayals and subsequent increases in suicide rates, particularly among youth (Gould, Jamieson, & Romer, 2003; for reviews, see Mann et al., 2005, and U.S. Department of Health and Human Services, 2001).

Mood Disorders: Causes and Treatments

Most theories of the causes of mood disorders, as well as treatments for mood disorders, have focused on depression because it is far more common than hypomania and mania. However, some theoretical perspectives have addressed bipolar disorder as well, and this section will discuss some of these. Among the general theoretical approaches to mood disorders, behavioral or interpersonal, cognitive, and neuroscience perspectives have had the greatest influence on understanding the causes of and generating treatments for mood disorders. Thus, we present these three perspectives in greater detail and then discuss the psychodynamic approach more briefly.

Interpersonal Perspective

Interpersonal theories of depression (e.g., Coyne, 1976; Giesler, Josephs, & Swann, 1996; Joiner, 2000) focus on the social context of depression. According to interpersonal formulations, depressed individuals engage in various maladaptive interpersonal strategies in an attempt to improve or regulate mood. But these strategies are typically unsuccessful.

Excessive Reassurance Seeking   Excessive reassurance seeking is an aversive behavioral style in which depressed individuals constantly seek reassurance that others care about and value them. Coyne (1976) stated that whereas the act of reassurance seeking is an individual's behavioral attempt at changing or improving their depressed state, the behavior actually serves to maintain the depression and worsens the individual's interpersonal environment. The excessive reassurance seeking irritates and drives away friends and family members, leaving the individual feeling rejected (Joiner, Metalsky, Katz, & Beach, 1999) and with a weakened social support network (Potthoff, Holahan, & Joiner, 1995). The depressed individual uses this withdrawal as evidence for depressive cognitions (e.g., "I'm unlovable"). The generated stress and further entrenchment of these depressive beliefs serves to deepen the depression in a self-perpetuating cycle (Joiner, 2000). Several studies have found support for the relationship between excessive reassurance seeking, generation of interpersonal stress, and depression (e.g., Joiner, Metalsky, Gencoz, & Gencoz, 2001). Indeed, excessive reassurance seeking predicts subsequent increases in depressive symptoms (Joiner et al., 1999).

Negative Feedback Seeking   Giesler et al. (1996) suggested that depressed individuals actually seek out rejection and negative feedback from others. They propose that depressed individuals find rejection and negative feedback more predictable and in line with their negative self-views. However, the presence of these negative stressors may deepen the depression rather than relieve it. Researchers have found support for the transactional relationship between negative feedback, rejection, and depression (Joiner et al., 1999; Pettit & Joiner, 2001).

Behavioral Perspective

Extinction   Early behavioral theories focused on the relationship between external reinforcers and behavior. Many behaviorists regard depression as a result of behavioral extinction (Fester, 1973; Jacobson, Martell, & Dimidjian, 2001; Lewinsohn, 1974). Generally, the behavioral theory of depression suggests that once behaviors are no longer rewarded (reinforced), individuals cease to perform these behaviors that were previously rewarded (extinction). Through the resulting withdrawal and inactivity, individuals become depressed. The behavioral theorists propose several reasons for the reduction in positive reinforcement that leads to the extinction of behaviors and subsequent depression. For example, Lewinsohn (1974) proposed that positive reinforcement is influenced by the number of available reinforcers in the environment, the range of stimuli that the individual finds reinforcing, and the ability of the individual to obtain reinforcement from the environment. In addition, Ferster (1973) proposed that changes in the environment and the increased passivity of the individual could influence the frequency of reinforcement of behaviors.

A number of studies have supported the extinction perspective on depression. Lewinsohn and colleagues conducted several studies supporting a direct correlation between the number of pleasurable activities engaged in and depression (Lewinsohn & Graf, 1973; MacPhillamy & Lewinsohn, 1974). In fact, one of the most prominent objections to this model of depression has been that depressed individuals may lack the ability to have a pleasurable response to positively reinforcing stimuli (anhedonia) rather than just lacking positively reinforcing stimuli themselves.

Behavioral Activation Therapy   In keeping with the extinction theory, behavioral activation (BA) treatment for depression is designed to increase activity and, in turn, develop more positively reinforcing behavior patterns in depressed individuals (Lewinsohn, Biglan, & Zeiss, 1976). Jacobson et al. (2001) found that even severely depressed people show an elevation in mood if they are more behaviorally active and, thus, experience increased positive reinforcement. The authors describe that in BA, therapists help clients engage in planned activities, creating positive reinforcement and alleviating depressed mood. In BA, the client and therapist identify specific activities (positively reinforcing behaviors) that the client deems to be most helpful. Clients are then asked to engage in the activity based on a predetermined schedule, whether they feel like it or not in the moment. Depending on the success of the behavior in alleviating mood or improving quality of life, clients are asked to continue engaging in the behavior. Over time, clients are asked to engage in progressively more difficult activities, from getting out of bed at a regularly scheduled time to engaging in positive interpersonal activities. These changes break and reverse the cycle of sad mood, decreased activity, and withdrawal.

Substantial research lends support for BA as a successful treatment for depression. BA therapy has been found both to reduce acute depression and prevent relapse over a 2-year follow-up

(Gortner, Gollan, Dobson, & Jacobson., 1998; Jacobson et al., 1996). Several recent meta-analyses supported the utility of BA in treating depression (Cuijpers, van Straten, & Warmerdam, 2007; Ekers, Richards, & Gilbody, 2008; Mazzucchelli, Kane, & Rees, 2009). In general, the reviews found that activity scheduling/BA treatments for depression were as effective as other interventions (e.g., cognitive therapy) and more effective than control conditions in alleviating depression. Cuijpers et al. (2007) reviewed randomized trials of BA. In the treatments reviewed, clients learned to monitor their mood and daily activities and were instructed to increase the number of pleasurable activities and positive interactions with the environment (positive reinforcement). The authors' analysis included 780 participants within 16 different studies. The authors found a large pooled effect size of 0.87 (95% confidence interval, 0.60–1.15) of the difference between BA intervention and control conditions after treatment. Both after treatment and at follow-up, individuals receiving BA did not significantly differ in their levels of depression from those receiving comparable treatments, such as cognitive therapy. Their analysis also found that overall BA gains were maintained over time.

A recent review of the BA literature assessed the different specific treatment components of BA and their effectiveness (Kanter et al., 2010). The identified components included activity monitoring, assessment of life goals and values, activity scheduling, skills training, relaxation training, contingency management, procedures targeting verbal behavior, and procedures targeting avoidance. The authors found that activity scheduling, relaxation, and skills training interventions received empirical support on their own. All other techniques were effective, but only within larger treatment packages. Thus, they found that the most important components of BA were activity monitoring and scheduling in line with the main extinction theory of depression.

Behavioral treatments for depression have also included social skills training, which is aimed at ameliorating the aversive interpersonal behavior such as reassurance seeking and negative feedback seeking. Social skills training teaches depressed clients basic techniques to engage in satisfying social interactions through modeling of positive interpersonal behaviors by the therapist and role playing by the client. Many behavioral treatments for depression are multifaceted, involving both BA and social skills training.

Cognitive Perspective

Depression and mania involve changes in emotional, motivational, cognitive, and physical functioning. Cognitive theories of mood disorders hold that the cognitive changes are the crucial factor. According to cognitive formulations, the way people think about themselves, the world, and the future gives rise to the other phenomena in depression and mania.

Helplessness and Hopelessness   The hopelessness theory of depression (Abramson, Metalsky, & Alloy, 1989) was derived from earlier work on learned helplessness (Seligman, 1975). Learned helplessness was first demonstrated with laboratory dogs. Seligman and his colleagues found that when dogs were exposed to inescapable electric shocks and then later were subjected to escapable shocks, they either did not try to escape or were slow and inept at escaping. The investigators concluded that when the shocks were inescapable, the dogs had learned that they were *uncontrollable*, a lesson they continued to act upon later even when it was possible to escape the shocks (Maier, Seligman, & Solomon, 1969; Peterson, Maier, & Seligman, 1993). Seligman (1975) noted that this phenomenon closely resembles depression—that depression is a reaction to seemingly inescapable stressors in which the person learns that he or she lacks control over reinforcement and as a result gives up. The learned helplessness model is consistent with the finding that uncontrollable loss events typically precipitate depressive episodes. Note the difference between the learned helplessness and extinction theories. The crucial factor in extinction theory is an objective environmental condition—the lack of positive reinforcement—whereas the crucial factor in learned helplessness is a subjective cognitive process, the *expectation* of lack of control over reinforcement.

Exposure to uncontrollable (versus controllable) stress results in neurobiological changes consistent with depression (Minor & Saade, 1997), and depressed patients who see themselves as helpless tend to show higher levels of MHPG (3-methoxy4-hydroxyphenylglycol), a product of norepinephrine metabolism (Samson, Mirin, Hauser, Fenton, & Schildkraut, 1992). Norepinephrine abnormalities are often found in depressed people. In addition, positron emission tomography (PET) scans of people doing unsolvable problems, which tend to produce learned helplessness, show that learned helplessness is associated with increased limbic system brain activity. The limbic system is also implicated in the processing of negative emotions such as depression (Schneider et al., 1996).

The original learned helplessness model had certain weaknesses. Although it explained the passivity characteristic of depression, it did not explain the equally characteristic sadness, guilt, and suicidal thoughts, or that different cases of depression vary considerably in severity and duration. Consequently, Abramson, Metalsky, and Alloy (1989) revised the helplessness model to a hopelessness theory. According to the hopelessness theory, depression depends not just on the belief that there is a lack of control over reinforcement (a *helplessness expectancy*), but also on the belief that negative events will persist or recur (a *negative outcome expectancy*). When a person holds both of these expectations—that bad things will happen and that there is nothing one can do about it—he or she develops hopelessness, and it is this hopelessness that is the immediate cause of the depression (Abramson et al., 1989).

Hopelessness, in turn, stems from the inferences people make regarding stressful life events, that is, the perceived causes and consequences of such events. People who see negative life events as due to causes that are (a) stable (permanent rather than temporary), (b) global (generalized over many areas of their life rather than specific to one area of their functioning), and (c) internal (part of their personalities, rather than external, or part of the environment) are at greatest risk for developing hopelessness and, in turn, severe and persistent depression. Similarly, people who infer that stressful events will have negative consequences for themselves or who infer that the occurrence of stressful events means that they are incompetent and unworthy are more likely to become hopeless and depressed. In fact, Abramson et al. (1989) proposed that *hopelessness depression* (HD) constitutes a distinct subtype of depression, with its own set of causes (negative inferential styles combined with stress), symptoms (passivity, sadness, suicidal tendencies, low self-esteem), and appropriate treatments. This theory also applies to suicide. Hopelessness is the best single predictor of suicide, even better than depression (Glanz, Haas, & Sweeney, 1995; Abramson et al., 2000).

The hopelessness theory has been extensively tested with mostly positive results. Depressed individuals are more likely than nondepressed individuals to attribute negative events to internal, stable, and global attributions (Joiner & Wagner, 1995; Sweeney, Anderson, & Bailey, 1986) and to exhibit expectations of low control or helplessness (Weisz, Southam-Gerow, & McCarty, 2001). Moreover, a negative inferential style is relatively stable over many years (Romens, Abramson, & Alloy, 2009) and predicts who has been depressed in the past (Alloy et al., 2000), who among never depressed individuals will develop a first onset of major depression and HD (Alloy, Abramson, Whitehouse, et al., 2006), who will become suicidal in the future (Abramson et al., 1998), and who, having recovered from depression, will relapse or have a recurrence (Alloy, Abramson, Whitehouse, et al., 2006; Illardi, Craighead, & Evans, 1997). It also predicts who will have a worse course of depression (Iacoviello, Alloy, Abramson, Whitehouse, & Hogan, 2006) and who, in a group of depressed people, will recover when exposed to positive events (Needles & Abramson, 1990).

Moreover, consistent with the vulnerability-stress hypothesis of the hopelessness theory, many studies have found that the combination of a negative inferential style (the vulnerability) and exposure to negative life events (the stress) predicts subsequent increases in depressive symptoms (e.g., Abela, Stolow, Mineka, Yao, & Zhu, 2011; Black et al., 2010; Gibb, Beevers, Andover, & Holleran, 2006; Hankin, Abramson, Miller, & Haeffel, 2004). Other studies have shown that the reason a combination of stress and negative inferential style predicts depression is that this combination predicts hopelessness. It is hopelessness that, in turn, predicts depression (Alloy & Clements, 1998; Iacoviello et al., 2010; Metalsky, Joiner, Hardin, & Abramson, 1993). Finally, people who show this combination also exhibit many of the symptoms hypothesized to be part of the HD subtype (Alloy & Clements, 1998; Alloy, Just, & Panzarella, 1997), and these symptoms cluster to form a distinct dimension of depression (Joiner, Streer et al., 2001). However, there is also conflicting evidence. For example, some researchers have found that the negative attributional style and stress combination does not necessarily lead to depression (Cole & Turner, 1993; Lewinsohn, Joiner, & Rohde, 2001).

Given that much evidence indicates that a negative inferential style does make people vulnerable to depression, it is important to discover the developmental origins of this cognitive vulnerability. Both social learning factors and a history of maltreatment may contribute to the development of negative inferential styles and depression. Individuals whose parents had negative cognitive styles, provided negative inferential feedback about the causes and consequences of stressful events in the individual's life (e.g., told their child, "You weren't invited to that party because you're unpopular, and now you'll be seen as a social outcast at school"), and whose parenting was low in warmth and affection are more likely to have negative cognitive styles as adults (Alloy et al., 2001; Garber & Flynn, 2001; Ingram & Ritter, 2000). In addition, people with childhood histories of emotional abuse from either parents or nonrelatives (peers, teachers, etc.) are also more likely to have negative cognitive styles as adults (Gibb, Abramson, & Alloy, 2004; Gibb et al., 2001). Emotional maltreatment also predicts onsets of depressive episodes (Liu, Alloy, Abramson, Iacoviello, & Whitehouse, 2009). Thus, a history of negative emotional feedback and abuse may lead to the development of later cognitive vulnerability to depression. However, prospective studies beginning in childhood are needed to test this hypothesis.

Negative Self-Schema   A second major cognitive theory of depression, Beck's (1967, 1987) negative self-schema model, evolved from his findings that the thoughts and dreams of depressed patients often contain themes of self-punishment, loss, and deprivation. Self-schemata are memory representations about the self that guide the way individuals process information from the environment such that their attention is directed toward information that is congruent with the content of their self-schemata. Beck hypothesized that individuals who have negative self-schemata involving themes of inadequacy, failure, loss, and worthlessness are vulnerable to depression. Such negative self-schemata are often represented as a set of dysfunctional attitudes, such as "I am nothing if I do not succeed at this job," in which the person believes that his or her self-worth is dependent on being perfect or on others' approval. Further, when confronted with a negative life event, individuals with this type of cognitive style are hypothesized to develop negatively biased perceptions of themselves (low self-esteem), their personal world, and their future (hopelessness). According to Beck, this negative bias—the tendency to see oneself as a "loser"—is the fundamental cause of depression. If childhood experiences lead someone to develop a cognitive schema in which the self, the world, and the future are viewed in a negative light, that person is then predisposed to depression. Stress can easily activate the negative schema, and the consequent negative perceptions merely strengthen the schema (Beck, 1987; Clark, Beck, & Alford, 1999).

Research supports Beck's claim that depressed individuals have unusually negative self-schemata (Dozois & Dobson, 2001; Mathews & Macleod, 2005) and that these schemata can be activated by negative cues. Negative self-schemata can also be activated by sad mood in people who have recovered from depression (Gemar, Segal, Sagrati, & Kennedy, 2001; Ingram, Miranda, & Segel, 1998), and such reactivated negative schemata predict later relapse and recurrence of depression (Segal, Gemar, & Williams, 1999). There is also strong evidence that depressed individuals recall negative material more easily than positive material (Mathews & MacLeod, 2005) and recall autobiographical memories that are overly general rather than specific (Williams et al., 2007). The evidence that depressed individuals exhibit attentional biases toward negative stimuli is much more mixed; however, recent findings provide stronger support for the notion that depressed individuals have difficulty inhibiting or disengaging their attention from negative material once they attend to it (Gotlib & Joorman, 2010; Koster, De Lissnyder, Derakshan, & De Raedt, 2011). This difficulty may underlie depressed individuals' tendency to persistently ruminate on their negative affect and the causes and consequences of their negative mood (Gotlib & Joorman, 2010; Koster et al., 2011). Rumination, in turn, has been found to predict a subsequent onset of major depressive episodes (Nolen-Hoeksema, 2000; Robinson & Alloy, 2003; Spasojevic & Alloy, 2001) and more severe depressions (Nolen-Hoeksema, Wisco, & Lyubomirsky, 2008).

Other studies indicate that people at high risk for depression, based on having negative cognitive styles, a history of major depression, or parents who are depressed, selectively attend to and remember more negative than positive information about themselves (Alloy, Abramson, Murray, Whitehouse, & Hogan, 1997; Ingram & Ritter, 2000; Taylor & Ingram, 1999). Still other research suggests that depressed individuals may have two distinct types of negative self-schemata, one centered on dependency and the other on self-criticism (Nietzel & Harris, 1990). For those with dependency self-schemata, stressful interpersonal events involving rejection or abandonment lead to depression. For those with self-criticism schemata, achievement failures should trigger depression. This hypothesis has been supported more strongly for dependency self-schemata and social events than for self-criticism schemata and failure (Coyne & Whiffen, 1995).

Although Beck's negative self-schema model of depression hypothesizes that depressed people exhibit systematic biases in their processing of negative information, some evidence suggests that depressed individuals' pessimism is sometimes realistic, a phenomenon known as "depressive realism" or the "sadder but wiser" effect (Alloy & Abramson, 1988; Alloy, Wagner, Black, Gerstein, & Abramson, 2010). For example, Lewinsohn, Mischel, Chaplin, and Barton (1980) found that depressed individuals' evaluations of the impression they had made on others were more accurate than those of two nondepressed groups, both of whom thought they had made more positive impressions than they actually had. Similarly, Alloy and Abramson (1979) found that depressed people were far more accurate in judging how much control they had over outcomes than were nondepressed participants, who tended to overestimate their control when they were doing well and to underestimate it when they were doing poorly. Thus, it may be that nondepressed people are optimistically biased and that such biases are essential for psychological health (Alloy & Abramson, 1988; Alloy, Wagner, Black, Gerstein, & Abramson, 2010; Haaga & Beck, 1995). Research supports this view. Alloy and Clements (1992), for example, found that individuals who were inaccurately optimistic about their personal control at baseline were less likely than more realistic participants to become depressed a month later in the face of stress.

Although most research on the cognitive theories of depression (both Beck's theory and the hopelessness theory) has focused on unipolar depression, recent findings suggest that cognitive models may be applicable to bipolar disorder as well. Individuals with bipolar disorders exhibit cognitive styles and self-schemata that are as negative as those with unipolar depression (Alloy, Abramson, Walshaw, Keyser, & Gerstain, 2006; Alloy, Abramson, Walshaw, & Neeren, 2006).

Moreover, negative cognitive styles combine with life events to predict subsequent increases in hypomanic or manic and depressive symptoms among people with bipolar disorder (Francis-Raniere et al., 2006; Reilly-Harrington, Alloy, Fresco, & Whitehouse, 1999). However, recent evidence suggests that the cognitive styles of individuals with bipolar spectrum disorders have a distinct character; they are specific to themes of high incentive motivation, goal striving, and reward sensitivity (Alloy, Abramson, Walshaw, et al., 2009; Lam, Wright, & Smith, 2004).

Behavioral Approach System Dysregulation   The distinctive nature of cognitive styles among bipolar individuals is consistent with the behavioral approach system (BAS) dysregulation model of bipolar spectrum disorders. The BAS dysregulation model is a motivational-cognitive theory of bipolar disorder, originally developed by Depue and Iacono (1989) and recently expanded by Alloy, Abramson, Urošević et al. (2009) and Urošević, Abramson, Harmon-Jones, and Alloy (2008). The BAS regulates approach motivation and goal-directed behavior. It is activated by rewards or external or internal goal-relevant cues. BAS activation is implicated in the generation of positive goal-striving emotions such as happiness (Gray, 1994). In addition, the BAS has been linked to a reward-sensitive neural network involving dopamine neurons that project between several emotion- and reward-relevant limbic and cortical brain systems (Depue & Iacono, 1989). According to the BAS dysregulation model, an overly sensitive BAS that is hyperreactive to relevant cues increases a person's vulnerability to bipolar disorder. When vulnerable individuals experience events involving rewards or goal striving and attainment, their hypersensitive BAS becomes excessively activated, leading to hypomanic or manic symptoms, such as increased energy, optimism, euphoria, decreased need for sleep, grandiosity, and excessive goal-directed behavior (Johnson, 2005). Alternatively, in response to events involving irreconcilable failures, losses, or nonattainment of goals, their overly sensitive BAS becomes excessively deactivated, leading to a shutdown of behavioral approach and depressive symptoms, such as decreased energy, sadness, loss of interest, hopelessness, and decreased motivation and goal-directed activity.

Recent evidence supports the BAS dysregulation model. Individuals with bipolar spectrum disorders exhibit significantly higher levels of self-reported BAS sensitivity and reward responsiveness on behavioral tasks than do individuals without mood disorders (see Alloy, Abramson, Urošević, , Nusslock, & Jager-Hyman, 2010; Urošević, Abramson, Harmon-Jones, & Alloy, 2008 for reviews). As noted above, they also exhibit BAS-relevant cognitive styles (Alloy et al., 2009) and overly ambitious goal striving and goal setting, as well as greater cognitive reactivity and positive generalization in response to success experiences (Johnson, 2005). Furthermore, they typically exhibit increased relative left frontal cortical activity on electroencephalography (EEG), a neurobiological indicator of BAS sensitivity and activation, both at rest and in response to rewards (Coan & Allen, 2004; Harmon-Jones et al., 2008). Moreover, high BAS sensitivity predicts first onset of bipolar spectrum disorders in individuals with no history of bipolar disorder (Alloy & Abramson, 2010), faster time to onset of hypomanic and manic episodes (Alloy et al., 2008), and a greater likelihood of progressing to a more severe bipolar diagnosis over follow-up among bipolar spectrum individuals (Alloy, Abramson et al., 2010). Finally, as noted previously, life events involving goal striving or attainment are especially likely to trigger hypomanic or manic episodes among bipolar spectrum individuals (Johnson et al., 2008; Nusslock et al., 2007), consistent with the BAS dysregulation model.

Cognitive-Behavioral Therapy   Beck and his colleagues developed a multifaceted therapy that includes behavioral assignments, modification of dysfunctional thinking, and attempts to change schemata (Beck, Rush, Shaw, & Emery, 1979). Cognitive-behavioral therapy (CBT) identifies, challenges, and ultimately aims to modify cognitive schemata to generate less negative information processing (Hollon, 2006). The alteration of schemata is considered most important and, according to Beck's theory, will immunize the patient against future depressions. First, however, the therapist attempts to remediate the current depression through "behavioral activation," that is, getting the patients to engage in pleasurable activities (see the discussion of BA therapy above) and by teaching them ways of testing and challenging their dysfunctional thoughts. Depressed patients are asked to record their negative thoughts, together with the events that preceded them. Then they are asked to counter such thoughts with rational responses and record the outcome. In addition, with the therapist's help, depressed patients are encouraged to conduct behavioral "experiments" that also allow them to test and challenge the veracity of their dysfunctional thoughts. CBT also includes *reattribution training*, which aims to correct negative attributional styles (Beck, Rush, Shaw, & Emery, 1979). Patients are taught to explain stressful events in more constructive ways ("It wasn't my fault—it was the circumstances," "It's not my whole personality that's wrong—it's just my way of reacting to strangers") and to seek out information consistent with these more hopeful attributions. A similar approach is used with suicidal patients. Beck and colleagues see this as a way of correcting negative bias and combating hopelessness.

In some encouraging evaluations, CBT has been shown to be at least as effective as medication (e.g., DeRubeis et al., 2005; DeRubeis, Siegle, & Hollon, 2008). A combination of CBT and pharmacotherapy may have a slight advantage when compared with either treatment by itself (DeRubeis et al., 2008; Kupfer & Frank, 2001). Moreover, recent studies have supported less relapse and recurrence for CBT than for pharmacotherapy (e.g., Dobson et al., 2008; Hollon et al., 2005; Jarrett et al., 2001). There is also some debate as to whether CBT works as well as medication for severely depressed patients (Blackburn & Moorhead, 2000; DeRubeis, Gelfand, Tang, & Simons, 1999), but recent studies suggest that it does (e.g., DeRubeis et al., 2005; Fournier et al., 2009).

Furthermore, there is controversy about the mechanisms by which CBT produces change. For example, there is evidence that CBT produces changes both in negative cognitions, as it is hypothesized to work, as well as in abnormal neurobiological processes (Blackburn & Moorhead, 2000; DeRubeis et al., 2008). So whether it works through the proposed cognitive mechanism or by changing biological processes is unclear. However, some recent studies indicate that much of the depression symptom improvement in CBT occurs in one between-session interval, called "sudden gains," and that these sudden gains appear to be associated with the correction of patients' negative beliefs in the immediately preceding therapy session, consistent with a cognitive mechanism of treatment efficacy (Tang, DeRubeis, Beberman, & Pham, 2005; Tang, DeRubeis, Hollon, Amsterdam, & Shelton, 2007). Also, as noted, Beck's CBT is multifaceted, including BA together with cognitive restructuring. Some studies found that the BA component of CBT worked as well as the entire treatment package, both at alleviating depression and at preventing relapse (Dobson et al., 2008; Gortner et al., 1998). Thus, it could be that CBT is just as effective without its cognitive components. Regardless of how it works, CBT does indeed work. Thus, recent efforts have extended this approach successfully to the prevention of depression in children and adolescents (e.g., Brunwasser, Gillham, & Kim, 2009; Garber et al., 2009). For example, the Penn Resiliency Program (PRP; Brunwasser et al., 2009) is a group intervention designed for late elementary and middle school students that teaches cognitive-behavioral and social problem-solving skills and is based on the Beck and hopelessness theories of depression. PRP has demonstrated some success in preventing symptoms of anxiety and depression among youth and its effects can be long-lasting (Gillham, Hamilton, Freres, Patton, & Gallop, 2006). CBT has also been extended to the treatment of patients with bipolar disorder as an adjunct to mood-stabilizing medications (Basco, 2000; Newman, Leahy, Beck, Reilly-Harrington, & Gyulai, 2002), with some success (see Nusslock, Abramson, Harmon-Jones, Alloy, & Coan,

2009, for a review). Nusslock et al. (2009) suggested that considering the implications of BAS dysregulation in bipolar disorder might further improve the effectiveness of CBT for bipolar conditions.

CBT also has been modified further to incorporate mindfulness techniques. Mindfulness was adopted from Eastern traditions such as Buddhism and refers to a mental state. The individual is said to harness his or her attention and focus on momentary somatic, sensory, environmental, and cognitive experience in an open and accepting manner (Bishop et al., 2004; Kabat-Zinn, 1994; Marlatt & Kristeller, 1999). Mindfulness involves the self-regulation of attention and the development of an open or accepting orientation to the present moment upon which that attention is focused. In mindfulness practice, meditation exercises are used to help individuals develop this skill to focus on bodily, cognitive, and emotional experiences. Segal, Williams, and Teasdale (2002) developed mindfulness-based cognitive therapy (MBCT) to help depressed individuals develop a decentered view of their thoughts, emotions, and sensations. They suggest that viewing these occurrences as mental events rather than reflections of reality helps break down some of the maladaptive thoughts and mental processes (rumination) that often maintain depression. Recent reviews suggest that MBCT is effective in treating depression and reducing relapse rates (Coelho, Canter, & Ernst, 2007; Hofmann, Sawyer, Witt, & Oh, 2010).

Acceptance and Commitment Therapy   Acceptance and commitment therapy (ACT; Hayes, Strosahl, & Wilson, 1999) is often referred to as a "third wave" of CBT. ACT, like CBT, combines cognitive and behavioral components, but it is based on relational frame theory (RFT; Hayes, Barnes-Holmes, & Roche, 2001), a contextual theory of language and cognition. The treatment aims to help individuals increase their acceptance of their subjective experiences. These experiences include distressing thoughts, beliefs, sensations, and feelings. Orienting behaviors toward living life in line with one's values (e.g., moving toward desired relationships or career goals) is thought to improve the individual's quality of life. A central feature of ACT is learning to view attempts to control unwanted experiences, such as negative emotions or thoughts, as ineffective. In fact, the model suggests that these attempts at controlling experiences actually serve to increase distress. Clients are encouraged to encounter their thoughts and feelings without the aim of controlling them. Instead, they are guided to focus on leading a values-oriented life. Thus, ACT promotes experiential acceptance and a commitment to one's actions to move toward this more valued life.

Psychodynamic Perspective

Loss and Attachment   Psychodynamic theorists have proposed several causes of depression. In his classic essay, "Mourning and Melancholia," Freud (1917/1994) likened the experience of depression to that of mourning for a lost object, either real or imagined. Although sadness is a natural response to a loss, Freud posited that depression is an overreaction to such an event. The individual is filled with conflicting feelings—love for this lost object, but simultaneously anger and resentment toward it. The anger soon turns into feelings of guilt because the individual feels responsible for the loss of the loved object and failing to live up to his or her own ideals. The depressive episode becomes a cry for love brought on by feelings of emotional insecurity (Rado, 1951). The finding that depression is frequently precipitated by life events involving interpersonal loss is consistent with this psychodynamic theory.

Another psychodynamic perspective on the etiology of depression comes from attachment theory, which offers an expansion of the idea of loss triggering depression. Bowlby (1982) and other attachment theorists proposed that the loss of an attachment figure would increase the likelihood of other stressors for the child and simultaneously decrease his or her resiliency to future adversity, which predisposes him or her to adult depression. It is also postulated that the child will have unresolved mourning due to his or her young age and inability to understand the experience of loss (Bowlby, 1980). In fact, research has shown that a strong predictor of adult depression is a history of a loss between age 5 and the second grade (Coffino, 2009).

Attachment theory posits that an infant's experiences with his or her caregiver will influence how he or she relates to others in the future, especially in intimate relationships (Bowlby, 1972; Hazan & Shaver, 1987). Children who view their caregiver as a secure base who will consistently respond to their distress will have better psychological outcomes such as higher self-esteem and lower levels of depression than those who have an unreliable, rejecting caregiver (Ainsworth, Blehar, Waters, & Wall, 1978). Research has found that both children and adults with this insecure attachment style tend to have higher levels of depressive symptoms than their securely attached counterparts (Bifulco, Mahon, Kwon, Moran, & Jacobs, 2003; Kobak, Sudler, & Gamble, 1991; Muris, Meesters, van Melick, & Zwambag, 2001).

Along with attachment, researchers have also focused on another important aspect of the parent–child relationship as a risk factor for depression—parenting itself. Studies have found that maternal depression is a strong predictor of childhood and adolescent depression (Hammen, Shih, & Brennan, 2004). Maternal depression decreases the quality of parenting and creates stressful life events for the family, both of which are risk factors for depression. One style of parenting, labeled *affectionless control*, is characterized by low parental warmth and high psychological control and has been shown to be an especially strong predictor of depression in children (Parker, 1983; Alloy, Abramson, Smith, Gibb, & Neeren, 2006).

Interpersonal Therapy   A common theme in these psychodynamic theories is how well an individual is able to relate to others. In the 1980s, Klerman (1988) and later Weissman (2006) developed a therapy based in part on this assumption called interpersonal therapy (IPT). This therapy was inspired by the work of Harry Stack Sullivan, who believed that interpersonal behaviors are of central importance to adaptive functioning as well as by the attachment theories of Bowlby. Unlike traditional psychodynamic therapy, which often is quite lengthy, IPT is a brief therapy (lasting 12 to 16 sessions) that focuses on the interpersonal issues that arise in depression. IPT seeks to address the issues surrounding grief, interpersonal disputes, role transitions, and a lack of social skills. Studies have shown that IPT is an efficacious treatment for depression across the lifespan and performs as well as medication (e.g., Hinrichsen, 2008; Mufson, Weissman, Moreau, & Garfinkel, 1999).

Neuroscience Perspective

Although mood disorders have a number of putative causes, including behavioral, cognitive, and environmental factors, an individual's underlying biology also significantly impacts whether he or she develops a mood disorder. This section discusses the genetic, neurophysiological, neuroimaging, hormonal, and neurotransmitter research on mood disorders, as well as biologically based treatments for these disorders.

Family and Genetic Studies   Some of the clearest evidence for the biological contribution to mood disorders comes from research examining genetics. For example, family studies have shown that an individual's risk of developing a mood disorder increases if there is a family history of mood disorder, and that the amount of genetic material in common relates to the elevation in the risk (i.e., higher risk for those with full siblings or parents with the disorder, lower but still elevated risk for those with grandparents, aunts, or uncles with the disorder). Individuals with a first-degree relative with MDD are almost 3 times more likely to develop the disorder, whereas those who have a first-degree relative with bipolar disorder are almost 10 times more likely to develop bipolar disorder, and the risk becomes even higher with early onset in the index case (Goodwin & Jamison, 2007; Sullivan, Neale, & Kendler, 2000). Although it is not uncommon to find a family history of unipolar depression among those with bipolar disorder, individuals with unipolar depression typically do not have a family history of bipolar disorder (Winokur, Coryell, Keller, Endicott, & Leon, 1995). This supports a conceptualization of mood disorders that specifies a unique etiology for bipolar disorder. More recent research exploring the heritability of bipolar I disorder versus unipolar depression has shown that upward of 71% of the genetic liability to mania is independent of the liability to depression, although bipolar II disorder may have more shared genetic factors with depression (McGuffin et al., 2003).

Family studies of MDD and bipolar disorder are sometimes difficult to interpret because genetic and environmental factors are conflated. For this reason, twin studies and adoption studies have been used to parse the contribution of genetics and shared environment to the etiology of the disorders. Twin studies examining bipolar disorder have found a concordance rate of 72% in monozygotic (MZ) twins, compared with 14% in dizygotic (DZ) twins, indicating that there is a significant contribution of genetics to this disorder (Allen, 1976). Similarly, the concordance of unipolar depression was approximately 43% in MZ twins and 28% in DZ twins, revealing that although genes do play an important role in the development of major depression, a genetic predisposition is less important in MDD than in bipolar disorder (Sullivan et al., 2000). These results did not depend on the gender of the twin pair.

Some of the limitations found in twin studies (i.e., the assumption of complete environmental sharing) have been addressed using adoption studies. Adoption studies have explored the relative incidence of mood disorder onset in the biological versus adoptive parents of children who were adopted at an early age. An early study found that 31% of adoptees with mood disorders had biological parents with a mood disorder, as compared to only 2% of adoptees who did not develop depression or mania or hypomania (Mendlewicz & Rainer, 1977). Wender et al. (1986) conducted a more comprehensive investigation of adoptees, their adoptive parents, and their biological parents, siblings, and half-siblings, and found that the prevalence of MDD was 8 times greater in the biological families of depressed individuals. The same study also found that the prevalence of suicide was over 15 times greater in the biological relatives of adoptees with depression.

Linkage and association studies, though not new to the field of mood disorders, have become much more prevalent due to the completion of the Human Genome Project and the use of genome-wide association data. These studies rely on the use of genetic sequencing to detect commonalities in populations with and without mood disorders. One of the earliest association studies examined an 81-member Amish clan, many of whom had been diagnosed with a mood disorder (primarily bipolar disorder). Genetic sequencing of each member's DNA revealed a genetic abnormality on chromosome 11 that discriminated those with psychopathology from those who had never had a mood episode (Egeland et al., 1987). More recent work examining chromosome 11 and bipolar disorder have found null results (e.g., Gill, McKeon, & Humphries, 1988; Hodgkinson et al., 1987), whereas other research has identified genetic alterations on specific regions of chromosome 17 and on the X chromosome, responsible for the transcription of the serotonin transporter protein and monoamine oxidase inhibitor A enzyme, respectively (e.g., Mundo, Walker, Cate, Macciardi, & Kennedy, 2001; Preisig et al., 2000). To complicate the genetic picture further, a recent meta-analysis of genome-wide association data (Liu et al., 2011) has implicated two regions on chromosomes 2 and 13 and several polymorphisms in genes responsible for the transcription of neuronal ion channels and structural components. Craddock and Forty (2006) stated that other meta-analyses of genome-wide linkage studies found a number of regions on chromosome 18 that may be influential in bipolar disorder. It is clear from these studies that the biological contribution to mood disorders cannot be represented as a single genetic abnormality. Rather, depression and mania are most likely the result of a complex integration of multiple genetic variations with multiple psychological and environmental factors.

Many of the other putative biological variables, such as alterations in neurotransmitter function and hormonal regulation, described below, are also seen in the children of those with mood disorders, even those who have never suffered from the disorder themselves. For example, a twin study examining the stress hormone cortisol, which has been shown to be elevated in individuals with mood disorders, found that "high-risk" twins (a psychopathology-free individual whose MZ twin had been diagnosed with a mood disorder) had higher levels of evening cortisol relative to low-risk (psychopathology-free MZ) twins (Vinberg, Bennike, Kyvik, Andersen, & Kessing, 2008). Finally, recent research has also found that functional polymorphisms that impact neurotransmitter systems implicated in mood disorders have been shown to interact with other well-established risk factors, specifically significant life stressors. These include functional polymorphisms for the serotonin transporter (responsible for recycling serotonin back into a presynaptic cell after its release into a synapse), the serotonin 2A receptor, tryptophan hydroxylase (an enzyme important in serotonin creation), as well as the enzyme catechol-O-methyltransferase (COMT), a chemical important in the regulation of dopamine levels within the synapse (Levinson, 2006). The functional polymorphism involving the serotonin transporter (HTTLPR) has garnered a great deal of attention due to recent evidence that the genotype involving the "short" allele (the genotype that leads to the production of a less efficient serotonin transporter) interacts with stressful life events to precipitate depression (Caspi et al., 2003). A recent meta-analysis supported the role of the 5-HTTLPR gene as a moderator of the relationship between stress and depression (Karg, Burmeister, Shedden & Sen, 2011).

Neurophysiological Research   Of particular interest to neurophysiological researchers is the role biological rhythms play in the onset and course of mood disorders. Sleep disruption is one of the most common symptoms of depression and bipolar disorder. Depressed individuals also consistently show abnormalities in their progression through the various stages of sleep (Emslie et al., 2001; Hasler, Buysse, Kupfer, & Germain, 2010; Steiger & Kimura, 2009). One of the most documented abnormalities is shortened rapid eye movement (REM) latency. In depressed individuals, the time between sleep onset and REM onset, the stage of sleep in which dreaming occurs, is much shorter than in healthy individuals (Kupfer, 1976; Kupfer & Foster, 1972). Shortened REM latency is predictive of differential response to antidepressant treatment over psychotherapy, persistence of shortened REM latency beyond episode recovery, familial history of shortened REM latency, and higher likelihood of relapse (Buysse & Kupfer, 1993; Giles, Kupfer, Rush, & Roffwarg, 1998). However, shortened REM latency may not be specific to depression, having also been observed in schizophrenia, panic disorder, obsessive-compulsive disorder, mania, and eating disorders (Steiger & Kimura, 2009). Sleep disruption is also a prominent feature of bipolar disorder (Harvey, Schmidt, Scarna, Semler, & Goodwin, 2005; Mehl et al., 2006).

The disruptions observed in the sleep cycles of individuals with mood disorders are suggestive of a flaw in the body's circadian system, or "biological clock." This circadian center is thought to reside in the suprachiasmatic nucleus (SCN) in the brain (Cermakian & Boivin, 2003). Many believe that abnormalities in this circadian pacemaker stem from genetic variations. Shi et al. (2008) reported a significant association between the interaction of three circadian genes and bipolar disorder, suggesting that this interaction contributes to genetic vulnerability to the disorder. Moreover, Benedetti et al. (2007) found that individual variations in circadian genes can influence sleep and activity symptoms in mood disorders, though one study suggests that a particular gene, 3111T/C CLOCK, may only have influence over these symptoms in bipolar disorder, not unipolar depression (Serretti et al., 2010).

Circadian disruption plays a central role in the social *zeitgeber* theory of mood disorders, a biopsychosocial theory developed by Ehlers, Frank, and Kupfer (1988). Social zeitgebers (translated from German as "time givers") are abundant in our everyday lives, routines, relationships, jobs, and so forth. These social "timing cues" are purported to possess the ability to entrain internal circadian rhythms, suggesting that disruption in social rhythms will lead to disruption in biological rhythms, resulting in affective symptoms (Ehlers et al., 1988). Life events play a crucial part in the social zeitgeber theory as they are thought to be the initiators of this chain of events leading to episode onset. The social zeitgeber theory has been most frequently applied to bipolar disorder. Shen et al. (2008) found significant irregularity of social rhythms among individuals with bipolar spectrum disorders. Additionally, this irregularity predicted shorter time to onset of major depressive and manic/hypomanic episodes. Substantial research also points to disruption in circadian rhythms in depression and bipolar disorder (Kennedy, Kutcher, Ralevski, & Brown, 1996; Leibenluft, Albert, Rosenthal, & Wehr, 1996; Shi et al., 2008). Jones, Hare, and Evershed (2005) found that circadian rhythm and sleep loss patterns were less stable among participants with bipolar disorder than those of control participants, even when the participants were not in a mood episode. Also consistent with the model, researchers have shown that stressful life events that disrupt social rhythms predict both manic and depressive episodes in bipolar disorder (Malkoff-Schwartz et al., 2000; Sylvia et al., 2009).

Treatment approaches aimed at stabilizing social and circadian rhythms have gained empirical support. Interpersonal and social rhythm therapy (IPSRT), a psychotherapy that combines elements of IPT (described above) with a sleep and social rhythm stabilizing regimen, has been shown to increase time to relapse in individuals with bipolar I disorder (Frank et al., 2005). Additionally, participants randomized to IPSRT had higher regularity of social rhythms than those in intensive clinical management, and this regularity was significantly associated with reduced likelihood of relapse during maintenance treatment (Frank et al., 2005). IPSRT is also showing promise as a treatment for individuals with bipolar II disorder (Swartz, Frank, Frankel, Novick, & Houck, 2009), as well as adolescent samples (Hlastala, Kotler, McClellan, & McCauley, 2010).

Another variant of depression with strong links to biological rhythm disturbance is seasonal affective disorder (SAD). Individuals with SAD experience depressive symptoms solely in the winter months. The *DSM–IV–TR* does not list SAD as its own separate disorder, but rather as a "course specifier" of depression. To meet criteria for this specification, the individual has to experience this pattern of seasonality for at least 2 years and report a history of seasonal mood episodes that outnumber nonseasonal episodes.

The predominant theory of the pathogenesis of SAD is that the disorder is precipitated by a lag in circadian rhythms, such that the individual experiences the kind of physical retardation during the day that should be taking place at night (Nurnberger et al., 2000; Teicher et al., 1997). Wehr et al. (2001) suggested that the circadian pacemaker, which regulates seasonal changes in behavior via the transmission of a "day length" signal to other sites in the body, may function differently in those with SAD compared to unaffected individuals. Moreover, genetic studies have revealed circadian clock-related polymorphisms in SAD, with these genetic influences impacting both susceptibility to SAD as well as diurnal preference (Johansson et al., 2003).

Roughly 75% of individuals with SAD report clinical improvements when treated with morning exposure to bright, artificial light (Oren & Rosenthal, 1992). Additionally, light therapy, when applied at the first sign of seasonal symptoms, may prevent progression to a full-blown episode (Meesters, Jansen, Beersma, Bouhuys, & van der Hoofdakker, 1993). This preference for morning exposure has support in the literature (Lewy et al., 1998), and one study has shown a positive correlation between circadian phase advance and improvement in depressive symptoms (Terman, Terman, Lo, & Cooper, 2001). Although light therapy remains the gold standard for treatment of SAD, recent pharmacological advances have resulted in a novel antidepressant, agomelatine, which serves as both a melatonergic receptor agonist and a serotonin 2C receptor antagonist and has been shown to restore disrupted circadian rhythms (Leproult, van Onderbergen, L'Hermite-Baleriaux, van Cauter, & Copinschi, 2005; Pirek et al., 2007; Rouillon, 2006; Quera Salva et al., 2007; Zupancic & Guilleminault, 2006).

Neuroimaging Research There has been a surge in studies investigating the neural substrates of mood disorders over the past 10 years. Taken together, results from these studies implicate key brain regions thought to underlie mood disorders and their respective core domains of psychopathology. These regions include areas associated with emotion processes and mood regulation such as amygdala, cingulate gyrus, ventral striatum, and ventromedial prefrontal cortex (Dalgeish, 2004), as well as areas that play a role in memory and the encoding of affect-related information, including the hippocampus (Scoville & Milner, 1957). For example, magnetic resonance imaging (MRI) studies report amygdala abnormalities in MDD and bipolar disorder (see Savitz & Drevets, 2009, for a review). Although reduced hippocampal volume has been consistently reported in elderly, middle-aged, and chronically ill individuals with MDD, few studies show volume reduction of this brain region in bipolar disorder. With regard to frontal and cingulate regions, volumetric decreases and functional abnormalities in orbital frontal cortex, dorsolateral prefrontal cortex, and anterior cingulate cortex have been detected in individuals with MDD and bipolar disorder. Additionally, because cortical and subcortical gray matter regions have been implicated in both MDD and bipolar disorder, recent work has also investigated white matter regions linking these areas. Frontal and subcortical white matter hyperintensities have been detected in major depression (Firbank, Lloyd, Ferrier, & O'Brien, 2004; Greenwald et al., 1998; Nobuhara et al., 2006; Taylor et al., 2005) and bipolar disorder (de Asis et al., 2006; Lyoo, Lee, Jung, Noam, & Renshaw, 2002; Silverstone, McPherson, Li, & Doyle, 2003). Diffusion tensor imaging (DTI), an MRI technique, provides evidence of altered white matter integrity in frontal, parietal, and occipitotemporal regions in MDD (Ma et al., 2007; Yang et al., 2007) as well as frontal, frontal-subcortical, and corpus callosum regions in bipolar disorder (Chaddock et al., 2009; Mahon et al., 2009; Sussmann et al., 2009; Zanetti et al., 2009).

Hormone Imbalance Hormonal abnormalities also have been associated with mood disorders, specifically with bipolar and unipolar depression. Hypersecretion of cortisol is one of the most consistent and robust findings in the depression literature. Individuals with severe depression have evidence of hypersecretion of corticotrophin-releasing hormone (CRH), exaggerated response to adrenocorticotropic hormone (ACTH), enlarged pituitary and adrenal glands, and elevated cortisol concentrations in plasma, urine, saliva, and cerebrospinal fluid (CSF) (Young, 2004). One of the most frequently used assessments for HPA axis dysregulation involves the administration of dexamethasone, a glucocorticoid agonist, which should inhibit cortisol production, and CRH, which should promote cortisol production. Individuals with severe or chronic depression experience what is called dexamethasone "nonsuppression," meaning that after being given even very high doses of dexamethasone, their bodies fail to inhibit cortisol secretion and their levels of circulating and salivary cortisol remain very high. Additionally, individuals with severe depression show reduced response to CRH, suggesting their bodies' ability to react appropriately (to promote or inhibit) to hormonal cues is severely impaired. Hypercortisolemia, once thought to be a trait-like characteristic of depression, has subsequently been shown to abate as mood symptoms remit (Deshauer, Duffy, Meany, Sharma, & Grof, 2006) and persists only in those who are at high risk of depressive episode relapse in the immediate future (DabanVieta, Mackin, & Young, 2005). Cortisol hypersecretion among healthy individuals has also been shown to be a risk factor for the first onset of MDD in prospective studies (Goodyer, Herbert, Tamplin, & Altham, 2000; Harris et al., 2000).

Hypercortisolemia has been associated with impairments in learning and memory, marked hippocampal atrophy, reductions in frontal lobe volume, and impairments in functions associated with these areas (Daban et al., 2005; Young, 2004). Many of the brain areas that are negatively impacted by elevated cortisol are those that contain high concentrations of glucocorticoid receptors, lending credence to the theory that elevated cortisol is the result of impaired production or inhibition and may be the cause of many of the cognitive deficits seen in depression. There is mixed evidence as to whether hormonal abnormalities are also present during mania and hypomania, although some work has shown that irritable mania and mixed mood episodes do demonstrate cortisol abnormalities similar to those seen during an MD episode (Daban et al., 2005).

Other hormones, such as thyroid hormone and gonadal or ovarian hormones, have also demonstrated dysregulation in mood disorders. Research has shown that individuals with unipolar and bipolar depression have both lower basal thyrotropin and thyroid-stimulating hormone (TSH) levels relative to euthymic individuals (Sassi et al., 2001). Individuals with particularly low thyroid levels have also been shown to be at greater risk of relapse (Joffe & Marriott, 2000). Additionally, a number of other studies have demonstrated a greatly increased risk for depression, mania, suicide, and even affective psychosis and psychiatric hospitalization during periods of drastic shifts in ovarian hormones (estrogen, progesterone), such as menarche, childbirth, and menopause in those individuals with a history of mood disorders (Rasgon, Bauer, Glenn, Elman, & Whybrow, 2003; Wieck et al., 1991). Estrogen's established influence on important neurotransmitters such as serotonin and dopamine (Joffe & Cohen, 1998; Kenna, Jiang, & Rasgon, 2009) could help explain its influence in mood disorders.

Neurotransmitter Dysfunction   A critical element in the neurobiology of mood disorders is the manner in which the creation, release, and metabolism of neurotransmitters, particularly serotonin (5-hydroxytryptamine, or 5-HT), norepinephrine (NE), and dopamine (DA), are dysregulated. Direct studies of neurotransmitter action within a living individual are prohibitively invasive and disruptive to the individual's biochemistry; thus, evidence for dysfunction in these systems is gathered from secondary sources, such as measures of neurotransmitter metabolites in blood, alterations of the genetics regulating neurotransmitter and receptor production and functioning, and studies of the efficacy of drugs that act on certain neurotransmitter systems.

The efficacy of selective serotonin reuptake inhibitors (SSRIs), such as fluoxetine (Prozac), sertraline (Zoloft), and paroxetine (Paxil), among others, has made these drugs the most common pharmacological treatment for depression and resulted in a great deal of research exploring the role of serotonin in mood. Research has shown that a reduction in 5-HT activity is associated with MD and suicide. For example, a depletion study in which the chemical precursor for 5-HT, l-tryptophan, was experimentally inhibited resulted in depressed mood (Ruhe, Mason & Schene, 2007). Other research has shown that individuals with MD have reductions in CSF levels of 5-HT metabolites, suggesting they have lower levels of 5-HT in their brains (Firk & Marcus, 2007). Genetic research has also demonstrated that presynaptic 5-HT reuptake transporters may also be altered, and that this alteration interacts with life stress to precipitate the onset of the disorder (Caspi et al., 2003; Kuzelova, Ptacek, & Macek, 2010). Investigations using PET scans have shown that depressed individuals show lower 5-HT receptor binding when compared with controls (Yaltham et al., 2000). Additionally, suicide completers present evidence of abnormally low 5-HT activity (Mann et al., 1992), including subnormal 5-HT levels and impaired 5-HT receptors in the brainstem and frontal cortex (Arango & Underwood, 1997; Meyer et al., 1999).

Catecholamines, including DA and NE, derived from the amino acid tyrosine, are thought to be critical to the phenomenology of mood disorders, particularly bipolar disorder. The DA neurons in the ventral tegmental area (VTA) of the brainstem project to reward and cognition centers, such as the nucleus accumbens and the prefrontal cortex. Reductions in DA in these brain areas have been associated with blunted reward response, anhedonia, decreased motivation, and difficulties in concentration, all of which are symptoms of both unipolar and bipolar depression (Naranjo, Tremblay, & Busto, 2001). In bipolar disorder, there is evidence that DA signaling is elevated during periods of mania and reduced during periods of depression (Berk et al., 2007), and such findings are consistent with the BAS dysregulation model of bipolar disorder, as discussed above. Other evidence for the role of DA in bipolar disorder includes the phenomenological similarities between mania and hypomania and amphetamine use (amphetamines increase DA in the synapse), high rates of comorbidities with bipolar disorder and other disorders impacted by DA (such as ADHD and substance abuse), structural abnormalities in dopaminergic brain structures in those with bipolar disorder, reduced CSF levels of DA metabolites (suggesting reduced DA volume), increased activity of enzymes responsible for DA break down (such as COMT), and decreased DA receptor binding in individuals with bipolar disorder (Cousins, Butts, & Young, 2009). All of these findings suggest that individuals with bipolar disorder may possess physical alterations to dopaminergic brain structures, reduced DA release, increased rates of DA breakdown when it is released, and impaired signaling when DA reaches the postsynaptic receptor.

Early studies posited a central role of NE, due in large part to the findings that experimentally increased levels of NE produce mania, whereas decreased levels produce depression (Delgado & Moreno, 2000; Schildkraut, 1965). Additionally, many of today's novel antidepressants, such as bupropion (Wellbutrin) and venlafaxine (Effexor), target NE signaling and disrupt reuptake of released neurotransmitter into the presynaptic neuron (Nutt et al., 2007). There is also evidence that other effective treatments, such as electroconvulsive therapy (ECT), may act by increasing the bioavailability of DA and NE (Nutt, 2006). A recent meta-analysis of monoamine depletion studies found that depletion of 5-HT, DA, and NE results in slightly lowered mood in those individuals with a family or personal history of depression, but not in normal controls (Ruhe et al., 2007). The authors of this analysis suggest that reductions in the bioavailability of these monoamines probably represents a vulnerability to depression, which then interacts with other environmental, social, and biological risk factors to actually lead to depression.

In addition to traditional neurotransmitter models of MD and bipolar disorder, there has also been investigation into other neurochemicals, such as glutamate, gamma aminobutyric acid (GABA), a variety of neuropeptides, and cell-signaling molecules, which may play a role in dysregulated affect (Kugaya & Sanacora, 2005). Pharmaceutical interventions targeting these novel neurobiological candidates are currently being explored (Matthew, Manji, & Charney, 2008). Finally, changes in plasticity (a neuron's ability to grow or shrink) and neuroarchitecture can result from treatment with antidepressants and mood stabilizers and are also theorized to play an important role in mood disorders (Sanacora, 2008; Frey et al., 2007).

Psychopharmacology Whatever the neuroscience perspective ultimately explains about the causes of mood disorders, it has contributed importantly to their treatment in the form of antidepressant and antimanic medications. The primary classes of antidepressant medication include the monoamine oxidase inhibitors (MAOIs), tricyclic antidepressants (TCAs), tetracyclic antidepressants (TeCAs), SSRIs, and serotonin-norepinephrine reuptake inhibitors (SNRIs). Newer types of antidepressants include noradrenergic and specific serotonergic antidepressants (NaSSAs), norepinephrine reuptake inhibitors (NRIs), norepinephrine-dopamine reuptake inhibitors (NDRIs), selective serotonin reuptake enhancers (SSREs), and norepinephrine-dopamine disinhibitors (NDDIs). Each of these classes seems to work by acting on certain neurotransmitters. For example, MAOIs interfere with an enzyme that breaks down 5-HT, DA, and NE; the tricyclics block the reuptake of 5-HT and NE; the TeCAs increase levels of NE and 5-HT; the SSRIs block the reuptake of 5-HT; and the SNRIs inhibit the reuptake of 5-HT and NE.

The choice of antidepressant depends on which drug provides the greatest symptom relief with the fewest side effects (Zimmerman et al., 2004). Additionally, treatment history, co-occurring psychiatric disorders, and particular clinical symptoms also should be taken into account. MAOIs, one of the older classes of antidepressant drugs, are not prescribed as frequently as the newer classes, given the adverse side effects associated with their use (including dangerous interactions with foods that contain high levels of tyramine, including particular types of meat, cheese, etc.). However, they are still used for certain types of depression, namely "atypical depression," characterized by excessive sleeping and/or eating (McGrath et al., 2000) and when other medications prove to be ineffective. TCAs, the oldest class of antidepressant medication, can also have negative side effects, including drowsiness, sexual dysfunction, blurred vision, and increased heart rate. Moreover, given their toxicity (10 times normal dosages), it is easy to overdose on TCAs and, thus, they must be prescribed with caution to suicidal patients. Nonetheless, TCAs have been shown to be significantly more effective than placebo (Arroll et al., 2005). Clinicians perceive the newer medications (e.g., SSRIs and SNRIs) to be more effective than TCAs (Petersen et al., 2002); thus, they have gradually displaced most other antidepressants. Importantly, however, efficacy of SSRIs for the treatment of depression remains controversial, as some studies report superior efficacy over placebo (Hollon, DeRubeis, Shelton, & Weiss, 2002; Thase, 2002), whereas others report that they may not be much more effective than placebos (Kirsch, Moore, Scoboria, & Nicholls, 2002). Two recent meta-analyses of clinical trials reported a small effect in mild and moderate depression, but a more robust effect in severe depression (Fournier et al., 2010; Kirsch et al., 2008). Further, SSRIs have the added advantage of fewer adverse effects than TCAs, and they act more quickly.

There is also a longstanding debate about whether pharmacotherapy or psychotherapy is a more effective approach to treating depression. Recent work comparing the two types of treatment found that antidepressants are as effective as psychotherapy for MDD, whereas medication yields better results for dysthymic disorder (Cuijpers, van Straten, van Oppen, & Andersson, 2008; Imel, Malterer, McKay, & Wampold, 2008). Further, SSRIs may be more efficacious than psychotherapy treatment initially, but more patients have been shown to discontinue antidepressants as compared with those in psychotherapy, perhaps due to medication side effects. Moreover, as discussed earlier, psychotherapies such as BA and CBT have been found to reduce relapses and recurrences of depression.

For bipolar disorder, mood stabilizer medications are typically the first choice of pharmacological treatment. Aside from lithium, most of these medications are anticonvulsants, such as sodium valproate (Macritchie et al., 2003). For patients with bipolar disorder experiencing more severe manic or mixed episodes, either lithium plus an antipsychotic or valproate plus an antipsychotic is typically prescribed. For patients with less severe symptoms, lithium, valproate, or an antipsychotic are prescribed. Lithium is among the most commonly prescribed mood-stabilizing medications for bipolar disorder. It works to control manic symptoms and prevent relapses of manic and depressive episodes. Nonetheless, it is important to note the difficulty in determining the maintenance dose, primarily because many times the effective dose is close to the toxic dose, which may lead to convulsions, delirium, and, in rare instances, death. Typically, an individual who has overdosed will experience warning signs, such as nausea, which will indicate he or she should discontinue use. One additional complication with lithium is that patients who stop taking it after approximately 2 years may experience a new depressive or manic episode and increased risk of suicide (Baldessarini, Tondo, & Viguera, 1999). As a result of the potential dangers associated with lithium, alternative treatment options have been introduced, including use of anticonvulsants, such as valproate, lamotrigine, gabapentin, topiramate, carbamazepine, and oxcarbazepine. Various psychotherapies are often used as an adjunctive treatment along with pharmacotherapy (Nusslock et al., 2009).

Electroconvulsive Therapy   Another longstanding biological treatment for mood disorders is ECT. Electric shock, when applied to the brain under controlled circumstances, has been shown to ameliorate symptoms of severe, refractory depression. ECT is conducted by administering a shock of approximately 70 to 130 V directly to the patient's brain, resulting in a convulsion similar to a seizure. The treatment is typically administered approximately 9 or 10 times, spaced over the period of several weeks. The patient is generally hospitalized prior to treatment and is anesthetized throughout the procedure.

ECT was first developed in the 1930s, and although it is clear that ECT *does* work (Bailine et al., 2000; 2010; Cohen et al., 2000), it is still relatively unclear *how* it works. Yatham et al. (2010) found that ECT functions to down-regulate 5-HT receptors, much in the same way as antidepressants. However, ECT is capable of further down-regulating the 5-HT receptors in individuals with treatment-resistant depression, thus perhaps shedding some light on why ECT is often efficacious in this difficult-to-treat subset of patients.

ECT is not without complications, however. The most common side effect is memory dysfunction, both anterograde (learning new material after treatment) and retrograde (recalling material from before treatment) amnesia. Anterograde memory deficits are temporary (Criado, Fernandez, & Ortiz, 2007; Hay & Hay, 1990), though retrograde memory deficits take longer to resolve, with most experiencing a marked loss 1 week following treatment and a nearly complete recovery within 7 months posttreatment. Longer-term follow-up studies of approximately 3.5 years posttreatment suggest that few permanent memory deficits remain (Cohen et al., 2000). In many cases, however, some subtle memory losses persist beyond the typical 7-month posttreatment period, particularly for events that occurred in the 1-year period prior to treatment and for interpersonal events (Lisanby, Maddox, Prudic, Devanand, & Sackeim, 2000). ECT confined to one hemisphere of the brain (ideally the right hemisphere) or ECT focused on the frontal rather than the temporal lobes is associated with decreased risk for cognitive impairment following treatment (Bailine et al., 2000; Sackeim et al., 2000).

A newer biological treatment for depression uses powerful magnetic fields to restore dysfunctional brain activity in depressed individuals. Transcranial magnetic stimulation (TMS) involves placing an electromagnetic coil on the scalp through which high-intensity current produces a brief magnetic field that induces electrical current in neurons, thus resulting in neural depolarization (George, Lisanby, & Sackeim, 1999). This is the same depolarization effect seen in ECT. An advantage of TMS lies in its ability to apply more finely tuned stimulation than ECT. Although occasional mild headache and discomfort at the stimulation site has been reported, patients receiving TMS generally report no other adverse side effects (George et al., 1999). Although the method has been approved for treatment-resistant depression in several countries, it has yet to gain approval in the United States, largely due to the U.S. Food and Drug Administration's concerns about the efficacy of TMS (Marangell, Martinez, Jurdi, & Zboyan, 2007). Tests of TMS using a sham control have yielded conflicting results and have been difficult to compare due to nonstandardized stimulation methods, thus making the true efficacy of the treatment difficult to determine (Burt, Lisanby, & Sackeim, 2002; Marangell et al., 2007). In a recent review of the randomized and nonrandomized controlled trials of TMS, Rasmussen

(2008) reported that only one of six randomized studies showed a higher number of responders to TMS versus ECT.

Conclusion

Although they have been recognized and studied for centuries, the mood disorders still remain something of a mystery. Although major advances in the understanding and treatment of mood disorders have been made over the past several decades, there are still gaps in our knowledge of these conditions. As discussed in this chapter, many different potential causes and treatments for the mood disorders have been suggested from a variety of theoretical perspectives. More recent theoretical models, such as the BAS dysregulation model or social zeitgeber theory, have attempted to integrate research across multiple perspectives. It is likely that a full understanding of the causes of mood disorders will require even further integration of cognitive, behavioral, psychosocial, and neurobiological mechanisms in the future.

References

Abela, J. R. Z., Stolow, D., Mineka, S., Yao, S., Zhu, X. Z., & Hankin, B. (2011). Cognitive vulnerability to depressive symptoms in adolescents in urban and rural Hunan, China: A multi-wave longitudinal study. *Journal of Abnormal Psychology*, DOI: 10.1037/a0025295.

Abramson, L. Y., Alloy, L. B., Hogan, M. E., Whitehouse, W. G., Cornette, M. M., Akhavan, S., & Chiara, A. (1998). Suicidality and cognitive vulnerability to depression among college students: A prospective study. *Journal of Adolescence, 21*, 473–487.

Abramson, L. Y., Alloy, L. B., Hogan, M. E., Whitehouse, W. G., Gibb, B. E., Hankin, B. L., & Cornette, M. M. (2000). The hopelessness theory of suicidality. In T. E. Joiner & M. D. Rudd (Eds.), *Suicide science: Expanding boundaries* (pp. 17–32). Boston: Kluwer Academic.

Abramson, L. Y., Metalsky, G. I., & Alloy, L. B. (1989). Hopelessness depression: A theory-based subtype of depression. *Psychological Review, 96*, 358–372.

Ainsworth, M. D. S., Blehar, M. C., Waters, E., & Wall, S. (1978). *Patterns of attachment: A psychological study of the strange situation*. Hillsdale, NJ: Erlbaum.

Akiskal, H. S., & Casano, G. B. (Eds.). (1997). *Dysthymia and the spectrum of chronic depressions*. New York: Guilford.

Akiskal, H. S., Djenderedjian, A. H., Rosenthal, R. H., & Khani, M. K. (1977). Cyclothymic disorder: Validating criteria for inclusion in the bipolar affective group. *American Journal of Psychiatry, 134*, 1227–1233.

Akiskal, H. S., Judd, L. L., Lemmi, H., & Gillin, J. C. (1997). Subthreshold depressions: Clinical and sleep EEG, validation of dysthymic, residual and masked forms. *Journal of Affective Disorders, 45*, 53–63.

Allen, M. G. (1976). Twin studies of affective illness. *Archives of General Psychiatry, 33*, 1476–1478.

Alloy, L. B., & Abramson, L. Y. (1979). The judgment of contingency in depressed and nondepressed students: Sadder but wiser? *Journal of Experimental Psychology: General, 108*, 441–485.

Alloy, L. B., & Abramson, L. Y. (1988). Depressive realism: Four theoretical perspectives. In L. B. Alloy (Ed.), *Cognitive processes in depression* (pp. 223–265). New York: Guilford.

Alloy, L. B., & Abramson, L. Y. (2010). The role of the behavioral approach system (BAS) in bipolar spectrum disorders. *Current Directions in Psychological Science, 19*, 189–194.

Alloy, L. B., Abramson, L. Y., Hogan, M. E., Whitehouse, W. G., Rose, D. T., Robinson, M. S., … Lapkin, J. B. (2000). The Temple–Wisconsin Cognitive Vulnerability to Depression (CVD) Project: Lifetime history of Axis I psychopathology in individuals at high and low cognitive risk for depression. *Journal of Abnormal Psychology, 109*, 403–418.

Alloy, L. B., Abramson, L. Y., Murray, L. A., Whitehouse, W. G., & Hogan, M. E. (1997). Self-referent information processing in individuals at high and low cognitive risk for depression. *Cognition and Emotion, 11*, 539–568.

Alloy, L. B., Abramson, L. Y., Smith, J. M., Gibb, B. E., & Neeren, A. M. (2006). Role of Parenting and maltreatment histories in unipolar and bipolar mood disorders: Mediation by cognitive vulnerability to depression. *Clinical Child and Family Psychology Review, 9*, 23–64.

Alloy, L. B., Abramson, L. Y., Tashman, N., Berrebbi, D. S., Hogan, M. E., Whitehouse, W. G., … Morocco, A. (2001). Developmental origins of cognitive vulnerability to depression: Parenting, cognitive, and inferential feedback styles of the parents of individuals at high and low cognitive risk for depression. *Cognitive Therapy and Research, 25*, 397–423.

Alloy, L. B., Abramson, L. Y., Urošević, S., Bender, R. E., & Wagner, C. A. (2009). Longitudinal predictors of bipolar spectrum disorders: A behavioral approach system (BAS) perspective. *Clinical Psychology: Science and Practice, 16*, 206–226.

Alloy, L. B., Abramson, L. Y., Urošević, S., Nusslock, R., & Jager-Hyman, S. (2010). Course of early-onset bipolar spectrum disorders during the college years: A behavioral approach system (BAS) dysregulation perspective. In D. J. Miklowitz & D. Cicchetti (Eds.), *Understanding bipolar disorder: A developmental psychopathology approach* (pp. 166–191). New York: Guilford.

Alloy, L. B., Abramson, L. Y., Walshaw, P. D., Cogswell, A., Sylvia, L. G., Hughes, M. E., ... Hogan, M. E. (2008). Behavioral approach system (BAS) and behavioral inhibition system (BIS) sensitivities and bipolar spectrum disorders: Prospective prediction of bipolar mood episodes. *Bipolar Disorders, 10*, 310–322.

Alloy, L. B., Abramson, L. Y., Walshaw, P. D., Gerstein, R. K., Keyser, J. D., Whitehouse, W. G., ... Harmon-Jones, E. (2009). Behavioral approach system (BAS)-relevant cognitive styles and bipolar spectrum disorders: Concurrent and prospective associations. *Journal of Abnormal Psychology, 118*, 459–471.

Alloy, L. B., Abramson, L. Y., Walshaw, P. D., Keyser, J., & Gerstein, R. K. (2006). A cognitive vulnerability-stress perspective on bipolar spectrum disorders in a normative adolescent brain, cognitive, and emotional development context. *Development and Psychopathology, 18*, 1055–1103.

Alloy, L. B., Abramson, L. Y., Walshaw, P. D., & Neeren, A. M. (2006). Cognitive vulnerability to unipolar and bipolar mood disorders. *Journal of Social and Clinical Psychology, 25*, 726–754.

Alloy, L. B., Abramson, L. Y., Whitehouse, W. G., Hogan, M. E., Panzarella, C., & Rose, D. T. (2006). Prospective incidence of first onsets and recurrences of depression in individuals at high and low cognitive risk for depression. *Journal of Abnormal Psychology, 115*, 145–156.

Alloy, L. B., & Clements, C. M. (1992). Illusion of control: Invulnerability to negative affect and depressive symptoms after laboratory and natural stressors. *Journal of Abnormal Psychology, 101*, 234–245.

Alloy, L. B., & Clements, C. M. (1998). Hopelessness theory of depression: Tests of the symptom component. *Cognitive Therapy and Research, 22*, 303–335.

Alloy, L. B., Just, N., & Panzarella, C. (1997). Attributional style, daily life events, and hopelessness depression: Subtype validation by prospective variability and specificity of symptoms. *Cognitive Therapy and Research, 21*, 321–344.

Alloy, L. B., Wagner, C. A., Black, S. K., Gerstein, R. K., & Abramson, L. Y. (2010). The breakdown of self-enhancement and self-protection in depression. In M. Alicke & C. Sedikides (Eds.), *The handbook of self-enhancement and self-protection* (pp. 358–379). New York: Guilford.

American Psychiatric Association. (2000). *Diagnostic and statistical manual of mental disorders* (4th rev. ed.). Washington, DC: Author.

Angst, J., Gamma, A., Gastpar, M., Lepine, J. P., Mendlewicz, J., & Tylee, A. (2002). Gender differences in depression: Epidemiological findings from the European DEPRES I and II studies. *European Archives of Psychiatry and Clinical Neuroscience, 252*(5), 201.

Arango, V., & Underwood, M. D. (1997). Serotonin chemistry in the brain of suicide victims. In R. W. Maris, M. M. Silverman, & S. S. Canetto (Eds.), *Review of suicidology* (pp. 237–250). New York: Guilford.

Arroll, B., Macgillivray, S., Ogston, S., Reid, I., Sullivan, F., Williams, B., & Crombie, I. (2005). Efficacy and tolerability of tricyclic antidepressants and SSRIs compared with placebo for treatment of depression in primary care: A meta-analysis. *Annals of Family Medicine, 3*, 449–456.

Bailine, S., Fink, M., Knapp, R., Petrides, G., Husain, M. M., Rasmussen, K., ... Kellner, C. H. (2010). Electroconvulsive therapy is equally effective in unipolar and bipolar depression. *Acta Psychiatrica Scandinavica, 121*, 431–436.

Bailine, S. H., Rifkin, A., Kayne, E., Selze, J. A., Vital-Herne, J., Blieka, M., & Pollack, S. (2000). Comparison of bifrontal and bitemporal ECT for major depression. *American Journal of Psychiatry, 157*, 121–123.

Baldessarini, R. J., Tondo, L., & Viguera, A. C. (1999). Discontinuing lithium maintenance treatment in bipolar disorders: Risks and implications. *Bipolar Disorders, 1*, 17–24.

Basco, M. R. (2000). Cognitive-behavioral therapy for bipolar I disorder. *Journal of Cognitive Psychotherapy: An International Quarterly, 14*, 287–304.

Beautrais, A. L., Joyce, P. R., Mulder, R. T., & Fergusson, D. M. (1996). Prevalence and comorbidity of mental disorders in persons making serious suicide attempts: A case-control study. *American Journal of Psychiatry, 153*(8), 1009–1014.

Beck, A. T. (1967). *Depression: Clinical, experimental, and theoretical aspects*. New York: Harper and Row.

Beck, A. T. (1987). Cognitive models of depression. *Journal of Cognitive Psychotherapy: An International Quarterly, 1*, 5–37.

Beck, A. T., Rush, A. J., Shaw, B. F., & Emery, G. (1979). *Cognitive theory of depression*. New York: Guilford.

Belsher, G., & Costello, C. G. (1988). Relapse after recovery from unipolar depression: A critical review. *Psychological Bulletin, 104*, 84–96.

Benazzi, F. (2000). Depression with DSM-IV atypical features: A marker for bipolar II disorder. *European Archives of Psychiatry and Clinical Neuroscience, 250*, 53–55.

Benazzi, F. (2001). The clinical picture of bipolar II outpatient depression in private practice. *Psychopathology, 34*, 81–84.

Benedetti F., Dallaspezia, S., Fulgosi, M. C., Lorenzi, C., Serretti, A., Barbini, B., ... Smeraldi, E. (2007). Actimetric evidence that CLOCK 3111 T/C SNP influences sleep and activity patterns in patients affected by bipolar depression. *American Journal of Medical Genetics Part B: Neuropsychiatric Genetics, 144B*(5), 631–635.

Berk, M., Dodd, S., Kauer-Sant'anna, M., Malhi, G. S., Bourin, M., Kapczinski, F., & Norman, T. (2007). Dopamine dysregulation syndrome: implications for a dopamine hypothesis of bipolar disorder. *Acta Psychiatrica Scandinavica—Supplement, 434*, 41–49.

Bifulco, A., Mahon, J., Kwon, J. H., Moran, P. M., & Jacobs, C. (2003). The Vulnerable Attachment Style Questionnaire (VASQ): An interview-based measure of attachment styles that predict depressive disorder. *Psychological Medicine, 33*(6), 1099–1110.

Birmaher, B., Axelson, D., Strober, M., Gill, M. K., Yang, M., Ryan, N., ... Leanard, H. (2009). Comparison of manic and depressive symptoms between children and adolescents with bipolar spectrum disorders. *Bipolar disorders, 11*, 52–62.

Bishop, S. R., Lau, M., Shapiro, S., Carlson, L., Anderson, N. D., Carmody, J., ... Devins, G. (2004). Mindfulness: A proposed operational definition. *Clinical Psychology Science and Practice, 11*, 230–241.

Black, S. K., Alloy, L. B., Klugman, J., Bender, R. E., Goldstein, K. E., & Abramson, L. Y. (2010). *Cognitive vulnerability—stress and stress generation models of depression: A prospective examination.* Manuscript under editorial review.

Blackburn, I. M., & Moorhead, S. (2000). Update in cognitive therapy for depression. *Journal of Cognitive Psychotherapy: An International Quarterly, 14*, 305–336.

Bora, E., Yucel, M., Fornito, A., Berk, M., & Pantelis, C. (2008). Major psychoses with mixed psychotic and mood symptoms: Are mixed psychoses associated with different neurobiological markers? *Acta Psychiatrica Scandinavica, 118*, 172–187.

Bowlby, J. (1972). *Attachment and loss:* Vol. 2. *Separation.* New York : Basic Books.

Bowlby, J. (1980). *Attachment and loss:* Vol. 3. *Loss.* New York: Basic Books.

Bowlby, J. (1982). Attachment and Loss: Retrospect and Prospect. *American Journal of Orthopsychiatry, 52*(4), 664–678.

Brunwasser, S. M., Gillham, J. E., & Kim, E. S. (2009). A meta-analytic review of the penn resiliency program's effect on depressive symptoms. *Journal of Consulting and Clinical Psychology, 77*(6), 1042–1054.

Burcusa, S. L. & Iacono, W. G. (2007). Risk for recurrence in depression. *Clinical Psychology Review, 27*, 959–985.

Burke, K. C., Burke, J. D., Rae, D. S., & Regier, D. A. (1991). Comparing age at onset of major depression and other psychiatric disorders by birth cohorts in five U.S. community populations. *Archives of General Psychiatry, 48*, 789–795.

Burt, T., Lisanby, S. H., & Sackeim, H. A. (2002). Neuropsychiatric applications of transcranial magnetic stimulation: a meta-analysis. *International Journal of Neuropsychopharmacology, 5*, 73–103.

Buysse, D. J., & Kupfer, D. J. (1993). Sleep disorders in depressive disorders. In J. J. Mann & D. J. Kupfer (Eds.), *Biology of depressive disorders:* Part A. *A systems perspective* (pp. 123–154). New York: Plenum.

Canuso, C. M., Bossie, C. A., Zhu, Y., Youssef, E., & Dunner, D. L. (2008). Psychotic symptoms in patients with bipolar mania. *Journal of Affective Disorders, 111*, 164–169.

Caspi, A., Sugdenm, K., Moffitt, T. E., Taylor, A., Craig, I. W., Harrington, H., ... Poulton, R. (2003). Influence of life stress on depression: Moderation by a polymorphism in the 5-HTT gene. *Science, 301*, 386–389.

Cassano, G. B., Dell'Osso, L., Frank, E., Miniati, M., Fagiolini, A., Shear, K., ... Maser, J. (1999). The bipolar spectrum: A clinical reality in search of diagnostic criteria and an assessment methodology. *Journal of Affective Disorders, 54*, 319–328.

Centers for Disease Control and Prevention. (2007). *Web-based inquiry statistics query and reporting system (WISQARS).* National Center for Injury Prevention and Control, CDC (producer). Retrieved from http://www.cdc.gov/injury/wisqars/index.html

Cermakian, N., & Boivin, B. (2003). A molecular perspective of human circadian rhythm disorders. *Brain Research Reviews, 42*, 204–220.

Chaddock, C. A., Barker, G. J., Marshall, N., Schulze, K., Hall, M. H., Fern, A., ... McDonald, C. (2009). White matter microstructural impairments and genetic liability to familial bipolar disorder. *British Journal of Psychiatry, 194*, 527–534.

Chiaroni, P., Hantouche, E., Gouvernet, J., Azorin, J., & Akiskal, H. S. (2005). The cyclothymic temperament in healthy controls and familially at risk individuals for mood disorder: Endophenotype for genetic studies? *Journal of Affective Disorders, 85*, 135–145.

Clark, D. A., Beck, A. T., & Alford, B. A. (1999). *Scientific foundations of cognitive theory and therapy of depression*. New York: Wiley.

Coan, J. A., & Allen, J. J. B. (2004). Frontal EEG asymmetry as a moderator and mediator of emotion. *Biological Psychology, 67*, 7–49.

Coelho, H., Canter, P., & Ernst, E. (2007). Mindfulness-based cognitive therapy: Evaluating current evidence and informing future research. *Journal of Consulting and Clinical Psychology, 75*(6), 1000–1005.

Coffino, B. (2009). The role of childhood parent figure loss in the etiology of adult depression: findings from a prospective longitudinal study. *Attachment and Human Development, 11*(5), 445–470.

Cohen, D., Taieb, O., Flament, M., Benoit, N., Chevret, S., Corcos, M., ... Basquin, M. (2000). Absence of cognitive impairment at long-term follow-up in adolescents treated with ECT for severe mood disorder. *American Journal of Psychiatry, 157*, 460–462.

Cole, D. A., & Turner, J. E. Jr. (1993). Models of cognitive mediation and moderation in child depression. *Journal of Abnormal Psychology, 102*, 271–281.

Compton, W. M., Conway, K. P., Stinson, F. S., & Grant, B. F. (2006). Changes in the prevalence of major depression and comorbid substance use disorders in the United States between 1991–1992 and 2001–2003. *American Journal of Psychiatry, 163*, 2141–2147.

Contreras, G., Menchon, J. M., Urretavizcaya, M., Navarro, M. A., Vallejo, J., & Parker, G. (2007). Hormonal differences between psychotic and non-psychotic melancholic depression. *Journal of Affective Disorders, 100*, 65–73.

Coryell, W., Akiskal, H. S., Leon, A. C., Winokur, G., Maser, J. D., Mueller, T. L., & Keller, M. B. (1994). The time course of nonchronic major depressive disorder: Uniformity across episodes and samples. *Archives of General Psychiatry, 51*, 405–410.

Coryell, W., & Young, E. A. (2005). Clinical predictors of suicide in primary major depressive disorder. *Journal of Clinical Psychiatry, 66*(4), 412–417.

Coryell, W., Young, E., & Carroll, B. (2006). Hyperactivity of the hypothalamic-pituitary-adrenal axis and mortality in major depressive disorder. *Psychiatry Research, 142*(1), 99–104.

Costello E. J., Erkanli A., & Angold, A. (2006). Is there an epidemic of child or adolescent depression? *Journal of Child Psychology and Psychiatry, 47*, 1263–1271.

Cousins, D. A., Butts, K., & Young, A. H. (2009). The role of dopamine in bipolar disorder. *Bipolar Disorders, 11*, 787–806.

Coyne, J. C. (1976). Toward an interactional description of depression. *Psychiatry, 39*, 28–40.

Coyne, J. C., & Whiffen, V. E. (1995). Issues in personality as diatheses for depression: The case of sociotropy-dependence and autonomy-self-criticism. *Psychological Bulletin, 118*, 358–378.

Craddock, N., & Forty, L. (2006). Genetics of affective (mood) disorders. *European Journal of Human Genetics, 14*, 660–668.

Crebbin, K., Mitford, E., Paxton, R., & Turkington, D. (2008). First-episode psychosis: An epidemiological survey comparing psychotic depression with schizophrenia. *Journal of Affective Disorders, 105*, 117–124.

Criado, J. M., Fernandez, A., & Ortiz, A. (2007). Long-term effects of electroconvulsive therapy on episodic memory. *Actas Espanolas d Psiquiatria, 35*, 40–46.

Cronkite, R. C., & Moos, R. H. (1995). Life context, coping process, and depression. In E. Beckham & B. Leber (Eds.), *Handbook of depression* (2nd ed., pp. 569–587). New York: Guilford.

Cuijpers, P., van Straten, A., van Oppen, P., & Andersson, G. (2008). Are psychological and pharmacologic interventions equally effective in the treatment of adult depressive disorders? A meta-analysis of comparative studies. *Journal of Clinical Psychiatry, 69*, 1675–1685.

Cuijpers, P., van Straten, A., & Warmerdam, L. (2007). Behavioral activation treatments of depression: A meta-analysis. *Clinical Psychology Review, 27*(3), 318–326.

Cusin, C., Serretti, A., Lattuada, E., Mandelli, L., & Smeraldi, E. (2000). Impact of clinical variables on illness time course in mood disorders. *Psychiatry Research, 97*, 217–227.

Cyranowski, J. M., Frank, E., Young, E., & Shear, M. K. (2000). Adolescent onset of the gender difference in lifetime rates of major depression: A theoretical model. *Archives of General Psychiatry, 57*(1), 21–27.

Daban, C., Vieta, E., Mackin, P., & Young, A. H. (2005). Hypothalamic-pituitary-adrenal axis and bipolar disorder. *Psychiatric Clinics of North America, 28,* 469–480.

Dagleish, T. (2004). The emotional brain. *Nature Reviews Neuroscience, 5,* 583–589.

Daley, S. E., Hammen, C., Burge, D., Davila, J., Paley, B., Lindberg, N., & Herzberg, D. S. (1997). Predictors of the generation of episodic stress: A longitudinal study of late adolescent women. *Journal of Abnormal Psychology, 106,* 251–259.

Danner, S., Fristad, M. A., Arnold, E., Youngstrom, E. A., Birmaher, B., Horwitz, S. M., … Kowatch, R. A. (2009). Early-onset bipolar spectrum disorders: Diagnostic issues. *Clinical Child and Family Psychological Review, 12,* 271–293.

deAsis, J. M., Greenwald, B. S., Alexopoulos, G. S., Klosses, D. N., Ashtari, M., … Young, P. C. (2006). Frontal signal hyperintensities in mania in old age. *American Journal of Geriatric Psychiatry, 14,* 598–604.

Delgado, P. L., & Moreno, F. A. (2000). Role of norepinephrine in depression. *Journal of Clinical Psychiatry, 61*(Suppl. 1), 5–12.

Depue, R. A., & Iacono, W. G. (1989). Neurobehavioral aspects of affective disorders. *Annual Review of Psychology, 40,* 457–492.

Depue, R. A., Slater, J., Wolfstetter-Kausch, H., Klein, D., Goplerud, E., & Farr, D. (1981). A behavioral paradigm for identifying persons at risk for bipolar depressive disorder: A conceptual framework and five validation studies [Monograph]. *Journal of Abnormal Psychology, 90,* 381–437.

DeRubeis, R. J., Gelfand, L. A., Tang, T. Z., & Simons, A. D. (1999). Medications versus cognitive behavior therapy for severely depressed outpatients: Mega-analysis of four randomized comparisons. *American Journal of Psychiatry, 156,* 1007–1015.

DeRubeis, R. J., Hollon, S. D., Amsterdam, J. D., Shelton, R. C., Young, P. R., Salomon, R. M., … Gallop, R. (2005). Cognitive therapy vs medications in the treatment of moderate to severe depression. *Archives of General Psychiatry, 62,* 409–416.

DeRubeis, R. J., Siegle, G. J., & Hollon, S. D. (2008). Cognitive therapy versus medication for depression: Treatment outcomes and neural mechanisms. *Nature Reviews Neuroscience, 9,* 788–796.

Deshauer, D., Duffy, A., Meany, M., Sharma, S., & Grof, P. (2006). Salivary cortisol secretion in remitted bipolar patients and offspring of bipolar patients. *Bipolar Disorders, 8,* 345–349.

Dilsaver, S. C., Chen, Y. R., Shoaih, A. M., & Swann, A. C. (1999). The phenomenology of mania: Evidence for distinct depressed, dysphoric, and euphoric presentations. *American Journal of Psychiatry, 156,* 426–430.

Dobson, K. S., Hollon, S. D., Dimidjian, S., Schmaling, K. B., Kohlenberg, R. J., Gallop, R., … Jacobson, N. S. (2008). Randomized trial of behavioral activation, cognitive therapy, and antidepressant medication in the prevention of relapse and recurrence in major depression. *Journal of Consulting and Clinical Psychology, 76,* 468–477.

Dozois, D. J. A., & Dobson, K. S. (2001). Information processing and cognitive organization in unipolar depression: Specificity and comorbidity issues. *Journal of Abnormal Psychology, 110,* 236–246.

Druss, B. G., Rosenbeck, R. A., & Sledge, W. H. (2000). Health and disability costs of depressive illness in a major U.S. corporation. *American Journal of Psychiatry, 157,* 1274–1278.

Edvardsen, J., Torgersen, S., Roysamb, E., Lygren, S., Skre, I., Onstad, S., & Oien, P. A. (2008). Heritability of bipolar spectrum disorders. Unity or heterogeneity? *Journal of Affective Disorders, 106,* 229–240.

Egeland, J. A., Gerhard, D. S., Pauls, D. L., Sussex, J. N., Kidd, K. K., Allen, C. R., … Housman, D. E. (1987). Bipolar affective disorders linked to DNA markers on chromosome 11. *Nature, 325,* 783–787.

Ehlers, C. L., Frank, E., & Kupfer, D. J. (1988). Social zeitgebers and biological rhythms. *Archives of General Psychiatry, 45,* 948–952.

Eisenberg, M. E., Ackard, D. M., & Resnick, M. D. (2007). Protective factors and suicide risk in adolescents with a history of sexual abuse. *Journal of Pediatrics, 151*(5), 482–487.

Ekers, D., Richards, D., & Gilbody, S. (2008). A meta-analysis of randomized trials of behavioural treatment of depression. *Psychological Medicine: A Journal of Research in Psychiatry and the Allied Sciences, 38*(5), 611–623.

Emslie, G. J., Armitage, R., Weinberg, W. A., Rush, A. J., Mayes, T. L., & Hoffman, R. F. (2001). Sleep polysomnography as a predictor of recurrence in children and adolescents with major depressive disorder. *International Journal of Neuropsychopharmacology, 4,* 159–168.

Ferster, C. (1973). A functional analysis of depression. *American Psychologist, 28*(10), 857–870.

Fiedorowicz, J. G., Leon, A. C., Keller, M. B., Solomon, D. A., Rice, J. P., & Coryell, W. H. (2009). Do risk factors for suicidal behavior differ by affective disorder polarity? *Psychological Medicine. A Journal of Research in Psychiatry and the Allied Sciences, 39*(5), 763–771.

Finch, J. R., Smith, J.-P., & Pokorny, A. D. (1970, May). *Vehicular studies*. Paper presented at the meeting of the American Psychiatric Association, San Francisco, CA.

Firbank, M. J., Lloyd, A. J., Ferrier, N., & O'Brien, J. T. (2004). A volumetric study of MRI signal hyperintensities in late-life depression. *American Journal of Geriatric Psychiatry, 12*, 606–612.

Firk, C., & Marcus, C. R. (2007). Serotonin by stress interaction: A susceptibility factor for the development of depression? *Journal of Psychopharmacology, 21*(5), 538–544.

Forty, L., Jones, L., Jones, I., Cooper, C., Russell, E., Farmer, A., … Craddock, N. (2009). Is depression severity the sole cause of psychotic symptoms during an episode of unipolar major depression? A study both between and within subjects. *Journal of Affective Disorders, 114*, 103–109.

Fountoulakis, K. N., Gonda, X., Siamouli, M., & Rihmer, Z. (2009). Psychotherapeutic intervention and suicide risk reduction in bipolar disorder: A review of the evidence. *Journal of Affective Disorders, 113*(1–2), 21–29.

Fournier, J. C., DeRubeis, R. J., Hollon, S. D., Dimidjian, S., Amsterdam, J. D., Shelton, R. C., & Fawcett, J. (2010). Antidepressant drug effects and depression severity. *Journal of the American Medical Association, 303*, 47–53.

Fournier, J. C., DeRubeis, R. J., Shelton, R. C., Hollon, S. D., Amsterdam, J. D., & Gallop, R. (2009). Prediction of response to medication and cognitive therapy in the treatment of moderate to severe depression. *Journal of Consulting and Clinical Psychology, 77*, 775–787.

Francis-Raniere, E. L., Alloy, L. B., & Abramson, L. Y. (2006). Depressive personality styles and bipolar spectrum disorders: Prospective tests of the event congruency hypothesis. *Bipolar Disorders, 8*, 382–399.

Frank, E., Kupfer, D. J., Thase, M. E., Malinger, A. G., Swartz, H. A., Fagiolini, A., … Monk, T. (2005). Two-year outcomes for individuals with bipolar I disorder. *Archives of General Psychiatry, 62*, 996–1004.

Freud, S. (1994). Mourning and melancholia. In R. V. Frankiel (Ed.), *Essential papers in psychoanalysis: The essential papers on object loss* (pp. 38–51). New York: New York University Press. (Original work published 1917).

Frey, B. N., Andreazza, A. C., Nery, F. G., Martins, M. R., Quevedo, J., Soares, J. C., & Kapczinski, F. (2007). The role of hippocampus in the pathophysiology of bipolar disorder. *Behavioral Pharmacology, 18*, 419–430.

Galfalvy, H., Huang, Y.-Y., Oquendo, M. A., Currier, D., & Mann, J. J. (2009). Increased risk of suicide attempt in mood disorders and tph1 genotype. *Journal of Affective Disorders, 115*(3), 331–338.

Garber, J., Clarke, G. N., Weersing, V. R., Beardslee, W. R., Brent, D. A., Gladstone, T. R. G., … Iyengar, S. (2009). Prevention of depression in at-risk adolescents: A randomized controlled trial. *Journal of the American Medical Association, 301*, 2215–2224.

Garber, J., & Flynn, C. (2001). Predictors of depressive cognitions in young adolescents. *Cognitive Therapy and Research, 25*, 353–376.

Gemar, M. C., Segal, Z. V., Sagrati, S., & Kennedy, S. J. (2001). Mood-induced changes on the implicit association test in recovered depressed patients. *Journal of Abnormal Psychology, 110*, 282–289.

George, M. S., Lisanby, S. H., & Sackeim, H. A. (1999). Transcranial magnetic stimulation: Applications in neuropsychiatry. *Archives of General Psychiatry, 56*, 300–311.

Gibb, B. E., Abramson, L. Y., & Alloy, L. B. (2004). Emotional maltreatment from parents, peer victimization, and cognitive vulnerability to depression. *Cognitive Therapy and Research, 28*, 1–21.

Gibb, B. E., Alloy, L. B., Abramson, L. Y., Rose, D. T., Whitehouse, W. G., Donovan, P., … Tierney, S. (2001). History of childhood maltreatment, negative cognitive styles, and episodes of depression in adulthood. *Cognitive Therapy and Research, 25*, 425–446.

Gibb, B. E., Beevers, C. G., Andover, M. S., & Holleran, K. (2006). The hopelessness theory of depression: A prospective multi-wave test of the vulnerability-stress hypothesis. *Cognitive Therapy and Research, 30*, 763–777.

Giesler, R., Josephs, R., & Swann, W. (1996). Self-verification in clinical depression: The desire for negative evaluation. *Journal of Abnormal Psychology, 105*(3), 358–368.

Giles, D. E., Kupfer, D. J., Rush, A. J., & Roffwarg, H. P. (1998). Controlled comparison of electrophysiological sleep in families of probands with unipolar depression. *American Journal of Psychiatry, 155*, 192–199.

Gill, M., McKeon, P., & Humphries, P. (1988). Linkage analysis of manic depression in an Irish family using H-ras 1 and INS DNA markers. *Journal of Medical Genetics, 25*, 634–635.

Gillham, J. E., Hamilton, J., Freres, D. R., Patton, K., & Gallop, R. (2006). Preventing depression among early adolescents in the primary care setting: A randomized controlled study of the penn resiliency program. *Journal of Abnormal Child Psychology, 34*(2), 203–219.

Glanz, L. M., Haas, G. L., & Sweeney, J. A. (1995). Assessment of hopelessness in suicidal patients. *Clinical Psychology Review, 15*, 49–64.

Goest, F. S., Sadler, B., Toolan, J., Zamoiski, R. D., Mondimore, F. M., MacKinnon, D. F., & Schweizer, B. (2007). Psychotic features in bipolar and unipolar depression. *Bipolar Disorders, 9,* 901–906.

Goldsmith, S. K., Pellmar, T. C., Kleinman, A. M., & Bunney, W. E. (2002). *Reducing suicide: A national imperative.* Washington, DC: National Academies Press.

Gonda, X., Fountoulakis, K. N., Kaprinis, G., & Rihmer, Z. (2007). Prediction and prevention of suicide in patients with unipolar depression and anxiety. *Annals of General Psychiatry, 6,* 23.

Goodwin, F. K., & Jamison, K. R. (2007). *Manic-depressive illness* (2nd ed.). New York: Oxford University Press.

Goodyer, I. M., Herbert, J., Tamplin, A., & Altham, P. M. (2000). FIrst-episode major depression in adolescents: Affective, cognitive and endocrine characteristics of risk status and predictors of onset. *British Journal of Psychiatry, 176,* 142–149.

Gortner, E. T., Gollan, J. K., Dobson, K. S., & Jacobson, N. S. (1998). Cognitive-behavioral treatment for depression: Relapse prevention. *Journal of Clinical and Consulting Psychology, 66,* 377–378.

Gotlib, I. H., & Joorman, J. (2010). Cognition and depression: Current status and future directions. *Annual Review of Clinical Psychology, 6,* 285–312.

Gould, M., Jamieson, P., & Romer, D. (2003). Media contagion and suicide among the young. *American Behavioral Scientist, 46*(9), 1269–1284.

Gray, J. A. (1994). Three fundamental emotion systems. In P. Eckman & R. J. Davidson (Eds.), *The nature of emotion: Fundamental questions* (pp. 243–247). New York: Oxford University Press.

Greenwald, B. S., Kramer-Ginsberg, E., Krishnan, K. R., Ashtari, M., Auerbach, C., … Patel, M. (1998). Neuroanatomic localization of magnetic resonance imaging signal hyperintensities in geriatric depression. *Stroke, 29,* 613–617.

Grunbaum, J. A., Kann, L., Kinchen, S. A., Williams, B., Ross, J. G., Lowry, R., & Kolbe, L. (2002). Youth risk behavior surveillance—United States, 2002. *Journal of School Health, 72*(8), 313–328.

Haaga, D. A. E., & Beck, A. T. (1995). Perspectives on depressive realism: Implications for cognitive theory of depression. *Behaviour Research and Therapy, 33,* 41–48.

Hammen, C. (2003). Interpersonal stress and depression in women. *Journal of Affective Disorders, 74*(1), 49–57.

Hammen, C. (2006). Stress generation in depression: Reflections on origins, research, and future directions. *Journal of Clinical Psychology, 62,* 1065–1082.

Hammen, C., Brennan, P. A., Keenan-Miller, D., & Herr, N. R. (2008). Early onset recurrent subtype of adolescent depression: Clinical and psychosocial correlates. *Journal of Child Psychology and Psychiatry, 49,* 433–440.

Hammen, C., Shih, J. H., & Brennan, P. A. (2004). Intergenerational transmission of depression: Test of an interpersonal stress model in a community sample. *Journal of Consulting and Clinical Psychology, 72*(3), 511–522.

Hankin, B. L., & Abramson, L. Y. (2001). Development of gender differences in depression: An elaborated cognitive vulnerability-transactional stress theory. *Psychological Bulletin, 127,* 773–796.

Hankin, B. L., Abramson, L. Y., Miller, N., & Haeffel, G. (2004). Cognitive vulnerability-stress theories of depression: Examining affective specificity in the prediction of depression versus anxiety in three prospective studies. *Cognitive Therapy and Research, 28,* 309–345.

Hankin, B. L., Fraley, C., Lahey, B. B., & Waldman, I. D. (2005). Is depression best viewed as a continuum or discrete category? A taxometric analysis of childhood and adolescent depression in a population-based sample. *Journal of Abnormal Psychology, 114,* 96–110.

Harmon-Jones, E., Abramson, L. Y., Nusslock, R., Sigelman, J. D., Urošević, S., Turonie, L., … Fearn, M. (2008). Effect of bipolar disorder on left frontal cortical responses to goals differing in valence and task difficulty. *Biological Psychiatry, 63,* 693–698.

Harris, T. O., Borsanyi, S., Messari, S., Stanford, K., Cleary, S. E., Shiers, H. M., … Herbert, J. (2000). Morning cortisol as a risk factor for subsequent major depressive disorder in adult women. *British Journal of Psychiatry, 177,* 505–510.

Hartlage, S., Alloy, L. B., Vazquez, V., & Dykman, B. (1993). Automatic and effortful processing in depression. *Psychological Bulletin, 113,* 247–278.

Harvey, A. G., Schmidt, D. A., Scarna, A., Semler, C. N., & Goodwin, G. M. (2005). Sleep-related functioning in euthymic patients with bipolar disorder, patients with insomnia, and subjects without sleep problems. *American Journal of Psychiatry, 162,* 50–57.

Hasler, B. P., Buysse, D. J., Kupfer, D. J., & Germain, A. (2010). Phase relationships between core body temperature, melatonin, and sleep are associated with depression severity: Further evidence for circadian misalignment in non-seasonal depression. *Psychiatry Research, 178,* 205–207.

Hay, D. P., & Hay, L. K. (1990). The role of ECT in the treatment of depression. In C. D. McCann & N. S. Endler (Eds.), *Depression: New directions in theory, research, and practice* (pp. 255–272). Toronto: Wall and Emerson.

Hayes, S., Barnes-Holmes, D., & Roche, B. (2001). Relational frame theory: A précis. In S. Hayes, D. Barnes-Holmes, & B. Roche (Eds.), *Relational frame theory: A post-Skinnerian account of human language and cognition* (pp. 141–154). New York: Kluwer Academic/Plenum.

Hayes, S., Strosahl, K., & Wilson, K. (1999). *Acceptance and commitment therapy: An experiential approach to behavior change*. New York: Guilford.

Hazan, C., & Shaver, P. (1987). Romantic love conceptualized as an attachment process. *Journal of Personality and Social Psychology, 52*(3), 511–524.

Hidalgo, M. P., Caumo, W., Posser, M., Coccaro, S. B., Camozzato, A. L., & Chaves, M. L. F. (2009). Relationship between depressive mood and chronotype in healthy subjects. *Psychiatry and Clinical Neurosciences, 63*, 283–290.

Hinrichsen, G. A. (2008). Interpersonal psychotherapy as a treatment for depression in later life. *Professional Psychology: Research and Practice, 39*(3), 306–312.

Hlastala, S. A., Kotler, J. S., McClellan, J. M., & McCauley, E. A. (2010). Interpersonal and social rhythm therapy for adolescents with bipolar disorder: Treatment development and results from an open trial. *Depression and Anxiety, 27*, 457–464.

Hodgkinson, S., Sherrington, R., Gurling, H., Marchbanks, R., Reeders, S., Mallet, J., … Brynjolfsson, J. (1987). Molecular genetic evidence for heterogeneity in manic depression. *Nature, 325*, 805–806.

Hofmann, S., Sawyer, A., Witt, A., & Oh, D. (2010). The effect of mindfulness-based therapy on anxiety and depression: A meta-analytic review. *Journal of Consulting and Clinical Psychology, 78*(2), 169–183.

Hollon, S. D. (2006). Cognitive therapy in the treatment and prevention of depression. In T. E. Joiner, J. S. Brown, & J. Kistner (Eds.), *The interpersonal, cognitive, and social nature of depression* (pp. 131–151). Mahwah, NJ: Erlbaum.

Hollon, S. D., DeRubeis, R. J., Shelton, R. C., Amsterdam, J. D., Salomon, R. M., O'Reardon, J. P., … Gallop, R. (2005). Prevention of relapse following cognitive therapy vs. medications in moderate to severe depression. *Archives of General Psychiatry, 62*, 417–422.

Hollon, S. D., DeRubeis, R. J., Shelton, R. C., & Weiss, B. (2002). The emperor's new drugs. Effect size and moderation effects. *Prevention and Treatment, 5*, Article 28. Retrieved October 12, 2011, from the PsycARTICLES database at http://www.apa.org/pubs/databases/psycarticles/index.aspx.

Hyde, J. S., Mezulis, A. H., & Abramson, L. Y. (2008). The ABCs of depression: Integrating affective, biological, and cognitive models to explain the emergence of the gender difference in depression. *Psychological Review, 115*(2), 291–313.

Iacoviello, B. M., Alloy, L. B., Abramson, L. Y., & Choi, J. Y. (2010). The early course of depression: A longitudinal investigation of prodromal symptoms and their relation to the symptomatic course of depressive episodes. *Journal of Abnormal Psychology, 119*, 459–467.

Iacoviello, B. M., Alloy, L. B., Abramson, L. Y., Whitehouse, W. G., & Hogan, M. E. (2006). The course of depression in individuals at high and low cognitive risk for depression: A prospective study. *Journal of Affective Disorders, 93*, 61–69.

Ilardi, S. S., Craighead, W. E., & Evans, D. D. (1997). Modeling relapse in unipolar depression: The effects of dysfunctional cognitions and personality disorders. *Journal of Consulting and Clinical Psychology, 65*, 381–391.

Imel, Z. E., Malterer, M. B., McKay, K. M., & Wampold, B. E. (2008). A meta-analysis of psychotherapy and medication in unipolar depression and dysthymia. *Journal of Affective Disorders, 110*, 197–206.

Ingram, R. E., Miranda, J., & Segal, Z. V. (1998). *Cognitive vulnerability to depression*. New York: Guilford.

Ingram, R. E., & Ritter, J. (2000). Vulnerability to depression: Cognitive reactivity and parental bonding in high-risk individuals. *Journal of Abnormal Psychology, 109*, 588–596.

Isometsä, E. T., Henriksson, M. M., Aro, H. M., & Heikkinen, M. E. (1994). Suicide in major depression. *American Journal of Psychiatry, 151*(4), 530–536.

Jackson, J., Cavanagh, J., & Scott, J. (2003). A systematic review of manic and depressive prodromes. *Journal of Affective Disorders, 74*, 209–217.

Jacobson, N. S., Dobson, K. S., Truax, P. A., Addis, M. E., Koerner, K., Gollan, J. K., … Prince, S. E. (1996). A component analysis of cognitive-behavioral treatment for depression. *Journal of Consulting and Clinical Psychology, 64*, 295–304.

Jacobson, N. S., Martell, C., & Dimidjian, S. (2001). Behavioral activation treatment for depression: Returning to contextual roots. *Clinical Psychology: Science and Practice, 8*(3), 255–270.

Jarrett, R. B., Kraft, D., Doyle, J., Foster, B. M., Eaves, G. G., & Silver, P. C. (2001). Preventing recurrent depression using cognitive therapy with and without a continuation phase: A randomized clinical trial. *Archives of General Psychiatry, 58*, 381–388.

Joffe, H., & Cohen, L. S. (1998). Estrogen, serotonin and mood disturbance: Where is the therapeutic bridge? *Biological Psychiatry, 44*, 798–811.

Joffe, R. T., & Marriott, M. (2000). Thyroid hormone levels and recurrence of major depression. *American Journal of Psychiatry, 157*, 1689–1691.

Johansson, C., Willeit, M., Smedh, C., Ekholm, J., Paunio, T., Kieseppa, T., ... Partonen, T. (2003). Circadian clock-related polymorphisms in seasonal affective disorder and their relevance to diurnal preference. *Neuropsychopharmacology, 28*, 734–739.

Johnson, J., Howarth, E., & Weissman, M. M. (1991). The validity of major depression with psychotic features based on a community study. *Archives of General Psychiatry, 45*, 1075–1081.

Johnson, S. L. (2005). Life events in bipolar disorder: Towards more specific models. *Clinical Psychology Review, 25*, 1008–1027.

Johnson, S. L., Cueller, A. K., Ruggero, C., Winett-Perlman, C., Goodnick, P., White, R., & Miller, I. (2008). Life events as predictors of mania and depression in bipolar I disorder. *Journal of Abnormal Psychology, 117*, 268–277.

Johnson, S. L., & Kizer, A. (2002). Bipolar and unipolar depression: A comparison of clinical phenomenology and psychosocial predictors. In I. H. Gotlib & C. L. Hammen (Eds.), *Handbook of depression* (pp. 141–165). New York: Guilford.

Joiner, T. (2000). Depression's vicious scree: Self-propagating and erosive processes in depression chronicity. *Clinical Psychology: Science and Practice, 7*(2), 203–218.

Joiner, T., Metalsky, G., Gencoz, F., & Gencoz, T. (2001). The relative specificity of excessive reassurance-seeking to depressive symptoms and diagnoses among clinical samples of adults and youth. *Journal of Psychopathology and Behavioral Assessment, 23*(1), 35–41.

Joiner, T., Metalsky, G., Katz, J., & Beach, S. (1999). Depression and excessive reassurance-seeking. *Psychological Inquiry, 10*(4), 269–278.

Joiner, T. E., Steer, R. A., Abramson, L. Y., Alloy, L. B., Metalsky, G. I., & Schmidt, N. B. (2001). Hopelessness depression as a distinct dimension of depressive symptoms among clinical and non-clinical samples. *Behaviour Research and Therapy, 39*, 523–536.

Joiner, T. E. Jr., & Wagner, K. D. (1995). Attributional style and depression in children and adolescents: A meta-analytic review. *Clinical Psychology Review, 15*, 777–798.

Jones, S. H., Hare, D. J., & Evershed, K. (2005). Actigraphic assessment of circadian activity and sleep patterns in bipolar disorder. *Bipolar Disorders, 7*, 176–186.

Judd, L. L. (1997). The clinical course of unipolar major depressive disorders. *Archives of General Psychiatry, 54*, 989–991.

Judd, L. L., Akiskal, H. S., Schettler, P. J., Endicott, J., Leon, A. C., Solomon, D. A., ... Keller, M. B. (2005). Psychosocial disability in the course of bipolar I and II disorders: A prospective, comparative, longitudinal study. *Archives of General Psychiatry, 62*, 1322–1330.

Judd, L. L., Akiskal, H. S., Zeller, P. J., Paulus, M., Leon, A. C., Maser, J. D., ... Keller, M. B. (2000). Psychosocial disability during the long-term course of unipolar major depressive disorder. *Archives of General Psychiatry, 57*, 375–380.

Kabat-Zinn, J. (1994). *Wherever you go, there you are: Mindfulness meditation in everyday life.* New York: Hyperion.

Kanter, J., Manos, R., Bowe, W., Baruch, D., Busch, A., & Rusch, L. (2010). What is behavioral activation? A review of the empirical literature. *Clinical Psychology Review, 30*(6), 608–620.

Karg, K., Burmeister, M., Shedden, K., & Sen, S. (2011). The serotonin transporter promoter variant (5-HTTLPR), stress, and depression meta-analysis revisited: Evidence of genetic moderation. *Archives of General Psychiatry, 68*(5), 444–454.

Kendler, K. S., Eaves, L. J., Walters, E. E., Neale, M. C., Heath, A. C., & Kessler, R. C. (1996). The identification and validation of distinct depressive syndromes in a population-based sample of female twins. *Archives of General Psychiatry, 53*, 391–399.

Kendler, K. S., Gardner, C. O., & Prescott, C. A. (2002). Toward a comprehensive developmental model for major depression in women. *American Journal of Psychiatry, 159*(7), 1133–1145.

Kendler, K. S., Karkowski, L. M., & Prescott, C. A. (1999). Causal relationship between stressful life events and the onset of major depression. *American Journal of Psychiatry, 156*, 837–841.

Kendler, K. S., Kuhn, J., & Prescott, C. A. (2004). The interrelationship of neuroticism, sex, and stressful life events in the prediction of episodes of major depression. *American Journal of Psychiatry, 161*(4), 631–636.

Kendler, K. S., Thornton, L. M., & Gardner, C. O. (2000). Stressful life events and previous episodes in the etiology of major depression in women: An evaluation of the "kindling" hypothesis. *American Journal of Psychiatry, 157*, 1243–1251.

Kenna, H. A., Jiang, B., & Rasgon, N. L. (2009). Reproductive and metabolic abnormalities associated with bipolar disorder and its treatment. *Harvard Review of Psychiatry, 17*, 138–146.

Kennard, B. D., Stewart, S. M., Hughes, J. L., Patel, P. G., & Emslie, G. J. (2006). Cognitions and depressive symptoms among ethnic minority adolescents. *Cultural Diversity and Ethnic Minority Psychology, 12*, 578–591.

Kennedy, S. H., Kutcher, S. P., Ralevski, E., & Brown, G. M. (1996). Nocturnal melatonin and 24-hour 6-sulphatoxymelatonin levels in various phases of bipolar affective disorder. *Psychiatry Research, 63*, 219–222.

Kessing, L. V. (2007). Epidemiology of subtypes of depression. *Acta Psychiatrica Scandinavica, 115*, 85–89.

Kessler, R. C. (2003). Epidemiology of women and depression. *Journal of Affective Disorders, 74*(1), 5–13.

Kessler, R. C., Akiskal, H. S., Ames, M., Birnbaum, H., Greenberg, P., Hirschfeld, R. M., … Wang, P. S. (2006). Prevalence and effects of mood disorders on work performance in a nationally representative sample of U.S. workers. *American Journal of Psychiatry, 163*, 1561–1568.

Kessler, R. C., Berglund, P., Demler, O., Jin, R., Koretz, D., Merikangas, K. R., … Wang, P. S. (2003). The epidemiology of major depressive disorder: results from the National Comorbidity Survey Replication (NCS-R). *Journal of the American Medical Association, 289*, 3095–3105.

Kessler, R. C., Borges, G., & Walters, E. E. (1999). Prevalence of and risk factors for lifetime suicide attempts in the national comorbidity survey. *Archives of General Psychiatry, 56*(7), 617–626.

Kirsch, I., Deacon, B. J., Huedo-Medina, T. B., Scoboria, A., Moore, T. J., & Johnson, B. T. (2008). Initial severity and antidepressant benefits: meta-analysis of data submitted to the Food and Drug Administration. *PLos Medicine, 5*, e45.

Kirsch, I., Moore, T. J., Scoboria, A., & Nicholls, S. S. (2002). The emperor's new drugs. An analysis of antidepressant medication data submitted to the U.S. Food and Drug Administration. *Prevention and Treatment, 5*, Article 23. Retrieved from http://alphachoices.com/repository/assets/pdf/EmperorsNewDrugs.pdf

Klein, D. N., Schatzberg, A. F., McCullough, J. P., Dowling, F., Goodman, D., Howland, R. H., … Keller, M. B. (1999). Age of onset in chronic major depression: Relation to demographic and clinical variables, family history, and treatment response. *Journal of Affective Disorders, 55*, 149–157.

Klein, D. N., Schwartz, J. E., Rose, S., & Leader, J. B. (2000). Five-year course and outcome of dysthymic disorder: A prospective, naturalistic follow-up study. *American Journal of Psychiatry, 157*, 931–939.

Klein, D. N., Shankman, S. A., & Rose, S. (2006). Ten-year prospective follow-up study of the naturalistic course of dysthymic disorder and double depression. *American Journal of Psychiatry, 163*, 872–880.

Klein, D. N., Taylor, E. B., Dickstein, S., & Harding, K. (1988). The early-late onset distinction in DSM-III-R dysthymia. *Journal of Affective Disorders, 14*, 25–33.

Klerman, G. L. (1988). The current age of youthful melancholia. *British Journal of Psychiatry, 152*, 4–14.

Kobak, R. R., Sudler, N., & Gamble, W. (1991). Attachment and depressive symptoms during adolescence: A developmental pathways analysis [Special issue]. *Journal of Development and Psychopathology, 3*, 461–474.

Kochman, F. J., Hantouche, E. G., Ferrari, P., Lancrenon, S., Bayart, D., & Akiskal, H. S. (2005). Cyclothymic temperament as a prospective predictor of bipolarity and suicidality in children and adolescents with major depressive disorder. *Journal of Affective Disorders, 85*, 181–189.

Koster, E. H. W., De Lissnyder, E., Derakshan, N., & De Raedt, R. (2011). Understanding depressive rumination from a cognitive science perspective: The impaired disengagement hypothesis. *Clinical Psychology Review, 31*(1), 138–145.

Kraepelin, E. (1921). *Manic-depressive insanity and paranoia*. Edinburgh, Scotland: E & S Livingstone.

Kuehner, C. (2003). Gender differences in unipolar depression: an update of epidemiological findings and possible explanations. *Acta Psychiatrica Scandinavica, 108*(3), 163–174.

Kugaya, A., & Sanacora, G. (2005). Beyond monoamines: glutamatergic function in mood disorders. *CNS Spectrum, 10*, 808–819.

Kupfer, D. J. (1976). REM latency: A psychobiologic marker for primary depressive disease. *Biological Psychiatry, 11*, 159–174.

Kupfer, D. J., & Foster, F. G. (1972). Interval between onset of sleep and rapid-eye movement sleep as an indicator of depression. *Lancet, 2*, 684–686.

Kupfer, D. J., & Frank, E. (2001). The interaction of drug- and psychotherapy in the long-term treatment of depression. *Journal of Affective Disorders, 62*, 131–137.

Kuzelova, H., Ptacek, R., & Macek, M. (2010). The serotonin transporter gene (5-HTT) variant and psychiatric disorders: Review of current literature. *Neuroendocrinology Letters, 1*, 4–10.

Lam, D., Wright, K., & Smith, N. (2004). Dysfunctional assumptions in bipolar disorder. *Journal of Affective Disorders, 79*, 193–199.

Leibenluft, E. (2000). Women and bipolar disorder: An update. *Bulletin of the Menninger Clinic, 64*, 5–17.

Leibenluft, E., Albert, P. S., Rosenthal, N. E., & Wehr, T. A. (1996). Relationship between sleep and mood in patients with rapid-cycling bipolar disorder. *Psychiatry Research, 63*, 161–168.

Leproult, R., van Onderbergen, A., L'Hermite-Baleriaux, M., van Cauter, E., & Copinschi, G. (2005). Phase-shifts of 24-h rhythms of hormonal release and body temperature following early evening administration of the melatonin agonist agomelatine in healthy older men. *Clinical Endocrinology, 63*, 298–304.

Levinson, D. F. (2006). The genetics of depression: A review. *Biological Psychiatry, 60*(2), 84–92.

Lewinsohn, P. M. (1974). A behavioral approach to depression. In R. J. Friedman & M. M. Katz (Eds.), *The psychology of depression: Contemporary theory and research* (pp. 157–185). Oxford, UK: Wiley.

Lewinsohn, P. M., Allen, N. B., Seeley, J. R., & Gotlib, I. H. (1999). First onset versus recurrence of depression: Differential processes of psychosocial risk. *Journal of Abnormal Psychology, 108*, 483–489.

Lewinsohn, P. M., Biglan, A., & Zeiss, A. M. (1976). Behavioral treatment of depression. In P. O. Davidson (Ed.), *The behavioral management of anxiety, depression and pain* (pp. 91–146). New York: Brunner/Mazel.

Lewinsohn, P. M., & Graf, M. (1973). Pleasant activities and depression. *Journal of Consulting and Clinical Psychology, 41*, 261–268.

Lewinsohn, P. M., Joiner, T. E., & Rohde, P. (2001). Evaluation of cognitive diathesis-stress models in predicting major depressive disorder in adolescents. *Journal of Abnormal Psychology, 110*, 203–215.

Lewinsohn, P. M., Mischel, W., Chaplin, W., & Barton, R. (1980). Social competence and depression: The role of illusory self-perceptions? *Journal of Abnormal Psychology, 89*, 203–212.

Lewinsohn, P. M., Rohde, P., Seeley, J. R., & Baldwin, C. L. (2001). Gender differences in suicide attempts from adolescence to young adulthood. *Journal of the American Academy of Child and Adolescent Psychiatry, 40*(4), 427–434.

Lewy, A. J., Bauer, V. K., Cutler, N. L., Sack, R. L., Ahmed, S., Thomase, K. H., … Jackson, J. M. (1998). Morning vs evening light treatment of patients with winter depression. *Archives of General Psychiatry, 55*, 890–896.

Lisanby, S. H., Maddox, J. H., Prudic, J., Devanand, D. P., & Sackeim, H. A. (2000). The effects of electroconvulsive therapy on memory of autobiographical and public events. *Archives of General Psychiatry, 57*, 581–590.

Liu, R. T., & Alloy, L. B. (2010). Stress generation in depression: A systematic review of the empirical literature and recommendations for future study. *Clinical Psychology Review, 30*, 582–593.

Liu, R. T., Alloy, L. B., Abramson, L. Y., Iacoviello, B. M., & Whitehouse, W. G. (2009). Emotional maltreatment and depression: Prospective prediction of depressive episodes. *Depression and Anxiety, 26*, 174–181.

Liu Y., Blackwood, D. H., Caesar, S., de Geus, E. J. C., Farmer, A., Ferreira, M. A. R., … Wellcome Trust Case-Control Consortium. (2011). Meta-analysis of genome-wide association data of bipolar disorder and major depressive disorder. *Molecular Psychiatry, 16*(1), 2–4.

Luby, J. L., & Navsaria, N. (2010). Pediatric bipolar disorder: Evidence for prodromal states and early markers. *Journal of Child Psychology and Psychiatry, 51*, 459–471.

Lyoo, I. K., Lee, H. K., Jung, J. H., Noam, G. G., & Renshaw, P. F. (2002). White matter hyperintensities on magnetic resonance imaging of the brain in children with psychiatric disorders. *Comprehensive Psychiatry, 43*, 361–368.

Ma, N., Li, L., Shu, N., Liu, J., Gong, G., He, Z., … Jiang, T. (2007). White matter abnormalities in first-episode, treatment-naïve young adults with major depressive disorder. *American Journal of Psychiatry, 164*, 823–826.

MacPhillamy, D. J., & Lewinsohn, P. M. (1974). Depression as a function of levels of desired and obtained pleasure. *Journal of Abnormal Psychology, 83*, 651–657.

Macritchie, K., Geddes, J. R., Scott, J., Haslam, D., de Lima, M., & Goodwin, G. (2003). Valproate for acute mood episodes in bipolar disorder. *Cochrane Database of Systematic Reviews, 1*, CD004052.

Madge, N., & Harvey, J. G. (1999). Suicide among the young: The size of the problem. *Journal of Adolescence, 22*(1), 145–155.

Mahon, K., Wu, J., Malhotra, A. K., Burdick, K. E., DeRosse, P., Ardekani, B. A., & Szeszko, P. R. (2009). A voxel-based diffusion tensor imaging study of white matter in bipolar disorder. *Neuropsychopharmacology, 34*, 1590–1600.

Maier, S. F., Seligman, M. E. P., & Solomon, R. L. (1969). Pavlovian fear conditioning and learned helplessness. In B. A. Campbell & R. M. Church (Eds.), *Punishment* (pp. 299–343). New York: Appleton.

Malkoff-Schwartz, S., Frank, E., Anderson, B. P., Hlastala, S. A., Luther, J. F., Sherrill, J. T., … Kupfer, D. J. (2000). Social rhythm disruption and stressful life events in the onset of bipolar and unipolar episodes. *Psychological Medicine, 30,* 1005–1016.

Malkoff-Schwartz, S., Frank, E., Anderson, B. P., Sherrill, J. F., Siegel, L., Patterson, D., & Kupfer, D. J. (1998). Stressful life events and social rhythm disruption in the onset of manic and depressive bipolar episodes. *Archives of General Psychiatry, 55,* 702–707.

Mann, J. J., Apter, A., Bertolote, J. M., Currier, D., Haas, A., Hegerl, U., … Hendin, H. (2005). Suicide prevention strategies: A systematic review. *Journal of the American Medical Association, 294,* 2064–2074.

Mann, J. J., Arango, V. A., Avenevoli, S., Brent, D. A., Champagne, F. A., Clayton, P., … Wenzel, A. (2009). Candidate endophenotypes for genetic studies of suicidal behavior. *Biological Psychiatry, 65*(7), 556–563.

Mann, J. J., McBride, A., Brown, R. P., Linnoila, M., Leon, A. C., DeMeo, M., … Stanley, M. (1992). Relationship between central and peripheral serotonin indexes in depressed and suicidal psychiatric inpatients. *Archives of General Psychiatry, 49,* 442–446.

Marangell, L. B., Martinez, M., Jurdi, R. A., & Zboyan, H. (2007). Neurostimulation therapies in depression: A review of new modalities. *Acta Psychiatrica Scandinavica, 116,* 174–181.

Marlatt, G. A., & Kristeller, J. L. (1999). Mindfulness and meditation. In W. R. Miller (Ed.), *Integrating spirituality in treatment* (pp. 67–84). Washington, DC: American Psychological Association.

Matthew, S. J., Manji, H. K., & Charney, D. S. (2008). Novel drugs and therapeutic targets for severe mood disorders. *Neuropsychopharmacology, 33,* 2080–2092.

Mathews, A., & MacLeod, C. (2005). Cognitive vulnerability to emotional disorders. *Annual Review of Clinical Psychology, 1,* 167–195.

Mazzucchelli, T., Kane, R., & Rees, C. (2009). Behavioral activation treatments for depression in adults: A meta-analysis and review. *Clinical Psychology: Science and Practice, 16*(4), 383–411.

McGrath, P. J., Stewart, J. W., Janal, M. N., Petkova, E., Quitkin, F. M., & Klein, D. F. (2000). A placebo-controlled study of fluoxetine versus imipramine in the acute treatment of atypical depression. *American Journal of Psychiatry, 157,* 344–350.

McGuffin, P., Rijsdijk, F., Andrew, M., Sham, P., Katz, R., & Cardno, A. (2003). The heritability of bipolar affective disorder and the genetic relationship to unipolar depression. *Archives General Psychiatry, 60,* 497–502.

McLaughlin, K. A., Hilt, L. M., & Nolen-Hoeksema, S. (2007). Racial/ethnic differences in internalizing and externalizing symptoms in adolescents. *Journal of Abnormal Child Psychology, 35,* 801–816.

Meadows, L. A., Kaslow, N. J., Thompson, M. P., & Jurkovic, G. J. (2005). Protective factors against suicide attempt risk among african american women experiencing intimate partner violence. *American Journal of Community Psychology, 36*(1–2), 109–121.

Meesters, Y., Jansen, J. H. C., Beersma, D. G. M., Bouhuys, A. L., & van der Hoofdakker, R. H. (1993). Early light treament can prevent an emerging winter depression from developing into a full-blown depression. *Journal of Affective Disorders, 29,* 41–47.

Mehl, R. C., O'Brien, L. M., Jones, J. H., Dreisbach, J. K., Mervis, C. B., & Gozal, D. (2006). Correlates of sleep and pediatric bipolar disorder. *Sleep, 29,* 193–197.

Mendlewicz, J., & Rainer, J. D. (1977). Adoption study supporting genetic transmission in manic-depressive illness. *Nature, 168,* 327–329.

Merikangas, K. R., Akiskal, H. S., Angst, J., Greenberg, P. E., Hirschfeld, R. M. A, Petukhova, M., & Kessler, R. C. (2007). Lifetime and 12-month prevalence of bipolar spectrum disorder in the national comorbidity survey replication. *Archives of General Psychiatry, 64,* 543–552.

Metalsky, G. I., Joiner, T. E., Hardin, T. S., & Abramson, L. Y. (1993). Depressive reactions to failure in a naturalistic setting: A test of the hopelessness and self-esteem theories of depression. *Journal of Abnormal Psychology, 102,* 101–109.

Meyer, J. H., Kapur, S., Houle, S., DaSilva, J., Owczarek, B., Brown, G. M., … Kennedy, S. H. (1999). Prefrontal cortex 5-HT$_2$ receptors in depression: An [^{18}F] Setoperone PET imaging study. *American Journal of Psychiatry, 156,* 1029–1034.

Miklowitz, D. J., & Johnson, S. L. (2006). The psychopathology and treatment of bipolar disorder. *Annual Review of Clinical Psychology, 4,* 33–52.

Mikolajczyk, R. T., Bredehorst, M., Khelaifat, N., Maier, C., & Maxwell, A. E. (2007). Correlates of depressive symptoms among Latino and non-Latino white adolescents: Findings from the 2003 California Health Interview Survey. *BioMed Central Public Health, 7,* 21.

Minor, T., & Saade, S. (1997). Poststress glucose mitigates behavioral impairment in rats in the "learned helplessness" model of psychopathology. *Biological Psychiatry, 42*, 324–334.

Mirowsky, J., & Ross, C. (2003). *Social causes of psychological distress.* New York: Aldine de Gruyter.

Monroe, S. M., & Harkness, K. L. (2005). Life stress, the "kindling" hypothesis, and the recurrence of depression: Considerations from a life stress perspective. *Psychological Review, 112*, 417–445.

Monroe, S. M., Rohde, P., Seeley, J. R., & Lewinsohn, P. M. (1999). Life events and depression in adolescence: Relationship loss as a prospective risk factor for first onset of major depressive disorder. *Journal of Abnormal Psychology, 108*, 606–614.

Moreno, C., Laje, G., Blanco, C., Huiping, J., Schmidt, A. B., & Olfson, M. (2007). National trends in the outpatient diagnosis and treatment of bipolar disorder in youth. *Archives of General Psychiatry, 64*, 1032–1039.

Morris, M. C., Ciesla, J. A., & Garber, J. (2010). A prospective study of stress autonomy versus stress sensitization in adolescents at varied risk for depression. *Journal of Abnormal Psychology, 2*, 341–354.

Mufson, L., Weissman, M. M., Moreau, D., & Garfinkel, R. (1999). Efficacy of interpersonal psychotherapy for depressed adolescents. *Archives of General Psychiatry, 56*(6), 573–579.

Mundo, E., Walker, M., Cate, T., Macciardi, F., & Kennedy, J. L. (2001). The role of serotonin transporter protein gene in antidepressant-induced mania in bipolar disorder: Preliminary findings. *Archives of General Psychiatry, 58*, 539–544.

Muris, P., Meesters, C., van Melick, M., & Zwambag, L. (2001). Self-reported attachment style, attachment quality, and symptoms of anxiety and depression in young adolescents. *Personality and Individual Differences, 30*(5), 809–818.

Murray, C. J. L., & Lopez, A. D. (Eds.). (1996). *The global burden of disease.* Geneva: World Health Organization.

Naranjo, C. A., Tremblay, L. K., & Busto, U. E. (2001). The role of the brain reward system in depression. *Progress in Neuro-Psychopharmacology and Biological Psychiatry, 25*, 781–823.

National Strategy for Suicide Prevention: Goals and Objectives for Action. (2001). Rockville, MD: U.S. Department of Health and Human Services.

Needles, D. J., & Abramson, L. Y. (1990). Positive life events, attributional style, and hopefulness: Testing a model of recovery from depression. *Journal of Abnormal Psychology, 99*, 156–165.

Newman, C. F., Leahy, R. L., Beck, A. T., Reilly-Harrington, N. A., & Gyulai, L. (2002). Bipolar disorder: A cognitive therapy approach. Washington, DC: American Psychological Association.

Nguyen, H. T., & Zonderman, A. B. (2006). Relationship between age and aspects of depression: Consistency and reliability across two longitudinal studies. *Psychology and Aging, 21*, 119–126.

Nietzel, M. T., & Harris, M. J. (1990). Relationship of dependency and achievement/autonomy to depression. *Clinical Psychology Review, 10*, 279–297.

Nobuhara, K., Okugawa, G., Sugimotor, T., Minami, T., Tamagaki, C., … Kinoshita, T. (2006). Frontal white matter anisotropy and symptom severity of late-life depression: A magnetic resonance diffusion tensor imaging study. *Journal of Neurology, Neurosurgery, and Psychiatry, 77*, 120–122.

Nock, M. K., Joiner, T. E. Jr., Gordon, K. H., Lloyd-Richardson, E., & Prinstein, M. J. (2006). Non-suicidal self-injury among adolescents: Diagnostic correlates and relation to suicide attempts. *Psychiatry Research, 144*(1), 65–72.

Nolen-Hoeksema, S. (1991). Responses to depression and their effects on the duration of depressive episodes. *Journal of Abnormal Psychology, 100*(4), 569–582.

Nolen-Hoeksema, S. (2000). The role of rumination in depressive disorders and mixed anxiety/depressive symptoms. *Journal of Abnormal Psychology, 109*, 504–511.

Nolen-Hoeksema, S. (2001). Gender differences in depression. *Current Directions in Psychological Science, 10*(5), 173–176.

Nolen-Hoeksema, S., & Girgus, J. S. (1994). The emergence of gender differences in depression during adolescence. *Psychological Bulletin, 115*(3), 424–443.

Nolen-Hoeksema, S., & Jackson, B. (2001). Mediators of the gender difference in rumination. *Psychology of Women Quarterly, 25*(1), 37.

Nolen-Hoeksema, S., Larson, J., & Grayson, C. (1999). Explaining the gender difference in depressive symptoms. *Journal of Personality and Social Psychology, 77*(5), 1061–1072.

Nolen-Hoeksema, S., Wisco, B. E., & Lyubomirsky, S. (2008). Rethinking rumination. *Perspectives in Psychological Science, 3*, 400–424.

Nurnberger, J. L., Adkins, S., Lahiri, D. K., Mayeda, A., Hu, K., Lewy, A., … Davis-Singh, D. (2000). Melatonin suppression by light in euthymic bipolar and unipolar patients. *Archives of General Psychiatry, 57*, 572–579.

Nusslock, R., Abramson, L. Y., Harmon-Jones, E., Alloy, L. B., & Coan, J. A. (2009). Psychosocial interventions for bipolar disorder: Perspective from the behavioral approach system (BAS) dysregulation theory. *Clinical Psychology: Science and Practice, 16*, 449–469.

Nusslock, R., Abramson, L. Y., Harmon-Jones, E., Alloy, L. B., & Hogan, M. E. (2007). A goal-striving life event and the onset of hypomanic and depressive episodes and symptoms: Perspective from the behavioral approach system (BAS) dysregulation theory. *Journal of Abnormal Psychology, 116*, 105–115.

Nutt, D. J. (2006). The role of dopamine and norepinephrine in depression and antidepressant treatment. *Journal of Clinical Psychiatry, 67*, 3–8.

Nutt, D., Demyttenaere, K., Janka, Z., Aarre, T., Bourin, M., Canonico, P. L., … Stahl, S. (2007). The other face of depression, reduced positive affect: the role of catecholamines in causation and cure. *Journal Psychopharmacology, 5*, 461–471.

O'Carroll, P. W., Berman, A., Maris, R. W., & Moscicki, E. K. (1996). Beyond the tower of babel: A nomenclature for suicidology. *Suicide and Life-Threatening Behavior, 26*(3), 237–252.

Oedegaard, K. J., Syrstad, V. E. G., Morken, G., Akiskal, H. S., & Fasmer, O. B. (2009). A study of age at onset of affective temperaments in a norwegian sample of patients with mood disorders. *Journal of Affective Disorders, 118*, 229–233.

Oquendo, M. A., Galfalvy, H., Russo, S., Ellis, S. P., Grunebaum, M. F., Burke, A., & Mann, J. J. (2004). Prospective study of clinical predictors of suicidal acts after a major depressive episode in patients with major depressive disorder or bipolar disorder. *American Journal of Psychiatry, 161*(8), 1433–1441.

Oquendo, M. A., Malone, K. M., Ellis, S. P., Sackeim, H. A., & Mann, J. J. (1999). Inadequacy of antidepressant treatment for patients with major depression who are at risk for suicidal behavior. *American Journal of Psychiatry, 156*(2), 190–194.

Oren, D. A., & Rosenthal, N. E. (1992). Seasonal affective disorders. In E. S. Paykel (Ed.), *Handbook of affective disorders* (2nd ed., pp. 551–568). New York: Guilford.

Ozyldirim, I., Cakir, S., & Yaziki, O. (2010). Impact of psychotic features on morbidity and course of illness in patients with bipolar disorder. *European Psychiatry, 25*, 47–51.

Paillere Martinot, M. L., Bragulat, V., Arriges, E., Dolle, F., Hinnen, F., Jouvent, R., & Martinot, J. L. (2001). Decreased presynaptic dopamine function in the left caudate of depressed patients with affective flattening and psychomotor retardation. *American Journal of Psychiatry, 158*, 314–316.

Panzarella, C., Alloy, L. B., & Whitehouse, W. G. (2006). Expanded hopelessness theory of depression: On the mechanisms by which social support protects against depression. *Cognitive Therapy and Research, 30*, 307–333.

Parker, G. (1983). Parental "affectionless control" as an antecedent to adult depression. A risk factor delineated. *Archives of General Psychiatry, 40*, 956–960.

Parker, G., Roy, K., Hadzi-Pavlovic, D., Mitchell, P., Wilhelm, K., Menkes, D. B., … Schweitzer, I. (2000). Subtyping depression by clinical features: The Australasian database. *Acta Psychiatrica Scandinavica, 101*, 21–28.

Pennix, B. W. J. H., Beekman, A. T. F., Honig, A., Deeg, D. J. H., Schoevers, R. A., van Eijk, J. T. M., & van Tilburg, W. (2001). Depression and cardiac mortality: Results from a community-based longitudinal study. *Archives of General Psychiatry, 58*, 221–227.

Perlis, R. H., Dennehy, E. B., Miklowitz, D. J., DelBello, M. P., Ostacher, M., Calabrese, J. R., … Sachs, G. (2009). Retrospective age at onset of bipolar disorder and outcome during two-year follow-up: Results from the STEP-BD study. *Bipolar Disorder, 11*, 391–400.

Petersen, T., Dording, C., Neault, N. B., Kornbluh, R., Alpert, J. E., Nierenberg, A. A., … Fava, M. (2002). A survey of prescribing practices in the treatment of depression. *Progress in Neuropsychopharmacology and Biological Psychiatry, 26*, 177–187.

Peterson, C., Maier, S. F., & Seligman, M. E. P. (1993). *Learned helplessness: A theory for the age of personal control*. New York: Oxford University Press.

Pettit, J., & Joiner, T. (2001). Negative-feedback seeking leads to depressive symptom increases under conditions of stress. *Journal of Psychopathology and Behavioral Assessment, 23*(1), 69–74.

Piccinelli, M., & Wilkinson, G. (2000). Gender differences in depression: Critical review. *British Journal of Psychiatry, 177*(6), 486–492.

Pirek, E., Winkler, D., Konstantinidis, A., Willeit, M., Praschak-Rieder, N., & Kasper, S. (2007). Agomelatine in the treatment of seasonal affective disorder. *Psychopharmachology, 190*, 575–579.

Post, R. M. (1992). Transduction of psychosocial stress into the neurobiology of recurrent affective disorder. *American Journal of Psychiatry, 149*, 999–1010.

Potthoff, J., Holahan, C., & Joiner, T. (1995). Reassurance seeking, stress generation, and depressive symptoms: An integrative model. *Journal of Personality and Social Psychology, 68*(4), 664–670.

Preisig, M., Bellivier, F., Fenton, B. T., Baud, P., Berney, A., Courtet, P., … Malafosse, A. (2000). Association between bipolar disorder and monoamine oxidase A gene polymorphisms: Results of a multicenter study. *American Journal of Psychiatry, 157,* 948–955.

Quera Salva, M. A., Vanier, B., Laredo, J., Hartley, S., Chapotot, F., Lofaso, C., & Guilleminault, C. (2007). Major depressive disorder, sleep EEG and agomelatine: An open-label study. *International Journal of Neuropsychopharmacology, 10,* 691–696.

Rado, S. (1951). Psychodynamics of depression from the etiologic point of view. *Psychosomatic Medicine, 13*(1), 51–55.

Rasgon, N., Bauer, M., Glenn, T., Elman, S., & Whybrow, P. C. (2003). Menstrual cycle related mood changes in women with bipolar disorder. *Bipolar Disorders, 5,* 48–52.

Rasmussen, K. G. (2008). Electroconvulsive therapy versus transcranial magnetic stimulation for major depression: A review with recommendations for future research. *Acta Neuropsychiatrica, 6,* 291–294.

Rehm, L. P., Wagner, A., & Ivens-Tyndal, C. (2001). Mood disorders: Unipolar and bipolar. In P. B. Sutker & H. E. Adams (Eds.), *Comprehensive handbook of psychopathology* (3rd ed., pp. 277–308). New York: Kluwer Academic/Plenum.

Reilly-Harrington, N., Alloy, L. B., Fresco, D. M., & Whitehouse, W. G. (1999). Cognitive styles and life events interact to predict bipolar and unipolar symptomatology. *Journal of Abnormal Psychology, 108,* 567–578.

Rende, R., Birmaher, B., Axelson, D., Strober, M., Gill, M. K., Valeri, S., … Keller, M. (2007). Childhood-onset bipolar disorder: Evidence for increased familial loading of psychiatric illness. *Journal of American Academy of Childhood and Adolescent Psychiatry, 46,* 197–204.

Rhebergen, D., Beekman, A. T. F., Graf, R., Nolen, W. A., Spijker, J., Hoogendijk, W. J., & Penninx, B. W. J. H. (2009). The three-year naturalistic course of major depressive disorder, dysthymic disorder, and double depression. *Journal of Affective Disorders, 115,* 450–459.

Rihmer, Z. (2007). Suicide risk in mood disorders. *Current Opinion in Psychiatry, 20*(1), 17–22.

Robinson, M. S., & Alloy, L. B. (2003). Negative cognitive styles and stress-reactive rumination interact to predict depression: A prospective study. *Cognitive Therapy and Research, 27,* 275–291.

Rockett, I. R. H., Samora, J. B., & Coben, J. H. (2006). The black-white suicide paradox: Possible effects of misclassification. *Social Science and Medicine, 63*(8), 2165–2175.

Romens, S. E., Abramson, L. Y., & Alloy, L. B. (2009). High and low cognitive risk for depression: Stability from late adolescence to early adulthood. *Cognitive Therapy and Research, 33,* 480–498.

Rouillon, F. (2006). Efficacy and tolerance profile of agomelatine and practical use in depressed patients. *International Clinical Psychopharmacology, 21*(Suppl. 1), S31–35.

Rudd, M. D., & Joiner, T. E. (1998). The assessment, management, and treatment of suicidality: Toward clinically informed and balanced standards of care. *Clinical Psychology: Science and Practice, 5,* 135–150.

Rudolph, K. D., & Conley, C. S. (2005). The socioemotional costs and benefits of social-evaluative concerns: Do girls care too much? *Journal of Personality, 73*(1), 115–138.

Rudolph, K. D., Hammen, C., Burge, D., Lindberg, N., Herzberg, D., & Daley, S. E. (2000). Toward an interpersonal life-stress model of depression: The developmental context of stress generation. *Development and Psychopathology, 12,* 215–234.

Ruhe, H. G., Mason, N. S., & Schene, A. H. (2007). Mood is indirectly related to serotonin, norepinephrine, and dopamine levels in humans: a meta-analysis of monoamine depletion studies. *Clinical Psychology Review, 12,* 331–359.

Rush, A. J., & Weissenburger, J. E. (1994). Melancholic symptom features and DSM-IV. *American Journal of Psychiatry, 151,* 489–498.

Rutz, W. (1996). Prevention of suicide and depression. *Nordic Journal of Psychiatry, 50*(Suppl. 37), 61–67.

Sachs, G. S., Baldassano, C. E., Truman, C. J., & Guillo, C. (2000). Comorbidity of attention deficit hyperactivity disorder with early- and late-onset bipolar disorder. *American Journal of Psychiatry, 157,* 469–471.

Sackeim, H. A., Prudic, J., Devanand, D. P., Nobler, M. S., Lisanby, S. H., Peyser, S., … Clark, J. (2000). A prospective, randomized, double-blind comparison of bilateral and right unilateral electroconvulsive therapy at different stimulus intensities. *Archives of General Psychiatry, 57,* 425–437.

Sainsbury, P., & Jenkins, J. S. (1982). The accuracy of officially reported suicide statistics for purposes of epidemiological research. *Journal of Epidemiological Community Health, 36*(1), 43–48.

Samson, J. A., Mirin, S. M., Hauser, S. T., Fenton, B. T., & Schildkraut, J. J. (1992). Learned helplessness and urinary MHPG levels in unipolar depression. *American Journal of Psychiatry, 149,* 806–809.

Sanacora, G. (2008). New understanding of mechanisms of action of bipolar medications. *Journal of Clinical Psychiatry, 69,* 22–27.

Sassi, R. B., Nicoletti, M., Brambilla, P., Harenski, K., Mallinger, A. G., Frank, E., ... Soares, J. C. (2001). Decreased pituitary volume in patients with bipolar disorder. *Biological Psychiatry, 50,* 271–280.

Savitz, J., & Drevets, W. C. (2009). Bipolar and major depressive disorder: Neuroimaging the developmental-degenerative divide. *Neuroscience Biobehavioral Reviews, 33,* 699–771.

Schildkraut, J. (1965). The catecholamine hypothesis of affective disorders: A review of supporting evidence. *American Journal of Psychiatry, 122,* 509–522.

Schleifer, S. J., Keller, S. E., Bartlett, J. A., Eckholdt, H. M., & Delaney, B. R. (1996). Immunity in young adults with major depressive disorder. *American Journal of Psychiatry, 153,* 477–482.

Schneider, F., Gur, R. E., Alavi, A., Seligman, M. E. P., Mozley, L. H., Smith, R. J., ... Gur, R. C. (1996). Cerebral blood flow changes in limbic regions induced by unsolvable anagram tasks. *American Journal of Psychiatry, 153,* 206–212.

Scoville, W. B., & Milner, B. (1957). Loss of recent memory after bilateral hippocampal lesions. *Journal of Neurology, Neurosurgery and Psychiatry, 20,* 11–21.

Segal, Z., Gemar, M., & Williams, S. (1999). Differential cognitive response to a mood challenge following successful cognitive therapy or pharmacotherapy for unipolar depression. *Journal of Abnormal Psychology, 108,* 3–10.

Segal, Z., Williams, J. M. G., & Teasdale, J. (2002). *Mindfulness-based cognitive therapy for depression: A new approach to preventing relapse.* New York: Guilford.

Seligman, M. E. P. (1975). *Helplessness: On depression, development, and death.* San Francisco: Freeman.

Serretti, A., Gaspar-Barba, E., Calati, R., Cruz-Fuentes, C. S., Gomez-Sanchez, A., Perez-Molina, A., & DeRonchi, D. (2010). 3111T/C CLOCK gene polymorphism is not associated with sleep disturbances in untreated patients. *Chronobiology International, 27,* 265–277.

Shen, G. C., Alloy, L. B., Abramson, L. Y., & Sylvia, L. G. (2008). Social rhythm regularity and the onset of affective episodes in bipolar spectrum individuals. *Bipolar Disorders, 10,* 520–529.

Shi, J., Wittke-Thompson, J. K., Badner, J. A., Hattori, E., Potash, J. B., Willour, V. L., ... Liu, C. (2008). Clock genes may influence bipolar disorder susceptibility and dysfunctional circadian rhythm. *American Journal of Medical Genetics Part B: Neuropsychiatric Genetics, 147B,* 1047–1055.

Siegel, J. M., Yancey, A. K., Aneshensel, C. S., & Schuler, R. (1999). Body image, perceived pubertal timing, and adolescent mental health. *Journal of Adolescent Health, 25,* 155–165.

Silverstone, T., McPherson, H., Li, Q., & Doyle, T. (2003). Deep white matter hyperintensities in patients with bipolar depression, unipolar depression and age-matched control subjects. *Bipolar Disorders, 5,* 53–57.

Sloan, D. M., Strauss, M. E., & Wisner, K. L. (2001). Diminished response to pleasant stimuli by depressed women. *Journal of Abnormal Psychology, 110,* 488–493.

Snowdon, D. A. (2001). *Aging with Grace.* New York: Bantam Books.

Solomon, D. A., Keller, M. B., Leon, A. C., Mueller, T. L., Shea, M. T., Warshaw, M., ... Endicott, J. (1997). Recovery from major depression: A 10-year prospective follow-up across multiple episodes. *Archives of General Psychiatry, 54,* 1001–1006.

Spasojevic, J., & Alloy, L. B. (2001). Rumination as a common mechanism relating depressive risk factors to depression. *Emotion, 1,* 25–37.

Steiger, A., & Kimura, M. (2009). Wake and sleep EEG provide biomarkers in depression. *Journal of Psychiatric Research, 44,* 242–252.

Subodh, B. N., Avasthi, A., & Chakrabarti, S. (2008). Psychosocial impact of dysthymia: A study among married patients. *Journal of Affective Disorders, 109,* 199–204.

Sullivan, P. E., Neale, M. C., & Kendler, K. S. (2000). Genetic epidemiology of major depression: Review and meta-analysis. *American Journal of Psychiatry, 157,* 1552–1562.

Suppes, T., Dennehy, E. B., & Gibbons, E. W. (2000). The longitudinal course of bipolar disorders. *Journal of Clinical Psychiatry, 61*(Suppl.), 23–30.

Sussmann, J. E., Lymer, G. K., McKirdy, J., Moorhead, T. W., Maniega, S. M., Job, D., ... McIntosh, A. M. (2009). White matter abnormalities in bipolar disorder and schizophrenia detected using diffusion tensor magnetic resonance imaging. *Bipolar Disorders, 11,* 11–18.

Swartz, H. A., Frank, E., Frankel, D. R., Novick, D., & Houck, P. (2009). Psychotherapy as monotherapy for bipolar II depression: A proof of concept study. *Bipolar Disorders, 11,* 89–94.

Sweeney, P. D., Anderson, K., & Bailey, S. (1986). Attributional style in depression: A meta-analytic review. *Journal of Personality and Social Psychology, 50,* 974–991.

Sylvia, L. G., Alloy, L. B., Hafner, J. A., Gauger, M. C., Verdon, K., & Abramson, L. Y. (2009). Life events and social rhythms in bipolar spectrum disorders: A prospective study. *Behavior Therapy, 40,* 131–141.

Tang, T. Z., DeRubeis, R. J., Beberman, R., & Pham, T. (2005). Cognitive changes, critical sessions, and sudden gains in cognitive-behavioral therapy for depression. *Journal of Consulting and Clinical Psychology, 73*, 168–172.

Tang, T. Z., DeRubeis, R. J., Hollon, S. D., Amsterdam, J., & Shelton, R. (2007). Sudden gains in cognitive therapy of depression and depression relapse/recurrence. *Journal of Consulting and Clinical Psychology, 75*, 404–408.

Taylor, L., & Ingram, R. E. (1999). Cognitive reactivity and depressotypic information processing in children of depressed mothers. *Journal of Abnormal Psychology, 108*, 202–210.

Taylor, W. D., MacFall, J. R., Payne, M. E., McQuoid, D. R., Steffens, D. C., Provenzale, J. M., & Krishnan, R. R. (2005). Greater MRI lesion volumes in elderly depressed subjects than in control subjects. *Psychiatry Research, 139*, 1–7.

Teicher, M. H., Glod, C. A., Magnus, E., Harper, D., Benson, G., Kruger, K., & McGreenery, C. E. (1997). Circadian rest-activity disturbances in seasonal affective disorder. *Archives of General Psychiatry, 54*, 124–130.

Terman, J. S., Terman, M., Lo, E. S., & Cooper, T. B. (2001). Circadian time of morning light administration and therapeutic response in winter depression. *Archives of General Psychiatry, 58*, 69–75.

Thase, M. E. (2002). Antidepressant effects: The suit may be small, but the fabric is real. Prevention and Treatment, 5, Article 32. Retrieved from http://www.mendeley.com/research/antidepressant-effects-suit-small-fabric-real-7/

Thase, M. E., & Denko, T. (2008). Pharmacotherapy of mood disorders. *Annual Review of Clinical Psychology, 4*, 53–91.

Thompson, A. H. (2008). Younger onset of depression is associated with greater suicidal intent. *Social Psychiatry and Psychiatric Epidemiology, 43*, 538–544.

Turner, R. J., & Lloyd, D. A. (1999). The stress process and the social distribution of depression. *Journal of Health and Social Behavior, 40*, 374–404.

Twenge, J., & Nolen-Hoeksema S. (2002). Age, gender, race, socioeconomic status, and birth cohort differences on the Children's Depression Inventory: A meta-analysis. *Journal of Abnormal Psychology, 111*, 578–588.

Urošević, S., Abramson, L. Y., Harmon-Jones, E., & Alloy, L. B. (2008). Dysregulation of the behavioral approach system (BAS) in bipolar spectrum disorders: Review of theory and evidence. *Clinical Psychology Review, 28*(7), 1188–1205.

U.S. Department of Health and Human Services. (2001). *National strategy for suicide prevention: Goals and objectives for action.* Rockville, MD: Author.

Ustin, T. B. (2001). The worldwide burden of depression in the 21st century. In M. M. Weissman (Ed.), *Treatment of depression: Bridging the 21st century* (pp. 35–45). Washington, DC: American Psychiatric Press.

Vinberg, M., Bennike, B., Kyvik, K. O., Andersen, P. K., & Kessing, L. V. (2008). Salivary cortisol in unaffected twins discordant for affective disorder. *Psychiatry Research, 161*, 292–301.

Walshaw, P. D., Alloy, L. B., & Sabb, F. W. (2010). Executive function in pediatric bipolar disorder and attention-deficit hyperactivity disorder: In search of distinct phenotypic profiles? *Neuropsychology Review, 20*, 103–120.

Wehr, T. A., Duncan, W. C., Sher, L., Aeschbach, D., Schwartz, P. J., Turner, E. H., ... Rosenthal, N. E. (2001). A circadian signal of change of season in patients with seasonal affective disorder. *Archives of General Psychiatry, 58*, 1108–1114.

Weiss, E. L., Longhurst, J. G., & Mazure, C. M. (1999). Childhood sexual abuse as a risk factor for depression in women: Psychosocial and neurobiological correlates. *American Journal of Psychiatry, 156*(6), 816–828.

Weissman, M. M. (2006). A brief history of interpersonal psychotherapy. *Psychiatric Annals, 8*, 553–557.

Weisz, J. R., Southam-Gerow, M. A., & McCarty, C. A. (2001). Control-related beliefs and depressive symptoms in clinic-referred children and adolescents: Developmental differences and model specificity. *Journal of Abnormal Psychology, 110*, 97–109.

Wells, K. B., & Sherbourne, C. D. (1999). Functioning and utility for current health of patients with depression or chronic medical conditions in managed, primary care practices. *Archives of General Psychiatry, 56*, 897–904.

Wender, P. H., Kety, S. S., Rosenthal, D., Schulsinger, F., Ortmann, J., & Lunde, I. (1986). Psychiatric disorders in the biological and adoptive families of adopted individuals with affective disorders. *Archives of General Psychiatry, 43*, 923–929.

Wieck, A., Kumar, R., Hist, A. D., Marks, M. N., Campbell, I. C., & Checkley, S. A. (1991). Increased sensitivity of dopamine receptors and recurrence of affective psychosis after childbirth. *British Medical Journal, 303*, 613–616.

Williams, J. M. G., Barnhofer, T., Crane, C., Herman, D., Raes, F., Watkins, E., & Dalgleish, T. (2007). Autobiographical memory specificity and emotional disorder. *Psychological Bulletin, 133*, 122–148.

Winokur, G., Coryell, W., Keller, M., Endicott, J., & Leon, A. (1995). A family study of manic-depressive (bipolar I) disease: Is it a distinct illness separable from primary unipolar depression? *Archives of General Psychiatry, 52*, 367–373.

World Health Organization. (2003). *The world health report 2003: Shaping the future.* Geneva: Author.

Yang, Q., Huang, X., Hong, N., & Yu, X. (2007). White matter microstructural abnormalities in late-life depression. *International Psychogeriatrics, 19*, 757–766.

Yatham, L. N., Liddle, P. F., Lam, R. W., Zis, A. P., Stoessl, A. J., Sossi, V., ... Ruth, J. T. (2010). Effect of electroconvulsive therapy on brain 5-HT2 receptors in major depression. *British Journal of Psychiatry, 196*, 474–479.

Yatham, L. N., Liddle, P. F., Shiah, I. S., Scarrow, G., Lam, R. W., Adam, M. J., ... Ruth, T. J. (2000). Brain serotonin 2 receptors in major depression: a positron emission tomography study. *Archives of General Psychiatry, 57*, 850–859.

Young, A. H. (2004). Cortisol in mood disorders. *Stress, 7*, 205–208.

Young, A. S., Kalp, R., Sherbourne, C. D., & Wells, K. R. (2001). The quality of care for depressive and anxiety disorders in the United States. *Archives of General Psychiatry, 58*, 55–61.

Youngstrom, E. A., Birmaher, B., & Findling, R. L. (2008). Pediatric bipolar disorder: Validity, phenomenology, and recommendations for diagnosis. *Bipolar Disorders, 10*, 194–214.

Zanetti, M. V., Jackowski, M. P., Versace, A., Almeida, J. R., Hassel, S., & Duran, F. L. (2009). State-dependent microstructural white matter changes in bipolar I depression. European *Archives of Psychiatry and Clinical Neuroscience, 259*, 36–328.

Zimmerman, M., Posternak, M., Friedman, M., Attiullah, N., Baymiller, S., Boland, R., ... Singer, S. (2004). Which factors influence psychiatrists' selection of antidepressants? *American Journal of Psychiatry, 161*, 1285–1289.

Zupancic, M., & Guilleminault, C. (2006). Agomelatine: A preliminary review of a new antidepressant. *CNS Drugs, 20*, 981–992.

10
Schizophrenia

LISA KESTLER

MedAvante, Inc.
Hamilton, New Jersey

ANNIE BOLLINI

Atlanta Veteran Affairs Medical Center
Atlanta, Georgia

KAREN HOCHMAN

Emory University
Atlanta, Georgia

VIJAY A. MITTAL

University of Colorado at Boulder
Boulder, Colorado

ELAINE WALKER

Emory University
Atlanta, Georgia

Schizophrenia is among the most debilitating of mental illnesses. It is typically diagnosed between 20 and 25 years of age, a stage of life when most people gain independence from parents, develop intimate romantic relationships, plan educational pursuits, and begin work or career endeavors (De Lisi, 1992). Because the clinical onset usually occurs during this pivotal time, the illness can have a profound negative impact on the individual's opportunities for attaining social and occupational success, and the consequences can be devastating for the patient's life course, as well as for family members (Addington & Addington, 2005). Further, the illness knows no national boundaries. Across cultures, estimates of the lifetime prevalence of schizophrenia range around 1% (1 of 100) (Arajarvi et al., 2005; Keith, Regier, & Rae, 1991; Kulhara, & Chakrabarti, 2001; Torrey, 1987), although the prognosis may differ among countries (Kulhara & Chakrabarti, 2001).

The origins of this devastating mental disorder have continued to elude researchers, despite many decades of scientific research. To date, no single factor has been found to characterize all patients with the illness. This holds for potential etiological factors as well as clinical phenomena. Schizophrenia patients vary in symptom profiles, developmental histories, family backgrounds, cognitive functions, and even brain morphology and neurochemistry. Although this has led some to express dismay at the chances of ever finding the cause of schizophrenia, there is reason to be optimistic. Research efforts have succeeded in revealing numerous pieces of what is now recognized as a complex puzzle of etiological processes.

The consensus in the field, based on findings from various lines of research, is that (a) schizophrenia is a brain disease, (b) its etiology involves the interplay between genetic and environmental factors, (c) multiple developmental pathways eventually lead to disease onset, and (d) brain maturational processes play a role in the etiological process. This chapter will provide an overview of the current state of our knowledge about schizophrenia. It will begin with a discussion of the history and phenomenology of the disorder and then proceed to a description of some of the key findings that have shed light on the illness.

History and Phenomenology

Written descriptions of patients experiencing psychotic symptoms have been recorded since antiquity. However, because psychotic symptoms can be a manifestation of a variety of disorders, it is unclear whether schizophrenia, as such, is an ancient or relatively new phenomenon. In the mid- to late 19th century, European psychiatrists were investigating the etiology, classification, and prognoses of various types of psychosis. At that time, the most common cause of psychosis was *tertiary syphilis*, although researchers were unaware that there was any link between psychosis and syphilis (Kohler & Johnson, 2005). The psychological symptoms of tertiary syphilis frequently overlap with symptoms of what is now called schizophrenia. The cause of syphilis was eventually traced to an infection with the spirochete *treponema pallidum*, and antibiotics were found to be effective for prevention and treatment of the disorder. This important discovery served to illustrate how a psychological syndrome can be produced by an infectious agent. It also sensitized researchers to the fact that similar syndromes might be the result of different causes.

Emil Kraepelin (1856–1926) was the medical director of the famous Heidelberg Clinic. He was the first to differentiate schizophrenia, which he referred to as "*dementia praecox*" (or dementia of the young) from manic-depressive psychosis (Kraepelin, 1913). He also lumped together "hebephrenia," "paranoia," and "catatonia" (previously thought to be distinct disorders), and classified all of them as variants of dementia praecox. He based this classification on their similarities in age of onset and the clinical feature of poor prognosis. Kraepelin did not believe that any one symptom was diagnostic of dementia praecox, but instead focused on the total clinical picture and changes in symptoms over time. If a psychotic patient deteriorated over an extended period of time (months or years), the condition was assumed to be dementia praecox.

Many contemporary mental health professionals continue to expect negative outcomes in those afflicted with schizophrenia, and this expectation infuses the mental health profession with an unfortunate sense of therapeutic nihilism. Yet, while it is true that the majority of patients manifest a chronic course that entails lifelong disability, this bleak scenario is not always the case (Carpenter & Buchanan, 1994). The story of Dr. John Nash, professor and mathematician at Princeton University, as told in the movie, *A Beautiful Mind* (Howard, 2001), illustrates this point quite well. Dr. Nash was able to function at a very high level in his academic field, despite his struggle with schizophrenia.

The term *schizophrenia* was introduced at the beginning of the 20th century by Eugen Bleuler (1857–1939), a Swiss psychiatrist and the medical director of a mental hospital in Zurich (Howells, 1991, pp. xii, 95). The word is derived from two Greek words: *schizo*, which means to tear or to split, and *phren*, which has several meanings: In ancient times, it meant "the intellect" or "the mind," but it also referred to the lungs and the diaphragm, which were believed to be the seat of emotions. Thus, the word schizophrenia literally means the splitting or tearing of the mind and emotional stability of the patient.

Bleuler classified the symptoms of schizophrenia into fundamental and accessory symptoms. The fundamental symptoms of schizophrenia are often reported in textbooks as the four A's, although, in fact, there are six A's and one D (Bleuler, 1950/1911). The fundamental symptoms

Table 10.1 Bleuler's Fundamental Symptoms of Schizophrenia

- Disturbances of **a**ssociation (loose, illogical thought processes)
- Disturbances of **a**ffect (indifference, apathy, or inappropriateness)
- **A**mbivalence (conflicting thoughts, emotions or impulses which are present simultaneously or in rapid succession)
- **A**utism (detachment from social life with inner preoccupation)
- **A**bulia (lack of drive or motivation)
- **D**ementia (irreversible change in personality)

Source: Bleuler, E. (1911/1950). *Dementia praecox or the group of schizophrenias*, p. 13. Translated by J. Zinkin. New York: International Universities Press.

are listed in Table 10.1. According to Bleuler, these symptoms are present in all patients, at all stages of the illness, and are *diagnostic* of schizophrenia.

Bleuler's "accessory symptoms" of schizophrenia included delusions, hallucinations, movement disturbances, somatic symptoms, and manic and melancholic states. In contrast to fundamental symptoms, he believed that these accessory symptoms were not present in all schizophrenia patients and often occurred in other illnesses. For these reasons, the accessory symptoms were not assumed to be as diagnostic of schizophrenia.

Further refinements in the diagnostic criteria for schizophrenia were proposed by Kurt Schneider in the mid-1900s. Like Bleuler, Kurt Schneider thought that certain 'key' symptoms were diagnostic of schizophrenia (Schneider, 1959). In his classification, he referred to these diagnostic symptoms as "first rank symptoms" (Schneider, 1959) (see Table 10.2). He believed that, after medical causes of psychosis were ruled out, one could make the diagnosis of schizophrenia if one or more first rank symptom was present. Schneider's descriptions of the symptoms were more detailed and specific than were Bleuler's fundamental symptoms. Subsequent diagnostic criteria for schizophrenia have been heavily influenced by Schneider's approach.

In subsequent years, investigators began to make a distinction between "positive" and "negative" symptoms of schizophrenia (Harvey & Walker, 1987). The positive symptoms are those that involve an excess of ideas, sensory experiences, or behavior. Hallucinations, delusions, and bizarre behaviors fall into this category. Most of the first rank symptoms described by Schneider are also considered to be positive symptoms. Negative symptoms, in contrast, involve a decrease in behavior, such as blunted or flat affect, anhedonia, and lack of motivation. These symptoms were highlighted by Bleuler.

During the middle of the 20th century, different diagnostic criteria for schizophrenia became popular in different parts of the world. The "Kraepelinian" tradition, with its longitudinal

Table 10.2 The Schneiderian "First Rank Symptoms"

- Thought echoing or audible thoughts (the patient hears his thoughts out loud)
- Thought broadcasting (patient believes that others can hear his thoughts out loud)
- Thought intrusion (patient feels that some of his thought are from outside; that is, not originating in his own mind)
- Thought withdrawal (patient believes that the cause of having lost track of a thought is that someone is taking his thoughts away)
- Somatic hallucinations (unusual, unexplained sensations in one's body)
- Passivity feelings (patient believes that his thoughts, feelings, or actions are controlled by another or others)
- Delusional perception (a sudden, fixed, false belief about a particular everyday occurrence or perception)

Source: Schneider, K. (1959). *Clinical psychopathology.* New York: Grune and Stratton.

requirements for diagnosis, identified patients with poorer long-term prognosis. In contrast, the Bleulerian and Schneiderian diagnostic systems allowed for a wider range of psychotic patients to be diagnosed with schizophrenia. Thus the patients diagnosed with these two systems tended to have a better prognosis than those diagnosed in the more stringent Kraepelinian tradition. Because of these discrepancies, the use of multiple diagnostic systems had a detrimental effect on research progress; research findings from countries using different diagnostic criteria were not comparable, thus limiting the generalizability of the results.

The next generation of diagnostic systems evolved with the intent of achieving uniformity in diagnostic criteria and improving diagnostic reliability. Among these were the Feighner or St. Louis diagnostic criteria (Feighner, Robins, & Guze, 1972), and the "research diagnostic criteria" developed by Spitzer, Endicott, and Robins (1978). These two approaches to the diagnosis of schizophrenia strongly influenced modern day diagnostic systems, most notably, the *Diagnostic and Statistical Manual of Mental Disorders* (*DSM*).

The *DSM* is now the most widely used system for diagnosing schizophrenia and other mental disorders. The current version of the *DSM* is the *DSM–IV–TR* (American Psychatric Association, 2000); however, the fifth edition (DSM–5) is in development and due for publication in 2013. It is anticipated that there will be some changes in the diagnostic categories and criteria for schizophrenia in the DSM–5, including better defined boundaries with schizoaffective disorder, dimensional assessment of symptoms in lieu of subtypes, and the inclusion of psychosis risk syndrome to identify individuals exhibiting early symptoms of psychotic disorder.

Using the current *DSM–IV–TR* criteria, schizophrenia can be diagnosed when signs and symptoms of the disorder have been present for 6 months or more (including prodromal and residual phases). The characteristic symptom criteria for schizophrenia include: (a) hallucinations, (b) delusions, (c) disorganized speech (e.g., frequent derailment or incoherence), (d) grossly disorganized or catatonic behavior, and (e) negative symptoms (i.e., affective flattening, alogia, or avolition).

At least two or more of these psychotic symptoms must be present for at least 1 month (or less if successfully treated). Only one of the symptoms is necessary if the delusions are bizarre or the hallucinated voices consist of a running commentary or of two voices conversing (both of these are derived from Schneider's first rank symptoms in Table 10.2). In addition to the clinical symptoms, there must be social or occupational dysfunction. Further, significant mood disorder, such as depression or manic symptoms, need not be present (this excludes individuals who meet the criteria for major depressive disorder with psychotic symptoms and bipolar disorder with psychotic symptoms). Finally, general medical conditions or substance abuse that might lead to psychotic symptoms must be ruled out.

The four subtypes of schizophrenia described in *DSM–IV–TR* are *paranoid*, *disorganized*, *catatonic*, and *undifferentiated* (Table 10.3). The paranoid type is characterized by a preoccupation with delusions or hallucinations, but there is no disorganized speech, disorganized or catatonic behavior, or flat or inappropriate affect. This subtype has the best prognosis. In the disorganized type, all of the following are prominent: disorganized speech, disorganized behavior, and flat or inappropriate affect, but the criteria for the catatonic subtype are not met. In terms of the course of illness this subtype is considered to have the worst prognosis. The catatonic type involves a clinical syndrome that is dominated by at least two of the following: motoric immobility, excessive, purposeless motor activity (catatonic excitement), extreme negativism (purposeless resistance to movement and/or all instructions), mutism (absence of speech), peculiar voluntary movements (voluntary assumption of bizarre or unusual postures), stereotyped movements (repetitive, nonfunctional, yet voluntary), prominent mannerisms (repetitive gestures or expressions), prominent facial grimacing, echolalia (repetition of another person's words or phrases), or echopraxia (repetition of another person's actions).

Table 10.3 Subtypes of Schizophrenia

Subtype	Prognosis
Paranoid	*Good*
• Well-organized delusional beliefs, frequently reflecting persecutory or grandiose beliefs • Frequent auditory hallucinations • Little or no negative (e.g., flat affect) or disorganized symptomatology	
Disorganized	*Poorest*
• Flat and inappropriate emotional expressions • Severely disorganized speech and behavior • Delusional ideas, hallucinations, and behavior characterized by fragmentation (i.e., not following a sequential course)	
Catatonic	*Poor*
• Highly irregular movements or actions (e.g., extreme excitement, bizarre postures or facial grimaces, complete immobility) • Echoing of words spoken by others, imitations of others movements	
Undifferentiated*	—
• Display of schizophrenic symptomatology in a pattern that does not fit other categories	

*Because the undifferentiated category is a bin for cases that do not fit within the other subtypes, it serves as a reminder that these labels are artificially constructed categories, rather than distinct diagnostic entities.

Finally, the undifferentiated subtype is diagnosed when the patient does not meet criteria for the previous subtypes, yet does meet the general criteria for schizophrenia. The inclusion of this subtype in the *DSM–IV–TR* serves to remind us that these are constructed categories, not distinct diagnostic entities with "natural" boundaries. Despite the clinical usefulness of subtypes to convey predominant symptoms, the DSM–5 task force has recommended elimination of these subtypes in light of the minimal utility and diagnostic stability of schizophrenia subtypes. Instead the DSM–5 may adopt a dimensional approach to assessment, rating the severity of symptoms across distinct psychopathological domains (Criterion A symptoms of schizophrenia, impaired cognition, depression, and mania).

Much research also supports the broader division of psychotic symptoms into positive and negative symptoms. This is based on research showing that these two patterns of symptoms may have distinct brain structure–function relationships (e.g., Lawrie & Abukmeil, 1998; Nestor et al., 2007), prognosis (Kirkpatrick, Fenton, Carpenter, & Marder, 2006), and treatment responses. For example, antipsychotics tend to relieve positive symptoms but are less effective with negative symptoms; this may be due to different brain pathology underlying the two types of symptoms (Kirkpatrick et al., 2006).

Two other diagnostic categories in the schizophrenia spectrum are worth noting. One is a category for individuals who have met criteria for schizophrenia in the past but no longer do. This is referred to as the *residual type*. This diagnosis is applied when there is a prominence of negative symptoms or two or more attenuated "characteristic" symptoms but no prominent delusions, hallucinations, catatonic symptoms, or disorganized behavior or speech. The other category, *schizophreniform disorder*, is for individuals whose symptoms do not meet the 6-month criterion. This diagnosis is frequently made as a prelude to the diagnosis of schizophrenia, when the patient presents for treatment early in the course of the disorder. Some individuals who fall into this category, however, will recover completely and not suffer further episodes of psychosis. The proposed psychosis risk syndrome for the DSM–5 will differ from schizophreniform disorder in that individuals meeting criteria for psychosis risk syndrome do not meet the full criteria for schizophrenia but may experience attenuated symptoms with intact reality testing. The proposal to include this diagnosis in the DSM–5 has been controversial with several issues that will need to be considered. Although there is a great deal of evidence for the effectiveness of detecting at risk individuals, critical issues to consider include accuracy of prediction, evidence for effective intervention, and issues related to stigma and potential harm of excessive treatment.

It is important to emphasize that, despite advances in diagnosis, the diagnostic boundaries of schizophrenia are still quite unclear (Wolff, 1991). Moreover, the boundaries between schizophrenia and mood disorders are sometimes obscure. Many individuals who meet the criteria for schizophrenia show marked signs of depression or manic tendencies. These symptoms are sometimes present before the onset of schizophrenia and frequently occur in combination with marked psychotic symptoms. As a result, the *DSM–IV–TR* includes a diagnostic category called *schizoaffective disorder*. This disorder can be conceived of, conceptually, as a hybrid between the mood disorders (bipolar disorder or major depression with psychotic features) and schizophrenia. The two subtypes of schizoaffective disorder are the depressive subtype (i.e., if the mood disturbance includes only depressive episodes) and the bipolar subtype (i.e., where the symptoms of the disorder have included either a manic or a mixed episode). Interestingly, the prognosis for patients with schizoaffective disorder is, on average, somewhere between that of schizophrenia and the mood disorders.

Cognitive and Emotional Aspects of Schizophrenia

Among the most well-established aspects of schizophrenia are the cognitive impairments that accompany the illness. In fact, some experts have argued that cognitive impairment should be added as a characteristic symptom in the upcoming DSM–5 (Keefe & Fenton, 2007); however, the DSM–5 task force has decided against making this recommendation because of its lack of diagnostic specificity. Schizophrenia patients manifest performance deficits on a broad range of cognitive tasks, from simple to complex (Bozikas, Kosmidis, Kiosseoglou, & Karavatos, 2006; Green, Kern, Braff, & Mintz, 2000). One of the most basic is the deficit in the very earliest stages of visual information processing. Using a laboratory procedure called backward masking, researchers have shown that compared to both healthy individuals and psychiatric controls, schizophrenia patients are slower in the initial processing of stimuli (Green, Nuechterlein, Breitmeyer, & Mintz, 1999, 2006). In addition to speed of processing, schizophrenia patients show deficits in attention or vigilance, working memory, verbal learning, visual learning, reasoning, and problem solving (Nuechterlein et al.,2004).

There are also deficits in thinking about social phenomena. Studies of social-cognitive abilities in schizophrenia patients have consistently shown that patients are impaired in their ability to comprehend and solve social problems, processing of emotions, social perception, and theory of mind (Green & Horan, 2010; Hooley, 2010; Penn, Corrigan, Bentall, Racenstein, & Newman, 1997). Deficits in social cognition may be partially due to limitations in more basic cognitive processes, such as memory and reasoning. However, basic cognitive impairments do not account completely for the more pervasive and persistent social-cognitive dysfunction observed in schizophrenia. There is also some evidence of a disconnection between fear and arousal networks in the brain that may contribute to social withdrawal and paranoia (Williams et al., 2007).

One of the diagnostic criteria for schizophrenia is blunted or inappropriate affect. It is not surprising, therefore, that patients show abnormalities in the expression of emotion in both their faces and in their verbal communications. These abnormalities include less positive and more negative emotion, as well as emotional expressions that seem inconsistent with the social context (Brozgold et al., 1998; Tremeau et al., 2005). Further, schizophrenia patients are less accurate than normal comparison patients in their ability to label facial expressions of emotion (Bigelow et al., 2006; Martin, Baudouin, Tiberghien, & Franck, 2005; Penn et al., 2000; Walker, 1981). Patients with more severe impairments in their abilities to recognize and express emotion also have more problems in social adjustment.

The Origins of Schizophrenia

Psychosocial Theories

In the early part of the 20th century, psychosocial theories of schizophrenia dominated the literature. For example, Sigmund Freud, the father of psychoanalysis, believed that psychological processes resulted in the development of psychotic symptoms (Howells, 1991). In 1948, Frieda Fromm-Reichmann proposed a theory of schizophrenia that postulated that the disorder arose in response to rearing by a "schizophrenogenic mother" (p. 263). Although this hypothesis has fallen in disfavor because of lack of support from empirical research, it caused considerable suffering for families. The theory added to the stigma and burden of family members seeking treatment for their ill family members. Subsequently, family interaction models of the etiology of schizophrenia were offered by various theorists (Howells, 1991). Again, these contributed relatively little to the understanding of the etiology of schizophrenia, although they did eventually serve to highlight the importance of considering the role of the family in providing support for the recovering patient.

Biological Theories

Kraepelin, Bleuler, and other early writers on schizophrenia did not offer specific theories about the origins of schizophrenia. They did suggest, however, that there might be a biological basis for at least some cases of the illness. Likewise, contemporary ideas about the origins of schizo phrenia focus on biological vulnerabilities that are assumed to be present in early development. Researchers have identified two sources of constitutional vulnerability: genetic factors and environmental factors (e.g., prenatal or obstetric complications, traumatic brain injury). Both appear to have implications for prenatal and postnatal brain development.

The Genetics of Schizophrenia   One of the most well-established findings in schizophrenia research is that a vulnerability to the illness can be inherited (Gottesman, 1991). Behavior genetic studies utilizing twin, adoption, and family history methods have all yielded evidence that the risk for schizophrenia is elevated in individuals who have a biological relative with the disorder; the closer the level of genetic relatedness, the greater the likelihood the relative will also suffer from schizophrenia.

In a review of family, twin, and adoption studies conducted from 1916 to 1989, Irving Gottesman (1991) outlined the compelling evidence for the role of genetic factors in schizophrenia. Monozygotic (MZ) twins, who essentially share 100% of their genes, have the highest concordance rate for schizophrenia. Among MZ co-twins of patients with schizophrenia, 25 to 50% will develop the illness. Dizygotic (DZ) twins and other siblings share, on average, only about half of their genes. About 10 to 15% of the DZ co-twins of patients are also diagnosed with the illness. Further, as genetic relatedness of the relative to the patient becomes more distant, such as from first-degree (parents and siblings) to second-degree relatives (grandparents, half-siblings, aunts, and uncles), the relative's lifetime risk for schizophrenia is reduced.

Adoption studies have provided evidence that the tendency for schizophrenia to run in families is primarily due to genetic factors, rather than the environmental stressor of growing up in close proximity to a mentally ill family member. In a seminal adoption study, Heston (1966) examined the rates of schizophrenia in adoptees with and without a biological parent who was diagnosed with the illness. He found higher rates of schizophrenia and other mental illnesses in the biological offspring of parents with schizophrenia when compared to adoptees with no mental illness in biological parents. Similarly, in a Danish sample, Kety (1988) examined the rates of mental illness in the relatives of adoptees with and without schizophrenia. He found that the biological relatives of adoptees who suffered from schizophrenia had a significantly higher rate of the disorder than the adoptive relatives who reared them. Also, the rate of schizophrenia in the biological relatives of adoptees with schizophrenia was higher than in the relatives (biological or adoptive) of healthy adoptees. These adoption studies provide ample evidence for a significant genetic component in the etiology of schizophrenia.

More recent findings from an adoption study indicate that the genetic influences often act in concert with environmental factors. Tienari, Wynne, Moring, and Lahti (1994) conducted an adoption study in Finland and found that the rate of psychosis and other severe disorders was significantly higher than in the matched control adoptees. However, the difference between the groups was only detected in adoptive families that were rated as dysfunctional. The genetic vulnerability was mainly expressed in association with a disruptive adoptive environment and was not detected in adoptees reared in a healthy, possibly protective, family environment. These findings, which highlight a genetic vulnerability interacting with environmental events, are consistent with the prevailing diathesis–stress models of etiology.

Taken together, the findings from behavioral genetic studies of schizophrenia lead to the conclusion that the disorder involves multiple genes, rather than a single gene (Gottesman, 1991). This conclusion is based on several observations, most notably the fact that the pattern of familial transmission does not conform to what would be expected from a single genetic locus, or even a small number of genes. Consistent with this assumption, attempts to identify a genetic locus that accounts for a significant proportion of cases of schizophrenia have not met with success. Instead, researchers using molecular genetic techniques have identified numerous genes that may account for a small proportion of cases. In the past decade, linkage studies using genome-wide scans have provided evidence for the involvement of several chromosomal regions, including 8p21-22, 22q11-12, and over 20 other regions with at least some likelihood of containing susceptibility genes for schizophrenia (Lewis et al., 2003; Tandon, Keshavan, & Nasrallah, 2008). Association studies compare variations in specific gene sequences between individuals with or without schizophrenia. Variants found with significantly different frequency among those with schizophrenia are considered to confer susceptibility to the disease. Results from association studies generally have very small effect sizes due to the large number of gene variants that can potentially be evaluated; thus replication is critical. Specific genes currently of interest in the etiology of schizophrenia include NRG1 (neuroregulin 1), DTNBP1 (dysbindin-1), DRD1–4 (dopamine receptors D1–D4), DISC1 (disrupted-in-schizophrenia-1), COMT (catechol-O-methyl-transferase), and GRM3 (metabotropic glutamate receptor 3) (Tandon et al., 2008). But the picture is quite complex; for example, because viral infection may play a role in the pathophysiology of schizophrenia, genes associated with the immune process are also likely candidates. Although this is only one direction in gene research, it serves as an illustrative example of the complexities and seemingly endless possibilities that genetic researchers face when interpreting results.

One of the most noteworthy genetic discoveries is a line of research concerning genetic abnormalities that affect dopamine activity (DA). The COMT gene creates the enzyme that breaks down DA. Although a majority of people inherit two copies, approximately 1 in 4,000 children are born with one copy of the COMT gene: this is referred to as 22q11 deletion or velocardiofacial syndrome. The 22q11 deletion occurs in about 0.025% of the general population, involves a microdeletion on chromosome 22q112, and is often accompanied by a physical syndrome that includes structural anomalies of the face, head, and heart. People with schizophrenia show a 40-fold increased prevalence of 22q11 deletion compared to the general population (Bassett & Chow, 2008) and roughly 30% of 22q11 deletion patients manifest schizophrenia (Murphy, Jones, & Owen, 1999). Furthermore, the rate of 22q11 deletion may be higher in patients with an earlier onset of schizophrenia (Bassett et al., 1998; Karayiorgou, Morris, & Morrow, 1995).

The advent of the biotechnology for conducting genome-wide scans has recently led to some other new perspectives on the genetics of schizophrenia. One concerns the role of the environment in altering the expression of genes. Studies of MZ twin pairs in which one has schizophrenia and the other does not indicate that there are also differences between the co-twins in patterns of gene expression (Kato, Iwamoto, Kakiuchi, Kuratomi, & Okazaki, 2005). Thus, it appears that environmental factors can alter the expression of vulnerability genes. Further, the occurrence of spontaneous mutations, including copy number variations and microdeletions, is much higher in schizophrenia patients than in healthy individuals (Sebat, Levy, & McCarthy, 2009; Stankiewicz & Lupski, 2010).

There are some ongoing controversies and concomitant shifting of paradigms concerning the genetics of schizophrenia. One of the controversies concerns the specificity of the genetic liability for schizophrenia. Early behavioral genetic studies led to the conclusion that there were separable genetic liabilities for schizophrenia and the major affective disorders, namely, bipolar disorder and psychotic depression. But more recent evidence indicates that this is not the case. Using quantitative genetic techniques with large twin samples, researchers have shown that there is significant overlap in the genes that contribute to schizophrenia, schizoaffective disorder, and manic syndromes (Cardno, Rijsdijk, Sham, Murray, & McGuffin, 2002; Fanous & Kendler, 2005). Based on these and other findings, many experts have concluded that genetic vulnerability does not conform to the diagnostic boundaries listed in *DSM* and other taxonomies (e.g., Boks, Leask, Vermunt, & Kahn, 2007). Rather, it appears that there is a genetic vulnerability to psychosis in general, and that the expression of this vulnerability can take the form of schizophrenia *or* an affective psychosis, depending on other genetic and acquired risk factors. In contrast, there is recent evidence suggesting that some susceptibility genes contribute to specific subtypes of schizophrenia, with symptomatic features and subtypes aggregating in families (Fanous & Kendler, 2008), suggesting specificity of inherited vulnerabilities. Clearly, more research is needed to understand the specificity for genetic liability for schizophrenia and mood disorders.

The second major controversy in the field concerns the magnitude and extent of the genetic vulnerability for schizophrenia. In other words, what is the relative importance of inherited vulnerability *versus* external factors that affect a developing individual? As mentioned above, we now know that the environment begins to have an impact before birth; prenatal events (some of which are discussed below) are linked with risk for schizophrenia. Thus, to index environmental events that contribute to nongenetic constitutional vulnerability, we must include both the prenatal and postnatal periods. At this point, however, researchers are not in a position to estimate the relative magnitude of the inherited and environmental contributors to the etiology of schizophrenia. Moreover, it is not yet known whether genetic vulnerability is present in all cases of schizophrenia. Some cases of the illness may be solely attributable to environmental risk factors.

Further, it is not known whether the genetic predisposition to schizophrenia is always expressed, though there is substantive evidence to indicate that it is not. It is well established that the concordance rate for schizophrenia in MZ twins is nowhere near 100%, suggesting that some genetically vulnerable individuals do not develop the illness. The genetic liability for schizophrenia may result from a mutation that occurs in only the affected member of discordant MZ pairs. But findings from studies of discordant MZ twins indicate that the rate of schizophrenia is similar, and elevated, in the offspring of both the affected *and* nonaffected co-twins (Gottesman & Bertelsen, 1989; Kringlen & Cramer, 1989). In other words, the offspring of the normal MZ twin have a rate of schizophrenia similar to the offspring of the ill co-twin, even though the former was not raised by a schizophrenic parent. This provides support for the notion that some individuals possess a genetic vulnerability for schizophrenia that they pass on to their offspring, despite the fact that they are never diagnosed with the illness. Thus, unexpressed genetic vulnerabilities for schizophrenia may be common in the general population. The presence of individuals who have an unexpressed genetic vulnerability to schizophrenia makes the work of genetic researchers much more difficult. At the same time, the evidence of unexpressed genotypes for schizophrenia leads us to inquire about factors that trigger the expression of illness in vulnerable individuals, and the hope is that this knowledge may, some day, lead to effective preventative interventions.

Prenatal and Perinatal Factors   In addition to the support it provides for hereditary influences on schizophrenia, the behavior genetic literature clearly illustrates the relevance of environmental factors. Identifying these factors is a primary focus of many investigators, and the prenatal period has received greater attention in recent years. There is extensive evidence that obstetrical complications (OCs) have an adverse impact on the developing fetal brain and may contribute to vulnerability for schizophrenia. Birth cohort studies have shown that schizophrenia patients are more likely to have a history of exposure to OCs (Buka, Tsuang, & Lipsitt, 1993; Dalman, Allebeck, Cullberg, Grunewald, & Koester, 1999; McNeil, 1988; Takagai et al., 2006). Included among these are prenatal conditions are toxemia and pre-eclampsia and labor and delivery complications. A meta-analysis of the OC literature by Cannon, Jones, and Murray (2002) concluded that, among the different types of OCs, complications of pregnancy (bleeding, pre-eclampsia, diabetes, and Rhesus factor incompatibility) were the most strongly linked with later schizophrenia, followed by abnormal fetal growth and development and complications of delivery. In the National Collaborative Perinatal Project, which involved over 9,000 children followed from birth through adulthood, the odds of developing adult-onset schizophrenia increased linearly with an increasing number of hypoxia-related OCs (Cannon, 1998; Zornberg, Buka, & Tsuang, 2000).

Another prenatal event that has been linked with increased risk for schizophrenia is maternal viral infection. The risk rate for schizophrenia is elevated for individuals born shortly after a flu epidemic (Barr, Mednick, & Munk-Jorgensen, 1990; Brown et al., 2004; Limosin, Rouillon, Payen, Cohen, & Strub, 2003; Murray, Jones, O'Callaghan, & Takei, 1992) or after being prenatally exposed to rubella (Brown, Cohen, Harkavy-Friedman, & Babulas, 2001). The critical period of exposure appears to be between the 4th and 6th months of pregnancy. The findings from research on prenatal maternal infection might be connected to the "season-of-birth" effect in schizophrenia. A meta-analysis has shown that a disproportionate number of schizophrenic patients are born during the winter months (Davies, Welham, Chant, Torrey, & McGrath, 2003). This timing may reflect seasonal exposure to viral infections, which are most common in late fall and early winter. Thus the fetus would have been exposed to the infection during the second trimester. The second trimester is an important time for brain development, and disruptions during this stage may lead to developmental abnormalities.

Studies of rodents and nonhuman primates have shown that prenatal maternal stress can interfere with fetal brain development and is associated with elevated glucocorticoid release and hippocampal abnormalities in the offspring (Charil, Laplante, Vaillancourt, & King, 2010; Coe et al., 2003). Along the same lines, in humans, there is evidence that stressful events during pregnancy are associated with greater risk for schizophrenia and other psychiatric disorders in adult offspring. Researchers have linked the incidence of schizophrenia to various maternal stressors during pregnancy, including bereavement (Huttunen, 1989), famine (Susser & Lin, 1992; St. Clair et al., 2005), military invasion (van Os & Selten, 1998), war (Malaspina et al., 2008), flood (Selten, Graaf, van Duursen, Gispen-de Wied, & Kahn, 1999), and earthquake (Watson, Mednick, Huttunen, & Wang, 1999). It is likely that prenatal stress triggers the release of maternal stress hormones, which have been found to disturb fetal neurodevelopment and subsequent functioning of the hypothalamic-pituitary-adrenal axis, which, in turn, influences behavior and cognition (Seckl & Holmes, 2007).

One of the chief questions confronting researchers is whether OCs act independently to increase risk for schizophrenia or have their effect in conjunction with a genetic vulnerability (Mittal, Ellman, & Cannon, 2008). One possibility is that the genetic vulnerability for schizophrenia involves an increased sensitivity to prenatal factors that interfere with fetal neurodevelopment (Cannon, 1998; Preti, 2005; Walshe et al., 2005). It is also plausible that obstetrical events act independently of genetic vulnerabilities, although such effects would likely entail complex interactions among factors (Susser, Brown, & Gorman, 1999). For example, to produce the neurodevelopmental abnormalities that confer risk for schizophrenia, it may be necessary for a specific OC to occur during a critical period of cellular migration or in conjunction with other factors such as maternal fever or immune response. Recent research has shown evidence that the presence of serious OCs may interact with certain genes, those that are regulated by hypoxia or involved in neurovascular function, to increase the risk for schizophrenia (Nicodemus et al., 2008).

Biological Indicators of Vulnerability

Having identified two likely sources of vulnerability for schizophrenia, genetic and obstetrical factors, we now turn to the *nature* of vulnerability. Where does the weakness lie? Since the turn of the century, writers in the field of psychopathology had suspected that schizophrenia involved some abnormality in the brain (Bleuler, 1965). This assumption was based, in part, on the severity of the symptoms and the deteriorating clinical course. However, it was not until the advent of neuroimaging techniques that solid, empirical data were gathered to support this assumption.

Abnormalities in Brain Structure

The first reports were based on computerized axial tomography (CAT) scans that showed that affected individuals had enlarged brain ventricles, especially increased volume of the lateral ventricles (Dennert & Andreasen, 1983). As new techniques for brain scanning were developed, these findings were replicated and additional abnormalities were detected (Henn & Braus, 1999). Magnetic resonance imaging (MRI) revealed decreased frontal, temporal, and whole brain volume among people with schizophrenia (Lawrie & Abukmeil, 1998; Tanskanen et al., 2010). More fine-grained analyses demonstrated reductions in the size of structures such as the thalamus and hippocampus. Diffuse tensor imaging (DTI) has allowed investigators to examine neuronal connections and white matter tracts in the brain and has shown that two networks of white matter tracts may be affected in schizophrenia, potentially influencing the connection between gray matter regions in the frontal and temporal lobes (Ellison-Wright & Bullmore, 2009).

A landmark study of MZ twins discordant for schizophrenia was the first to demonstrate that these brain abnormalities were not solely attributable to genetic factors (Suddath, Christison, Torrey, Casanova, & Weinberger, 1990). When compared to their healthy identical co-twins, twins with schizophrenia were found to have smaller temporal lobe volumes, with the hippocampal region showing the most dramatic difference between the affected and nonaffected co-twins. Subsequent studies have confirmed smaller brain volumes among affected twins than among their healthy identical co-twins (Baare et al., 2001). These studies lend support to the hypothesis that the brain abnormalities observed in schizophrenia are at least partially due to factors that interfere with prenatal brain development.

There is also a wealth of evidence to suggest that irregularities in neural development during the adolescent period (immediately before mean age of onset) contribute to the abnormalities of structural and connective tissue observed in adults with schizophrenia. Among healthy adolescents, researchers have observed a normative change in cerebral white matter proportion that was significantly greater than the change in total cerebral gray matter proportion over the adolescent period, suggesting that the relative gray matter reduction may correspond with significant increases in white matter (Bartzokis et al., 2001; Sowell et al., 2003). Because researchers have observed gray and white matter abnormalities (e.g., irregular elements of white matter including myelin and oligodendroglia abnormalities) in frontal regions (Foong et al., 2001; Hoptman et al., 2002) of adults with psychotic illness, researchers have begun to wonder if disruptions in this normative maturational pattern may be contributing to the etiology of psychosis. Although few longitudinal studies of high-risk individuals (prospective designs) have been conducted, results suggest a developmental pattern of declining gray matter structures in left inferior fontal, medial temporal, cerebral, and cingulate regions (Job, Whalley, Johnstone, & Lawrie, 2005; Pantelis et al., 2007). Researchers have also observed DTI evidence that, across age, patients failed to show a normal pattern of increasing white matter integrity with age in the temporal lobe (Karlsgodt, Niendam, Bearden, & Cannon, 2009). Taken together, this accumulating evidence points to a prominent role of abnormal adolescent neurodevelopment and conductivity in the pathogenesis of schizophrenia and suggests that many of the noted structural and connective deficits may have been present prior to the formal onset of illness.

Despite the plethora of research findings indicating the presence of abnormalities in the brains of patients with schizophrenia, no specific abnormality has yet been shown to be definitely pathognomonic. In other words, there is no evidence that a specific morphological abnormality is unique to schizophrenia or characterizes all schizophrenia patients. The structural brain abnormalities observed in schizophrenia are, therefore, gross manifestations of the occurrence of a deviation in neurodevelopment that has implications for the functioning of neurocircuitry.

Neurotransmitters

The idea that schizophrenia involves an abnormality in neurotransmission has a long history. Initial neurotransmitter theories focused on epinephrine and norepinephrine. Subsequent approaches have hypothesized that serotonin, glutamate, and/or gamma aminobutyric acid (GABA) abnormalities are involved in schizophrenia. But, compared to other neurotransmitters, dopamine has played a more enduring role in theorizing about the biochemical basis of schizophrenia. This section will review the major neurotransmitter theories of schizophrenia, with an emphasis on dopamine.

In the early 1950s, investigators began to suspect that dopamine might play a central role in schizophrenia. Dopamine is widely distributed in the brain and is one of the neurotransmitters that enables communication in the circuits that link subcortical with cortical brain regions (Jentsch, Roth, & Taylor, 2000). Since the 1950s, support for this idea has waxed and waned. Since 2000, however, there has been a resurgence of interest in dopamine, largely because research findings have offered a new perspective.

The initial support for the role of dopamine in schizophrenia was based on two indirect pieces of evidence (Carlsson, 1988): (1) drugs that reduce dopamine activity also serve to diminish psychotic symptoms, and (2) drugs that heighten dopamine activity exacerbate or trigger psychotic episodes. It was eventually shown that standard antipsychotic drugs had their effect by blocking dopamine receptors, especially the D_2 subtype, which is prevalent in subcortical regions of the brain. The newer antipsychotic drugs, or "atypical" antipsychotics, have the advantage of causing fewer motor side effects. Nonetheless, they also act on the dopamine system by blocking various subtypes of dopamine receptors.

The relationship between DA and psychotic symptomology can be demonstrated by studies examining compounds such as levodopa that are used to treat Parkinson's disease by increasing DA transmission. For example, motor abnormalities associated with Parkinson's disease (i.e., hypokinesias; slow jerking movements, rigidity) are related to low levels of dopamine characteristic of the disease. However, patients with Parkinson's disease, who are being treated with dopamine agonists (i.e., levodopa induced elevated striatal DA) show drug-induced dyskinesias (Hoff, Plas, Wagemans, & van Hilten, 2001) and, in extreme cases, psychotic symptomatology (Papapetropoulos & Mash, 2005). In a similar vein, other amphetamines, such as cocaine, increase DA and can cause both hyperkinesias and psychotic symptoms (Weiner, Rabinstein, Levin, Weiner, & Shulman, 2001). The interplay between DA and movement can also been seen in research examining genetics and drug responsivity in schizophrenia. For example, schizophrenia patients with the type *3 or *4 alleles of the CYP2D6 gene related to poor metabolization of neuroleptic drugs show a heightened rate of dyskinesias (Ellingrod, Schultz, & Arndt, 2002).

Early studies of dopamine in schizophrenia sought to determine whether there was evidence of excess neurotransmitter in schizophrenia patients. But concentrations of dopamine and its metabolites were generally found not to be elevated in body fluids from schizophrenia patients. When investigators examined dopamine receptors, however, there was some evidence of increased densities. Both postmortem and functional MRI studies of patients' brains yielded evidence that the number of dopamine D_2 receptors tends to be greater in patients than normal controls (Kestler, Walker, & Vega, 2001). Controversy has surrounded this literature because antipsychotic drugs can change dopamine receptor density. Nonetheless, even studies of never-medicated patients with schizophrenia have shown elevations in dopamine receptors (Kestler et al., 2001).

Other abnormalities in dopamine transmission have also been found. It appears, for example, that dopamine synthesis and release may be more pronounced in the brains of people with schizophrenia than among normals (Lindström et al., 1999). When schizophrenia patients and normal controls are given amphetamine, a drug that enhances dopamine release, the patients show more augmented dopamine release (Abi-Dargham et al., 1998; Soeares & Innis, 1999).

Glutamate, an excitatory neurotransmitter, may also play an important role in the neurochemistry of schizophrenia. Glutamatergic neurons are part of the pathways that connect the hippocampus, prefrontal cortex, and thalamus, all regions that have been implicated in schizophrenia. There is evidence of diminished activity at glutamatergic receptors among schizophrenia patients in these brain regions (Carlsson, Hansson, Waters, & Carlsson, 1999; Coyle, 2006; Ghose, Gleason, Potts, Lewis-Amezcua, & Tamminga, 2009). One of the chief receptors for glutamate in the brain is the N-methyl-d-aspartic acid (NMDA) subtype of receptor. Blockade of NMDA receptors produces the symptomatic manifestations of schizophrenia in normal subjects, including negative symptoms and cognitive impairments. For example, administration of NMDA receptor antagonists, such as phencyclidine (PCP) or ketamine, induces a broad range of schizophrenic-like symptomatology in humans, and these findings have contributed to a hypoglutamatergic hypothesis of schizophrenia (Coyle, 2006). Conversely, drugs that indirectly enhance NMDA receptor function can reduce negative symptoms and improve cognitive functioning in schizophrenia patients. It is important to note that the idea of dysfunction of glutamatergic transmission is not inconsistent with the dopamine hypothesis of schizophrenia because there are reciprocal connections between forebrain dopamine projections and systems that use glutamate (Grace, 2010). Thus dysregulation of one system would be expected to alter neurotransmission in the other (Stone, Morrison, & Pilowsky, 2007).

There also is evidence of abnormalities in GABA neurotransmission in the dorsolateral prefrontal cortex (Lewis & Hashimoto, 2007). Disruptions in GABA, an inhibitory neurotransmitter, may underlie the reduced capacity for working memory in schizophrenia. Current theories about the role of GABA in schizophrenia assume that it is important because cortical processes require an optimal balance between GABA inhibition and glutamatergic excitation (Costa et al., 2004).

The true picture of the neurochemical abnormalities in schizophrenia may be more complex than we assume. All neurotransmitter systems interact in intricate ways at multiple levels in the brain's circuitry (Carlsson et al., 2001). Consequently, an alteration in the synthesis, reuptake or receptor density, or affinity for any one of the neurotransmitter systems would be expected to have implications for one or more of the other neurotransmitter systems. Further, because neural circuits involve multiple segments that rely on different transmitters, it is easy to imagine how an abnormality in even one specific subgroup of receptors could result in the dysfunction of all the brain regions linked by a particular brain circuit.

Course and Prognosis

Assuming that genetic and obstetrical factors confer the vulnerability for schizophrenia, the diathesis must be present at birth. Yet, schizophrenia is typically diagnosed in late adolescence or early adulthood, with the average age of diagnosis in males about 4 years earlier than for females (Riecher-Rossler & Hafner, 2000). This raises intriguing questions about the developmental course prior to the clinical onset.

Premorbid Development

There is compelling evidence that there are signs of schizophrenia long before the illness is diagnosed. Most of these signs are subtle and do not reach the severity of clinical disorder. Nonetheless, when compared to children with healthy adult outcomes, children who later develop schizophrenia manifest deficits in multiple domains. In some of these domains, the deficits are apparent as early as infancy.

In the area of cognitive functioning, children who later develop schizophrenia tend to perform below their healthy siblings and classmates. These cognitive deficits are reflected in lower scores on measures of intelligence and achievement and poorer grades in school (Aylward, Walker, & Bettes, 1984; Jones, Rodgers, Murray, & Marmot, 1994). Preschizophrenic children also show abnormalities in social behavior. They are less responsive in social situations, show less positive emotion (Walker, Grimes, Davis, & Smith, 1993; Walker & Lewine, 1990), and have poorer social adjustment than children with healthy adult outcomes (Done, Crow, Johnstone, & Sacker, 1994). In studies of the childhood home movies of schizophrenia patients, preschizophrenic children showed more negative facial expression of emotion than did their siblings as early as the first year of life, indicating that the vulnerability for schizophrenia is subtly manifested in the earliest interpersonal interactions (Walker et al., 1993).

Vulnerability to schizophrenia is also apparent in motor functions. When compared to their siblings with healthy adult outcomes, preschizophrenic children show more delays and abnormalities in motor development, including deficits in the acquisition of early motor milestones such as bimanual manipulation and walking (Walker, Savoie, & Davis, 1994). Deficits in motor function extend throughout the premorbid period (Walker, Lewis, Loewy, & Palyo, 1999) and persist after the onset of the clinical illness (McNeil, Cantor-Graae, & Weinberger, 2000). Furthermore, abnormal gesture behavior has been observed in both premorbid (Mittal et al., 2006; Mittal et al., 2010) and unmedicated individuals with schizophrenia (Troisi, Spalletta, & Pasini, 1998). These data imply that the movement abnormalities recognized in schizophrenia are likely to have complex interactions with language and motor planning centers.

It is important to note that neuromotor abnormalities are not pathognomonic for schizophrenia, in that they are observed in children at risk for a variety of disorders, including learning disabilities and conduct and mood disorders. But they are one of several important clues pointing to the involvement of brain dysfunction in schizophrenia. Further, although medication-induced movement abnormalities, such as tardive dyskinesia, involve characteristic motor signs, these are not to be confused with involuntary movements that have been demonstrated to be present in drug-free groups such as at-risk infants (Fish, 1987), at-risk adolescents (Walker et al., 1999), and never medically treated schizophrenia patients (Khot & Wyatt, 1991).

Despite the subtle signs of abnormality that have been identified in children at risk for schizophrenia, most of these children do not manifest diagnosable mental disorders in childhood. Thus, while their parents may recall some irregularities in their development, most preschizophrenic children were not viewed as clinically disturbed. But the picture often changes in adolescence. Many adolescents who go on to develop schizophrenia show a pattern of escalating adjustment problems (Walker & Baum, 1998). They show a gradual increase in feelings of depression, social withdrawal, irritability, and noncompliance. This developmental pattern is not unique to schizophrenia; adolescence is also the critical period for the expression of the first signs of mood disorders, substance abuse, and some other mental disorders. As a result, researchers view adolescence as a critical period for the emergence of various kinds of behavioral dysfunction (Walker, 2002; Corcoran et al., 2003).

Among the behavioral risk indicators sometimes observed in preschizophrenic adolescents are "subclinical" signs of psychotic symptoms. These signs are also the defining features of a *DSM* Axis II disorder, namely, *schizotypal personality disorder* (SPD). The diagnostic criteria for SPD include social anxiety or withdrawal, affective abnormalities, eccentric behavior, unusual ideas (e.g., persistent belief in extrasensory perception, aliens, extrasensory phenomena, etc.), and unusual sensory experiences (e.g., repeated experiences with confusing noises with people's voices or seeing objects move). Although the individual's unusual ideas and perceptions are not severe or persistent enough to meet criteria for delusions or hallucinations, they are recurring and atypical of the person's cultural context. An extensive body of research demonstrates genetic and developmental links between schizophrenia and SPD. The genetic link between SPD and schizophrenia has been documented in twin and family history studies (Kendler, McGuire, Gruenberg, & Walsh, 1995; Kendler, Neale, & Walsh, 1995; Raine & Mednick, 1995). The developmental transition from schizotypal signs to schizophrenia in young adulthood has been followed in several recent longitudinal studies, with researchers reporting that 20 to 40% of schizotypal youth eventually show an Axis I schizophrenia spectrum disorder (Cannon et al., 2008; Miller et al., 2002; Yung et al., 1998). Other young adults with SPD either go on to develop other adjustment problems or to a complete remission of symptoms. Given the high rate of progression to schizophrenia, researchers are now attempting to determine whether schizotypal youth who will eventually manifest schizophrenia can be identified prior to the onset of the illness.

Since the 1990s, investigations have revealed that adolescents with SPD manifest some of the same functional abnormalities observed in patients with schizophrenia. For example, SPD youth show motor abnormalities (Neumann & Walker, 2003; Mittal et al., 2006; Walker et al., 1999), cognitive deficits (Diforio, Kestler, & Walker, 2000; Harvey, Reichenberg, Romero, Granholm, & Siever, 2006; Mittal et al., 2010), and an increase in cortisol, a stress hormone that is elevated in several psychiatric disorders (Mittal, Dhruv, Tessner, Walder, & Walker, 2007; Mitropoulou et al., 2004; Walker, Walder, & Reynolds, 2001; Weinstein, Diforio, Schiffman, Walker, & Bonsall, 1999). These new findings may eventually aid in the identification of SPD adolescents who are at greatest risk for developing schizophrenia.

The Illness Onset

The onset of the first episode of schizophrenia may be sudden or gradual. But as mentioned above, it is usually preceded by escalating adjustment problems, a period referred to as the *prodromal* phase (Lencz, Smith, Auther, Correll, & Cornblatt, 2003; Lieberman et al., 2001). There is some evidence that longer untreated psychotic episodes may be harmful for schizophrenia patients and may result in a worse course of illness (Davidson & McGlashan, 1997; Harris et al.,

2005; Perkins et al., 2004). However, this conclusion is controversial, and some researchers suggest that the relation between longer duration of untreated psychosis and worse prognosis may be a product of poorer premorbid functioning and an insidious onset (Larsen et al., 2001).

People with schizophrenia vary in their course of illness and prognosis. Being male, having a gradual onset, an early age of onset, poor premorbid functioning, and a family history of schizophrenia are all associated with poorer prognosis (Gottesman, 1991). In addition, some environmental factors contribute to a worse outcome. For example, schizophrenia patients who live in homes where family members express more negative emotion are more likely than those with supportive families to have more frequent relapses (Butzlaff & Hooley, 1998; Rosenfarb, Bellack, & Aziz, 2006). Also, exposure to stress can exacerbate schizophrenia symptoms. Researchers have found an increase in the number of stressful events in the months immediately preceding a schizophrenia relapse (Horan et al., 2005; Ventura, Neuchterlein, Hardesty, & Gitlin, 1992). Finally, there is a rapidly accumulating body of research indicating that cannabis use is associated with an increase in risk for psychotic disorders, earlier onset of disorder in vulnerable individuals, and exacerbation of psychotic symptoms (Rey, Martin, & Krabman, 2004).

As outlined, the prognosis for many schizophrenia patients is poor. Only 20 to 30% of patients are able to lead somewhat normal lives, meaning they can live independently and maintain a job (Grebb & Cancro, 1989). The majority experience a more debilitating course, with 20 to 30% manifesting continued moderate symptoms and over half experiencing significant impairment the rest of their lives. Further, patients with schizophrenia often suffer from other comorbid (i.e., co-occurring) conditions. For example, the rate of substance abuse among schizophrenia patients is very high, with as many as 47% in the community and 90% in prison settings meeting lifetime *DSM–IV* criteria for substance abuse or dependence (Regier et al., 1990).

Suicide is the leading cause of death among people with schizophrenia. It has been estimated that 25 to 50% of schizophrenia patients attempt suicide and 4 to 13% successfully commit suicide (Meltzer, 2001). Risk factors associated with suicide in this population include more severe depressive symptoms, being male, having an earlier onset, and suffering recent traumatic events (Schwartz & Cohen, 2001).

The Treatment of Schizophrenia

Researchers have not yet identified any biological or psychological cures for schizophrenia. However, significant progress has been made in treatments that greatly improve the prognosis of the illness. As a result of this research progress, the quality of life for individuals with schizophrenia is dramatically better than it was at the turn of the 21st century.

The first issue to be addressed in the evaluation and treatment of schizophrenia is safety. The risk of self-harm and potential for violence must be assessed (McGirr et al., 2006; Siris, 2001). A medical examination is typically conducted to rule out other illnesses that can cause or exacerbate psychotic symptoms. This examination includes a review of the medical history, a physical examination, and laboratory tests. Many patients with schizophrenia have untreated or undertreated medical conditions such as nutritional deficiencies and infections that are a result of their psychological or socioeconomic limitations (Goff, Heckers, & Freudenreich, 2001).

If a patient is not an acute risk to self or others, the next consideration becomes the type of treatment that would be most beneficial. There are several factors to consider. These include the person's living situation (many patients with schizophrenia are homeless), level of insight, willingness to accept treatment, treatment history, financial resources including health insurance, and family and other available social support. To increase the chances of successful treatment, the patient with schizophrenia should be encouraged to talk openly about their treatment preferences, beliefs about medication, and concerns about side effects or changes.

The treatment of schizophrenia can be divided into three phases: acute, stabilization, and maintenance phases (Sadock & Sadock, 2000). In the acute phase, the goal of treatment is to reduce the severity of symptoms. This phase usually lasts 4 to 8 weeks. In the stabilization phase, the goal is to consolidate treatment gains. This usually takes about 6 months. Finally, during the maintenance phase, the symptoms are in remission (partial or complete). At this point, the goal of treatment is to prevent relapse and improve functioning.

Antipsychotic Medication

The mainstay of the biological treatment of schizophrenia is antipsychotic medication. First developed in the 1950s, these medications had an enormous impact on the lives of people afflicted with schizophrenia. Their psychotic symptoms improved and many were able to leave psychiatric hospitals (deinstitutionalization). The first effective biological treatment for schizophrenia, chlorpromazine (Thorazine), was the first in a line of medications now referred to as the "typical" antipsychotics or neuroleptics. All of these medications act by blocking activity in the dopamine systems. The typical antipsychotic medications are classified as high, medium, and low potency and differ from one another in side-effect profiles (Table 10.4). *High potency* neuroleptics tend to carry a higher risk of extrapyramidal side effects (e.g., motor abnormalities) and are prescribed in low dosages. Some examples of high potency agents are Prolixin (fluphenazine), Stelazine (trifluoperazine), and Haldol (haloperidol). *Low potency* neuroleptics are prescribed in higher milligram doses and have lower risk of motor side effects, but a higher risk of inducing seizures, antihistaminic effects (including sedation and weight gain), anticholinergic effects (including cognitive dulling, dry mouth, blurry vision, urinary hesitancy, and constipation), and antiadrenergic effects (including postural hypotension and sexual dysfunction). Examples of low potency neuroleptics include Thorazine (chlorpromazine) and Mellaril (thioridazine). *Medium potency* agents tend to have intermediate side effects, between the low and high potency drugs. Examples of these include Trilafon (perphenazine) and Loxapac (loxapine).

In the 1990s a new generation of antipsychotic medications became available for therapeutic use in Europe and North America. The new class of medication is commonly referred to as "the atypical" or "second-generation" antipsychotics. Medications in this class share a lower risk of both the early occurring and the late emerging (or tardive) movement disorders. The atypical antipsychotics include Risperdal (risperidone), Zyprexa (olanzapine), Seroquel (quetiapine),

Table 10.4 Selected Antipsychotic Drugs

Drug	Route of Administration	Usual Daily Oral Dose (mg)	Sedation	Autonomic	Extrapyramidal Adverse Effects
Chlorpromazine	Oral, IM	200–600	+++	+++	++
Fluphenazine	Oral, IM, depot	2–20	+	+	+++
Trifluoperazine	Oral, IM	5–30	++	+	+++
Perphenazine	Oral, IM	8–64	++	+	+++
Haloperidol	Oral, IM, depot	5–20	+	+	+++
Loxapine	Oral, IM	20–100	++	+	++
Olanzapine	Oral	7.5–25	+	++	0?
Quetiapine	Oral	150–750	++	++	0?
Risperidone	Oral	2–16	+	++	+
Clozapine	Oral	150–900	+++	+++	0?

IM, intramuscular; + = low; ++ = medium; +++ = high; 0? = possibly none.
From Sadock & Sadock, 2000, p. 1204, with permission.

Geodon (ziprasidone), Abilify (aripiprazole), Invega (paliperidone), and Clozaril (clozapine). The individual medications differ significantly from one another in the neurotransmitter receptors that they occupy. Although all block dopamine neurotransmission to some extent, they vary in the extent to which they affect serotonin, glutamate, and other neurotransmitters. These atypical antipsychotics have become first-line treatment for schizophrenia. The efficacy of the atypical antipsychotics for the treatment of positive symptoms is at least equivalent to that of the typical antipsychotics, and some studies suggest that they are more effective for negative symptoms and the cognitive impairments associated with the disorder (Forster, Buckley, & Phelps, 1999; Sadock & Sadock, 2000). Of practical and clinical significance, however, is the substantial risk of developing a "metabolic syndrome" related to the use of this class of medicines. Recent research has revealed that the atypical antipsychotics may carry an elevated risk, causing substantial weight gain, new onset or worsening diabetes mellitus, and lipid abnormalities (Newcomer, 2005).

Antipsychotic medications are usually administered orally. For patients who are not compliant with oral medication, injectable, long-lasting (depot) antipsychotic medication may be administered (usually every 2 to 4 weeks). Three depot neuroleptics are commercially available in the United States. Two are first-generation or "typical" antipsychotics: Prolixin (fluphenazine decanoate) and Haldol (haloperidol decanoate). The third is a second-generation or atypical agent: Risperdal Consta (risperidone). Benefits of depot neuroleptics include the ease of use for the patient and the fact that compliance is easily monitored by the clinician. The risks are similar to the risks of all of the typical antipsychotics. The only additional risk is that of localized pain or swelling at the injection site.

Drug-induced movement disorders can be divided into early and late emerging syndromes (Saddock & Sadock, 2000, p. 1207, Table 12.8-3). Early emerging motor symptoms include pseudo-parkinsonism, bradykinesias (decreased movement), rigidity, and dystonic reactions (sudden onset of sustained intense, uncontrollable muscle contraction commonly occurring in the facial and neck muscles). Tardive dyskinesia is a late emerging syndrome that includes irregular choreiform (twisting or worm-like) movements that usually involve the facial muscles, but can involve any voluntary muscle group. It is fortunate that the rate of tardive dyskinesia has declined since the introduction of atypical neuroleptics. It is important to note the these drug-induced movement abnormalities are a distinct and separate entity from the spontaneous movement abnormalities noted earlier, which occur as a natural correlate of schizophrenia.

Mention should also be made of the neuroleptic malignant syndrome (NMS). This is a rare, idiopathic, life-threatening complication of neuroleptic medication. It is characterized by mental status changes (delirium), immobility, rigidity, tremulousness, staring, fever, sweating, and autonomic instability (labile blood pressure and tachycardia). Laboratory investigations often reveal an elevated white blood cell count (in the absence of infection) and an elevated creatine phosphokinase (CPK) level. Treatment involves discontinuation of neuroleptic medication, supportive medical treatment, a peripheral muscle relaxant, and bromocriptine (a D_2 receptor agonist; Rosebush & Mazurek, 2001).

Antipsychotic Medication for Prodromal Populations Several reports indicate that antipsychotics may be effective in reducing the progression of prodromal syndromes into *DSM* Axis I psychotic disorders. Prodromal signs are typically defined as subclinical psychotic symptoms. A review of several recently completed randomized clinical trials with antipsychotic medication reports that following the end of treatment, antipsychotic medication as a prepsychotic intervention may delay the onset of psychosis or ameliorate prepsychotic symptoms (De Koning et al., 2009). However, most studies find no significant differences at the end of follow-up

1 to 4 years later. Although the onset may be delayed, there is no indication that psychosis is prevented.

It is also important to acknowledge the potential risks of antipsychotic medications when used as a preventative intervention (Corcoran, First, & Cornblatt, 2010). The side effects of second-generation antipsychotics include extrapyramidal symptoms, weight gain, and metabolic complications. With no proven long-term effects, the benefit–risk ratio of using antipsychotics as a prepsychotic intervention must be weighed carefully. It is also not yet known what the effects of these medications are on prodromal adolescents. The increased use of psychotropic medication for other behavioral or emotional problems in children presents a valuable opportunity to study a population of youth less likely to meet the restrictive inclusion criteria of preventive clinical trials, but more likely to represent children and adolescents who are currently being seen in actual clinical practice. Thus, it would be advantageous to conduct naturalistic prospective studies aimed at elucidating the developmental course of symptoms in these children and adolescents (Simeon, Milin, & Walker, 2002). As knowledge of the effects of psychotropic medication on adolescent growth and development increases, physicians will be in a better position to weigh any adverse effects against potential benefits, both short term and long term (Jensen et al., 1999).

Psychosocial Treatments of Schizophrenia

Although administering antipsychotic medication is the crucial first step in the treatment of schizophrenia, there is substantial evidence that psychosocial interventions can also be beneficial for both the patient and his or her family. It is unfortunate that such treatments are not always available because of limited mental health resources. Nonetheless, it is generally agreed that the optimal treatment approach is one that integrates pharmacologic and psychosocial interventions.

Research supports the use of family therapy, which includes psychoeducational and behavioral components, in treatment programs for schizophrenia (Bustillo, Lauriello, Horan, & Keith, 2001). Family therapy has been shown to reduce the risk of relapse, reduce family burden, and improve family members' knowledge of and coping with schizophrenia.

Comprehensive programs for supporting the patient's transition back into the community have been effective in enhancing recovery and reducing relapse. One such program, called assertive community treatment (ACT), was originally developed in the 1970s by researchers in Madison, Wisconsin (Udechuku et al., 2005; see also Bustillo et al., 2001; Saddock & Sadock, 2000). ACT is a comprehensive treatment approach for the seriously mentally ill who are living in the community. Patients are assigned to a multidisciplinary team (nurse, case manager, general physician, and psychiatrist) that has a fixed caseload and a high staff to patient ratio (1:12). The team delivers all services to the patient when and where he or she needs it and is available to the patient at all times. Services include home delivery of medication, monitoring of physical and mental health status, in vivo social skills training, and frequent contact with family members. Studies suggest that ACT can reduce time spent in a hospital, improve housing stability, and increase patient and family satisfaction.

Social skills training seeks to improve the overall functioning of patients by teaching the skills necessary to improve performance of activities of daily living, employment-related skills, and interaction with others. Research indicates that social skills training can improve social competence in the laboratory and in the clinic (Bustillo et al., 2001; Penn & Mueser, 1996). However, it remains unclear to what extent this improvement in social competence translates into better functioning in the community.

The rate of competitive employment for the severely mentally ill has been estimated at less than 20% (Lehman, 1995); thus, vocational rehabilitation has been a major focus of many treatment programs. Vocational rehabilitation programs have a positive influence on work-related activities, although they have not yet been shown to have a substantial impact on patients' abilities to obtain employment in the community (Lehman, 1995). Some evidence suggests that supported employment programs produce better results than traditional vocational rehabilitation programs as measured by patients' ability to obtain competitive, independent employment. Nonetheless, job retention remains a significant problem (Lehman et al., 2002), and little evidence supports the contention that employment improves self-esteem or quality of life (Bustillo et al., 2001).

Finally, cognitive behavior therapy for schizophrenia draws on the principles of cognitive therapy that were originally developed by Beck (1976) and Ellis (1986). The theory is that normal psychological processes can help maintain or reduce specific psychotic symptoms. Cognitive-behavioral therapy (CBT) for psychosis challenges the notion of a discontinuity between psychotic and normal thinking. The normal cognitive mechanisms that are already being used in the nonpsychotic aspects of the patient's thinking can be used to help the psychotic individuals deal directly with their symptoms (Kingdon & Turkington, 2005). Individual CBT emphasizes a collaborative relationship between patient and therapist. The therapist and patient jointly examine the patient's specific symptoms. The choice of target symptoms is based on the patient's preference or severity of the problems created by the psychotic symptom in question. Psychotic beliefs are never directly confronted, although specific psychotic symptoms such as hallucinations, delusions, and related problems are targeted for intervention (Dickerson, 2000). The few published randomized controlled trials available for review suggest that CBT is at least somewhat effective in reducing hallucinations and delusions in medication-resistant patients and as a complement to pharmacotherapy in acute psychosis (Bustillo et al., 2001; Wykes et al., 2005). A recent meta analysis examining 14 studies including 1,484 patients concluded that, compared to other adjunctive therapies (supplementing medication), CBT was more effective; this finding was significantly more robust for acute patients in comparison to those suffering from chronic schizophrenia (Zimmerman, Favrod, Trieu, & Pomini, 2005). However, these authors noted that many moderating factors still need to be evaluated, including the therapeutic alliance as well as the extent of neurocognitive deficits.

Summary

This chapter reviewed a broad range of scientific research on the nature and origins of schizophrenia. Spanning over a century, the efforts of investigators have yielded, piece by piece, a clearer view of the illness. The puzzle is not solved, but we can certainly claim progress toward a solution. The picture that has emerged is best described in the framework of the *diathesis-stress* model that has dominated the field for several decades (Walker & Diforio, 1997; Walker, Mittal, & Tessner, 2008).

Figure 10.1 illustrates a contemporary version of the diathesis-stress model. This particular model postulates that constitutional vulnerability (i.e., the diathesis) emanates from both inherited and acquired constitutional factors. The inherited factors are genetically determined characteristics of the brain that influence its structure and function. Acquired vulnerabilities arise mainly from prenatal events that compromise fetal neurodevelopment.

Whether the constitutional vulnerability is a consequence of genetic factors, environmental factors, or a combination of both, the model assumes that vulnerability is, in most cases, congenital. But the assumption that vulnerability is present at birth does not imply that it will be clinically expressed at any point in the lifespan. Rather, the model posits that two sets of factors determine the postnatal course of the vulnerable individual. First, external stressors influence the expression of the vulnerability. Although this is a longstanding assumption among theorists, it is important to clarify it. Empirical research has provided evidence that episodes

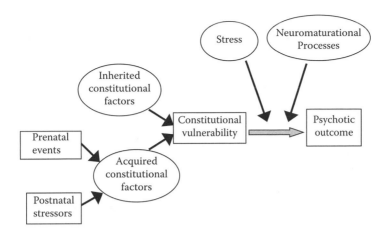

Figure 10.1 A Diathesis-Stress Model of the Etiology of Schizophrenia.

of schizophrenia follow periods of increased life stress (Horan et al., 2005; Ventura et al., 1992). Nonetheless, there is no evidence that individuals affected by schizophrenia experience more stress than nonschizophrenic persons, but rather that they are more sensitive to stress when it occurs. This assumption is the essence of the model; the interaction between vulnerability and stress is critical.

Diathesis-stress models have incorporated mechanisms to account for the adverse impact of stress on brain function (Walker & Diforio, 1997; Walker et al., 2008). The hypothalamic-pituitary-adrenal (HPA) axis, which is responsible for the release of cortisol and other stress hormones, has been examined as one of the primary neural systems triggered by stress exposure, leading to the expression of vulnerability for schizophrenia (Walder, Walker, & Lewine, 2000). Results from this research indicate that psychotic disorders are associated with elevated baseline and challenge-induced HPA activity, that antipsychotic medications reduce HPA activation, and that agents that augment stress hormone release exacerbate psychotic symptoms (Walker et al., 2008).

In addition, the model assumes that neuromaturation is a key element. In particular, adolescence to early adulthood appears to be a critical period for the expression of the vulnerability for schizophrenia. Thus some aspects(s) of brain maturational processes during the postpubertal period are likely playing an important role in triggering the clinical expression of latent liabilities (Corcoran et al., 2003; Walker, Kestler, Bollini, & Hochman, 2004).

In summary, although not all the pieces of the puzzle have been found, there has been significant progress in moving toward a comprehensive account of the etiology of schizophrenia. Among the mental disorders, schizophrenia remains a clear illustration of the complex interaction that take place between the individual and his or her environment. In the coming years, it is expected that research will yield important information about the precise nature of the brain's vulnerabilities associated with schizophrenia and the mechanisms involved in the interaction of congenital vulnerability with subsequent life stress and neuromaturation. Genetic data and research into gene expression will provide insight into this etiology, as well as further the understanding of the role of neurotransmitter abnormalities in schizophrenia. Longitudinal studies conducted during the prodromal period hold strong promise to elucidate the complicated interactions between development (e.g., hormones, neural maturation) and latent constitutional vulnerabilities. Furthermore, research during this period holds strong potential to inform the next generation of psychosocial and pharmacological preventive interventions.

References

Abi-Dargham, A., Gil, R., Krystal, J., Baldwin, R. M., Seibyl, J. P., Bowers, M., … Laruelle, M. (1998). Increased striatal dopamine transmission in schizophrenia: Confirmation in a second cohort. *American Journal of Psychiatry, 155*(6), 761–767.

Addington, J., & Addington, D. (2005). Patterns of premorbid functioning in first episode psychosis: Relationship to 2-year outcome. *Acta Psychiatrica Scandinavica, 112*, 40–46.

American Psychiatric Association. (2000). *Diagnostic and statistical manual of mental disorders* (4th rev. ed.). Washington, DC: Author.

Arajärvi, R., Suvisaari, J., Suokas, J., Schreck, M., Haukka, J., Hintikka, J., … Lönnqvist, J. (2005). Prevalence and diagnosis of schizophrenia based on register, case record and interview data in an isolated Finnish birth cohort born 1940–1969. *Social Psychiatry and Psychiatric Epidemiology, 40*(10), 808–816.

Aylward, E., Walker, E., & Bettes, B. (1984). Intelligence in schizophrenia: meta-analysis of the research. *Schizophrenia Bulletin, 10*, 430–459.

Baare, W. F., van Oel, C. J., Pol, H. E., Schnack, H. G., Durston, S., Sitskoorn, M. M., & Kahn, R. S. (2001). Volumes of brain structures in twins discordant for schizophrenia. *Archives of General Psychiatry, 58*(1), 33–40.

Barr, C. E., Mednick, S. A., & Munk-Jorgensen, P. (1990). Exposure to influenza epidemics during gestation and adult schizophrenia: A 40-year study. *Archives of General Psychiatry, 47*, 869–874.

Bartzokis, G., Beckson, M., Lu, P. H., Nuechterlein, K. H., Edwards, N., & Mintz, J. (2001). Age-related changes in frontal and temporal lobe volumes in men: a magnetic resonance imaging study. *Archives of General Psychiatry, 58*(5), 461–465.

Bassett, A. S., & Chow, E. W. C. (2008). Schizophrenia and 22q11.2 deletion syndrome. *Current Psychiatry Reports, 10*, 148–157.

Bassett, A. S., Hodgkinson, K., Chow, E. W., Correia, S., Scutt, L. E., & Weksberg, R. (1998). 22q11 deletion syndrome in adults with schizophrenia. *American Journal of Medical Genetics, 81*(4), 328–337.

Beck, Aaron T. (1976). *Cognitive therapy and the emotional disorders*. Oxford, England: International Universities Press.

Bigelow, N. O., Paradiso, S., Adolphs, R., Moser, D. J., Arndt, S., Heberlein, A., & Andreasen, N. C. (2006). Perception of socially relevant stimuli in schizophrenia. *Schizophrenia Research, 83*(2–3), 257–267.

Bleuler, E. (1950). *Dementia praecox or the group of schizophrenias* (J. Zinkin, Trans.). New York: International Universities Press. (Original work published in 1911.)

Bleuler, M. (1965). Conception of schizophrenia within the last fifty years and today. *International Journal of Psychiatry, 1*(4), 501–523.

Boks, M. P. M., Leask, S., Vermunt, J. K., & Kahn, R. S. (2007) The structure of psychosis revisited: The role of mood symptoms. *Schizophrenia Research, 93*, 178–185.

Bozikas, V. P., Kosmidis, M. H., Kiosseoglou, G., & Karavatos, A. (2006). Neuropsychological profile of cognitively impaired patients with schizophrenia. *Comprehensive Psychiatry, 47*(2), 136–143.

Brown, A. S., Begg, M. D., Gravenstein, S., Schaefer, C. A., Wyatt, R. J., Bresnahan, M., & Susser, E. S. (2004). Serologic evidence of prenatal influenza in the etiology of schizophrenia. *Archives of General Psychiatry, 61*(8), 774–780.

Brown, A. S., Cohen, P., Harkavy-Friedman, J., & Babulas, V. (2001). Prenatal rubella, premorbid abnormalities, and adult schizophrenia. *Biological Psychiatry, 49*, 473–486.

Brozgold, A. Z., Borod, J. C., Martin, C. C., Pick, L. H., Alpert, M., & Welkowitz, J. (1998). Social functioning and facial emotional expression in neurological and psychiatric disorders. *Applied Neuropsychology, 5*(1), 15–23.

Buka, S. L., Tsuang, M. T., & Lipsitt, L. P. (1993). Pregnancy/delivery complications and psychiatric diagnosis: A prospective study. *Archives of General Psychiatry, 50*, 151–156.

Bustillo, J. R., Lauriello, J., Horan, W. P., & Keith, S. J. (2001). The psychosocial treatment of schizophrenia: An update. *American Journal of Psychiatry, 158*(2), 163–175.

Butzlaff, R. L., & Hooley, J. M. (1998). Expressed emotion and psychiatric relapse. *Archives of General Psychiatry, 55*(6), 547–552.

Cannon, M., Jones, P. B., & Murray, R. M. (2002). Obstetric complications and schizophrenia: Historical and meta-analytic review. *American Journal of Psychiatry, 159*, 1080–1092.

Cannon, T. D. (1998). Genetic and perinatal influences in the etiology of schizophrenia: A neurodevelopmental model. In M. F. Lenzenweger & R. H. Dworkin (Eds.), *Origins and development of schizophrenia* (pp. 67–92). Washington, DC: American Psychological Association.

Cannon, T. D., Cadenhead, K., Cornblatt, B., Woods, S. W., Addington, J., Walker, E., … Heinssen, R. (2008). Prediction of psychosis in youth at high clinical risk: a multisite longitudinal study in North America. *Archives of General Psychiatry, 65*, 28–37.

Cardno, A. G., Rijsdijk, F. V., Sham, P. C., Murray, R. M., & McGuffin, P. (2002). A twin study of genetic relationships between psychotic symptoms. *American Journal of Psychiatry, 159*(4), 539–545.

Carlsson, A. (1988). The current status of the dopamine hypothesis of schizophrenia. *Neuropsychopharmacology, 1*(3), 179–186.

Carlsson, A., Hansson, L. O., Waters, N., & Carlsson, M. L. (1999). A glutamatergic deficiency model of schizophrenia. *British Journal of Psychiatry, 37*, 2–6.

Carlsson, A., Waters, N., Holm-Waters, S., Tedroff, J., Nilsson, M., & Carlsson, M. L. (2001). Interactions between monoamines, glutamate, and GABA in schizophrenia: new evidence. *Annual Review of Pharmacology and Toxicology, 41*, 237–260.

Carpenter, W. T., & Buchanan, R. W. (1994). Schizophrenia. *New England Journal of Medicine, 330*(10), 681–690.

Charil, A., Laplante, D. P., Vaillancourt, C., & King, S. (2010). Prenatal stress and brain development. *Brain Research Reviews, 65*, 56–79.

Coe, C. L., Kramer, M., Czéh, B., Gould, E., Reeves, A. J., Kirschbaum, C., & Fuchs, E. (2003). Prenatal stress diminishes neurogenesis in the dentate gyrus of juvenile rhesus monkeys. *Biological Psychiatry, 54*(10), 1025–1034.

Corcoran, C. M., First, M. B., & Cornblatt, B. (2010). The psychosis risk syndrome and its proposed inclusion in the DSM-V: A risk–benefit analysis. *Schizophrenia Research, 120*(1), 16–22.

Corcoran, C., Walker, E. F., Huot, R., Mittal, V. A., Tessner, K., Kestler, K., & Malaspina, D. (2003). The stress cascade and schizophrenia: Etiology and onset. *Schizophrenia Bulletin, 29*(4), 671–692.

Costa, E., Davis, J. M., Dong, E., Grayson, D. R., Guidotti, A., Tremolizzo, L., & Veldic, M. (2004). A GABAergic cortical deficit dominates schizophrenia pathophysiology. *Critical Reviews of Neurobiology, 16*, 1–23.

Coyle, J. T. (2006). Glutamate and schizophrenia: beyond the dopamine hypothesis. *Cellular and Molecular Neurobiology, 26*, 365–384.

Dalman, C., Allebeck, P., Cullberg, J., Grunewald, C., & Koester, M. (1999). Obstetric complications and the risk of schizophrenia: A longitudinal study of a national birth cohort. *Archives of General Psychiatry, 56*(3), 234–240.

Davidson, L., & McGlashan, T. H. (1997). The varied outcomes of schizophrenia. *Canadian Journal of Psychiatry, 42*, 34–43.

Davies, G., Welham, J., Chant, D., Torrey, E. F., & McGrath, J. (2003). A systematic review and meta-analysis of Northern Hemisphere season of birth studies in schizophrenia. *Schizophrenia Bulletin, 29*, 587–593.

De Koning, M. B., Bloemen, O. J. N., Van Amelsvoort, T. A. M. J., Becker, H. E., Nieman, D. H., Van Der Gaag, M., & Linszen, D. H. (2009). Early intervention in patients at ultra high risk of psychosis: benefits and risks. *Acta Psychiatrica Scandinavica, 119*, 426–442.

De Lisi, L. E. (1992). The significance of age of onset for schizophrenia. *Schizophrenia Bulletin, 18*, 209–215.

Dennert, J. W., & Andreasen, N. C. (1983). CT scanning and schizophrenia: A review. *Psychiatric Developments, 1*(1), 105–122.

Dickerson, F. B. (2000). Cognitive behavioral psychotherapy for schizophrenia: A review of recent empirical studies. *Schizophrenia Research, 43*, 71–90.

Diforio, D., Kestler, L., & Walker, E. (2000). Executive functions in adolescents with schizotypal personality disorder. *Schizophrenia Research, 42*, 125–134.

Done, D. J., Crow, T. J., Johnstone, E. C., & Sacker, A. (1994). Childhood antecedents of schizophrenia and affective illness: Social adjustment at ages 7 and 11. *British Medical Journal, 309*(6956), 699–703.

Ellingrod, V. L., Schultz, S. K., & Arndt, S. (2002). Abnormal movements and tardive dyskinesia in smokers and nonsmokers with schizophrenia genotyped for cytochrome P450 2D6. *Pharmacotherapy, 22*, 1416–1419.

Ellis, A. (1986). Rational-emotive therapy and cognitive-behavioral therapy: Similarities and differences. In A. Ellis & R. Grieger (Eds.), *Handbook of rational-emotive therapy* (Vol. 2, pp. 31–45). New York: Springer.

Ellison-Wright, I., & Bullmore, E. (2009). Meta-analysis of diffusion tensor imaging studies in schizophrenia. *Schizophrenia Research, 108*(1–3), 3–10.

Fanous, A. H., & Kendler, K. S. (2005). Genetic heterogeneity, modifier genes, and quantitative phenotypes in psychiatric illness: searching for a framework. *Molecular Psychiatry, 10*, 6–13.

Fanous, A. H., & Kendler, K. S. (2008). Genetics of clinical features and subtypes of schizophrenia: a review of the recent literature. *Current Psychiatry Reports, 10*, 164–170.

Feighner, J. P., Robins, E., & Guze, S. B. (1972). Diagnostic criteria for use in psychiatric research. *Archives of General Psychiatry, 26*, 57–63.

Fish, B. (1987). Infant predictors of the longitudinal course of schizophrenic development. *Schizophrenia Bulletin, 13*(3), 395–409.

Foong, J., Symms, M. R., Barker, G. J., Maier, M., Woermann, F. G., Miller, D. H., & Ron, M. A. (2001). Neuropathological abnormalities in schizophrenia: evidence from magnetization transfer imaging. *Brain, 124*(Pt. 5), 882–892.

Forster, P. L., Buckley, R., & Phelps, M. A. (1999). Phenomenology and treatment of psychotic disorders in the psychiatric emergency service. *Psychiatric Clinics of North America, 22*(4), 735–754.

Fromm-Reichmann, F. (1948). Notes on the treatment of schizophrenia by psychoanalytic psychotherapy. *Psychiatry, 11*, 263.

Ghose, S., Gleason, K. A., Potts, B. W., Lewis-Amezcua, K., & Tamminga, C. A. (2009). Differential expression of metabotropic glutamate receptors 2 and 3 in schizophrenia: A mechanism for antipsychotic drug action? *American Journal of Psychiatry, 166*, 812–820.

Goff, D. C., Heckers, S., & Freudenreich, O. (2001). Advances in the pathophysiology and treatment of psychiatric disorders: Implications for internal medicine. *Medical Clinics of North America, 85*(3), 663–689.

Gottesman, I. (1991). *Schizophrenia genesis: The origins of madness.* New York: Freeman.

Gottesman, I. I., & Bertelsen, A. (1989). Confirming unexpressed genotypes for schizophrenia: Risks in the offspring of Fischer's Danish identical and fraternal discordant twins. *Archives of General Psychiatry, 46*(10), 867–872.

Grace, A. A. (2010). Ventral hippocampus, interneurons, and schizophrenia: A new understanding of the pathophysiology of schizophrenia and its implications for treatment and prevention. *Current Directions in Psychological Science, 19*, 232–237.

Grebb, J. A., & Cancro, R. (1989). Schizophrenia: Clinical features. In J. I. Kaplan & B. J. Sadock (Eds.), *Synopsis of psychiatry: behavioral sciences, clinical psychiatry* (5th ed., pp. 757–777). Baltimore: Williams and Wilkins.

Green, M. F., & Horan, W. P. (2010). Social cognition in schizophrenia. *Current Directions in Psychological Science, 19*, 243–248.

Green, M. F., Kern, R. S., Braff, D. L., & Mintz, J. (2000). Neurocognitive deficits and functional outcome in schizophrenia: Are we measuring the "right stuff"? *Schizophrenia Bulletin, 26*(1), 119–136.

Green, M. F., Nuechterlein, K. H., Breitmeyer, B., & Mintz, J. (1999). Backward masking in unmedicated schizophrenic patients in psychotic remission: Possible reflection of aberrant cortical oscillation. *American Journal of Psychiatry, 156*(9), 1367–1373.

Green, M. F., Nuechterlein, K. H., Breitmeyer, B., & Mintz, J. (2006). Forward and backward visual masking in unaffected siblings of schizophrenic patients. *Biological Psychiatry, 59*(5), 446–451.

Harris, M. G., Henry, L. P., Harrigan, S. M., Purcell, R., Schwartz, O. S., Farrelly, S. E., … McGorry, P. D. (2005). The relationship between duration of untreated psychosis and outcome: An eight-year prospective study. *Schizophrenia Research, 79*(1), 85–93.

Harvey, P. D., Reichenberg, A., Romero, M., Granholm, E., & Siever, L. J. (2006). Dual-task information processing in schizotypal personality disorder: Evidence of impaired processing capacity. *Neuropsychology, 20*(4), 453–460.

Harvey, P. D., & Walker, E. F. (Eds.). (1987). *Positive and negative symptoms of psychosis: Description, research, and future directions.* Hillsdale, UK: Erlbaum.

Henn, F. A., & Braus, D. F. (1999). Structural neuro-imaging in schizophrenia. An integrative view of neuromorphology. *European Archives of Psychiatry and Clinical Neuroscience, 249*(Suppl. 4), 48–56.

Heston, L. L. (1966). Psychiatric disorders in foster home reared children of schizophrenic mothers. *British Journal of Psychiatry, 112*, 819–825.

Hoff, J. I., van den Plas, A. A., Wagemans, E. A., & van Hilten, J. J. (2001). Accelerometric assessment of levodopa-induced dyskinesias in Parkinson's disease. *Movement Disorders, 16*(1), 58–61.

Hooley, J. M. (2010). Social factors in schizophrenia. *Current Directions in Psychological Science, 19*, 238–242.

Hoptman, M. J., Volavka, J., Johnson, G., Weiss, E., Bilder, R. M., & Lim, K. O. (2002). Frontal white matter microstructure, aggression, and impulsivity in men with schizophrenia: a preliminary study. *Biological Psychiatry, 52*(1), 9–14.

Horan, W. P., Ventura, J., Nuechterlein, K. H., Subotnik, K. L., Hwang, S. S., & Mintz, J. (2005). Stressful life events in recent-onset schizophrenia: Reduced frequencies and altered subjective appraisals. *Schizophrenia Research, 75* (2), 363–374.

Howard, R. (Director). (2001). *A beautiful mind.* Universal City, CA: Universal Studios and Dreamworks LLC.

Howells, J. G. (1991). *The concept of schizophrenia: Historical perspectives*. Washington, DC: American Psychiatric Press.

Huttunen, M. (1989). Maternal stress during pregnancy and the behavior of the offspring. In S. Doxiadis & S. Stewart (Eds.), *Early influences shaping the individual. NATO Advanced Science Institute Series: Life sciences* (Vol. 160, pp. 175–182). New York: Plenum.

Jensen, P. S., Bhatara, V. S., Vitiello, B., Hoagwood, K., Feil, M., & Burke, L. B. (1999). Psychoactive medication prescribing practices for U.S. children: Gaps between research and clinical practice. *Journal of the American Academy of Child and Adolescent Psychiatry, 38*(5), 557–65.

Jentsch, J. D., Roth, R. H., & Taylor, J. R. (2000). Role for dopamine in the behavioral functions of the prefrontal corticostriatal system: Implications for mental disorders and psychotropic drug action. *Progress in Brain Research, 126*, 433–453.

Job, D. E., Whalley, H. C., Johnstone, E. C., & Lawrie, S. M. (2005). Grey matter changes over time in high risk subjects developing schizophrenia. *Neuroimage, 25*(4), 1023–1030.

Jones, P., Rodgers, B., Murray, R., & Marmot, M. (1994). Child developmental risk factors for adult schizophrenia in the British 1946 birth cohort. *Lancet, 344*, 1398–1402.

Karayiorgou, M., Morris, M. A., & Morrow, B. (1995). Schizophrenia susceptibility associated with interstitial deletions of chromosome 22q11. *Proceedings of the National Academy of Science, 92*, 7612–7616.

Karlsgodt, K. H., Niendam, T. A., Bearden, C. E., & Cannon, T. D. (2009). White matter integrity and prediction of social and role functioning in subjects at ultra-high risk for psychosis. *Biological Psychiatry, 66*(6), 562–569.

Kato, T., Iwamoto, K., Kakiuchi, C., Kuratomi, G., & Okazaki, Y. (2005). Genetic or epigenetic difference causing discordance between monozygotic twins as a clue to molecular basis of mental disorders. *Molecular Psychiatry, 10*, 622–630.

Keefe, R. S. E., & Fenton, W. S. (2007). How should DSM-V criteria for schizophrenia include cognitive impairment? *Schizophrenia Bulletin 33*(4): 912–920.

Keith, S. J., Regier, D. A., & Rae, D. S. (1991). Schizophrenic disorders. In L. N. Robins & D. A. Regier (Eds.), *Psychiatric disorders in America: The Epidemiologic Catchment Area study* (pp. 33–52). New York: Free Press.

Kendler, K. S., McGuire, M., Gruenberg, A. M., & Walsh, D. (1995). Schizotypal symptoms and signs in the Roscommon family study: Their factor structure and familial relationship with psychotic and affective disorders. *Archives of General Psychiatry, 52*, 296–303.

Kendler, K. S., Neale, M. C., & Walsh, D. (1995). Evaluating the spectrum concept of schizophrenia in the Roscommon family study. *American Journal of Psychiatry, 152*, 749–754.

Kestler, L. P., Walker, E., & Vega, E. M. (2001). Dopamine receptors in the brains of schizophrenia patients: a meta-analysis of the findings. *Behavioural Pharmacology, 12*(5), 355–371.

Kety, S. S. (1988). Schizophrenic illness in the families of schizophrenic adoptees: Findings from the Danish national sample. *Schizophrenia Bulletin, 14*, 217–222.

Khot, V., & Wyatt, R. J. (1991). Not all that moves is tardive dyskinesia. *American Journal of Psychiatry, 148*, 661–666.

Kingdon, D. G., & Turkington, D. (2005). *Cognitive therapy of schizophrenia*. (J. B. Persons, series editor). New York: Guilford.

Kirkpatrick, B., Fenton, W. S., Carpenter, W. T., & Marder, S. R. (2006). The NIMH-MATRICS consensus statement on negative symptoms. *Schizophrenia Bulletin, 32*, 214–219.

Kohler, C. G., & Johnson, C. (2005). Neurosyphilis, HIV, and psychosis. In H. Fatemi (Ed.), *Neuropsychiatric disorders and infection* (pp. 51–59). London: Taylor and Francis.

Kraepelin E. (1913). *Psychiatrie* (8th ed.). (Translated by R. M. Barclay (1919) from vol. 3, part 2, as Dementia Praecox and Paraphrenia). Edinburgh: Livingstone.

Kringlen, E., & Cramer, G. (1989). Offspring of monozygotic twins discordant for schizophrenia. *Archives of General Psychiatry, 46*(10), 873–877.

Kulhara, P., & Chakrabarti, S. (2001). Culture and schizophrenia and other psychotic disorders. *Psychiatric Clinics of North America, 24*(3), 449–464.

Larsen, T. K., Friis, S., Haahr, U., Joa, I., Johannessen, J. O., Melle, I., Opjordsmoen, S., … Vaglum, P. (2001). Early detection and intervention in first-episode schizophrenia: A critical review. *Acta Psychiatrica Scandinavic, 103*(5), 323–334.

Lawrie, S. M., & Abukmeil, S. S. (1998). Brain abnormality in schizophrenia: A systematic and quantitative review of volumetric magnetic resonance imaging studies. *British Journal of Psychiatry, 172*, 110–120.

Lehman, A. F. (1995). Vocational rehabilitation in schizophrenia. *Schizophrenia Bulletin, 21*(4), 64–56.

Lehman, A. F., Goldberg, R., Dixon, L., McNary, S., Postrado, L., Hackman, A., & McDonnell, K. (2002). Improving employment outcomes for persons with severe mental illnesses. *Archives of General Psychiatry, 59*(2), 165–172.

Lencz, T., Smith, C. W., Auther, A. M., Correll, C. U., & Cornblatt, B. A. (2003). The assessment of "prodromal schizophrenia": Unresolved issues and future directions. *Schizophrenia Bulletin, 29*(4), 717–728.

Lewis, D. A., & Hashimoto, T. (2007). Deciphering the disease process of schizophrenia: The contribution of cortical GABA neurons. *International Review of Neurobiology, 78*, 109–131.

Lewis, C. M., Levinson, D. F., Wise, L. H., DeLisi, L. E., Straub, R. E., Hovatta, I., … Helgason, T. (2003). Genome scan meta-analysis of schizophrenia and bipolar disorder, part II: schizophrenia. *American Journal of Human Genetics, 73*, 34–48.

Lieberman, J. A., Perkins, D., Belger, A., Chakos, M., Jarskog, F., Boteva, K., & Gilmore, J. (2001). The early stages of schizophrenia: Speculations on pathogenesis, pathophysiology, and therapeutic approaches. *Biological Psychiatry, 50*(11), 884–897.

Limosin, F., Rouillon, F., Payan, C., Cohen, J., & Strub, N. (2003). Prenatal exposure to influenza as a risk factor for adult schizophrenia. *Acta Psychiatrica Scandinavica, 107*(5), 331–335.

Lindström, L. H., Gefvert, O., Hagberg, G., Lundberg, T., Bergström, M., Hartvig, P., & Långström, B. (1999). Increased dopamine synthesis rate in medial prefrontal cortex and striatum in schizophrenia indicated by L-(beta-11C) DOPA and PET. *Biological Psychiatry, 46*(5), 681–688.

Malaspina, D., Corcoran, C., Kleinhaus, K. R., Perrin, M. C., Fennig, S., Nahon, D., … Harlap, S. (2008). Acute maternal stress in pregnancy and schizophrenia in offspring: A cohort prospective study. *BMC Psychiatry, 8*, 71–80.

Martin, F., Baudouin, J.-Y., Tiberghien, G., & Franck, N. (2005). Processing emotional expression and facial identity in schizophrenia. *Psychiatry Research, 134*(1), 43–53.

McGirr, A., Tousignant, M., Routhier, D., Pouliot, L., Chawky, N., Margolese, H., & Turecki, G. (2006). Risk factors for completed suicide in schizophrenia and other chronic psychotic disorders: A case-control study. *Schizophrenia Research, 84*(1), 132–143.

McNeil, T. F. (1988). Obstetric factors and perinatal injuries. In M. T. Tsuang & J. C. Simpson (Eds.), *Handbook of schizophrenia: Nosology, epidemiology and genetics* (Vol. 3, pp. 319–343). Amsterdam: Elsevier Science.

McNeil, T. F., Cantor-Graae, E., & Weinberger, D. R. (2000). Relationship of obstetric complications and differences in size of brain structures in monozygotic twin pairs discordant for schizophrenia. *American Journal of Psychiatry, 157*(2), 203–212.

Meltzer, H. J. (2001). Treatment of suicidality in schizophrenia. In H. Hendin & J. J. Mann (Eds.), *The clinical science of suicide prevention. Annals of the New York Academy of Sciences* (Vol. 932, pp. 44–60). New York: New York Academy of Sciences.

Miller, T. J., McGlashan, T. H., Rosen, J. L., Somjee, L., Markovich, P. J., Stein, K., & Woods, S. W. (2002). Prospective diagnosis of the initial prodrome for schizophrenia based on the Structured Interview for Prodromal Syndromes: Preliminary evidence of interrater reliability and predictive validity. *American Journal of Psychiatry, 159*(5), 863–865.

Mitropoulou, V., Goodman, M., Sevy, S., Elman, I., New, A. S., Iskander, E. G., … Siever, L. J. (2004). Effects of acute metabolic stress on the dopaminergic and pituitary-adrenal axis activity in patients with schizotypal personality disorder. *Schizophrenia Research, 70*(1), 27–31.

Mittal, V. A., Dhruv, S., Tessner, K. D., Walder, D. J., & Walker, E. F. (2007). The relations among putative bio risk markers in schizotypal adolescents: minor physical anomalies, movement abnormalities and salivary cortisol. *Biological Psychiatry, 61*, 1179–1186.

Mittal, V. A., Ellman, L. M., & Cannon, T. D. (2008). Gene-environment interaction and covariation in schizophrenia: The role of obstetric complications. *Schizophrenia Bulletin, 34*, 1083–1094.

Mittal, V. A., Tessner, K., Sabuwalla, Z., McMillan, A., Trottman, H., & Walker, E. F. (2006). Gesture behavior in unmedicated schizotypal adolescents. *Journal of Abnormal Psychology, 115*(2), 351–358.

Mittal, V. A., Walker, E. F., Walder, D., Trottman, H., Bearden, C. E., Daley, M., … Cannon, T. D. (2010). Markers of basal ganglia dysfunction and conversion to psychosis: Neurocognitive deficits and dyskinesias in the prodromal period. *Biological Psychiatry, 68*, 93–99.

Murphy K. C., Jones, L. A., & Owen, M. J. (1999). High rates of schizophrenia in adults with velo-cardio-facial syndrome. *Archives of General Psychiatry, 56*, 940–945.

Murray, R. M., Jones, P. B., O'Callaghan, E., & Takei, N. (1992). Genes, viruses and neurodevelopmental schizophrenia. *Journal of Psychiatric Research, 26*, 225–235.

Nestor, P. G., Onitsuka, T., Gurrera, R. J., Niznikiewicz, M., Frumin, M., Shenton, M. E., & McCarley, R. W. (2007). Dissociable contributions of MRI volume reductions of superior temporal and fusiform gyri to symptoms and neuropsychology in schizophrenia. *Schizophrenia Research, 91*(1–3), 103–106.

Neumann, C. S., & Walker, E. F. (2003). Neuromotor functioning in adolescents with schizotypal personality disorder: Associations with symptoms and neurocognition. *Schizophrenia Bulletin, 29*(2), 285–298.

Newcomer, J. W. (2005). Second-generation (atypical) antipsychotics and metabolic effects: A comprehensive literature review. *CNS Drugs, 19,* 1–93.

Nicodemus, K. K., Marenco, S., Batten, A. J., Vakkalanka, R., Egan, M. F., Straub, R. E., & Weinberger, D. R. (2008). Serious obstetric complications interact with hypoxia-regulated/vascular-expression genes to influence schizophrenia risk. *Molecular Psychiatry, 13,* 873–877.

Nuechterlein, K. H., Barch, D. M., Gold, J. M., Goldberg, T. E., Green, M. F., & Heaton, R. K. (2004). Identification of separable cognitive factors in schizophrenia. *Schizophrenia Research, 72,* 29–39.

Pantelis, C., Velakoulis, D., Wood, S. J., Yucel, M., Yung, A. R., Phillips, L. J., … McGorry, P. D. (2007). Neuroimaging and emerging psychotic disorders: the Melbourne ultra-high risk studies. *International Review of Psychiatry, 19*(4), 371–381.

Papapetropoulos, S., & Mash, D. C. (2005). Psychotic symptoms in Parkinson's disease: From description to etiology. *Journal of Neurology, 252*(7), 753–764.

Penn, D. L., Combs, D. R., Ritchie, M., Francis, J., Cassisi, J., Morris, S., & Townsend, M. (2000). Emotion recognition in schizophrenia: Further investigation of generalized versus specific deficit models. *Journal of Abnormal Psychology, 109,* 512–516.

Penn, D. L., Corrigan, P. W., Bentall, R. P., Racenstein, J. M., & Newman, L. (1997). Social cognition in schizophrenia. *Psychological Bulletin, 121*(1), 114–132.

Penn, D. L., & Mueser, K. T. (1996). Research update on the psychosocial treatment of schizophrenia. *American Journal of Psychiatry, 153*(5), 607–617.

Perkins, D. O., Lieberman, J. A., Gu, H., Tohen, M., McEvoy, J., Green, A. I., … HGDH Research Group. (2004). Predictors of antipsychotic treatment response in patients with first-episode schizophrenia, schizoaffective and schizophreniform disorders. *British Journal of Psychiatry, 185*(1), 18–24.

Preti, A. (2005). Obstetric complications, genetics and schizophrenia. *European Psychiatry, 20*(4), 354.

Raine, A., & Mednick, S. (Eds.). (1995). *Schizotypal personality disorder.* London: Cambridge University.

Regier, D. A., Farmer, M. E., Rae, D. S., Locke, B. Z., Keith, S. J., Judd, L. L., & Goodwin, F. K. (1990). Comorbidity of mental disorders with alcohol and other drug abuse. Results from the Epidemiologic Catchment Area (ECA) study. *Journal of the American Medical Association, 264,* 2511–2518.

Rey, J. M., Martin, A., & Krabman, P. (2004). Is the party over? Cannabis and juvenile psychiatric disorder: The past 10 years. *Journal of the American Academy of Child and Adolescent Psychiatry, 43*(10), 1194–1205.

Riecher-Rossler, A., & Hafner, H. (2000). Gender aspects in schizophrenia: bridging the border between social and biological psychiatry. *Acta Psychiatrica Scandinavica, 102*(407, Suppl.), 58–62.

Rosebush, P. I., & Mazurek, M. F. (2001). Identification and treatment of neuroleptic malignant syndrome. *Child and Adolescent Psychopharmacology News, 6*(3), 4.

Rosenfarb, I. S., Bellack, A. S., & Aziz, N. (2006). Family interactions and the course of schizophrenia in African American and White patients. *Journal of Abnormal Psychology, 115*(1), 112–120.

Sadock, B. J., & Sadock, V. A. (Eds.). (2000). *Kaplan and Sadock's comprehensive textbook of psychiatry* (Vol. 1, 7th ed.). New York: Lippincott Williams and Wilkins.

Schneider, K. (1959). *Clinical psychopathology.* New York: Grune and Stratton.

Schwartz, R. C., & Cohen, B. N. (2001). Risk factors for suicidality among clients with schizophrenia. *Journal of Counseling and Development, 79*(3), 314–319.

Siris, S. G. (2001). Suicide and schizophrenia. *Journal of Psychopharmacology, 1*(2), 127–135.

Sebat, J., Levy, D. L., & McCarthy, S. E. (2009). Rare structural variants in schizophrenia: one disorder, multiple mutations; one mutation, multiple disorders. *Trends in Genetics, 25,* 528–535.

Seckl, J. R., & Holmes, M. C. (2007). Mechanisms of disease: glucocorticoids, their placental metabolism and fetal 'programming' of adult pathophysiology. *Nature Clinical Practice, 3,* 479–488.

Selten, J. P., Graaf, Y., van Duursen, R., Gispen-de Wied, C. C., & Kahn, R. S. (1999). Psychotic illness after prenatal exposure to the 1953 Dutch flood disaster. *Schizophrenia Research, 35,* 243–245.

Simeon, J., Milin, R., & Walker, S. (2002). A retrospective chart review of risperidone use in treatment-resistant children and adolescents with psychiatric disorders. *Progress in Neuropsychopharmacology and Biological Psychiatry, 26*(2), 267–275.

Sowell, E. R., Peterson, B. S., Thompson, P. M., Welcome, S. E., Henkenius, A. L., & Toga, A. W. (2003). Mapping cortical change across the human life span. *Natural Neuroscience, 6*(3), 309–315.

Soares, J. C., & Innis, R. B. (1999). Neurochemical brain imaging investigations of schizophrenia. *Biological Psychiatry, 46*(5), 600–615.

Spitzer, R. L., Endicott, J., & Robins, E. (1978). *Research diagnostic criteria (RDC) for a selected group of functional disorders*. New York: Biometrics Research.

Stankiewicz, P., & Lupski, J. R. (2010). Structural variation in the human genome and its role in disease. *Annual Review of Medicine, 61*, 437–455.

St. Clair, D., Xu, M., Wang, P., Yu, Y., Fang, Y., Zhang, F., … He, L. (2005). Rates of adult schizophrenia following prenatal exposure to the Chinese famine of 1959–1961. *Journal of the American Medical Association, 294*, 557–562.

Stone, J. M., Morrison, P. D., & Pilowsky, L. S. (2007). Glutamate and dopamine dysregulation in schizophrenia—a synthesis and selective review. *Journal of Psychopharmacology, 21*, 440–452.

Suddath, R. L., Christison, G. W., Torrey, E. F., Casanova, M. F., & Weinberger, D. R. (1990). Anatomical abnormalities in the brains of monozygotic twins discordant for schizophrenia. *New England Journal of Medicine, 322*(12), 789–794.

Susser, E. S., Brown, A. S., & Gorman, J. M. (Eds.). (1999). *Prenatal exposures in schizophrenia. Progress in psychiatry*. Washington, DC: American Psychiatric Press.

Susser, E. S., & Lin, S. P. (1992). Schizophrenia after prenatal exposure to the Dutch Hunger Winter of 1944–1945. *Archives of General Psychiatry, 49*, 983–988.

Takagai, S., Kawai, M., Tsuchiya, K. J., Mori, N., Toulopoulou, T., & Takei, N. (2006). Increased rate of birth complications and small head size at birth in winter-born male patients with schizophrenia. *Schizophrenia Research, 83*(2–3), 303–305.

Tandon, R., Keshavan, M. S., & Nasrallah, H. A. (2008). Schizophrenia, "Just the facts": What we know in 2008. 2. *Epidemiology and etiology, Schizophrenia Research, 102*(1), 1–18.

Tanskanen, P., Ridler, K., Murray, G. K., Haapea, M., Veijola, J. M., Jääskeläinen, E., … Isohanni, M. K. (2010). Morphometric brain abnormalities in schizophrenia in a population-based sample: relationship to duration of illness. *Schizophrenia Bulletin, 36*, 766–777.

Tienari, P., Wynne, L. C., Moring, J., & Lahti, I. (1994). The Finnish adoptive family study of schizophrenia: Implications for family research. *British Journal of Psychiatry, 164*(Suppl. 23), 20–26.

Torrey, E. F. (1987). Prevalence studies in schizophrenia. *British Journal of Psychiatry, 150*, 598–608.

Tremeau, F., Malaspina, D., Duval, F., Correa, H., Hager-Budny, M., Coin-Bariou, L., … Gorman, J. M. (2005). Facial expressiveness in patients with schizophrenia compared to depressed patients and nonpatient comparison subjects. *American Journal of Psychiatry, 162*(1), 92–101.

Troisi, A., Spalletta, G., & Pasini, A. (1998). Non-verbal behavior deficits in schizophrenia: An ethological study of drug-free patients. *Acta Psychiatrica Scandinavica, 97*, 109–115.

Udechuku, A., Olver, J., Hallam, K., Blyth, F., Leslie, M., Nasso, M., … Burrows, G. (2005). Assertive community treatment of the mentally ill: Service model and effectiveness. *Australasian Psychiatry, 13*(2), 129–134.

van Os, J., & Selten, J. (1998). Prenatal exposure to maternal stress and subsequent schizophrenia: The May 1940 invasion of the Netherlands. *British Journal of Psychiatry, 172*, 324–326.

Ventura, J., Nuechterlein, K. H., Hardesty, J. P., & Gitlin, M. (1992). Life events and schizophrenic relapse after withdrawal of medication. *British Journal of Psychiatry, 161*, 615–620.

Walder, D., Walker, E., & Lewine, R. J. (2000). The relations among cortisol release, cognitive function and symptom severity in psychotic patients. *Biological Psychiatry, 48*, 1121–1132.

Walker, E. (1981). Emotion recognition in disturbed and normal children: A research note. *Journal of Child Psychology and Psychiatry, 22*, 263–268.

Walker, E. (2002). Adolescent neurodevelopment and psychopathology. *Current Directions in Psychological Science, 11*, 24–28.

Walker, E., & Baum, K. (1998). Developmental changes in the behavioral expression of the vulnerability for schizophrenia. In M. Lenzenweger & R. Dworkin (Eds.), *Origins and development of schizophrenia: Advances in experimental psychopathology* (pp. 469–491). Washington, DC: American Psychological Association.

Walker E., & Diforio, D. (1997). Schizophrenia: A neural diathesis-stress model. *Psychological Review, 104*, 1–19.

Walker, E., Grimes, K., Davis, D., & Smith, A. (1993). Childhood precursors of schizophrenia; Facial expressions of emotion. *American Journal of Psychiatry, 150*, 1654–1660.

Walker, E., Kestler, L., Bollini, A., & Hochman, K. M. (2004). Schizophrenia: Etiology and course. *Annual Review of Psychology, 55*, 401–430.

Walker, E., & Lewine, R. J. (1990). Prediction of adult-onset schizophrenia from childhood home movies of the patients. *American Journal of Psychiatry, 147*, 1052–1056.

Walker, E., Lewis, N., Loewy, R., & Palyo, S. (1999). Motor dysfunction and risk for schizophrenia. *Development and Psychopathology, 11*, 509–523.

Walker, E., Mittal, V., & Tessner, K. (2008). Stress and the hypothalamic pituitary adrenal axis in the developmental course of schizophrenia. *Annual Review of Clinical Psychology, 4*, 189–216.

Walker, E., Savoie, T., & Davis, D. (1994). Neuromotor precursors of schizophrenia. *Schizophrenia Bulletin, 20*, 441–452.

Walker, E., Walder, D., & Reynolds, F. (2001). Developmental changes in cortisol secretion in normal and at-risk youth. *Development and Psychopathology, 13*, 719–730.

Walshe, M., McDonald, C., Taylor, M., Zhao, J., Sham, P., Grech, A., … Murray, R. M. (2005). Obstetric complications in patients with schizophrenia and their unaffected siblings. *European Psychiatry, 20*(1), 28–34.

Watson, J. B., Mednick, S. A., Huttunen, M., & Wang, X. (1999). Prenatal teratogens and the development of adult mental illness. *Development and Psychopathology, 11*, 457–466.

Weiner, W. J., Rabinstein, A., Levin, B., Weiner, C., & Shulman, L. (2001). Cocaine-induced persistent dyskinesias. *Neurology, 56*(7), 964–965.

Weinstein, D., Diforio, D., Schiffman, J., Walker, E., & Bonsall, B. (1999). Minor physical anomalies, dermatoglyphic asymmetries and cortisol levels in adolescents with schizotypal personality disorder. *American Journal of Psychiatry, 156*, 617–623.

Williams, L. M., Das, P., Liddell, B. J., Olivieri, G., Peduto, A. S., David, A. S., … Harris, A. W. F. (2007). Fronto-limbic and autonomic disjunctions to negative emotion distinguish schizophrenia subtypes. *Psychiatry Research: Neuroimaging, 155*, 29–44.

Wolff, S. (1991). "Schizoid" personality in childhood and adult life I: The vagaries of diagnostic labeling. *British Journal of Psychiatry, 159*, 615–620.

Wykes, T., Hayward, P., Thomas, N., Green, N., Surguladze, S., Fannon, D., & Landue, S. (2005). What are the effects of group cognitive behaviour therapy for voices? A randomised control trial. *Schizophrenia Research, 77*(2–3), 201–210.

Yung, A. R., Phillips, L. J., McGorry, P. D., Hallgren, M. A., McFarlane, C. A., Francey, S., … Jackson, H. J. (1998). Prediction of psychosis: A step towards indicated prevention of schizophrenia. *British Journal of Psychiatry, 172*(Suppl. 33), 14–20.

Zimmerman, G., Favrod, J., Trieu, V., & Pomini, V. (2005). The effect of cognitive behavioral treatment on the positive symptoms of schizophrenia spectrum disorders: A meta-analysis. *Schizophrenia Research, 77*(1), 1–9.

Zornberg, G. L., Buka, S. L., & Tsuang, M. T. (2000). Hypoxic-ischemia-related fetal/neonatal complications and risk of schizophrenia and other nonaffective psychoses: A 19-year longitudinal study. *American Journal of Psychiatry, 157*(2), 196–202.

11

Personality Disorders

JENNIFER RUTH PRESNALL and THOMAS A. WIDIGER

University of Kentucky
Lexington, Kentucky

In 1980, the American Psychiatric Association (APA) published the third edition of the *Diagnostic and Statistical Manual of Mental Disorders* (*DSM–III*), which introduced the innovative multi-axial classification system. Axis II was devoted primarily to personality dysfunction, due to the prevalence of maladaptive personality traits in general clinical practice and the substantial impact of these traits on the course and treatment of other mental disorders (Frances, 1980). The current version of this diagnostic manual, *DSM–IV–TR* (APA, 2000) includes 10 personality disorders organized into three clusters: (1) paranoid, schizoid, and schizotypal (the odd-eccentric cluster); (2) antisocial, borderline, histrionic, and narcissistic (dramatic-emotional-erratic cluster); and (3) avoidant, dependent, and obsessive-compulsive (anxious-fearful cluster). However, the diagnosis of personality disorders is likely to undergo a major revision within the next edition (i.e., DSM–5), including a shift to Axis I, deletion of up to half of the diagnoses, replacement of diagnostic criterion sets with prototype matching, and the inclusion of a supplementary dimensional model of patient description (see http://www.dsm5.org). This chapter will begin with a discussion of personality disorders in general, followed by a consideration of five disorders in particular. Throughout we describe and discuss the revisions likely to occur with DSM–5, as well as provide an alternative model for the diagnosis and classification of maladaptive personality functioning, the five-factor model (FFM; Widiger & Trull, 2007).

Personality Disorder in General

Everyone, including those with psychological problems, has a characteristic manner of thinking, feeling, behaving, and relating to others that would have been present prior to the onset of any anxiety, mood, substance use, or other mental disorder, and, for many of these individuals, these personality traits will be so maladaptive that they would constitute a personality disorder. A personality disorder is defined in *DSM–IV–TR* as "an enduring pattern of inner experience and behavior that deviates markedly from the expectations of the individual's culture, is pervasive and inflexible, has an onset in adolescence or early adulthood, is stable over time, and leads to distress or impairment" (APA, 2000, p. 686).

It is estimated that 10–15% of the general population would meet the criteria for one of the 10 *DSM–IV–TR* personality disorders (Mattia & Zimmerman, 2001; Torgersen, 2005a). Table 11.1 provides data reported by the best available studies to date for estimating the prevalence of individual personality disorders within the community. These prevalence estimates are generally close to those provided in *DSM–IV–TR*. The prevalence of personality disorders within clinical settings is estimated to be well above 50% (Mattia & Zimmerman, 2001). As many as 60% of inpatients within some clinical settings are diagnosed with borderline personality disorder (APA, 2000; Gunderson, 2001). Antisocial personality disorder may be diagnosed in up to 50% of inmates within a correctional setting (Derefinko & Widiger,

Table 11.1 Epidemiology of Personality Disorders

Study	Sample	N	DSM	PRN	SZD	STP	ATS	BDL	HST	NCS	AVD	DPD	OCP
Drake et al. (1988)	Men	369	III	1.1	4.1	2.4	0.8	0.5	3.8	3.5	1.6	10.3	0.5
Coryell et al. (1989)	R-HN	185	II	0.5	1.6	2.2	1.6	1.1	1.6	0.0	1.6	0.5	3.2
Maier et al. (1992)	Comm	452	III–R	1.8	0.4	0.7	0.2	1.1	1.3	0.0	1.1	1.5	2.2
Black et al. (1993)	R-HN	127	III	1.6	0.0	3.9	0.0	5.5	3.9	0.0	3.2	2.4	7.9
Black et al. (1993)	R-OCD	120	III	1.7	0.0	2.5	0.8	0.8	2.5	0.0	0.8	0.8	10.8
Molden et al. (1994)	HN	302	III–R	0.0	0.0	0.7	2.6	2.0	0.3	0.0	0.7	1.0	0.7
Samuels et al. (1994)	Comm	762	III	0.0	0.0	0.1	1.5	0.4	2.1	0.0	0.0	0.1	1.7
Klein et al. (1995)	R-DP	258	III–R	1.7	0.9	0.0	2.2	1.7	1.7	3.9	5.2	0.4	2.6
Lenzenweger (1997)	Stdts	1,646	III–R	0.4	0.4	0.0	0.8	0.0	1.9	1.2	0.4	0.4	0.0
Torgersen et al.(2001)	Comm	2,053	III–R	2.4	1.7	0.6	0.7	0.7	2.0	0.8	5.0	1.5	2.0
Samuels et al. (2002)	Comm	742	IV	0.7	0.7	1.8	4.5	1.2	0.4	0.1	1.4	0.3	1.2
Median				1.1	0.4	0.7	0.8	1.1	1.9	0.0	1.6	0.8	2.2
DSM–IV estimates				0.5–2.5	uncm	3	2	2	2–3	<1	0.5–1	—	1

Note: N, number of people in study; DSM, edition of *Diagnostic and Statistical Manual* that was used; PRN, paranoid; SZD, schizoid; STP, schizotypal; ATS, antisocial; BDL, borderline; HST, histrionic; NCS, narcissistic; AVD, avoidant; DPD, dependent; OCP, obsessive-compulsive; R-HN, relatives of hypernormal (those without history of mental disorder); R-OCD, relatives of those with obsessive-compulsive anxiety disorder; R-DP, relatives of those with depression; Stdts, students; Comm, community; uncm, uncommon.

2008). The prevalence of personality disorder is generally underestimated in clinical practice due to a lack of time to provide systematic or comprehensive evaluations of personality functioning (Widiger & Boyd, 2009) and perhaps due as well to a reluctance to diagnose the disorders because insurance companies may consider them to be untreatable (Zimmerman & Mattia, 1999).

Personality disorders are among the most difficult disorders to treat because they involve well-established behaviors that can be integral to a client's self-image (Stone, 1993). Nevertheless, much has been written on the treatment of personality disorders (e.g., Beck, Freeman, & Associates, 1990; Benjamin, 2004; Clarkin, Fonagy, & Gabbard, 2010; Critchfield & Benjamin, 2006; Gunderson & Gabbard, 2000; Livesley, 2001, 2003; Magnavita, 2010; Young, Klosko, & Weishaar, 2003), and there is empirical support for clinically and socially meaningful changes in response to psychosocial and pharmacologic treatments (Livesley, 2001; Magnavita, 2010). The development of an ideal or fully healthy personality structure is unlikely to occur through the course of treatment, but given the considerable social, public health, and personal costs associated with some personality disorders, such as the antisocial and borderline, even moderate adjustments to personality functioning can represent socially and clinically significant improvements.

The major innovation of *DSM–III* was the inclusion of specific and explicit criterion sets to facilitate the obtainment of reliable diagnoses. However, it is likely that the personality disorders will be the only class of disorders in DSM–5 to no longer include diagnostic criterion sets (Skodol, 2010). The DSM–5 personality disorders work group has recommended a return to the method used in *DSM–II* (APA, 1968), in which clinicians match their global perception of a patient to a paragraph description, considering the narrative "as a whole rather than counting individual symptoms" (Westen, Shedler, & Bradley, 2006, p. 847). Gestalt matching to paragraph narratives is preferred by clinicians, largely because it is much easier than having to systematically assess each individual diagnostic criterion (Spitzer, First, Shedler, Westen, & Skodol, 2008). Nevertheless, the reliability and validity of this approach is questionable, at best (Block, 2008; Widiger, 2007a; Wood, Garb, Nezworski, & Koren, 2007; Zimmerman, 2011).

An additional DSM–5 revision will be the inclusion of a supplementary *dimensional model*, the precise content of which is difficult to predict as it has been revised a number of times. Watson, Clark, and Chmielewski (2008) first proposed a six-factor model based on a factor analysis they had conducted, consisting of neuroticism, introversion, antagonism, conscientiousness, openness, and oddity. However, Clark and Krueger (2010) revised this proposal to a different six-factor model consisting of negative emotionality, introversion, antagonism, compulsivity, disinhibition, and schizotypy, with 37 underlying traits. Krueger et al. (2011) have revised it once again on the basis of their latest factor analysis to a five-dimensional model (emotional dysregulation, detachment, antagonism, disinhibition, and peculiarity), with 25 underlying traits. The 25 (or 37) traits can be used in two different ways. First, one can use the traits as diagnostic criteria for one of the five personality disorders (e.g., callousness, aggression, manipulativeness, hostility, deceitfulness, narcissism, irresponsibility, recklessness, and impulsivity are suggested for the diagnosis of antisocial personality disorder). However, few clinicians are likely to use the traits in this manner because the narrative paragraphs will be much easier to use (e.g., clinicians are unlikely to assess for the presence of 37 traits in favor of simply matching to a narrative gestalt).

A second possible use of the traits is to provide an alternative means for patient description. One general goal of DSM–5 is to shift psychiatry toward a dimensional classification of psychopathology (Regier, Narrow, Kuhl, & Kupfer, 2010; see also Widiger, this volume). The personality disorder field is clearly moving in this direction (Widiger & Simonson, 2005). One approach to converting the personality disorder nomenclature of psychiatry to a dimensional model is to integrate it with the FFM of general personality structure developed within psychology (Mullins-Sweatt & Widiger, 2006). Five broad domains of personality functioning have been identified empirically through the study of the languages of a number of different cultures (Ashton & Lee, 2001). Language can be understood as a sedimentary deposit of the observations of people over the thousands of years of the language's development and transformation. The most important domains of personality functioning would be those with the greatest number of terms to describe and differentiate their various manifestations and nuances, and the structure of personality would be evident in the empirical relationship among the trait terms (Goldberg, 1993). Such lexical analyses of languages have typically identified five fundamental dimensions of personality: neuroticism (or negative affectivity) versus emotional stability, introversion versus extraversion, closedness versus openness to experience, antagonism versus agreeableness, and conscientiousness (constraint) versus disinhibition. These five broad domains align well with the five (or six) to be included in DSM–5: FFM neuroticism aligns with DSM–5 emotional dysregulation, FFM introversion aligns with DSM–5 detachment, FFM antagonism aligns with DSM–5 antagonism, FFM low conscientiousness aligns with DSM–5 disinhibition, and FFM openness aligns with DSM–5 schizotypy (and FFM high conscientiousness aligns with DSM–5 compulsivity, if that domain is included; Widiger, 2011).

Each of the five broad domains of the FFM can be differentiated further in terms of underlying facets. For example, the facets of antagonism versus agreeableness include suspiciousness versus trusting gullibility, callous tough mindedness versus tender mindedness, confidence and arrogance versus modesty and meekness, exploitation versus altruism and sacrifice, oppositionalism and aggression versus compliance, and deception and manipulation versus straightforwardness and honesty (Costa & McCrae, 1992).

Each of the *DSM–IV–TR* personality disorders can be readily understood as maladaptive or extreme variants of the FFM domains and facets (Lynam & Widiger, 2001; Samuel & Widiger, 2004). For example, *DSM–IV–TR* obsessive-compulsive personality disorder is primarily a disorder of maladaptively extreme conscientiousness, including the facets of deliberation (rumination), self-discipline, achievement striving (workaholism), dutifulness (overconscientiousness, scrupulousness about matters of ethics and morality), order (preoccupation with details), and competence (perfectionism). The FFM description also goes beyond the *DSM–IV–TR* diagnostic criteria by including high anxiousness, low impulsiveness, low excitement seeking, and closed mindedness to feelings, values, ideas, and actions. Table 11.2 indicates how each of the *DSM–IV–TR* personality disorders can be understood from the perspective of the FFM. (It may be noted that the FFM conceptualizations in Table 11.2 are, in part, based on the *NEO PI-R* [Costa & McCrae, 1992]. The potential impact of instrument choice is discussed later in this chapter.) Figure 11.1 indicates how each of the 37 maladaptive traits proposed for inclusion in DSM–5 would be organized with respect to the FFM.

There are a number of advantages of an FFM of personality disorder (Widiger & Mullins-Sweatt, 2009; Widiger & Trull, 2007). The dimensional model addresses the many fundamental limitations of the categorical system (e.g., heterogeneity within diagnoses, inadequate coverage, lack of consistent diagnostic thresholds, and excessive diagnostic co-occurrence). It provides a description of abnormal personality functioning within the same model and language used to describe general personality structure, allowing for a more comprehensive system that would enable clinicians to identify personality strengths as well as deficits (Widiger & Lowe, 2007). It would transfer to the psychiatric nomenclature a wealth of knowledge concerning the origins, development, universality, and stability of personality structure (Widiger & Trull, 2007). Finally, it would represent a significant step toward rapprochement and integration of psychiatry with psychology. Empirical support for the integration of the *DSM–IV–TR* personality nomenclature with the FFM is summarized by Clark (2007), Samuel and Widiger (2008a), and Widiger and Cosa (2002).

Table 11.2 *DSM-IV* Personality Disorders From the Perspective of the Five-Factor Model of General Personality Structure

	PRN	SZD	SZT	ATS	BDL	HST	NCS	AVD	DPD	OCP
Neuroticism (vs. emotional stability)										
Anxiousness			H	L	H			H	H	H
Angry Hostility	H			H	H		H			
Depressiveness					H			H		
Self-Consciousness			H	L		L	L	H	H	
Impulsivity				H	H	H		L		L
Vulnerability					H			H	H	
Extraversion (vs. introversion)										
Warmth (vs. coldness)	L	L	L			H	L			
Gregariousness (vs. withdrawal)	L	L	L			H		L		
Assertiveness (vs submissiveness)		L		H		H	H	L	L	
Activity (vs. passivity)		L		H	L	H		L		
Excitement-seeking		L		H		H	H	L	L	L
Positive Emotionality (vs. anhedonia)	L	L	L			H		L		
Openness (vs closedness)										
Fantasy						H				
Aesthetics										
Feelings (vs. alexithymia)		L			H	H	L			L
Actions	L	L		H	H	H	H	L		L
Ideas			H					L		
Values	L							L		
Agreeableness (vs. antagonism)										
Trust (vs. mistrust)	L		L	L	L	H	L		H	
Straightforwardness (vs. deception)	L			L	L		L			
Altruism (vs. aggression)	L			L			L		H	
Compliance (vs. aggression)	L			L	L		L		H	
Modesty (vs. arrogance)					L		L	H	H	
Tender-mindedness (vs. tough-minded)	L			L			L			
Conscientiousness (vs. disinhibition)										
Competence (vs. laxness)										H
Order (vs. disordered)			L							H
Dutifulness (vs. irresponsibility)					L					H
Achievement-striving										H
Self-discipline (vs, negligence)					L		L			H
Deliberation (vs. rashness)				L	L	L				H

Note: PRN, paranoid; SZD, schizoid; SZT, schizotypal; ATS, antisocial; BDL, borderline; HST, histrionic; NCS, narcissistic; AVD, avoidant; DPD, dependent; OCP, obsessive-compulsive; L, low; H, high. Adapted from Lynam and Widiger (2001) and Samuel and Widiger (2004).

Five Personality Disorders and Their Five-Factor Formulations

Space limitations prohibit detailed coverage of all 10 *DSM–IV–TR* personality disorders; but that would seem worthless because up to half are likely to be deleted in DSM–5 (Skodol, 2010). However, the five discussed here are not the same five likely to be retained in DSM–5. We discuss the five personality disorders for which there has been the most research: antisocial, borderline,

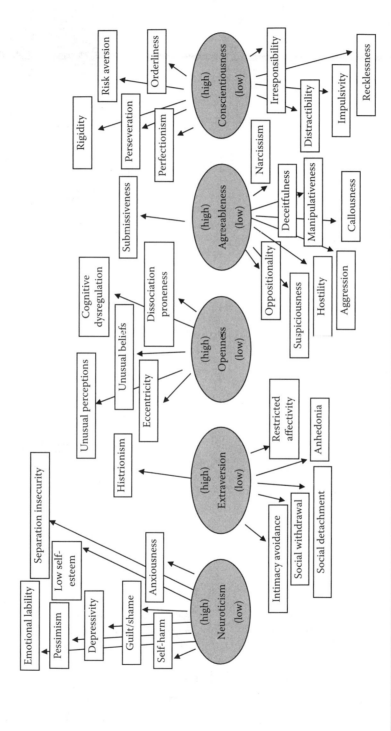

Figure 11.1 Proposed DSM-5 Traits Arranged With Respect to the Five-Factor Model of Personality.

narcissistic, schizotypal, and dependent. The narcissistic and dependent are currently slated for deletion, in favor of the avoidant and obsessive-compulsive, although this may not be the final decision in DSM–5.

The primary rationale for deleting half of the disorders is to address the problematic diagnostic co-occurrence among the 10 disorders (Skodol, 2010). Most patients meet the diagnostic criteria for more than one personality disorder (Clark, 2007; Widiger & Trull, 2007); simply deleting half of the disorders seems a rather draconian solution to this problem (Widiger, 2011). Lack of coverage has also been a problem, and with these deletions this will become much worse. There will still be those with paranoid, schizoid, histrionic, narcissistic, and dependent personality traits even if the diagnoses are not included. Objections have also been raised with respect to which particular diagnoses have been slated for deletion, as there does appear to be more research and clinical utility for narcissistic (Miller, Widiger, & Campbell, 2010; Ronningstam, 2011) and dependency (Bornstein, 2011; Widiger, 2011) than for the avoidant or obsessive-compulsive personality disorders. In any case, for each of the five diagnoses discussed in this chapter, we describe what is known about their etiology, pathology, differential diagnosis, comorbidity, course, and treatment. We also indicate how each of the diagnoses can be understood from the perspective of the FFM of general personality functioning and how this conceptualization can also help to address one or more issues that have been problematic for that personality disorder.

Antisocial Personality Disorder

Antisocial personality disorder (ASPD) has been included within every edition of the *DSM*. One might even characterize ASPD as the prototypic personality disorder as the term *psychopath* originally referred to all cases of personality disorder (Schneider, 1923). Psychopathy now refers to a particularly severe variant of ASPD (Derefinko & Widiger, 2008). Much of the current research on ASPD is being conducted with regard to this more severe variant, as assessed, for instance, by the Psychopathy Checklist-Revised (PCL-R; Hare, 2003; Hare & Neumann, 2008).

Definition DSM–IV–TR defines ASPD as a pervasive pattern of disregard for and violation of the rights of others (APA, 2000). Its primary diagnostic criteria include criminal activity, deceitfulness, impulsivity, recklessness, aggressiveness, irresponsibility, and indifference to the mistreatment of others. *DSM–IV–TR* overlaps substantially with PCL-R psychopathy. The primary differences are the inclusion of glib charm, arrogance, lack of empathy, and shallow affect within the PCL-R, and the requirement within *DSM–IV–TR* for the evidence of conduct disorder within childhood (Widiger, 2006). In DSM–5, the name of the disorder is likely to make reference to both antisocial and psychopathy, and the narrative description for its diagnosis will include additional traits of psychopathy.

Etiology and Pathology Twin, family, and adoption studies have provided substantial support for a genetic contribution to the etiology of the criminal, delinquent tendencies of those meeting criteria for ASPD, accounting for approximately 50% of the variance in antisocial behavior (Waldman & Rhee, 2006). Exactly what is inherited in ASPD, however, is not known. It could be an impulsivity, an antagonistic callousness, an abnormally low anxiousness, or all of these dispositions combined.

Numerous environmental factors have also been implicated in the etiology of antisocial behavior. Shared, or common, environmental influences account for 15–20% of variation in criminality or delinquency (Rhee & Waldman, 2002). Not surprisingly, shared environmental factors such as low family income, inner-city residence, poor parental supervision, single-parent households, rearing by antisocial parents, delinquent siblings, parental conflict, harsh discipline, neglect, large family size, and young mother have all been implicated as risk factors for antisocial behavior (Farrington, 2006). Nonshared environmental influences (30%) comprise the remaining variance not accounted for by the genetic (50%) or shared environmental (20%) influences. Nonshared environmental factors may include delinquent peers, individual social and academic experiences, or sexual or physical abuse (Moffitt, 2005).

The interactive effects of genetic and environmental influences are difficult to separate and likely create confusion about what these estimates mean in terms of causation. For example, the individual who is genetically predisposed to antisocial behavior will likely elicit experiences that can in turn contribute to the development of antisocial behavior, such as peer problems, academic difficulty, and harsh discipline from parents. In other words, the person genetically disposed to antisocial behavior can help create an environment that would reinforce antisocial behavior. In addition, antisocial individuals receive their genes from antisocial parents who had also exhibited delinquent and irresponsible behavior, thus creating a home environment that would model and reinforce instability and criminality. In sum, it can be difficult to disentangle what is really genetic and what is really environmental. Studies that explicitly address these issues have found that environmental factors continue to play a large part in the etiology of antisocial behavior beyond genetic factors alone. For instance, after controlling for the genetic component of physical maltreatment, Jaffee, Caspi, Moffitt, and Taylor (2004) found that the environmental etiological effect of physical maltreatment remained.

Considerable research effort has been focused on the pathology of psychopathy. This extensive research base indicates that many deficits can be involved, leading to a very complex picture. Historically, the psychopathic individual was said to suffer from superego lacunae or a semantic dementia (Cleckley, 1941), which involved a deficit of conscience or, more generally, a deficient processing of feelings and emotion. Laboratory research is now providing support for this theoretical model in studies assessing the psychopath's autonomic reaction to emotional words and fearful images (Blackburn, 2006).

Many psychophysiological deficits have also been associated with psychopathy, including, for example, a low level of physiological arousal or fear response (Fowles & Dindo, 2006). Support for this hypothesis has included abnormally low physiological responses (reduced skin conductance) to a conditioned stimulus paired with electric shock, indicating that a person with psychopathy may not develop the expected anticipatory arousal from threat of physical punishment. Additional autonomic arousal assessments include low resting heart rate levels and startle response deficits (Derefinko & Widiger, 2008). There is also the suggestion that those with ASPD may have abnormally low levels of anxiousness. Some distress proneness (FFM anxiousness or neuroticism) and attentional self-regulation (FFM constraint or conscientiousness) may be necessary to develop an adequate sense of guilt or conscience. Normal levels of neuroticism will promote the internalization of a conscience by associating wrongdoing or misbehavior with distress and anxiety, and the temperament of self-regulation will help modulate impulses into socially acceptable channels (Fowles & Kochanska, 2000).

Cognitive functioning deficits have been implicated. The psychopath's notorious failure to accurately anticipate negative consequences suggests a cognitive deficit (Hiatt & Newman, 2006). Existing research indicates that the psychopath experiences stable deficits in the cognitive domains of attention and response modulation (Gao, Glenn, Schug, Yang, & Raine, 2009). According to this research, psychopaths continue to engage in behaviors that are initially interpreted as positively reinforcing, even when additional information is presented indicating substantial overall costs (Newman & Lorenz, 2003).

Differential Diagnosis ASPD is most closely associated with narcissistic personality traits, the differentiation of which will be discussed later in this chapter. At times, ASPD may be difficult to differentiate from a substance dependence disorder because many with ASPD develop a substance-related disorder, and many with substance dependence engage in antisocial acts. However, the requirement that a conduct disorder be present prior to the age of 15 will usually ensure the onset of ASPD prior to the onset of a substance-related disorder. If both were evident prior to the age of 15, then it is likely that both disorders are present and both diagnoses should be given (Widiger, 2006). Often, ASPD and substance dependence will interact, exacerbating each other's development (Sutker & Allain, 2001).

Epidemiology   The National Institute of Mental Health Epidemiologic Catchment Area (ECA) study estimated that 3% of males and 1% of females meet *DSM* criteria for ASPD (Sutker & Allain, 2001). Subsequent studies have replicated this rate, but it has also been suggested that the ECA finding may have underestimated the prevalence in males due to a failure to consider the full range of ASPD features. Other estimates have been as high as 6% in males (Kessler et al., 1994). Within prison and forensic settings, the rate of ASPD has been estimated to be 50% (Hare, 2003). However, the ASPD criteria may inflate the prevalence within such settings due to the emphasis on overt acts of criminality, delinquency, and irresponsibility (Sutker & Allain, 2001). More specific criteria for psychopathy provided by the PCL-R obtain a more conservative estimate of 20–30% of male prisoners meeting criteria for ASPD (Hare, 2003), by placing relatively less emphasis on the history of criminal behavior and more emphasis on personality traits associated with this criminal history (e.g., callousness and arrogance).

ASPD is much more common in men than in women (Verona & Vitale, 2006). A sociobiological explanation for the differential gender prevalence is the presence of a genetic advantage for social irresponsibility, infidelity, superficial charm, and deceit in men but not women. These traits may be related to reproductive success for men (having more offspring) but also contribute to a higher likelihood of developing features of ASPD (Sutker & Allain, 2001).

Course   ASPD is the only personality disorder for which much is known about childhood antecedents. Approximately 40% of the children with conduct disorder grow up to meet criteria for ASPD, and the presence of conduct disorder is required for the diagnosis of ASPD (APA, 2000). There are also compelling data to indicate that ASPD is a relatively chronic disorder that persists into adulthood, although research suggests that as the person reaches middle to older age, the frequency of criminal acts decreases. Nevertheless, the core personality traits may remain largely stable (Hare, 2003).

Five-Factor Model Reformulation   ASPD can be understood primarily as excessive, maladaptively low conscientiousness and high antagonism (see Table 11.2). Specifically, these individuals would be described as aimless, unreliable, lax, negligent, and hedonistic (low in the facets of self-discipline and deliberation), as well as manipulative, exploitative, aggressive, and ruthless (low in straightforwardness, altruism, compliance, and tender mindedness). Additional facets of the FFM would be seen in prototypic cases of ASPD, including low anxiousness, low self-consciousness (glib charm), low vulnerability (fearlessness), high impulsivity, high angry hostility, and high gregariousness (Lynam & Widiger, 2007a).

An ongoing issue surrounding the *DSM* diagnosis of ASPD has been the failure to include all of the personality traits of psychopathy identified originally by Cleckley (1941), emphasizing instead those traits that could most easily be identified by objectively observed behaviors (e.g., irresponsible or illegal acts). An advantage of the FFM conceptualization of psychopathy is that it includes all of the traits that are common to both ASPD and the PCL-R, including deception, exploitation, aggression, irresponsibility, negligence, rashness, angry hostility, impulsivity, excitement seeking, and assertiveness (see Table 11.2). However, the FFM also includes many of the traits that are unique to the PCL-R, including glib charm (low self-consciousness), arrogance, and lack of empathy (tough-minded callousness). In addition, the FFM includes those traits of psychopathy that had been emphasized originally by Cleckely (1941) but were not included in either the *DSM–IV–TR* or the PCL-R (i.e., low anxiousness and fearlessness). Considerable evidence supports the FFM conceptualization of ASPD (Lynam & Widiger, 2007a). Miller and Lynam (2003) have shown that the extent to which an individual's FFM profile matches the FFM profile for a prototypic case of psychopathy (see Table 11.2) can itself be used as a quantitative indication of the likelihood that a person would be diagnosed as psychopathic.

An FFM conceptualization of ASPD also provides some clarity in regard to the often discussed but poorly understood concept of the "successful psychopath" (Hall & Benning, 2006). Systematic research has been confined largely to the study of the "unsuccessful" psychopath, which typically means the incarcerated criminal (Sutker & Allain, 2001). However, there is considerable social and theoretical interest in understanding those with psychopathy who are equally exploitative, callous, and ruthless, but they either manage never to get arrested or convicted or pursue a white-collar career that only flirts with the edges of the legal system (Hall & Benning, 2006). From the perspective of the FFM, these individuals share many of the traits of the prototypic psychopath (i.e., low anxiousness, high fearlessness, high assertiveness and gregariousness, and high exploitativeness, deceptiveness, and callousness of antagonism), but are high rather than low in the facets of conscientiousness (Mullins-Sweatt, Glover, Derefinko, Miller, & Widiger, 2010). These individuals would be even more dangerous than most of the incarcerated psychopaths because they share the disposition to engage in behavior harmful to others but also possess the traits (deliberation, competence, and self-discipline) that contribute to a more "successful" criminal career. A potential case illustration of such a "successful" psychopath is that of the infamous serial killer Theodore "Ted" Bundy (Samuel & Widiger, 2006).

For many years researchers have attempted to identify the single, core pathology of psychopathy, and a variety of compelling but inconsistent models have been proposed. These alternative conceptualizations can be integrated and their inconsistencies addressed by the FFM (Lynam & Widiger, 2007a). Their apparent inconsistency may reflect that each alternative model of pathology is focusing on a different facet and at times even a different domain of the FFM. Poor fear conditioning and electrodermal hypoarousal (Fowles & Dindo, 2006) would place particular emphasis on low neuroticism (i.e., low anxiousness or low vulnerability). Lack of response modulation, or an inability to refrain from acting on first impulse (Hiatt & Newman, 2006), would focus within the FFM domain of conscientiousness. A deficit in empathy or the processing of affective language (Blackburn, 2006) can be understood in terms of the antagonism facet of callous tough mindedness. In sum, the personality profile for the prototypic psychopath involves a constellation of personality traits that together provides a virulent and at times even lethal mix (i.e., high antagonism, low conscientiousness, low vulnerability, low anxiousness, high assertiveness, high gregariousness, and high excitement seeking). Researchers are approaching this constellation like the blind men from Indostan, each interpreting the elephant upon which they are laying their hands in a much different manner, depending on which component of the FFM is the focus of their attention (Lynam & Widiger, 2007a).

Treatment   ASPD is considered to be the most difficult personality disorder to treat (Gunderson & Gabbard, 2000; Stone, 1993). Individuals with ASPD can be seductively charming and declare a commitment to change, but they often lack sufficient motivation. Their declarations of desire to change might even be dishonest. They will also fail to appreciate the future costs associated with antisocial acts (e.g., imprisonment and lack of meaningful interpersonal relationships), and may stay in treatment only as required by an external source, such as a parole requirement. Residential programs that provide a carefully controlled environment of structure and supervision, combined with peer confrontation, have been recommended (Gunderson &

Gabbard, 2000). However, it is unknown what benefits may be sustained after the ASPD individual leaves this environment. When in inpatient treatment, individuals with ASPD may manipulate and exploit staff and fellow patients. Studies have indicated that outpatient therapy is not likely to be successful, although the extent to which those with ASPD are entirely unresponsive to treatment may have been somewhat exaggerated (Salekin, 2002).

Therapists of individuals with ASPD should anticipate that they may have considerable negative feelings toward clients with extensive histories of aggressive, exploitative, and abusive behaviors (Gunderson & Gabbard, 2000). Rather than attempt to develop a sense of conscience in these individuals, therapeutic techniques should perhaps be focused on rational and utilitarian arguments against repeating past mistakes. These approaches would focus on the tangible, material value of prosocial behavior (Young et al., 2003).

Narcissistic Personality Disorder

This personality disorder was first included in *DSM–III* (APA, 1980). Its inclusion "was suggested by an increasing psychoanalytic literature and by the isolation of narcissism as a personality factor in a variety of psychological studies" (Frances, 1980, p. 1053). However, it is still not included in the World Health Organization's (WHO) *International Classification of Diseases* (*ICD–10*; WHO, 1992), despite its presence in the *DSM* since 1980, as it has been perceived internationally as largely an American concept. It is currently slated for deletion in DSM–5 (Skodol, 2010).

Definition   Narcissistic personality disorder (NPD) is defined in *DSM–IV–TR* as a pervasive pattern of grandiosity (in fantasy or behavior), need for admiration or adulation, and lack of empathy (APA, 2000). Its primary diagnostic criteria include a grandiose sense of self-importance; preoccupation with success, power, brilliance, or beauty; the belief that he or she is special and can only be understood by high-status individuals; a demand for excessive admiration; a strong sense of entitlement; an exploitation of others; a lack of empathy; and arrogance (APA, 2000).

Etiology and Pathology   There has been little systematic research on the etiology of narcissism. Twin studies have supported heritability for narcissistic personality traits (Reichborn-Kjennerud, 2008; Torgersen et al., 2000), although given the trait complexity of narcissism (Fossatti et al., 2005; Morf & Rhodewalt, 2000; Ronningstam, 2005), it is not entirely clear what precisely is being inherited. The predominant models for the etiology of narcissism have been largely social learning or psychodynamic (Ronningstam, 2005). One model proposes that narcissism develops through an excessive idealization by parental figures, which is then incorporated by the child into his or her self-image (Millon et al., 1996). Narcissism may also develop through unempathic, neglectful, inconsistent, or even devaluing parental figures who have failed to adequately mirror a child's natural need for idealization (Kohut, 1977). The child may find that the attention, interest, and perceived love of a parent are contingent largely on achievements or successes. They may fail to perceive the parents as valuing or loving them for their own sake, but may instead recognize that the love and attention are largely conditional on successful accomplishments. They might then develop the belief that their own feelings of self-worth are dependent on a continued recognition by others of such achievements, status, or success. The character armor of arrogant self-confidence then masks a vulnerability and at times rage over the feeling of having been so neglected, and perhaps even mistreated and denigrated, as a child.

Conflicts and deficits with respect to self-esteem are central to the pathology of the disorder (Ronninstam, 2005), and there is considerable empirical support for this pathology in studies published within the general personality literature (Miller et al., 2010; Morf & Rhodewalt, 2001; Pincus & Lukowitsky, 2010). Narcissistic individuals must continually seek and obtain signs and symbols of recognition to compensate for conscious or perhaps even unconscious feelings of inadequacy. Narcissism is not simply arrogant self-confidence, as it is more highly correlated with an instability in self-esteem rather than a consistently high self-confidence. Their feelings of insecurity will at times be evident but may also be masked by a disdainful indifference to criticism or even by overt expressions of anger, rage, or aggression (Miller et al., 2010). Narcissistic individuals may at times claim that it is not narcissism if they are in fact brilliant, talented, and successful. However, the pathology would still be evident by the excessive need for the recognition of their achievements. They are uncomfortable when they are not being adequately appreciated for their accomplishments, and they may in fact feel grossly insulted or enraged when they feel unjustly slighted.

Differential Diagnosis   NPD overlaps substantially with psychopathy (Widiger, 2006). To help differentiate the narcissistic and antisocial personality disorders, it has been suggested that "narcissists are usually more grandiose, while ASPD patients are exploitative, have a superficial value system, and are involved in recurrent antisocial activities" (Ronningstam, 1999, p. 681). It is also suggested that "exploitiveness in antisocial patients is probably more likely to be consciously and actively related to materialistic or sexual gain, while exploitive behavior in narcissistic patients is more passive, serving to enhance self-image by attaining praise or power" (Ronningstam, 1999, p. 681). An alternative view is that these are not in fact qualitatively distinct disorders, but represent instead overlapping constellations of maladaptive personality traits (Lynam & Widiger, 2001). Prototypic cases of narcissism and psychopathy will share the features of lack of empathy, exploitation of others, and arrogance, but most cases will have varying degrees of these traits. Rather than try to determine which diagnosis is the correct one, it might be best simply to describe the extent to which each respective narcissistic or psychopathic trait is present within any particular person (Widiger & Lowe, 2007).

Epidemiology   NPD is among the least frequently diagnosed personality disorders within clinical settings, with estimates of prevalence as low as 2% (APA, 2000). A curious finding is that many community studies that have used a semistructured interview have not even been able to identify one single case (see Table 11.1), despite the substantial amount of research on maladaptive narcissistic personality traits within normal community and college samples (Morf & Rhodewalt, 2001; Pincus & Lukowitsky, 2010; Ronningstam, 2005). It may be that the *DSM–IV–TR* diagnostic criteria do not fully capture all of the important features of NPD or place too much emphasis on a grandiosity that is rarely actually present (Pincus & Lukowitsky, 2010). *DSM–IV–TR* NPD is diagnosed more frequently in males (APA, 2000), consistent with the finding within general personality research that men tend to be, on average, more arrogant than women (Lynam & Widiger, 2007b).

Course   NPD does not generally abate with age and may even become more evident into middle or older age. Those with this disorder might be seemingly well adjusted and even successful as a young adult, having experienced substantial achievements in education, career, and perhaps even within relationships (Ronningstam, 2005). However, there is a considerable body of research demonstrating an association of narcissism with relationship failure (Miller et al., 2010). Relationships with colleagues, peers, and intimates can become strained over time as their lack of consideration for and even exploitative use of others becomes cumulatively evident. Successes might also become more infrequent with age as their inability to accurately perceive or address criticism and setback contributes to a mounting number of defeats. Those with this disorder may at times not recognize their pathology until they have had a substantial number of setbacks or they have finally recognized that the excessive importance they have given to achievement, success, and status has led to an emptiness and loneliness in their older age (Stone, 1993). As a result, mid-life and late-life transitions may be particularly difficult.

Five-Factor Model Reformulation   One of the facets of FFM antagonism is arrogance, the central trait of NPD (APA, 2000; Millon et al., 1996). However, as indicated in Table 11.2, additional traits of narcissism can also be described in terms of the FFM. An advantage of the FFM dimensional classification is the ability to distinguish between arrogant individuals who are high versus low in neuroticism (Samuel & Widiger, 2008b). A longstanding concern within the clinical literature on narcissism is the distinction between the narcissistic person who is consistently self-confident, arrogant, and conceited (described as the arrogant or grandiose narcissist; Pincus & Lukowitsky, 2010; Ronningstam, 2005) versus the narcissistic person who is quite insecure and self-conscious (referred to as the shy or vulnerable narcissist). The dimensional perspective of the FFM would not create a further subtyping of a diagnostic category to account for this variation but would simply describe the extent to which a person who is high in arrogance is also low in the anxiousness, self-consciousness, and vulnerability facets of neuroticism. Further distinctions would be provided by the extent to which the person is low in extraversion (the shy narcissist) versus high in extraversion (the outgoing, interpersonally engaging narcissist), or high in conscientiousness (the narcissist who is relatively successful in school, college, and career).

Treatment   Those with NPD rarely seek treatment for their narcissism. Individuals with NPD usually enter treatment to seek assistance for another mental disorder, such as substance abuse (secondary to career stress), mood disorder (secondary to career setback), or even something quite specific, such as test anxiety. One may at times find narcissistic individuals who seek treatment for a growing sense of discontent and futility with their lives (Ronningstam, 2005). Once an individual with NPD is in treatment, he or she will have difficulty perceiving the relationship as collaborative and will likely attempt to dominate, impress, or devalue the therapist. They can idealize their therapists (to affirm that the therapist is indeed of sufficient status or quality to be treating them), but they may also devalue the therapist to affirm to themselves that they are of greater intelligence, capacity, and quality to reject the insights they have failed to identify themselves or to indicate they warrant or deserve an even better therapist. How best to respond is often unclear, as the establishment and maintenance of rapport will be an early and ongoing issue. It may at times be preferable to simply accept the praise or criticism, particularly when exploration will likely be unsuccessful, whereas at other times it is preferable to confront and discuss the motivation for the devaluation (or the idealization). Therapists must be careful not to become embroiled within intellectual conflicts and competitions. Narcissistic individuals can be acutely aware of the self-esteem conflicts of their therapist, and it is best for the therapist to model a comfortable indifference to losing disputes or conflicts.

Borderline Personality Disorder

Borderline personality disorder (BPD) was a new edition to *DSM–III* (Spitzer, Endicott, & Gibbon, 1979). However, it has since become the single most frequently diagnosed (Gunderson, 2001) and studied (Blashfield & Intoccia, 2000) personality disorder.

Definition   BPD is a pervasive pattern of impulsivity and instability in interpersonal relationships, affect, and self-image (APA, 2000). Its primary diagnostic criteria include frantic efforts to avoid abandonment, unstable and intense relationships, impulsivity (e.g., substance abuse, binge eating, or sexual promiscuity), recurrent suicidal thoughts and gestures, self-mutilation, and episodes of rage and anger.

Etiology and Pathology   There are studies supportive of BPD as a disorder with a distinct genetic disposition, but many studies have also suggested a shared genetic association with mood and impulse control disorders (Torgersen, 2005b). There is also substantial empirical support for a childhood history of physical or sexual abuse, parental conflict, loss, and neglect (Silk, Wolf, Ben-Ami, & Poortinga, 2005). Past traumatic events are present in many (if not most) cases of BPD, contributing to the comorbidity with posttraumatic stress and dissociative disorders (Gunderson, 2001; Hefferman & Cloitre, 2000). BPD is perhaps best understood as an interaction of an emotionally unstable temperament with a cumulative and evolving series of intensely pathogenic relationships (Gunderson, 2001; Widiger, 2005b).

The pathogenic mechanisms of BPD are addressed in numerous theories. Most concern issues of abandonment, separation, or exploitative abuse. Those with BPD will often describe quite intense, disturbed, or abusive relationships with significant individuals in their past (Gunderson, 2001). The development of malevolent perceptions and expectations of others is not surprising (Ornduff, 2000). These malevolent expectations and lingering feelings of bitterness and rage, along with an impairment in the ability to regulate affect (Linehan, 1993), may contribute to the perpetuation of intense, hostile, and unstable relationships.

Differential Diagnosis   Most individuals with BPD develop quite a number of Axis I mental disorders, including mood, dissociative, eating, substance use, and anxiety disorders (Pfohl, 2005). It can be difficult to differentiate BPD from these disorders if the assessment is confined to current symptomatology (Gunderson, 2001). The diagnostic criteria for BPD require that the symptomatology be evident since adolescence, which should differentiate BPD from Axis I disorder in all cases other than a chronic mood disorder. If a chronic mood disorder is present, then the additional features of transient, stress-related paranoid ideation, dissociative experiences, impulsivity, and anger dyscontrol of BPD should be emphasized in the diagnosis (Gunderson, 2001).

Epidemiology   It is estimated that 1–2% of the general population would meet the *DSM–IV–TR* criteria for BPD (see Table 11.1). BPD is the most prevalent personality disorder within most clinical settings (although perhaps not the most prevalent in community settings; see Table 11.1). Approximately 15% of all inpatients (51% of inpatients with a personality disorder) and 8% of all outpatients (27% of outpatients with a personality disorder) will meet the criteria for BPD. Approximately 75% of those diagnosed with BPD are female (Lynam & Widiger, 2007b).

Course   Individuals with BPD are likely to report having been emotionally unstable, impulsive, and hostile as children; however, there is little longitudinal research on the childhood antecedents of BPD (Gunderson, 2001; Silk et al., 2005). As adolescents, their intense affectivity and impulsivity may contribute to involvement with rebellious groups, along with a variety of Axis I disorders, including eating, substance, and mood disorders. BPD is at times diagnosed in children and adolescents, but considerable caution should be used when doing so, as some of the symptoms of BPD (e.g., identity disturbance, hostility, and unstable relationships) could be confused with a normal adolescent rebellion or identity crisis (Ad-Dab'bagh & Greenfield, 2001; Gunderson, 2001).

Adults with BPD may be repeatedly hospitalized due to their affect and impulse dyscontrol, psychotic-like and dissociative symptomatology, and suicide attempts (Gunderson, 2001). The risk of suicide is increased with a comorbid mood disorder and substance-related disorder. It is estimated that 3–10% of those with BPD will commit suicide by the age of 30 (Gunderson, 2001). Intimate relationships tend to be unstable and explosive, and employment history is generally poor (Stone, 2001). As the person reaches the age of 30, affective lability and impulsivity may begin to diminish. These symptoms may lessen earlier if the person becomes involved with a supportive and patient sexual partner (Stone, 2001). Some, however, may achieve stability only by abandoning the effort to obtain a relationship, opting instead for a lonelier but less volatile life. Occurrence of a severe stressor, however, can easily disrupt the lessening of symptomatology, resulting in a brief psychotic, dissociative, or mood disorder episode.

A controversy within the research literature is the rate of remission of BPD. Two longitudinal studies provide quite high estimates for remission (Skodol et al., 2005; Zanarini, Frankenburg, Hennen, Reich, & Silk, 2005). However, a considerable portion of these findings may have simply represented diagnostic errors (Widiger, 2005a). Gunderson et al. (2003) provided details concerning the recent history for many of the 18 borderlines described as experiencing sudden, dramatic remissions within the first 6 months of the onset of the Collaborative Longitudinal Personality Disorders study (Skodol et al., 2005). For one of the participants, the symptoms were attributed to the use of a stimulant for weight reduction during the year prior to the beginning of the study:

> [T]he most dramatic improvement following a treatment intervention occurred when a subject discontinued a psychostimulant she had used the year prior to baseline for purposes of weight loss.... Discontinuation was followed by a dramatic reduction of her depression, panic, abandonment fears, and self-destructiveness. (Gunderson et al., 2003, p. 116)

Five of the 18 remissions "had the dramatic reduction of BPD criteria at the same time as the remission of a coexisting Axis I disorder.... In these five cases, the remission of the Axis I disorder was judged to be the most likely cause for the sudden BPD improvement" (Gunderson et al., 2003, p. 114). The remission for the rest of the cases involved gaining relief from severely stressful situations they were in at the time of the baseline assessment.

Warner et al. (2004), using data from the Collaborative Longitudinal Personality Disorders study, considered the role of FFM personality traits in accounting for the symptoms of BPD over time. They first indicated that BPD features, as diagnosed according to *DSM–IV–TR*, do change over time, but that there appears to be common latent variables underlying the personality traits and BPD symptoms. Most important:

> the results indicate that there is a specific temporal relationship between traits and disorder whereby changes in the [FFM] personality traits hypothesized to underlie personality disorders lead to subsequent changes in the disorder [but] this relationship does not seem to hold in the opposite direction, which supports the contention that personality disorders stem from particular constellations of personality traits. (Warner et al., 2004, pp. 222–223)

Five-Factor Model Reformulation   BPD is primarily composed of excessively high neuroticism. In particular, these individuals are at the very highest range of anxiousness, angry hostility, depressiveness, impulsiveness, and vulnerability (see Table 11.2). Borderline clients will also likely be low in the agreeableness facets of trust and compliance and low on the conscientiousness facet of competence. Describing individuals with BPD as being high in neuroticism may not convey well the severity of this personality disorder, as the term *neuroticism* refers to the normal range of the domain. Those diagnosed with BPD will be at the very highest levels within the population for angry hostility (e.g., episodes of rage), vulnerability (frantic efforts to avoid abandonment), depressiveness (suicidal ideation), and anxiousness (panicked reactions to stress). The correlation of FFM neuroticism with BPD (Samuel & Widiger, 2008a) is almost as high as any two borderline measures correlate with another (Widiger & Boyd, 2009).

Morey and Zanarini (2000) provided FFM data on 290 patients who met the diagnostic criteria for BPD. They reported that the FFM did account well for BPD symptoms, particularly the domain of neuroticism. They concluded:

[T]he FFM could indicate a temperamental vulnerability to a disorder that is then triggered by developmental events (such as childhood neglect or abuse), resulting in functional levels that may be quite variable in response to situational elements even while the underlying traits remain relatively stable. (Morey & Zanarini, 2000, p. 737)

Trull, Widiger, Lynam, and Costa (2003) replicated and extended the findings of Morey and Zanarini (2000). They developed an FFM borderline index by correlating each participant's FFM profile, as assessed by the *NEO PI-R* (Costa & McCrae, 1992), with the prototypic FFM trait profile provided by Lynam and Widiger (2001). The correlation of each participant's actual FFM trait profile with the profile of a prototypic case was then used as a numerical index of the extent to which the participant had a BPD from the perspective of the FFM. They reported that this FFM borderline index correlated with self-report measures of BPD as highly as these self-report measures correlated with one another.

The FFM conceptualization of BPD is helpful in explaining its substantial prevalence within clinical settings and its excessive diagnostic comorbidity. Those with BPD are likely to meet the *DSM–IV–TR* criteria for at least one other personality disorder, particularly histrionic, dependent, antisocial, schizotypal, or passive aggressive (Gunderson, 2001). A diagnostic category defined primarily by all of the facets of neuroticism (i.e., vulnerability to stress, impulse dyscontrol, anxiousness, depressiveness, and other components of negative affectivity) should be highly prevalent within clinical settings. In addition, all of the other *DSM–IV–TR* personality disorders include at least some components of neuroticism. Lynam and Widiger (2001) demonstrated that much of the diagnostic co-occurrence of BPD with other personality disorders can be explained by the facets of neuroticism held in common.

Treatment   Clients with BPD form relationships with therapists that are similar to their other significant relationships; that is, the therapeutic relationship can often be tremendously unstable, intense, and volatile. Ongoing consultation with colleagues is recommended to address the therapist's negative reactions toward the client (e.g., distancing, rejecting, or abandoning the patient in response to feelings of anger or frustration) as well as positive reactions (e.g., fantasies of being the therapist who in fact rescues or cures the patient or romantic, sexual feelings in response to a seductive patient). Sessions should emphasize the building of a strong therapeutic alliance, monitoring self-destructive and suicidal behaviors, validation of suffering and abusive experience (but also helping the client take responsibility for actions), promotion of self-reflection rather than impulsive action, and setting limits on self-destructive behavior (Gunderson, 2001). The tendency of borderline patients to engage in "splitting" (polarization of an emotional response) should also be carefully monitored and addressed (e.g., devaluation of prior therapists, coupled with idealization of current therapist).

The APA (2001) has published practice guidelines for the psychotherapeutic and pharmacologic treatment of those with BPD. Because borderline patients can present with significant suicide risk, a thorough evaluation of the potential for suicidal ideation and activity should have the initial priority. Also, many patients with BPD will have comorbid Axis I disorders, some of which might take priority (e.g., major depressive disorder, substance dependence, or dissociative disorder).

There is empirical support for both psychodynamic and cognitive-behavioral treatments of BPD (APA, 2001; Paris, 2009). The most common version of the former approach is mentalization-based treatment (MBT; Bateman & Fonagy, 2010). MBT uses many structured techniques to help those with BPD to mentalize, or stand outside their feelings, and more accurately observe the feelings within themselves and others. The most common form of cognitive-behavioral BPD treatment is dialectical behavior therapy (DBT; Lynch, Trost, Salsman, & Linehan, 2007). The dialectical component of DBT was derived largely from Zen Buddhist principles of overcoming suffering through acceptance (Linehan, 1993). Mastery of conflict is achieved in part through no longer struggling or fighting adversity; pain is overcome when it is accepted as an inevitable, fundamental part of life. This principle is taught in part through the meditative technique of mindfulness, in which one attempts to empty one's mind of all thoughts, but accepts whenever and wherever the mind naturally travels. DBT initially focuses on reducing self-harm and parasuicidal behaviors that are disruptive to treatment. Contracts may be implemented, where time with the therapist is limited secondary to treatment for disruptive behavior. This can even go so far as to include suspension of treatment secondary to suicidal behavior. After mastery of treatment for disruptive behavior, DBT teaches coping skills focused on emotional control and interpersonal relatedness. Individuals in DBT attend regular sessions with an individual therapist and discuss problems in applying the new skills. These sessions are augmented with a didactic skills-training group.

Schizotypal Personality Disorder

Schizotypal personality disorder (STPD) was a new addition to *DSM–III*. It was developed through the process of constructing BPD, both being gleaned from broad clinical and research literature discussing cases of "borderline schizophrenia," "borderline personality," "latent schizophrenia," and similar constructs (Spitzer et al., 1979).

Definition   STPD is characterized by a pervasive pattern of social and interpersonal deficits marked by an acute discomfort with close relationships, eccentricities of behavior, and cognitive-perceptual aberrations. Its diagnostic criterion set was developed originally from studies of biological relatives of those diagnosed with schizophrenia (Spitzer et al., 1979). Diagnostic criteria for STPD include odd beliefs, magical thinking, social withdrawal, unusual perceptual experiences, odd speech, inappropriate or constricted affect, social anxiety, and social withdrawal.

Etiology and Pathology   STPD is not included within the personality disorder section of the *ICD–10*, where it is classified instead as a form of schizophrenia (WHO, 1992). There is compelling empirical support for a genetic association of STPD with schizophrenia (Fanous, Gardner, Walsh, & Kendler, 2001), which is not surprising given that the diagnostic criteria were obtained from the observations of biological relatives of those with schizophrenia (Miller, Useda, Trull, Burr, & Minks-Brown, 2001; Siever & Davis, 2004).

A predominant model for the psychopathology of STPD is deficits or defects in the attention and selection processes that organize a person's cognitive-perceptual evaluation of and relatedness to his or her environment (Raine, 2006). These deficits may lead to discomfort within social situations, misperceptions and suspicions, and a coping strategy of social isolation. Correlates of central nervous system dysfunction seen in those with schizophrenia have been observed in STPD laboratory studies, including performance on tests of visual and auditory attention (e.g., backward masking and sensory gating tests) and smooth pursuit eye movement (Parnas, Licht, & Bovet, 2005). This dysfunction may be the result of dysregulation along dopaminergic pathways, which could be serving to modulate the expression of an underlying schizotypal genotype.

Differential Diagnosis   An initial concern for many clinicians when confronted with a person with STPD is whether the more appropriate diagnosis might be schizophrenia. Those with more severe variants of STPD can closely resemble individuals within the prodromal (or residual) phase of schizophrenia (APA, 2000). A differentiation of the two conditions can be guided in part by age of onset and whether there is a recent deterioration in functioning. Those with STPD will have evidenced their social anxiety, social withdrawal, magical thinking, odd behavior, and perceptual aberrations since childhood and will not typically be characterized by any recent deterioration in functioning. Longitudinal follow-up would provide the conclusive differentiation, as a prodromal phase of schizophrenia will eventually be followed by an active psychotic episode.

The close relationship of STPD to the phenomenology, genetics, and pathology of schizophrenia has suggested that perhaps it should in fact be classified in future editions of the *DSM* as a variant of schizophrenia rather than a personality disorder (First et al., 2002). However, contrary to this proposal are the findings that schizophrenia itself may have polygenetic determinants (not all of which will be evident in those with schizotypia), STPD is much more comorbid with other personality disorders than with psychotic disorders, and schizotypal symptomatology appears to be evident within the general population with no apparent relationship to schizophrenia (Raine, 2006).

The more problematic differential diagnoses for STPD will often be other personality disorders, particularly the schizoid and avoidant. The schizoid personality disorder shares the feature of social withdrawal but is distinguished from the schizotypal by the absence of social anxiety and the cognitive-perceptual aberrations. Central to schizoid personality disorder is an anhedonia that provides the temperament basis for the social withdrawal (Parnas et al., 2005). Just as STPD might represent subsyndromal positive symptoms of schizophrenia (e.g., cognitive-perceptual aberrations and magical thinking), the schizoid may represent subsyndromal negative symptoms (social and physical anhedonia). Avoidant personality disorder also shares the feature of social withdrawal, as well as social anxiety, but the social anxiety of STPD does not diminish with familiarity, and the anxiety of the avoidant is concerned primarily with the initiation of a relationship (APA, 2000). STPD is also a more severe disorder that includes the cognitive and perceptual aberrations that are not seen in those with avoidant personality disorder.

Epidemiology STPD may occur in as much as 3% of the general population, although most studies with semistructured interviews have suggested a somewhat lower percentage (see Table 11.1). STPD might occur somewhat more often in males (Parnas et al., 2005; Raine, 2006). Common Axis I disorders are major depressive disorder and generalized social phobia (Miller et al., 2001).

Course There is insufficient research to describe the childhood precursors of adult STPD (Widiger, De Clerq, & De Fruyt, 2009). There are studies on infant and childhood neurodevelopmental abnormalities of those with STPD (Parnas et al., 2005; Raine, 2006). They would be expected to appear peculiar and odd to their peers and may have been teased or ostracized. Achievement in school might be impaired, and they may have been heavily involved in esoteric fantasies and peculiar interests. As adults, they may drift toward esoteric, fringe groups that support their magical thinking and aberrant beliefs. These activities can provide structure for some with STPD, but they can also contribute to a further loosening and deterioration if there is an encouragement of aberrant experiences. The symptomatology of STPD does not appear to remit with age (Miller et al., 2001; Raine, 2006). The course appears to be relatively stable, with some proportion of schizotypal individuals remaining marginally employed, withdrawn, and transient throughout their lives. Some who meet *DSM–IV–TR* criteria for STPD do eventually go on to develop schizophrenia (Walker, Kestler, Bollini, & Hochman, 2004). However, the vast majority of cases do not (Raine, 2006). Schizotypal symptomatology, as measured in scales assessing cognitive-perceptual aberrations, magical thinking, and social and physical anhedonia, have been studied longitudinally in a number of community samples, and the findings to date do not suggest any meaningful likelihood of the development of schizophrenia (Gooding, Tallent, & Matts, 2005).

Five-Factor Model Reformulation   The FFM conceptualization of STPD proposes it as a disorder of personality, including introversion (social withdrawal) and the anxiousness facet of neuroticism. Key to STPD are the magical ideation, cognitive-perceptual aberrations, and eccentric behaviors, which are considered within the FFM of personality disorder to be maladaptive variants of openness to ideas, fantasies, and actions (Widiger, Trull, Clarkin, Sanderson, & Costa, 2002), as supported in a number of empirical studies (e.g., Camisa et al., 2005; Kwapil, Barrantes-Vidas, & Silvia, 2008; Ross, Lutz, & Bailey, 2002).

The relationship of FFM general personality structure to maladaptive personality functioning has not been as strong for openness as it has been for the other domains of the FFM (Samuel & Widiger, 2008a; Widiger, 2011). This may be due in part to a limitation of the *NEO PI-R* (Costa & McCrae, 1992), the predominately used measure of the FFM. Haigler and Widiger (2001) reported insignificant correlations of *NEO PI-R* (Costa & McCrae, 1992) openness with three measures of STPD. They revised *NEO PI-R* openness items by inserting words to indicate that the behavior described within the item was excessive, extreme, or maladaptive. The content of the items was not otherwise altered. This experimentally revised openness scale then obtained significant correlations with all three measures of STPD. Haigler and Widiger (2001) concluded that their findings

> offer further support for the hypothesis that personality disorders are maladaptive variants of normal personality traits by indicating that correlations of NEO PI-R [openness with schizotypal symptomatology] would ... be obtained by simply altering existing NEO PI-R ... items that describe desirable, adaptive behaviors or traits into items that describe undesirable, maladaptive variants of the same traits. (p. 356)

Their findings also suggest a limitation of the *NEO PI-R* as a measure of maladaptive personality functioning.

Treatment   Those with STPD may seek treatment for anxiousness, perceptual disturbances, or depression. Treatment of those with STPD should include cognitive, behavioral, supportive, or pharmacologic options, as they will often find the intimacy and emotionality of reflective, exploratory psychotherapy to be too stressful, and they have the potential for psychotic decompensation (Stone, 1993).

Those with STPD will often fail to consider their social isolation and aberrant cognitions and perceptions to be particularly problematic or maladaptive. They may consider themselves to be simply eccentric, creative, or nonconformist. Rapport can be difficult to develop, as increasing familiarity and intimacy may only increase their level of discomfort and anxiety (Millon et al., 1996). They are unlikely to be responsive to informality or playful humor. The sessions should be well structured to curb loose and tangential ideation.

Practical advice is usually helpful and often necessary (Beck et al., 1990). The therapist should serve as the patient's counselor or guide to more adaptive decisions with respect to everyday problems (e.g., finding an apartment, interviewing for a job, and personal appearance). Those with STPD should also receive social skills training directed at their awkward and odd behavior, mannerisms, dress, and speech. There should be specific, concrete discussions on what to expect and do in various social situations (e.g., formal meetings, casual encounters, and dates; Stone, 1993).

Most of the systematic empirical research on the treatment of STPD has been confined to pharmacologic interventions. Low doses of neuroleptic medications (e.g., thiothixene) have shown some effectiveness in the treatment of schizotypal symptoms, particularly the perceptual aberrations and social anxiousness (Markovitz, 2001). Group therapy has also been recommended for those with STPD, but only when the group is highly structured and supportive (Millon et al., 1996). The emotional intensity and intimacy of unstructured groups will usually be too stressful. Schizotypal patients with predominant paranoid symptoms may even have difficulty in highly structured groups.

Dependent Personality Disorder

A diagnosis of dependent personality disorder (DPD) was, technically speaking, a new addition to *DSM–III*. However, a diagnosis of passive-dependent personality trait disturbance was included in *DSM–I*. This diagnosis is slated for deletion in DSM–5 (Skodol, 2010).

Definition   DPD involves a pervasive and excessive need to be taken care of that leads to submissiveness, clinging, and fears of separation (APA, 2000; Bornstein, 2005; Pincus & Wilson, 2001). Its primary diagnostic criteria include extreme difficulty making decisions without others' input, need for others to assume responsibility for most aspects of daily life, extreme difficulty disagreeing with others, inability to initiate projects due to lack of self-confidence, and going to excessive lengths to obtain the approval of others.

Etiology and Pathology   Insecure interpersonal attachment is considered to be central to the etiology and pathology of DPD (Bornstein, 2005; Pincus & Wilson, 2001; Stone, 1993), although there is actually limited empirical research concerning the etiology and pathology of DPD. Insecure attachment and helplessness may be generated through a parent–child relationship, perhaps by a clinging parent or by continued infantilization during a time in which individuation and separation normally occurs (Gabbard, 2000). However, the combination of an anxious or inhibited temperament with inconsistent or overprotective parenting may also generate and exacerbate dependent personality traits (Bornstein, 2005). Unable to generate feelings of security and confidence for themselves, dependent individuals may rely on a parental figure for constant reassurance of their worth. Eventually, those with DPD may come to believe that their self-worth is defined by their importance to another person (Beck et al., 1990).

Differential Diagnosis   Excessively dependent behavior may be seen in those who have developed debilitating mental and physical conditions, such as agoraphobia, schizophrenia, dementia, or following severe injuries. However, a diagnosis of DPD requires the presence of the dependent traits to be present since late childhood or adolescence (APA, 2000). One can diagnose the presence of a personality disorder at any age during a person's lifetime, but if (for example) a DPD diagnosis is given to a person at the age of 75, this presumes that the dependent behavior was evident since the age of approximately 18 (i.e., predates the onset of a comorbid physical disorder secondary to aging).

Differences in personality due to differing cultural norms should not be confused with the presence of a personality disorder (Bornstein, 2005; Millon & Grossman, 2005). Cultural groups will differ greatly in the degree of importance attached to deferent behavior, politeness, and passivity. The diagnosis of DPD requires that the dependent behavior result in clinically significant functional impairment or distress.

Epidemiology   DPD is one of the more prevalent personality disorders, and it is estimated to occur in 5–30% of patients and 2–4% of the general community (Mattia & Zimmerman, 2001).

Studies have indicated that dependent personality traits are a risk factor for the development of depression in response to interpersonal loss (Blatt, 2004; Bornstein, 2005; Hammen, 2005; Zuroff, Mongrain, & Santor, 2004).

Course   To the extent that independent responsibility and initiative are required, job functioning will be impaired or unsatisfactory. Individuals with DPD are prone to mood disorders throughout life, particularly major depression and dysthymia, and to anxiety disorders, particularly agoraphobia, social phobia, and panic disorder (Bornstein, 2005). However, the severity of the symptomatology will tend to lessen with age, particularly if the person has obtained a reliable, empathic partner.

The self-esteem of someone with DPD is said to depend substantially on the maintenance of a supportive and nurturing relationship (Blatt, 2004; Bornstein, 2005), yet these intense needs for reassurance can have the paradoxical effect of driving the needed person away. The dependent person's worst fears are then realized (i.e., he or she is abandoned and alone), and his or her sense of self-worth, meaning, or value is then furthered injured, perhaps even crushed by the rejection (Shahar, Joiner, Zuroff, & Blatt, 2004). The dependent person might then indiscriminately select a readily available but unreliable (and perhaps even abusive) person simply to be with someone (Widiger & Lowe, in press). This partner would again reaffirm the worst fears through the abuse, derogation, and denigration (i.e., conveying to the dependent person that he or she is indeed undesirable and unlovable and that the relationship is again tenuous). In other words, a combination of evocative, reactive, and then proactive transactions with the environment are the means by which a dependent personality style can lead to depression.

Research on the relationship of dependency to depression, however, is not without fundamental concerns (Coyne, Thompson, & Whiffen, 2004). An important focus of future research will be a further articulation of the precise process or mechanism through which this association occurs. In theory, dependent personality traits contribute to the instability of intimate and supportive relationships through the expression of excessive needs for reassurance or a premorbid emotional instability and pathogenic cognitions that contribute to intense feelings of helplessness and neediness. However, it is also possible that the emotional instability and pathologic attitudes are themselves the result of unstable interpersonal relationships. Dependency is a personality disposition that is seen much more often in women than in men (Lynam & Widiger, 2007b). A provocative reformulation of dependency in women is that the apparent feelings of insecurity may say less about the women than the individuals with whom the women are involved. "Men and women may differ in what they seek from relationships, but they may also differ in what they provide to each other" (Coyne & Whiffen, 1995, p. 368). In other words, "women might appear (and be) less dependent if they weren't involved with such undependable men" (Widiger & Anderson, 2003, p. 63).

Five-Factor Model Reformulation   Dependent personality is characterized in terms of the FFM by maladaptively high levels of agreeableness (meek, gullible, and compliant) and the neuroticism facets of anxiousness, self-consciousness, and vulnerability (see Table 11.2). McCrae and Costa (1987) stated that extremely high scores on the *NEO PI-R* agreeableness may describe a "dependent and fawning" (p. 88) person, and researchers have verified an association between the FFM domain of agreeableness and dependent personality disorder symptomatology (Samuel & Widiger, 2008a). Some studies have failed to confirm the association (Bornstein & Cecero, 2000), but this again appears to be due to the finding that the most commonly used measure of the FFM, the *NEO PI-R*, does not adequately assess maladaptively high levels of agreeableness (Lowe, Edmundson, & Widiger, 2009).

A controversial issue in the diagnosis of DPD is its differential gender prevalence (Morey, Alexander, & Boggs, 2005; Widiger, 2007b). DPD is diagnosed much more frequently in females (APA, 2000), and some have argued that this may reflect a masculine bias toward what constitutes a personality disorder (Kaplan, 1983; Morey et al., 2005) or a failure of males to acknowledge the presence of dependency needs (Bornstein, 2005). One difficulty in resolving this issue is the absence of any gold standard or even theoretical basis for hypothesizing, let alone determining, whether there should in fact be a differential gender prevalence rate. Understanding the *DSM–IV–TR* personality disorders from the perspective of the FFM, however, does provide a theoretical basis for gender difference expectations (Lynam & Widiger, 2007b). Researchers have consistently found that women tend to score higher than men on the domains of agreeableness and neuroticism (Costa & McCrae, 1992). Costa, Terracciano, and McCrae (2001) found these differences to be consistent across 26 cultures, ranging from very traditional (Pakistan) to modern (the Netherlands). Thus, to the extent that DPD is a maladaptive variant of FFM agreeableness and neuroticism, one should then expect to obtain a differential gender prevalence rate. This is not to suggest, however, that no gender bias operates in clinical assessments. Gender stereotyping could occur in clinical settings, due in part to the relationship of DPD to common gender differences.

Studies have indicated that some self-report inventories are providing gender-biased assessments of DPD (Lindsay, Sankis, & Widiger, 2000). The Millon Clinical Multiaxial Inventory (MCMI–III; Millon, Millon, Davis, & Grossman, 2009) and the Minnesota Multiphasic Personality Inventory (MMPI-2; Colligan, Morey, & Offord, 1994) are personality disorder inventories that include gender-related items that are keyed in the direction of adaptive rather than maladaptive functioning. An item need not assess for dysfunction to contribute to a valid assessment of personality disorders. For example, items assessing for gregariousness can identify histrionic individuals, items assessing for confidence can identify narcissistic individuals, and items assessing conscientiousness can identify obsessive-compulsive individuals (Millon et al., 2009). Items keyed in the direction of adaptive rather than maladaptive functioning can also be helpful in countering the tendency of some respondents to deny or minimize personality disorder symptomatology. However, these items will not be useful in differentiating abnormal from normal personality functioning, and they are likely to contribute to an overdiagnosis of personality disorders in normal or minimally dysfunctional populations, such as seen in student counseling centers, child custody disputes, and personnel selection (Widiger & Boyd, 2009).

Treatment   There are no empirically validated treatments for DPD. Treatment recommendations are based essentially on anecdotal clinical experience. Those with DPD will often be in treatment for one or more Axis I disorders, particularly a mood (depressive) or an anxiety disorder. These individuals will tend to be very agreeable, compliant, and grateful, at times to excess (Bornstein, 2005). Many with DPD will find that the therapeutic relationship itself satisfies their need for support and concern and they may then desist from seeking a partner. The therapist can be perceived as the caring partner who will always be there. The dependent client might then even fear success in the treatment because termination may shortly follow (Gabbard, 2000). Thus, the client may remain excessively compliant and agreeable to be a patient that the therapist would continue to treat. Therapists should be careful neither to encourage unwittingly this submissiveness to maintain a "peaceful" therapeutic milieu nor to reject the client to be rid of his or her clinging dependency.

An important component of treatment will often be a thorough exploration of the need for support and its root causes. Cognitive-behavioral techniques can be useful to address feelings of inadequacy and helplessness and to provide training in assertiveness and problem-solving techniques (Beck et al., 1990; Young et al., 2003). Group therapy may be useful for those with

DPD, providing interpersonal feedback and modeling autonomous behavior. DPD is not known to respond to pharmacotherapy.

Conclusions

Maladaptive personality traits can be the focus of clinical treatment and will often impair or impede the treatment of other mental disorders. Reviews of practitioners' clinical records suggest that personality disorders are not being diagnosed as frequently as they in fact occur, perhaps because it can be difficult to obtain insurance coverage for their treatment. This is regrettable because some maladaptive personality traits (e.g., borderline and antisocial) have substantial social and public health care costs.

The five-factor model offers a compelling alternative to the categorical diagnosis of personality disorders as provided in *DSM–IV–TR*. Advantages of understanding personality disorders in terms of this dimensional model are the provision of more specific descriptions of individual patients (including adaptive as well as maladaptive personality functioning), the avoidance of arbitrary categorical distinctions, and the ability to bring to bear the extensive amount of research on the heritability, temperament, development, and course of general personality functioning to an understanding of personality disorders.

The proposals posted by the DSM–5 work group are radical, to say the least, including the deletion of half of the diagnoses, the removal of diagnostic criterion sets for prototype matching, and the provision of a newly developed dimensional model that will have no official coding recognition within a patient's medical record. The DSM–5 work group's proposals may gut and cripple personality disorder diagnosis. The gutting is the deletion of fully half its coverage. The work group is well into the process of dismantling the home for maladaptive personality functioning without actually having secured a new residence. The crippling is the shift to a method of diagnosis (prototype matching) that has long been recognized as unreliable. These changes are so severe that the future of personality disorders is, at best, shaky.

References

Ad-Dab'bagh, Y., & Greenfield, B. (2001). Multiple complex developmental disorder: The "multiple and complex" evolution of the "childhood borderline syndrome" construct. *Journal of American Academic Child and Adolescent Psychiatry, 40*, 954–964.

American Psychiatric Association. (1968). *Diagnostic and statistical manual of mental disorders* (2nd ed.). Washington, DC: Author.

American Psychiatric Association. (1980). *Diagnostic and statistical manual of mental disorders* (3rd ed.). Washington, DC: Author.

American Psychiatric Association. (2000). *Diagnostic and statistical manual of mental disorders* (4th ed., text rev.). Washington, DC: Author.

American Psychiatric Association. (2001). *Practice guidelines for the treatment of patients with borderline personality disorder.* Washington, DC: Author.

Ashton, M. C., & Lee, K. (2001). A theoretical basis for the major dimensions of personality. *European Journal of Personality, 15*, 327–353.

Bateman, A., & Fonagy, P. (2010). Mentalization-based treatment and borderline personality disorder. In J. F. Clarkin, P. Fonagy, & G. O. Gabbard (Eds.), *Psychodynamic psychotherapy for personality disorders: A clinical handbook* (pp. 187–208). Arlington, VA: American Psychiatric Publishing.

Beck, A. T., Freeman, A., and Associates. (1990). *Cognitive therapy of personality disorders.* New York: Guilford.

Benjamin, L. S. (2004). Interpersonal reconstructive therapy (IRT) for individuals with personality disorder. In J. Magnavita (Ed.), *Handbook of personality disorders: Theory and practice* (pp. 151–168). Hoboken, NJ: Wiley.

Black, D. W., Noyes, R., Pfohl, B., Goldstein, R. B., & Blum, N. (1993). Personality disorder in obsessive-compulsive volunteers, well comparison subjects, and their first degree relatives. *American Journal of Psychiatry, 150*, 1226–1232.

Blackburn, R. (2006). Other theoretical models of psychopathy. In C. Patrick (Ed.), *Handbook of psychopathy* (pp. 35–57). New York: Guilford.

Blashfield, R. K., & Intoccia, V. (2000). Growth of the literature on the topic of personality disorders. *American Journal of Psychiatry, 157,* 472–473.

Blatt, S. J. (2004). *Experiences of depression: Theoretical, clinical, and research perspectives.* Washington, DC: American Psychological Association.

Block, J. (2008). *The Q-sort in character appraisal: Encoding subjective impressions of persons quantitatively.* Washington, DC: American Psychological Association.

Bornstein, R. F. (2005). *The dependent patient. A practitioner's guide.* Washington, DC: American Psychological Association.

Bornstein, R. F. (2011). Reconceptualizing personality pathology in DSM-5: Limitations in evidence for eliminating dependent personality disorder and other DSM-IV syndromes. *Journal of Personality Disorders, 25*(2), 235–247.

Bornstein, R. F., & Cecero, J. J. (2000). Deconstructing dependency in a five-factor world: A meta-analytic review. *Journal of Personality Assessment, 74,* 324–343.

Camisa, K. M., Bockbrader, M. A., Lysaker, P., Rae, L. L., Brenner, C. A., & O'Donnell, B. F. (2005). Personality traits in schizophrenia and related personality disorders. *Psychiatry Research, 133,* 23–33.

Clark, L. A. (2007). Assessment and diagnosis of personality disorder. Perennial issues and an emerging reconceptualization. *Annual Review of Psychology, 57,* 277–257.

Clark, L. A., & Krueger, R. F. (2010, February 10). *Rationale for a six-domain trait dimensional diagnostic system for personality disorder.* Retrieved from http://www.dsm5.org/ProposedRevisions/Pages/RationaleforaSix-DomainTraitDimensionalDiagnosticSystemforPersonalityDisorder.aspx

Clarkin, J. F., Fonagy, F., & Gabbard, G. O. (Eds.). (2010). *Psychodynamic psychotherapy for personality disorders: A clinical handbook.* Arlington, VA: American Psychiatric Publishing.

Cleckley, H. (1941). *The mask of sanity.* St. Louis, MO: Mosby.

Colligan, R. C., Morey, L. C., & Offord, K. P. (1994). MMPI/MMPI-2 personality disorder scales. Contemporary norms for adults and adolescents. *Journal of Clinical Psychology, 50,* 168–200.

Coryell, W. H., & Zimmerman, M. (1989). Personality disorder in the families of depressed, schizophrenic, and never-ill probands. *American Journal of Psychiatry, 146,* 496–502.

Costa, P. T. Jr., & McCrae, R. R. (1992). *Revised NEO Personality Inventory (NEO-PI-R) and NEO Five Factor Inventory (NEO-FFI) professional manual.* Odessa, FL: Psychological Assessment Resources.

Costa, P. T. Jr., Terracciano, A., & McCrae, R. R. (2001). Gender differences in personality traits across cultures: Robust and surprising findings. *Journal of Personality and Social Psychology, 81,* 322–331.

Coyne, J. C., Thompson, R., & Whiffen, V. (2004). Is the promissory note of personality as vulnerability to depression in default? Reply to Zuroff, Mongrain, and Santor (2004). *Psychological Bulletin, 130,* 512–517.

Coyne, J. C., & Whiffen, V. E. (1995). Issues in personality as diathesis for depression: The case of sociotropy dependency and autonomy self criticism. *Psychological Bulletin, 118,* 358–378.

Critchfield, K. K., & Benjamin, L. S. (2006). Principles for psychosocial treatment of personality disorders: Summary of the APA Division 12 task force/NASPR review. *Journal of Clinical Psychology, 62,* 661–674.

Derefinko, K. J., & Widiger, T. A. (2008). Antisocial personality disorder. In S. H. Fatemi & P. Clayton (Eds.), *The medical basis of psychiatry* (3rd ed., pp. 213–226). Totowa, NJ: Humana.

Drake, R. E., Adler, D. A., & Vaillant, G. E. (1988). Antecedents of personality disorders in a community sample of men. *Journal of Personality Disorders, 2,* 60–68.

Fanous, A., Gardner, C., Walsh, D., & Kendler, K. (2001). Relationship between positive and negative symptoms of schizophrenia and schizotypal symptoms in nonpsychotic relatives. *Archives of General Psychiatry, 58,* 669–673.

Farrington, D. P. (2006). Family background and psychopathy. In C. J. Patrick (Ed.), *Handbook of psychopathy* (pp. 229–250). New York: Guilford.

First, M. B., Bell, C. B., Cuthbert, B., Krystal, J. H., Malison, R., Offord, D. R., … Wisner, K. L. (2002). Personality disorders and relational disorders: A research agenda for addressing crucial gaps in DSM. In D. J. Kupfer, M. B. First, & D. A. Regier (Eds.), *A research agenda for DSM-V* (pp. 123–199). Washington, DC: American Psychiatric Association.

Fossati, A., Beauchaine, T. P., Grazioli, F., Carretta, I., Cortinovis, F., & Maffei, C. (2005). A latent structure analysis of *Diagnostic and Statistical Manual of Mental Disorders,* fourth edition, narcissistic personality disorder criteria. *Comprehensive Psychiatry, 46,* 361–367.

Fowles, D. C., & Dindo, L. (2006). A dual-deficit model of psychopathy. In C. Patrick (Ed.), *Handbook of psychopathy* (pp. 14–34). New York: Guilford.

Fowles, D. C., & Kochanska, G. (2000). Temperament as a moderator of pathways to conscience in children: The contribution of electrodermal activity. *Psychophysiology, 37*, 788–795.

Frances, A. J. (1980). The DSM-III personality disorders section: A commentary. *American Journal of Psychiatry, 137*, 1050–1054.

Gabbard, G. O. (2000) *Psychodynamic Psychiatry in Clinical Practice* (3rd ed.). Washington, DC: American Psychiatric Press.

Gao, Y., Glenn, A. L., Schug, R. A., Yang, Y., & Raine, A. (2009). The neurobiology of psychopathy: A neuro-developmental perspective. *Canadian Journal of Psychiatry, 54*, 813–823.

Goldberg, L. R. (1993). The structure of phenotypic personality traits. *American Psychologist, 48*, 26–34.

Gooding, D. C., Tallent, K. A., & Matts, C. W. (2005). Clinical status of at-risk individuals 5 years later: further validation of the psychometric high-risk strategy. *Journal of Abnormal Psychology, 114*, 170–175.

Gunderson, J. G. (2001). *Borderline personality disorder: A clinical guide*. Washington, DC: American Psychiatric Press.

Gunderson, J. G., Bender, D., Sanislow, C., Yen, S., Rettew, J. B., Dolan Sewell, R., ... Skodol, A. E. (2003). Plausibility and possible determinants of sudden "remissions" in borderline patients. *Psychiatry, 66*, 111–119.

Gunderson, J. G., & Gabbard, G. O. (Eds.). (2000). *Psychotherapy for personality disorders*. Washington, DC: American Psychiatric Press.

Haigler, E. D., & Widiger, T. A. (2001). Experimental manipulation of NEO-PI-R items. *Journal of Personality Assessment, 77*, 339–358.

Hall, J. R., & Benning, S. D. (2006). The "successful" psychopath: adaptive and subclinical manifestations of psychopathy in the general population. In C. Patrick (Ed.), *Handbook of psychopathy* (pp. 459–478). New York: Guilford.

Hammen, C. (2005). Stress and depression. *Annual Review of Clinical Psychology, 1*, 293–319.

Hare, R. D. (2003). *Hare Psychopathy Checklist Revised (PCL-R). Technical manual*. North Tonawanda, NY: Multi-Health Systems.

Hare, R. D., & Neumann, C. S. (2008). Psychopathy as a clinical and empirical construct. *Annual Review of Clinical Psychology, 4*, 217–246.

Hefferman, K., & Cloitre, M. (2000). A comparison of posttraumatic stress disorder with and without borderline personality disorder among women with a history of childhood sexual abuse: Etiological and clinical characteristics. *Journal of Nervous and Mental Disorder, 188*, 589–595.

Hiatt, K. D., & Newman, J. P. (2006). Understanding psychopathy: The cognitive side. In C. J. Patrick (Ed.), *Handbook of psychopathy* (pp. 156–171). New York: Guilford.

Jaffee, S. R., Caspi, A., Moffitt, T. E., & Taylor, A. (2004). Physical maltreatment victim to antisocial child: Evidence of an environmentally mediated process. *Journal of Abnormal Psychology, 113*, 44–55.

Kaplan, M. (1983). A woman's view of DSM-III. *American Psychologist, 38*, 786–792.

Kessler, R. C., McGonagle, K. A., Zhao S., Nelson, C. B., Hughes, M., Eshleman, S., ... Kendler, K. S. (1994). Lifetime and 12-month prevalence of DSM-III-R psychiatric disorders in the United States: Results from the national comorbidity survey. *Archives of General Psychiatry, 51*, 8–19.

Klein, D. N., Riso, L. P., Donaldson, S. K., Schwartz, J. E., Anderson, R. L., Oiumette, P. C., ... Aronson, T. A. (1995). Family study of early-onset dysthymia: Mood and personality disorders in relatives of outpatients with dysthymia and episodic major depressive and normal controls. *Archives of General Psychiatry, 52*, 487–496.

Kohut, H. (1977). *The restoration of the self*. New York: International Universities Press.

Krueger, R. F., Eaton, N. R., Derringer, J., Markon, K., Watson, D., & Skodol, A. E. (2011). Personality in DSM-5: Helping delineate personality disorder content and framing the meta-structure. *Journal of Personality Assessment, 93*(4), 325–331.

Kwapil, T. R., Barrantes-Vidal, N., & Silvia, P. J. (2008). The dimensional structure of the Wisconsin Schizotypy Scales: Factor identification and construct validity. *Schizophrenia Bulletin, 34*, 444–457.

Lenzenweger, M. F., Loranger, A. W., Korfine, L., & Neff, C. (1997). Detecting personality disorders in a nonclinical population. *Archives of General Psychiatry, 54*, 345–351.

Lindsay, K. A., Sankis, L. M., & Widiger, T. A. (2000). Gender bias in self-report personality disorder inventories. *Journal of Personality Disorders, 14*, 218–232.

Linehan, M. M. (1993). *Cognitive-behavioral treatment of borderline personality disorder*. New York: Guilford.

Livesley, W. J. (Ed.). (2001). *Handbook of personality disorders. Theory, research, and treatment*. New York: Guilford.

Livesley, W. J. (2003). *Practical management of personality disorder*. New York: Guilford.

Lowe, J. R., Edmundson, M., & Widiger, T. A. (2009). Assessment of dependency, agreeableness, and their relationship. *Psychological Assessment, 21*, 543–553.

Lynam, D. R., & Widiger, T. A. (2001). Using the five-factor model to represent the personality disorders. *Journal of Abnormal Psychology, 110*, 401–412.

Lynam, D. R., & Widiger, T. A. (2007a). Using a general model of personality to identify the basic elements of psychopathy. *Journal of Personality Disorders, 21*, 160–178.

Lynam, D. R., & Widiger, T. A. (2007b). Using a general model of personality to understand sex differences in the personality disorders. *Journal of Personality Disorders, 21*, 583–602.

Lynch, T. R., Trost, W. T., Salsman, N., & Linehan, M. M. (2007). Dialectical behavior therapy for borderline personality disorder. *Annual Review of Clinical Psychology, 3*, 181–206.

Magnavita, J. J. (Ed.). (2010). *Evidence-based treatment of personality dysfunction: Principles, processes, and strategies.* Washington, DC: American Psychological Association.

Maier, W., Lichtermann, D., Klinger, T., & Heun, R. (1992). Prevalences of personality disorders (DSM-III-R) in the community. *Journal of Personality Disorders, 6*, 187–196.

Markovitz, P. (2001). Pharmacotherapy. In W. J. Livesley (Ed.), *Handbook of personality disorders* (pp. 475–493). New York: Guilford.

Mattia, J. I., & Zimmerman, M. (2001). Epidemiology. In W. J. Livesley (Ed.), *Handbook of personality disorders* (pp. 107–123). New York: Guilford.

McCrae, R. R., & Costa, P. T. Jr. (1987). Validation of the five-factor model of personality across instruments and observers. *Journal of Personality and Social Psychology, 52*, 81–90.

Miller, J. D., & Lynam, D. R. (2003). Psychopathy and the five-factor model of personality: A replication and extension. *Journal of Personality Assessment, 81*, 168–178.

Miller, M. B., Useda, J. D., Trull, T. J., Burr, R. M., & Minks-Brown, C. (2001). Paranoid, schizoid, and schizotypal personality disorders. In H. E. Adams & P. B. Sutker (Eds.), *Comprehensive handbook of psychopathology* (3rd ed., pp. 535–558). New York: Plenum.

Miller, J. D., Widiger, T. A., & Campbell, W. K. (2010). Narcissistic personality disorder and the DSM-V. *Journal of Abnormal Psychology, 119*(4), 640–649.

Millon, T., Davis, R. D., Millon, C. M., Wenger, A., Van Zullen, M. H., Fuchs, M., & Millon, R. B. (1996). *Disorders of personality. DSM-IV and beyond* (2nd. ed.). New York. Wiley.

Millon, T., & Grossman, S. D. (2005). Sociocultural factors. In J. M. Oldham, A. E. Skodol, & D. S. Bender (Eds.), *Textbook of personality disorders* (pp. 223–235). Washington, DC: American Psychiatric Publishing.

Millon, T., Millon, C., Davis, R., & Grossman, S. (2009). *MCMI-III manual* (4th ed.). Minneapolis: Pearson.

Moffitt, T. E. (2005). The new look of behavioral genetics in developmental psychopathology: Gene-environment interplay in antisocial behaviors. *Psychological Bulletin, 131*, 533–554.

Moldin, S. O., Rice, J. P., Erlenmeyer-Kimling, L., & Squires-Wheeler, E. (1994). Latent structure of DSM-III-R Axis II psychopathology in a normal sample. *Journal of Abnormal Psychology, 103*, 259–266.

Morey, L. C., Alexander, G. M., & Boggs, C. (2005). Gender and personality disorder. In J. Oldham, A. Skodol, & D. Bender (Eds.), *Textbook of personality disorders* (pp. 541–554). Washington, DC: American Psychiatric Press.

Morey, L. C., & Zanarini, M. C. (2000). Borderline personality: traits and disorder. *Journal of Abnormal Psychology, 109*, 733–737.

Morf, C. C., & Rhodewalt, F. (2001). Unraveling the paradoxes of narcissism: A dynamic self-regulatory processing model. *Psychological Inquiry, 12*, 177–196.

Mullins-Sweatt, S. N., Glover, N., Derefinko, K. J., Miller, J. D., & Widiger, T. A. (2010). The search for the successful psychopath. *Journal of Research in Personality, 44*, 559–563.

Mullins-Sweatt, S. N., & Widiger, T. A. (2006). The five-factor model of personality disorder: A translation across science and practice. In R. Krueger & J. Tackett (Eds.), *Personality and psychopathology: Building bridges* (pp. 39–70). New York: Guilford.

Newman, J. P., & Lorenz, A. R. (2003). Response modulation and emotion processing: Implications for psychopathy and other dysregulatory psychopathology. In R. J. Davidson, K. Scherer, & H. H. Goldsmith (Eds.), *Handbook of affective sciences* (pp. 1043–1067). New York: Oxford University Press.

Ornduff, S. R. (2000). Childhood maltreatment and malevolence: quantitative research findings. *Clinical Psychology Review, 20*, 991–1018.

Paris, J. (2009). The treatment of borderline personality disorder: implications of research on diagnosis, etiology, and outcome. *Annual Review of Clinical Psychology, 5*, 277–290.

Parnas, J., Licht, D., & Bovet, P. (2005). Cluster A personality disorders: A review. In M. Maj, H. S. Akiskal, J. E. Mezzich, & A. Okasha (Eds.), *Personality disorders* (pp. 1–74). New York: Wiley.

Pfohl, B. (2005). Comorbidity and borderline personality disorder. In M. Zanarini (Ed.), *Borderline personality disorder* (pp. 135–153). Washington, DC: American Psychiatric Press.

Pincus, A. L., & Lukowitsky, M. R. (2010). Pathological narcissism and narcissistic personality disorder. *Annual Review of Clinical Psychology, 6*, 421–446.

Pincus, A. L., & Wilson, K. R. (2001). Interpersonal variability in dependent personality. *Journal of Personality, 69*, 223–252.

Raine, A. (2006). Schizotypal personality: neurodevelopmental and psychosocial trajectories. *Annual Review of Clinical Psychology, 2*, 291–326.

Regier, D. A., Narrow, W. E., Kuhl, E. A., & Kupfer, D. J. (2010). The conceptual development of DSM-V. *American Journal of Psychiatry, 166*, 645–655.

Reichborn-Kjennerud, T. (2008). Genetics of personality disorders. *Psychiatric Clinics of North America, 31*, 421–440.

Rhee, S. H., & Waldman, I. D. (2002). Genetic and environmental influences on antisocial behavior: A meta-analysis of twin and adoption studies. *Psychological Bulletin, 128*, 490–529.

Ronningstam, E. (1999). Narcissistic personality disorder. In T. Millon, P. H. Blaney, & R. D. Davis (Eds.), *Oxford textbook of psychopathology* (pp. 674–693). New York: Oxford University Press.

Ronningstam, E. (2005). Narcissistic personality disorder: A review. In M. Maj, H. S. Akiskal, J. E. Mezzich, & A. Okasha (Eds.), *Personality disorders* (pp. 278–327). New York: Wiley.

Ronningstam, E. (2011). Narcissistic personality disorder in DSM-5—in support of retaining a significant diagnosis. *Journal of Personality Disorders, 25*(2), 248–259.

Ross, S. R., Lutz, C. J., & Bailey, S. E. (2002). Positive and negative symptoms of schizotypy and the five-factor model: A domain and facet level analysis. *Journal of Personality Assessment, 79*, 53–72.

Salekin, R. T. (2002). Psychopathy and therapeutic pessimism: Clinical lore or clinical reality? *Clinical Psychology Review, 22*, 79–112.

Samuel, D. B., & Widiger, T. A. (2004). Clinicians' personality descriptions of prototypic personality disorders. *Journal of Personality Disorders, 18*, 286–308.

Samuel, D. B., & Widiger, T. A. (2006). Clinicians' judgments of clinical utility: A comparison of the DSM-IV and five factor models. *Journal of Abnormal Psychology, 115*, 298–308.

Samuel, D. B., & Widiger, T. A. (2008a). A meta-analytic review of the relationships between the five-factor model and DSM-IV-TR personality disorders: a facet level analysis. *Clinical Psychology Review, 28*, 1326–1342.

Samuel, D. B., & Widiger, T. A. (2008b). Convergence of narcissism measures from the perspective of general personality functioning. *Assessment, 15*, 364–374.

Samuels, J. F., Eaton, W. W., Bienvenu, O. J., Brown, C., Costa, P. T., & Nestadt, G. (2002). Prevalence and correlates of personality disorders in a community sample. *British Journal of Psychiatry, 180*, 536–542.

Samuels, J. F., Nestadt, G., & Romanoski, A. J. (1994). DSM-III personality disorders in the community. *American Journal of Psychiatry, 151*, 1055–1062.

Schneider, K. (1923). *Psychopathic personalities*. Springfield, IL: Charles C. Thomas.

Shahar, G., Joiner, T. E., Zuroff, D. C., & Blatt, S. J. (2004). Personality, interpersonal behavior, and depression: Co-existence of stress-specific moderating and mediating effects. *Personality and Individual Differences, 36*, 1583–1596.

Siever, L. J., & Davis, K. L. (2004). The pathophysiology of schizophrenia disorders: perspectives from the spectrum. *American Journal of Psychiatry, 161*, 398–403.

Silk, K. R., Wolf, T. L., Ben-Ami, D., & Poortinga, E. W. (2005). Environmental factors in the etiology of borderline personality disorder. In M. Zanarini (Ed.), *Borderline personality disorder* (pp. 41–62). Washington, DC: American Psychiatric Press.

Skodol, A. (2010, February 10). *Rationale for proposing five specific personality types*. Retrieved from http://www.dsm5.org/ProposedRevisions/Pages/RationaleforProposingFiveSpecificPersonalityDisorderTypes.aspx

Skodol, A. E., Gunderson, J. G., Shea, M. T., McGlashan, T. H., Morey, L. C., Sanislow, C. A., ... Stout, R. L. (2005). The Collaborative Longitudinal Personality Disorders study (CLPS): Overview and implications. *Journal of Personality Disorders, 19*, 487–504.

Spitzer, R. L., Endicott, J., & Gibbon, M. (1979). Crossing the border into borderline personality and borderline schizophrenia. *Archives of General Psychiatry, 36*, 17–24.

Spitzer, R. L., First, M. B., Shedler, J., Westen, D., & Skodol, A. (2008). Clinical utility of five dimensional systems for personality diagnosis. *Journal of Nervous and Mental Disease, 196*, 356–374.

Stone, M. H. (1993). *Abnormalities of personality: Within and beyond the realm of treatment*. New York: Norton.

Stone, M. H. (2001). Natural history and long-term outcome. In W. J. Livesley (Ed.), *Handbook of personality disorders* (pp. 259–273). New York: Guilford.

Sutker, P. B., & Allain, A. N. (2001). Antisocial personality disorder. In P. B. Sutker & H. E. Adams (Eds.), *Comprehensive textbook of psychopathology* (3rd ed., pp. 445–490). New York: Plenum.

Torgersen, S. (2005a). Epidemiology. In J. M. Oldham, A. E. Skodol, & D. S. Bender (Eds.), *Textbook of personality disorders* (pp. 129–141). Washington, DC: American Psychiatric Publishing.

Torgersen, S. (2005b). Genetics of borderline personality disorder. In M. Zanarini (Ed.), *Borderline personality disorder* (pp. 127–134). Washington, DC: American Psychiatric Press.

Torgersen, S., Kringlen, E., & Cramer, V. (2001). The prevalence of personality disorders in a community sample. *Archives of General Psychiatry, 58,* 590–596.

Torgersen, S., Lygren, S., Oien, P. A., Skre, I., Onstad, S., Edvardson, E., … Kringeln, E. (2000). A twin study of personality disorders. *Comprehensive Psychiatry, 41,* 416–425.

Trull, T. J., Widiger, T. A., Lynam, D. R., & Costa, P. T. (2003). Borderline personality disorder from the perspective of general personality functioning. *Journal of Abnormal Psychology, 112,* 193–202.

Verona, E., & Vitale, J. (2006). Psychopathy in women: Assessment, manifestations, and etiology. In C. J. Patrick (Ed.), *Handbook of psychopathy* (pp. 415–436). New York: Guilford.

Waldman, I. D., & Rhee, S. H. (2006). Genetic and environmental influences on psychopathy and antisocial behavior. In C. J. Patrick (Ed.), *Handbook of psychopathy* (pp. 205–228). New York: Guilford.

Walker, E., Kestler, L., Bollini, A., & Hochman, K. M. (2004). Schizophrenia: Etiology and course. *Annual Review of Psychology, 55,* 401–430.

Warner, M. B., Morey, L. C., Finch, J. F., Gunderson, J. G., Skodol, A. E., Sanislow, C. A., … Grilo, C. M. (2004). The longitudinal relationship of personality traits and disorders. *Journal of Abnormal Psychology, 113,* 217–227.

Watson, D., Clark, L. A., & Chmielewski, M. (2008). Structures of personality and their relevant to psychopathology: II. Further articulation of a comprehensive unified trait structure. *Journal of Personality, 76,* 1485–1522.

Westen, D., Shedler, J., & Bradley, R. (2006). A prototype approach to personality disorder diagnosis. *American Journal of Psychiatry, 163,* 846–856.

Widiger, T. A. (2005a). CIC, CLPS, and MSAD. *Journal of Personality Disorders, 19,* 586–593.

Widiger, T. A. (2005b). A temperament model of borderline personality disorder. In M. Zanarini (Ed.), *Borderline personality disorder* (pp. 63–81). Washington, DC: American Psychiatric Press.

Widiger, T. A. (2006). Psychopathy and DSM-IV psychopathology. In C. Patrick (Ed.), *Handbook of psychopathy* (pp. 156–171). New York: Guilford.

Widiger, T. A. (2007a). Alternatives to DSM-IV Axis II. In W. O'Donohue, K. A. Fowler, & S. O. Lilienfeld (Eds.), *Personality disorders. Toward the DSM-V* (pp. 21–40). Los Angeles: Sage.

Widiger, T. A. (2007b). DSM's approach to gender: history and controversies. In W. E. Narrow, M. B. First, P. J. Sirovatka, & D. A. Regier (Eds.), *Age and gender considerations in psychiatric diagnosis: A research agenda for DSM-V* (pp. 19–29) Washington, DC: American Psychiatric Association.

Widiger, T. A. (2011). A shaky future for personality disorders. *Personality Disorders: Theory, Research, and Treatment, 2*(1), 54–67.

Widiger, T. A., & Anderson, K. G. (2003). Personality and depression in women. *Journal of Affective Disorders, 74,* 59–66.

Widiger, T. A., & Boyd, S. (2009). Personality disorders assessment instruments. In J. N. Butcher (Ed.), *Oxford handbook of personality assessment* (pp. 336–363). New York: Oxford University Press.

Widiger, T. A., & Costa, P. T. Jr. (2002). FFM personality disorder research. In P. T. Costa Jr. & T. A. Widiger (Eds.), *Personality disorders and the five-factor model of personality* (pp. 59–87). Washington, DC: American Psychological Association.

Widiger, T. A., De Clerq, B., & De Fruyt, F. (2009). Childhood antecedents of personality disorder: an alternative perspective. *Development and Psychopathology, 21,* 771–791.

Widiger, T. A., & Lowe, J. (2007). Five factor model assessment of personality disorder. *Journal of Personality Assessment, 89,* 16–29.

Widiger, T. A., & Lowe, J. R. in press. Pathological altruism and personality disorder. In B. Oakley (Ed.), *Pathological altruism.* New York: Springer.

Widiger, T. A., & Mullins-Sweatt, S. N. (2009). Five-factor model of personality disorder: A proposal for DSM-V. *Annual Review of Clinical Psychology, 5,* 115–138.

Widiger, T. A., & Simonsen, E. (2005). The American Psychiatric Association's research agenda for the DSM-V. *Journal of Personality Disorders, 19,* 103–109.

Widiger, T. A., & Trull, T. J. (2007). Plate tectonics in the classification of personality disorder: Shifting to a dimensional model. *American Psychologist, 62,* 71–83.

Widiger, T. A., Trull, T. J., Clarkin, J. F., Sanderson, C., & Costa, P. T. Jr. (2002). A description of the DSM-IV personality disorders with the five-factor model of personality. In P. T. Costa Jr. & T. A. Widiger (Eds.), *Personality disorders and the five-factor model of personality* (pp. 89–99). Washington, DC: American Psychological Association.

Wood, J. M., Garb, H. N., Nezworski, M. T., & Koren, D. (2007). The Shedler-Westen Assessment Procedure-200 as a basis for modifying DSM personality disorder categories. *Journal of Abnormal Psychology, 116,* 823–836.

World Health Organization. (1992). *The ICD-10 classification of mental and behavioural disorders: Clinical descriptions and diagnostic guidelines.* Geneva: Author.

Young, J. E., Klosko, J. S., & Weishaar, M. E. (2003). *Schema therapy: A practitioner's guide.* New York: Guilford.

Zanarini, M. C., Frankenburg, F. R., Hennen, R., Reich, D. B., & Silk, K. R. (2005). The McLean Study of Adult Development (MSAD): Overview and implications of the first six years of prospective follow-up. *Journal of Personality Disorders, 19,* 505–523.

Zimmerman, M. (2011). A critique of the proposed prototype rating system for personality disorders in DSM-5. *Journal of Personality Disorders, 25*(2), 206–221.

Zimmerman, M., & Mattia, J. I. (1999). Differences between clinical and research practices in diagnosing borderline personality disorder. *American Journal of Psychiatry, 156,* 1570–1574.

Zuroff, D. C., Mongrain, M., & Santor, D. A. (2004). Conceptualizing and measuring personality vulnerability to depression: Comment on Coyne and Whiffen (1995). *Psychological Bulletin, 130,* 489–511.

12
Sexual Dysfunctions and Disorders

JENNIFER T. GOSSELIN

Sacred Heart University
Fairfield, Connecticut

Sexual behavior has a long history of emotionally charged social and cultural expectations, rules, taboos, myths, and misconceptions. "Normal" versus "dysfunctional" or "deviant" sexual behaviors are determined arbitrarily and are tied to the social norms of a particular time and place (Marecek, Crawford, & Popp, 2004). The social construction of appropriate and inappropriate sexual behavior is best reflected by the historical and cultural changes in what has been considered normal and abnormal. In ancient Greece, for example, a male mentor might have sex with his male adolescent student as part of their relationship, which was relatively accepted at that time as a way to demonstrate social standing or hierarchy (King, 1996; Plante, 2006). In the Sambian tribe in New Guinea, an important rite involves younger boys performing oral sex on older boys in order to ingest semen, which is believed to provide strength and masculinity; when they get older, they transition into heterosexual adults (Stoller, 1985). In contrast, the Victorian era in England (during most of the 1800s) was a time of sexual conservatism, although like the Sambians, beliefs about sex were rigid and based on misconceptions about semen. The purpose of sex during this era was to produce children, not to experience pleasure. Masturbation was believed to be a cause of mental or physical illness (including blindness; King, 1996). In some cases, treatment for masturbation included clitoridectomy (removal of the clitoris), male circumcision, or castration (King, 1996; Lips, 2006). Throughout history, we find that today's deviance was yesterday's normalcy, and vice versa.

In many nations around the world, major developments and changes have occurred, such as improved methods of contraception and movements for the rights of women and homosexuals. Homosexuality was included as a disorder in older editions of the American Psychiatric Association's (APA) *Diagnostic and Statistical Manual of Mental Disorders* (*DSM*), but was downgraded to "ego dystonic homosexuality" in the third edition in 1980 and was removed as a disorder in the *DSM–III–R* (APA, 1987) due to political pressure and the lack of empirical evidence for homosexuality as a psychological disorder. Many societies—particularly in Europe and the West in general—have become more open about presenting sexual matters in the media. With this acceptance of sex, however, have come new ways to define and treat problems related to sex. Expectations about sexual performance and satisfaction may be unrealistic in part due to how sex is commonly portrayed in television and film—as completely spontaneous and intensely and entirely satisfying for both partners, often without discussion or use of condoms or contraception, without distractions or body image concerns, and without communication about what is permissible and pleasurable for each partner (Dune & Shuttleworth, 2009).

Sex researchers today owe a great deal to the pioneers in this field, such as Alfred Kinsey, William Masters, Virginia Johnson, Katharine Davis, Havelock Ellis, Gilbert Hamilton, and many others (Irvine, 1990; Kimmel & Plante, 2004). These early researchers paved the way for later researchers by challenging social norms to study the taboo topic of sex. Kinsey gathered data through surveys, beginning his work in the late 1930s, to learn about typical sexual behavior and experiences. His data normalized many sexual practices that were thought to be very rare or deviant. Masters and Johnson studied sexual behavior in the laboratory, using volunteers who would masturbate or married couples who would have sex. In the 1960s and 1970s, Masters and Johnson's best-sellers *Human Sexual Response* (1966) and *Human Sexual Inadequacy* (1970) dispelled many myths about sexual function. Their human sexual response cycle has been a widely used model of normal sexual functioning and would later be used as a framework for the sexual dysfunction categories in the *DSM* (Masters, Johnson, & Kolodny, 1985).

Categories of Sexual Disorders

The current nomenclature, the *DSM–IV–TR* (APA, 2000) identifies two primary categories of sexual disorders: sexual dysfunction (such as erectile dysfunction) and paraphilias (such as sexual fetishism). Although most people have had occasional experiences that fall into a sexual dysfunction category—such as the inability to reach orgasm when so desired—sexual difficulties that are more frequent and distressing than an incidental occurrence are considered to be sexual dysfunctions, according to the *DSM–IV–TR*. For ease of understanding, this chapter will use the term *sexual dysfunction* to indicate problems associated with sexual desire, arousal, orgasm, and pain during sex, while *sexual disorders* will refer to the paraphilias, such as exhibitionism, fetishism, frotteurism, pedophilia, sexual masochism, sexual sadism, transvestic fetishism, and voyeurism. This chapter will also address gender identity disorder, although this disorder is concerned with gender identification, rather than a sexual dysfunction or a sexual disorder. Additionally, compulsive sexual behavior or hypersexuality will be presented with the paraphilias, despite its omission from the current *DSM*. Diagnostic descriptions, prevalence, etiological or causal factors, and treatment approaches will be discussed for each dysfunction or disorder presented.

Sexual Dysfunctions

Defining and Describing Sexual Dysfunctions

The *DSM–IV–TR* defines sexual dysfunction as "a disturbance in the processes that characterize the sexual response cycle or by pain associated with sexual intercourse" (APA, 2000, p. 535). The sexual response cycle indicated in this definition follows Masters and Johnson's model, including Kaplan's (1979) addition of the initial stage of desire, followed by excitement, plateau, orgasm, and resolution (Masters et al., 1985). Sexual desire involves sexual thoughts and fantasies; sexual excitement involves the physiological arousal of the sex organs; plateau involves physiological changes that may lead to orgasm; the next stage is orgasm; and finally, during the resolution phase, the body returns to its unaroused state (Masters et al., 1985).

The types of sexual dysfunction, according to the *DSM–IV–TR*, are:

- *Sexual desire disorders*: deficiency or absence of sexual fantasies and desire for sexual activity that causes marked distress or interpersonal difficulty. These include hypoactive sexual desire disorder (absence of sexual fantasies and desire for sex) and sexual aversion disorder (extreme avoidance of sex with a partner).
- *Sexual arousal disorders*: female sexual arousal disorder (persistent or recurrent inability to attain or maintain an adequate lubrication-swelling response of sexual excitement in females) and male erectile disorder (persistent or recurrent inability to attain or to maintain an adequate erection during sexual activity).
- *Orgasmic disorders*: persistent or recurrent delay in, or absence of, orgasm following a normal sexual excitement phase. These disorders include female orgasmic disorder,

male orgasmic disorder, and premature ejaculation (onset of orgasm and ejaculation with minimal stimulation or before the person wishes it).

- *Sexual pain disorders*: dyspareunia (genital pain that is associated with sexual intercourse in males and females and is not due to lack of lubrication) and vaginismus (recurrent or persistent involuntary contraction of the perineal muscles surrounding the outer third of the vagina when vaginal penetration is attempted by self or others with an item such as a tampon, speculum, penis, or finger).

The *DSM–IV–TR* also includes several subtypes of sexual dysfunction. The clinician indicates whether the dysfunction has been acquired after a period of normal functioning or if it has been lifelong; whether the dysfunction is limited to particular partners, types of stimulation, or situations, or if it generalizes across these factors; and whether the dysfunction is due to psychological or both psychological and medical (combined) factors. Sexual difficulties must be considered "persistent or recurrent" by the clinician to be considered a disorder, and they cannot be due exclusively to a substance, medication, or medical condition, in which case the clinician should use the diagnosis of sexual dysfunction due to a particular medical condition or substance-induced sexual dysfunction. To distinguish between sexual impairment that is not considered a disorder and sexual impairment that is diagnosable, significant distress or interpersonal difficulty or impairment is required for diagnosis.

Criticisms of Sexual Dysfunction Diagnostic Categories

Most of the criticisms of the *DSM*'s sexual dysfunction categories stem from its reliance on the human sexual response cycle as a model, which deemphasizes psychological factors in favor of physiological changes. Critics argue that sexual experience is presented in this model as a relationship- and context-independent phenomenon (Tiefer, 2001). They further argue that the human sexual response cycle is a linear model with seemingly discrete stages, which does not necessarily reflect real sexual experience (Basson, 2005; Basson et al., 2004). Researchers also assert that the model is based on male sexual response, and that it superimposes the male cycle onto the female response (Basson, 2005; Basson et al., 2004). Further, the research conducted to establish the model was based on carefully selected participants who, for example, could reach orgasm through masturbation and coitus, which is considered a biased sample (Tiefer, 1991). In place of the existing model, researchers have proposed a circular model—particularly to reflect female sexual experience—that includes emotional intimacy and responsiveness to sexual stimuli as motivating factors, instead of sexual fantasies and spontaneous desire as the primary motivating forces (Basson, 2002).

Researchers following a diagnostic system similar to the field of medicine (e.g., either one has the diagnosis or not) have generally attempted to create two categories of individuals with respect to sexual functioning: (1) those who are sexually satisfied and have "normal" sexual functioning, and (2) those who are sexually dissatisfied and are sexually "dysfunctional." Both qualitative and quantitative studies, however, do not support this dichotomy. Sexual dysfunctions and consistency of orgasm tend to be poor predictors of sexual satisfaction (Frank, Anderson, & Rubinstein, 1978; Lavie-Ajayi, 2005; McConaghy, 1993). Over half of the women in one study who had difficulty reaching orgasm reported that it did not concern them (Lavie-Ajayi, 2005). Some of these inorgasmic women found their lack of orgasm problematic only to the extent that it resulted in their male partners' feelings of inadequacy. Other research suggests that women's distress about their sexual relationship is better predicted by their feelings toward their partners during sex and their subjective state of well-being than by their physical sexual response (Bancroft, Loftus, & Long, 2003). In addition, hypoactive sexual desire disorder is virtually always the result of one partner having a stronger desire for sex than the other partner

(Gehring, 2003). Particularly given that hyperactive sexual desire disorder is not included in the current *DSM*, the diagnostic category of hypoactive sexual desire disorder therefore implicitly includes a value judgment that the partner with a lower desire for sex should rise to meet the level of desire of his or her partner, rather than vice versa or considering alternative solutions to this discrepancy in sexual desire.

Dissatisfaction with the sexual dysfunction categories has not led to major revisions to the *DSM* thus far, although some changes, particularly with respect to sexual arousal disorder subtypes, are anticipated for the DSM–5 ("Responses to the Proposed DSM-V Changes," 2010), and these are discussed in the final section of this chapter. Alternatively, the 10th edition of the *International Classification of Diseases* (*ICD-10*), created by the World Health Organization, defines sexual dysfunction as "the various ways in which an individual is unable to participate in a sexual relationship as he or she would wish," and explains that "Sexual response is a psychosomatic process and both psychological and somatic processes are usually involved in the causation of sexual dysfunction" (2006, section F52). Although both the *ICD-10* and the *DSM–IV–TR* use the human sexual response cycle as their diagnostic structure, the definition used by the *ICD-10* emphasizes the subjective nature of the sexual experience, rather than emphasizing genital response.

Epidemiology of Sexual Dysfunctions

Rates of sexual dysfunctions vary greatly from study to study due to different measures used, methodological differences, the considerable degree of clinical judgment involved in the diagnostic categories themselves, and the use of different samples (Rosen & Laumann, 2003). Research indicates that 40–45% of women and 20–31% of men have one or more sexual dysfunctions (Laumann, Paik, & Rosen, 1999; Lewis et al., 2004, 2010). Rates of female sexual dysfunction vary from 27% (Kadri, Alami, & Tahiri, 2002) to as high as 55% (Fisher, Boroditsky, & Morris, 2004). When researchers include both sexual problems and overall sexual dissatisfaction, however, only about 14% of women report both concerns (Lutfey, Link, Rosen, Wiegel, & McKinlay, 2009).

The most common sexual dysfunctions among women tend to be hypoactive sexual desire disorder, female sexual arousal disorder (Nicolosi et al., 2006; Utian et al., 2005), and female orgasmic disorder (Fisher et al., 2004; West, Vinikoor, & Zolnoun, 2004). The most common sexual dysfunctions among men are premature ejaculation and erectile dysfunction (Dunn, Croft, & Hackett, 1999; Nicolosi et al., 2004, 2006). Rates of premature ejaculation range from 4 to 26% (Laumann, Glasser, Neves, & Moreira, 2009; Simons & Carey, 2001), and rates of erectile dysfunction vary greatly with age. More specifically, less than 10% of men under 40 years of age, 49% of men 40 to 88 years old, and 76% of men 50 to 75 years old in separate studies report erectile dysfunction, with an overall rate of 18% for men aged 20 to 75 years of age or older (Feldman, Goldstein, Hatzichristou, Krane, & McKinlay, 1994; Grover et al., 2006; Lewis et al., 2004; Prins, Blanker, Bohnen, Thomas, & Bosch, 2002; Saigal, Wessells, Pace, Schonlau, & Wilt, 2006; Shiri et al., 2003; Simons & Carey, 2001).

The wide variation in prevalence estimates of sexual dysfunction is a source of ongoing debate (see Derogatis & Burnett, 2007, for a review). Prevalence estimates may be inflated because many studies do not include diagnostic interviews, and they often do not assess significant personal or interpersonal distress associated with the dysfunction, which are criteria for *DSM* diagnosis. Similar to the large variability in prevalence based on measurement differences, incidence rates of sexual dysfunction for men and women reported within the past year is 11%, while 68% of men and 69% of women report subclinical sexual difficulties over the previous year (Christensen et al., 2011). The suggestion that the majority of men and women have a sexual difficulty is inconsistent with the finding that the majority of people around the world report that they are satisfied with their sexual functioning, including approximately 80% of men and women in Western nations and 42–90% of men and women in mostly South American and Eastern countries (Laumann et al., 2006). Further, research repeatedly shows that among women with sexual difficulties, the overwhelming majority are still satisfied with their sex lives or are not distressed by their sexual difficulties (Ferenidou et al., 2008; King, Holt, & Nazareth, 2007).

Etiology of Sexual Dysfunctions

Sexual desire, arousal, and behavior can be explained using a *biopsychosocial model*, meaning that internal processes, such as one's physiological systems, thoughts, and feelings, interact with one's behaviors and with external factors, such as environmental, interpersonal, and social forces (Althof et al., 2005; Fagan, 2004). This interactionist approach provides a multidimensional explanation for problems that usually do not have a clear, singular causal factor (King et al., 2007). Sexual difficulties can have multiple etiologies, and these factors tend to be inextricably linked.

Biological Factors in Sexual Dysfunctions   Sexual dysfunctions can be due to a variety of biological factors, including a wide range of vascular (blood vessel) and related medical, neurological, and anatomical conditions, as well as biochemical factors (Pfaus, 2009; Reffelmann & Kloner, 2010). Sex hormones (produced by the ovaries and testes) play a role in sexual interest and functioning in men and women (Berman, Berman, & Goldstein, 1999). Low levels of androgens, particularly testosterone, have been linked in some studies to loss of sexual arousal and orgasm in women (see Shifren, 2004, for a review), although other studies contradict this finding (Davis, Davison, Donath, & Bell, 2005; Nyunt et al., 2005). In men, testosterone has more consistently been associated with sexual desire and activity, with low testosterone leading to decreased desire and function (Bradford, 2001; Goldstein, 2004; Rowland, 2006). Similarly, low levels of estrogens in women also may be related to diminished sexual desire and sexual functioning, although it is likely that sexual functioning in women is the result of a combination of estrogens and androgens (Berman & Bassuk, 2002; Rowland, 2006).

Neurotransmitters, such as serotonin and dopamine, also play a role in sexual function, a finding that is supported by animal and human research as well as by the sexual side effects of medications that affect levels of these neurotransmitters in the synapse (Basson, 2005; Kafka, 1997b; Pfaus, 2009; Rowland, 2006). Serotonin influences a wide range of physiological, behavioral, and mood-related phenomena, including appetite, nausea, sleep, body temperature, anxiety, depression, suicidality, and impulsivity (Carlson, 2001; Pinel, 2003). Increased levels of serotonin (due to antidepressant medications that block reuptake of serotonin, for example) tend to inhibit sexual activity and delay orgasm in both humans and rats (McMahon, 2004). Further, researchers have identified genetic variants involving specific serotonin receptors that predict sexual dysfunction in certain individuals taking selective serotonin reuptake inhibitors (SSRIs) compared to other individuals taking SSRIs (Bishop, Moline, Ellingrod, Schultz, & Clayton, 2006). Similarly, other genetic variations that affect the production of serotonin transporters (which enable serotonin reuptake) are associated with lifelong premature ejaculation (Janssen et al., 2009).

Dopamine is involved in motivation and the experience of pleasure or reward, leading to the repetition of rewarding experiences, such as eating and having sex. (Dopaminergic pathways are thus also important in addictive behaviors.) The connection between dopamine and sexual behavior has been established, in part, through research on individuals who suffer from conditions involving dopaminergic pathways, such as Parkinson's disease and schizophrenia. For example, on the one hand, Parkinson's disease (which involves a depletion of dopamine) commonly includes diminished sexual interest or functioning, and patients who are treated with medications that facilitate dopamine transmission also tend to report an increase in impulse control difficulties, including hypersexual behavior (Weintraub et al., 2010). Schizophrenia, on the other hand, seems to involve excess dopaminergic transmission, and patients who are treated with medications that inhibit dopamine transmission often report diminished sexual desire and may experience sexual dysfunction (Dominguez & Hull, 2005; Miclutia, Popescu, & Macrea, 2008). In addition to the monoamines, nitric oxide (a neurotransmitter in the form of a soluble gas) plays a role in physiological sexual responses, such as erection, by relaxing smooth muscle tissue and allowing blood flow to the genitals. Medications such as sildenafil (Viagra) increase erectile functioning by influencing the signaling of nitric oxide (Trussell, Anastasiadis, Padma-Nathan, & Shabsigh, 2004).

In men and women, a proposed cause of limited physiological arousal is insufficient blood flow to the genitalia. This physiological problem, in turn, may have a number of causes, including illnesses that involve vascular impairment, such as cardiovascular disease. More specifically, sexual dysfunction in men and women is associated with chronic diseases, particularly hypertension, cardiovascular and heart disease, and diabetes, as well as genitourinary disease (such as disease or dysfunctions involving the kidneys, prostate, urethra, or bladder), and spinal cord injuries (Kriston, Gunzler, Agycmang, Bengel, & Berner, 2010; Lewis et al., 2004, 2010; Sipski, 2002). Sexual dysfunction in men is predicted by obesity, endocrine disorders (such as hypogonadism or dysfunction of the testes, thyroid disorders, and diabetes), smoking, hyperlipidemia (elevated lipids in the blood), Peyronie's disease (extreme curvature of the penile shaft), bicycle riding, and chronic prostatitis or chronic pelvic pain syndrome (Larsen, Wagner, & Heitmann, 2007; Lewis et al., 2004, 2010; Reffelmann & Kloner, 2010; Smith, Pukall, Tripp, & Nickel, 2007; Sommer, Goldstein, & Korda, 2010).

Among women, breast cancer and its treatment, urinary incontinence (and particularly *coital incontinence* or involuntary urination during intercourse), and cervical and endometrial cancer treatment have been linked with sexual dysfunction (Brotto, Heiman et al., 2008; Carbone & Seftel 2004; Garrusi & Faezee, 2008). Research on the link between hysterectomies and sexual dysfunction is mixed, with some women experiencing decreased orgasm or sexual arousal due to scar tissue or nerve damage, although sexual difficulties tend to abate over time, particularly after the patient has fully recovered from surgery (Bayram & Beji, 2010; Meston, 2004). In addition, women who have suffered pelvic trauma, surgical or obstetrical complications, those who have endometriosis or similar health conditions, or those who have undergone female circumcision or female genital mutilation (a cultural practice in certain regions, particularly in northern Africa) are more likely to experience dyspareunia (Berman et al., 1999; Committee on Bioethics, 1998; Elgaali, Strevens, & Mardh, 2005).

Age and Sexual Dysfunctions Sexual dysfunction is also often associated with older age in Western and Eastern samples around the world (Lewis et al., 2004; Nicolosi et al., 2003; Turkistani, 2004). Research findings are mixed, however, with respect to the specific sexual dysfunction and its relationship with age. For example, some researchers have reported that among women, sexual difficulties actually decrease with age (Kadri et al., 2002; Laumann et al., 1999), although other research contradicts this finding (Lutfey et al., 2009). In cases in which sexual function improves with age, a possible explanation is that older women tend to have the same sexual partner for a longer period of time than do younger women, which may allow for more consistent sexual behavior and orgasm (Laumann et al., 1999), particularly since women do not report masturbating at the same rates as men (Meston & Ahrold, 2010). Although some women may experience more pain during sex as they enter menopause, sexual satisfaction does not appear to be related to menopause status (Cain et al., 2003). Other research shows that sexual difficulties have similar prevalence rates among women aged 30–49 (approximately 32–35%), but by age 50, sexual difficulties increase to 53% and increase further to 63% among women aged 60–79 (Lutfey et al., 2009), with vaginal dryness in particular tending to increase with age (Laumann et al., 1999; Nicolosi et al., 2004, 2006).

Similarly, sexual interest or desire declines with age for both men and women (Bancroft et al., 2003; Bitzer, Platano, Tschudin, & Alder, 2008; Eplov, Giraldi, Davidsen, Garde, & Kamper-Jorgensen, 2007; Laumann et al., 1999; Lewis et al., 2004; Nicolosi et al., 2004). Also, among males, the ability to maintain and sustain an erection and to fully ejaculate tends to decrease with age (Blanker et al., 2001; Helgason et al., 1996; Laumann et al., 1999; Nicolosi et al., 2003). Hypogonadism (diminished function of the testes) is relatively common as men reach older age, and its symptoms (such as fatigue, diminished strength, and diminished sexual desire) can be difficult to separate from normal aging (Stanworth & Jones, 2008).

Medication-Induced Sexual Dysfunctions   A wide range of medications can influence sexual functioning by affecting the release of neurotransmitters or their receptors or by influencing the vascular system. Antidepressant medications, such as SSRIs, monoamine oxidase inhibitors (MAOIs), and tricyclic antidepressants (TCAs), are associated with sexual dysfunction (Montgomery, Baldwin, & Riley, 2002). A potential confounding variable is that diminished sexual desire or arousal may be a symptom of depression, rather than a side effect. Although research suggests that a substantial portion (about 40–50%) of nonmedicated individuals with depression have decreased sexual desire or sexual difficulties (Kennedy, Dickens, Eisfeld, & Bagby, 1999), research comparing treatment and control groups indicates that antidepressants also contribute to sexual impairment, particularly delayed or absent orgasm (Montgomery et al., 2002). A host of other medications have been associated with diminished sexual functioning, including anxiolytics (antianxiety medications), such as benzodiazepines; beta-blockers, which lower blood pressure; antipsychotic medications, which increase levels of prolactin; oral contraceptives; antiretroviral treatment for HIV; and chemotherapy and other treatments for cancer (Asboe et al., 2007; Bishop, Ellingrod, Akroush, & Moline, 2009; Gruszecki, Forchuk, & Fisher, 2005; Kao et al., 2003; Knegtering, van der Moolen, Castelein, Kluiter, & van den Bosch, 2003; Murthy & Wylie, 2007; Rowland, 2006; Segraves, 2002; Trotta et al., 2008).

Among experts in the area of sexual side effects due to antidepressants, the most common strategies used to minimize sexual side effects were switching antidepressant medications, adding medications to the existing SSRI treatment regimen, or reducing the dose of the antidepressant (Balon & Segraves, 2008). When switching the patient to an antidepressant with fewer sexual side effects, physicians may choose antidepressants that enhance neurotransmission of both serotonin and norepinephrine, such as milnacipran or mirtazapine (Baldwin, Moreno, & Briley, 2008; Osvath, Fekete, Voros, & Almasi, 2007; Segraves, 2002; Serretti & Chiesa, 2009), or they may choose medications that enhance transmission of dopamine and norepinephrine, such as bupropion (Dhillon, Yang, & Curran, 2008; Zisook, Rush, Haight, Clines, & Rockett, 2006). Instead of replacing the patient's medications, physicians may choose to add a medication that enhances sexual functioning, such as sildenafil.

Psychological, Interpersonal, and Sociocultural Factors in Sexual Dysfunctions   Previous sexual experiences, beliefs and knowledge about sex, as well as current levels of stress, depression, anxiety, relationship issues, and many other factors may play a role in the development of sexual difficulties and dysfunction (Araujo, Durante, Feldman, Goldstein, & McKinlay, 1998; Bancroft et al., 2003; Bodenmann, Ledermann, Blattner, & Galluzzo, 2006; Laumann et al., 1999; van Lankveld & Grotjohann, 2000). For example, an individual may learn to associate sex with pain or fear due to past traumatic experiences. In some studies, male and female survivors of childhood sexual abuse or female sexual assault survivors were more likely to experience sexual dysfunction (Laumann et al., 1999; Oberg, Fugl-Meyer, & Fugl-Meyer, 2002), although not all studies demonstrate the same findings (Dennerstein, Guthrie, & Alford, 2004). Research does show, however, that vaginismus is more likely among females who were sexually abused as children (Reissing, Binik, Khalife, Cohen, & Amsel, 2003), and both vaginismus and sexual avoidance are more common among sexual assault survivors who have been treated for alcohol or other drug abuse (Sanjuan, Langenbucher, & Labouvie, 2009).

Cultural and religious beliefs, practices, and expectations may also play a role in sexual difficulties, such as views that women should be subordinate to men and should not enjoy sex, the discouragement of body exploration, and the prearranged marriage of young girls. In some regions of Asia, individuals may complain of a sudden fear that the penis (or vulva and nipples in females) will retreat into the body; this fear is called *koro* (APA, 2000). Beliefs about the origin of sexual difficulties also vary by culture; for example, over 80% of Moroccan women experiencing sexual dysfunction reported that their dysfunction was due to sorcery by someone who wished them harm (Kadri et al., 2002). More broadly, individuals and their sexual beliefs may be influenced by cultural values conveyed explicitly or implicitly through the media. For example, greater exposure to sexual objectification of the body through television and magazines is related to greater body self-consciousness during physical intimacy (Aubrey, 2007). Satisfaction with one's body and perceived sexual attractiveness, in turn, predict sexual satisfaction among women (Pujols, Seal, & Meston, 2010).

From a social cognitive perspective, individuals have a cognitive framework that reflects their perception of themselves as sexual beings, termed *sexual self-schemas*, which guide attention and information processing in sexual situations (Cyranowski, Aarestad, & Andersen, 1999; Reissing, Laliberte, & Davis, 2005). Individuals also hold sexual self-efficacy beliefs, meaning beliefs about their ability to perform certain sexual behaviors in a given situation (Cyranowski et al., 1999). Negative self-perceptions in terms of sexual schematic representations and low self-efficacy for sexual behaviors interact with particular situations (such as one's partner not reaching orgasm) to result in particular thoughts in the moment (such as "I'm a failure" or "My partner doesn't find me sexually appealing"). These thoughts influence and interact with feelings, behaviors, and physiology, including one's sexual response (Nobre & Pinto-Gouveia, 2009). Research has demonstrated that individuals with erectile disorder, as compared to those without this disorder, are more likely to explain negative sexual events—such as loss of an erection—as the result of something that is wrong with them (internal attribution) and as something that is likely to continue (stable attribution; Scepkowski et al., 2004). Diminished erectile response can also be evoked among sexually functional males by providing them with prior, bogus, negative erectile feedback and an internal, stable attribution of their supposed diminished erectile response (Weisberg, Brown, Wincze, & Barlow, 2001).

In addition to beliefs about oneself and one's sexual functioning, research has highlighted the important role of attention as a mechanism that directly impacts sexual arousal and performance (de Jong, 2009). Experimental research shows that individuals can manipulate their physiological, sexual arousal by shifting their attentional focus (Beck & Baldwin, 1994; Koukounas & Over, 2001). For example, focusing on sexual fantasies can increase arousal, while focusing on sexually irrelevant thoughts can decrease arousal. Similarly, attending to one's own body and experience by focusing on enjoyable sexual sensations creates a positive feedback loop of increasing sexual arousal, while focusing on one's body or sexual performance from a judgmental, other-oriented perspective creates a feedback loop of increasing attention to sexually inhibiting thoughts, thereby decreasing arousal (de Jong, 2009). Physiological sexual processes thus cannot be separated from psychosocial factors, including cognitive processes, beliefs about the self, previous sexual experiences, interpersonal relationship issues, and the context of the sexual behavior.

Treatment of Sexual Dysfunctions

Psychotherapy Treatments for Sexual Dysfunctions   Sexual difficulties may go untreated because these difficulties are one of the most challenging problems for people to discuss with a doctor, therapist, or even with their partners. Moreover, without education about sex, individuals' anxiety and misconceptions about their difficulties may exacerbate the problem (Kadri et al., 2002; Turkistani, 2004). Treatment of sexual dysfunctions involves a learning process; clients must learn not only about sexual functioning in general, but also about their own bodies and the connection between their own psychological and physiological processes. They also must learn about their partners' bodies and preferences. Just as the etiology of sexual dysfunctions can be explained using a biopsychosocial approach, the same, integrative approach applies to treatment of sexual dysfunctions (Gambescia, Sendak, & Weeks, 2009).

Rather than adopting a model of focusing treatment on the "disease" (called a disease-centered approach), physicians and clinicians may better serve their patients (or clients) by adopting a *patient-centered approach* to treatment (Hatzichristou et al., 2004). This approach involves an empathic understanding of the patient's perspective of the problem, as well as patient education and active inclusion of the patient (and his or her partner, if possible) in exploring treatment options. Treatment providers should obtain a thorough account of past and present psychosocial, romantic relationship, sexual, and physical health functioning, as well as a physical examination and relevant laboratory tests when indicated (Basson et al., 2004; Hatzichristou et al., 2004). This process of data gathering may involve collaboration between multiple specialists in different fields. Throughout assessment and treatment, open, reciprocal communication between the patient and treatment provider is paramount for effective treatment of sexual dysfunctions (Hatzichristou et al., 2004).

Couples Approaches to Therapy   Sexual dysfunctions are virtually always interpersonal difficulties by definition and should be addressed as such, including facilitation of interpersonal communication and a sense of trust and shared involvement in treatment, as well as shared consideration of treatment options. Another reason for shared treatment participation is that when one partner in a relationship has a sexual difficulty or dysfunction, the likelihood increases that the other partner has or will develop a sexual difficulty or decreased sexual desire (Fugl-Meyer & Fugl-Meyer, 2002; Greenstein, Abramov, Matzkin, & Chen, 2006; Lewis et al., 2004). Further, labeling the partner with the sexual difficulty as the "dysfunctional" partner discounts the importance of the couple's relationship as well as the interactional, interpersonal nature of sexual behavior and may lead to further diminishment of the individual's sexual self-confidence, potentially resulting in the development of a self-fulfilling prophecy of sexual inadequacy (Betchen, 2009).

Clinicians should gather detailed information about the couple's relationship, as well as their sexual functioning and sexual scripts. *Sexual scripts* generally refer to expectations about sexual thoughts, plans, and behaviors, including with whom it is acceptable to have sex, the appropriate reasons for sex, and where and when sexual activity can take place (Gagnon, Rosen, & Leiblum, 1982). Sexual scripts can more specifically refer to a particular couple's implicit rules, expectations, and sequences of sexual activity, including the roles each partner takes on during the sexual activity, such as the "initiator," the "resister," or the "passive participant" (Gagnon et al., 1982; Lips, 2006; Matlin, 2000; McCormick, 1987). Through education and communication, modifications to the script can be made to satisfy both partners and allow more flexibility of the couple's sexual roles and sexual activities (Foley, 1994; Gagnon et al., 1982).

Behavioral Therapy   Sexual problems are also behavioral problems, and research suggests that addressing the specific sexual difficulty is a critical part of therapy, above and beyond enhancing the couple's relationship in general (Baucom, Shoham, Mueser, Daiuto, & Stickle, 1998; see also Gambescia & Weeks, 2006, for a review of behavioral therapy techniques). Effective behavioral techniques include learning about and practicing masturbation for treatment of orgasmic disorder (LoPiccolo & Lobitz, 1972), as well as progressive dilation using fingers or plastic dilators for vaginismus (Masters & Johnson, 1970). In some cases, vaginal muscle biofeedback for dyspareunia and vaginismus can be helpful (Basson et al., 2004; Lechtenberg & Ohl, 1994). Women who experience pain in their vaginal opening when touched (termed *provoked vestibulodynia*) were generally successfully treated with a combination of psychosexual education, psychological counseling, and progressive steps completed at home involving touching the sensitive area, pelvic floor contraction and relaxation, and penetration (Backman, Widenbrant, Bohm-Starke, & Dahlof, 2008; see also Stinson, 2009, for a review of treatments for female sexual dysfunction). Pelvic floor exercises have also been used to successfully treat coital incontinence, which is linked to sexual aversion, lack of desire or arousal, dyspareunia, and anorgasmia (Salonia et al., 2004; see also Moore, 2010, and Serati, Salvatore, Uccella, Nappi, & Bolis, 2009, for reviews on treatment of urinary incontinence and sexual function).

Sexual difficulties may also be due to distraction (Barlow, 1986; Beck & Barlow, 1986). One can become distracted by one's thoughts about sexual performance, the appearance of one's own body, possible intrusion by others during sex, and many other concerns. The term *spectatoring* or the *spectator role* refers to heightened self-focused attention that interferes with arousal due to concomitant thoughts of performance failure and negative self-evaluation (Masters et al., 1985). Couples techniques, such as sensate focus, have been used to treat arousal difficulties and spectatoring. *Sensate focus* involves removing the psychological pressure involved in sexual performance by instead engaging in relaxed, sensual touch without the goal of intercourse or orgasm (Masters & Johnson, 1970). Another couples' technique is the treatment of premature ejaculation through starting and stopping sexual activity to allow the man to better control and delay ejaculation, as well as through use of the *squeeze technique*, which involves repeatedly squeezing the penis for a few seconds either at the frenulum (near the ridge at the top of the penis) or at the base of the penis to deter ejaculation until desired (Masters & Johnson, 1970; Masters et al., 1985).

Individuals who have come to associate sex with trauma or anxiety can unlearn this association through gradual exposure to sexual activity at home with their partners, which is an application of Wolpe's *systematic desensitization* (Janata & Kingsberg, 2005; Wolpe, 1958). The individual learns relaxation techniques and may start with sexual imagery before moving on to in vivo sexual exercises. He or she should have a sense of control over what occurs (unlike past traumatic experiences, if that is the case), and the exposure should begin with less threatening situations, such as nonsexual touching, and progress to increasingly more potentially anxiety-provoking stimuli as he or she feels comfortable. Systematic desensitization has generally shown positive results for erectile disorder and sexual anxiety, although women with orgasmic difficulties seem to be better treated by masturbation exercises (Heiman & Meston, 1997). In most cases, however, much of the outcome of therapy rests on the couple's ability to communicate clearly, openly, and specifically. Miscommunication about sex is common among couples due to the use of confusing euphemisms and reluctance to be specific about anatomy and behavior (Gambescia et al., 2009). Couples need to talk to each other about what each finds pleasurable; verbal as well as nonverbal techniques may be used to guide one's partner during sexual activity (Lechtenberg & Ohl, 1994). Providing feedback to one's partner is also likely to increase his or her self-efficacy for sexual activity (Reissing et al., 2005).

Cognitive-Behavioral Therapy   Cognitive-behavioral therapy has also received empirical support as an effective treatment for sexual dysfunctions (McCabe, 2001; see ter Kuile, Both, & van Lankveld, 2010, for a review). The cognitive-behavioral approach to sexual dysfunction treatment involves facilitating the couple's communication, practicing sexual skills, and identifying and modifying maladaptive beliefs about sex that may be exacerbating or even causing the difficulty. For example, men who believe that a man must be ready for sex at any moment and that failure to sustain an erection is indicative of personal failure or that impotence is an affront to a man's masculinity will likely experience more debilitating anxiety and self-doubt when faced with loss of an erection, compared to men who do not add special significance to their body's functioning (Nobre & Pinto-Gouveia, 2006). Unrealistic expectations can also impede women's sexual functioning, such as the belief that women should be able to have an orgasm through intercourse during every sexual encounter, as well as beliefs that virtuous women, mothers, and older women should not be sexual (Nobre & Pinto-Gouveia, 2006). Dysfunctional automatic thoughts, such as thoughts of sexual performance failure or negative thoughts about one's partner, lead to decreases in arousal and sexual function for men and women (Carvalho & Nobre, 2010; Nobre & Pinto-Gouveia, 2006). Cognitive-behavioral therapists undermine these erroneous beliefs, dysfunctional automatic thoughts, and their negative effects through psychoeducation, cognitive restructuring, and homework assignments involving behavioral techniques, such as sensate focus (McCabe, 2001). Similarly, individuals seem to benefit from learning *mindfulness* techniques, which assist individuals in attending to and enjoying their moment-to-moment sexual experience while also learning to relax (Brotto, Basson, & Luria, 2008; Brotto, Heiman et al., 2008).

Medical Treatments for Sexual Dysfunctions   The use of medication to treat sexual dysfunctions is generally accepted for men but remains controversial for the treatment of female sexual dysfunctions (Tiefer, 2001). Most researchers recommend addressing relationship concerns for both men and women before considering medication (Basson et al., 2004; Hatzichristou et al., 2004). Since sexual functioning may decline with age, along with reproductive capacity, some researchers advocate an acceptance of these natural changes, rather than an emphasis on artificial maintenance of abilities associated with youth (Potts, Grace, Vares, & Gavey, 2006). The use of medication to treat sexual dysfunction, particularly erectile disorder, however, has become exceedingly popular. This popularity has overshadowed both the acceptance of sexual changes that occur over time and psychological explanations and treatments of sexual dysfunction. Patients therefore readily seek medication as a simple solution to their difficulties (Tiefer, 2006), and physicians—many of whom have received minimal training in terms of assessing and treating sexual dysfunctions—are often willing to simply write a prescription, rather than discuss psychosocial components of sexual functioning or to schedule an additional appointment with the patient and his or her partner (McCarthy & McDonald, 2009; Wiggins, Wood, Granai, & Dizon, 2007). Research has also moved away from psychotherapeutic approaches to treating sexual dysfunction and instead moved toward medical approaches, which tend to be better funded (Baucom et al., 1998).

Anatomically, sexual arousal in men and women is a similar process overall, involving the nervous and vascular systems, such as the dilation of blood vessels and flow of blood to the genitals, although this process has been studied more thoroughly in men than in women, as described subsequently (Segraves, 2002). Most medical treatments for men involve maximizing blood flow to the genitals or relaxing smooth muscle tissue. Popular treatments for erectile dysfunction include phosphodiesterase-5 inhibitors, such as sildenafil, tadalafil (Cialis), and vardenafil (Levitra). Rather than targeting blood flow to the penis, another strategy is to target areas of the brain believed to be involved in sexual functioning. Apomorphine, a medication that is often prescribed for Parkinson's disease, has been shown to be beneficial to men with erectile dysfunction because of its action on dopamine receptors (Wylie & MacInnes, 2005). Other, less commonly used treatments include the use of a vacuum constriction device that increases blood flow to the penis, intracavernosal injections (injections of medications into the penis), urethral suppository (depositing medication into the urethra), and surgically implanted prostheses (Archer, Gragasin, Webster, Bochinski, & Michelakis, 2005; Sadeghi-Nejad & Seftel, 2004). Low testosterone, which can lead to erectile dysfunction, has recently been successfully treated with subcutaneous (under the skin) injections of pellets into the back (Cavender & Fairall, 2009).

The usually undesirable sexual side effect of delayed orgasm from antidepressants and other medications is the desired effect for men with premature ejaculation, who may be effectively treated with these medications, such as SSRIs (Heiman & Meston, 1997; Waldinger, Zwinderman, Schweitzer, & Olivier, 2004). Antidepressants are not a panacea for premature ejaculation, however, as they can also cause unwanted side effects, such as diminished sexual desire (Barnes & Eardley, 2007). Although it may seem counterintuitive, research has provided some support for treatment of premature ejaculation with sildenafil, partly because it may facilitate additional, consecutive sexual encounters and a therefore longer total sexual experience (Barnes & Eardley, 2007). Simply becoming healthier, through exercising, losing extra weight, and quitting smoking, can also improve sexual functioning, including erectile function (Archer et al., 2005; Larsen et al., 2007).

For women, many treatments have targeted hormones that are thought to be etiological factors in female sexual dysfunction, particularly disorders involving desire and arousal (see Brotto, Bitzer, Laan, Leiblum, & Luria, 2010, for a review). Androgen therapy—such as treatment with testosterone creams and testosterone transdermal (absorbed through the skin) patches—has shown some success in increasing sexual desire and arousal among postmenopausal women and women who have had their ovaries and uterus removed (Berman et al., 1999; Braunstein et al., 2005; Shifren, 2004; Shifren et al., 2000, 2006). Testosterone is not recommended as a long-term treatment at high doses, however, due to masculinizing effects (such as facial hair growth, deepening of one's voice, and acne), and it is not approved by the U.S. Food and Drug Administration to treat female sexual dysfunction (Shifren, 2004). Hormone replacement therapy to increase estrogen levels has also been used, although there may be significant health risks associated with these medications, including blood clots, stroke, heart attack, and breast cancer, and findings about its sexual benefits are mixed (Archer et al., 2005; Basson et al., 2004; Gonzalez, Viafara, Caba, & Molina, 2004). Recent findings suggest that hormone therapies such as tibolone (available in Europe) and a transdermal patch that releases estradiol combined with norethisterone acetate may be effective in improving sexual function among postmenopausal women, although these medications also include potential health risks that are associated with hormone therapies (Nijland et al., 2008).

Given their general success with men, vasoactive drugs, such as sildenafil (taken orally) and alprostadil (applied as a topical cream to the genital area) have been tested among women, although findings are either nonsignificant (Basson, McInnes, Smith, Hodgson, & Koppiker, 2002), mixed, or should be interpreted cautiously due to a substantial placebo effect (see Bradford & Meston, 2009, for a meta-analysis; Heiman, 2002; Heiman et al., 2006). In addition, even when these medications do result in the desired physiological response, women's subjective sense of sexual desire tends to remain unchanged. For example, a recent study of treatment with sildenafil showed improvement in orgasm among premenopausal women with sexual dysfunction due to SSRIs, although these women did not show improvements in sexual desire, arousal, or sexual pain above placebo effects (Stulberg & Ewigman, 2008). Dopaminergic drugs, such as bupropion and apomorphine, have resulted in some success in treating female sexual dysfunction (Caruso et al., 2004; Segraves, Clayton, Croft, Wolf, & Warnock, 2004). Despite successful outcomes with some medications, there does not seem to be a "magic pill" to treat female sexual dysfunction (Bradford & Meston, 2009).

Medical approaches other than medication include surgery to correct existing physiological problems, such as urinary incontinence (Sertai et al., 2009). Similar to devices created to assist male sexual arousal, there are also female sexual arousal devices, such as the U.S. Food and Drug Administration–approved clitoral vacuum device called the EROS Clitoral Therapy Device (UroMetrics, St. Paul, Minnesota), which uses a gentle suction to increase blood flow to the clitoris (Billups et al., 2001).

Paraphilias and Hypersexual Behavior

Defining and Describing the Paraphilias

Paraphilia, literally meaning "lover" (*phile*) of that which is "beyond" or "abnormal" (*para*), can include a wide range of sexual activities, objects, and situations. According to the *DSM–IV–TR*, the paraphilias are "recurrent, intense sexually arousing fantasies, sexual urges, or behaviors generally involving (1) nonhuman objects, (2) the suffering or humiliation of oneself or one's partner, or (3) children or other nonconsenting persons that occur over a period of at least 6 months" (APA, 2000, p. 566). The paraphilias include fetishism, transvestic fetishism, voyeurism, exhibitionism, frotteurism, pedophilia, sexual masochism, and sexual sadism. Unlike sexual dysfunctions, some of the paraphilias—specifically those involving nonconsenting partners, including pedophilia, voyeurism, exhibitionism, frotteurism, and sexual sadism with a nonconsenting partner—do not require the criterion of significant personal distress or impairment to be diagnosed according to the *DSM–IV–TR*. The following descriptions of the paraphilias are based on the *DSM–IV–TR* diagnostic features.

Sexual fetishism involves sexual focus on a specific object to the extent that it leads to personal distress or impairment, such as relationship difficulties. Examples of fetish objects include underwear, shoes, stockings, belts, and perfume. Although many people find certain objects or items of clothing sexy, an individual with a sexual fetish is different in that the object usually must be rubbed or smelled during nearly every sexual activity for sexual satisfaction. Partialism (categorized under "paraphilia not otherwise specified" in the *DSM–IV–TR*) is similar to fetishism, although the item that elicits arousal is a part of the body, such as feet, rather than an inanimate object. Although common fetish objects are female undergarments, transvestic fetishism involves sexual arousal from wearing attire of the opposite sex, which usually means men wearing women's clothing. The idea of the self as a woman is often the paraphilic focus. Cross-dressing can range from a single item of clothing to a head-to-toe cross-gendered appearance. Typically, the individual is heterosexual, and the cross-dressing is not due to gender dysphoria (discomfort with one's gender). To meet the diagnostic criteria for transvestic fetishism, the individual must be significantly distressed or impaired by the cross-dressing.

Voyeurism involves observing individuals undress or have sex, through a window, for example, without the individuals' knowledge. The voyeur often masturbates while observing. *Exhibitionism*—unlike the inconspicuous activities of voyeurism—is the exposure of one's genitals to a stranger in an inappropriate place and without the observer's consent. This may be performed to shock the observer or with the intent to elicit arousal in the observer. Although the exhibitionist may masturbate during exposure, he or she usually does not attempt to sexually assault the observer. The most commonly reported method of exposure in one study was while driving a car (Grant, 2005). Like exhibitionism, *frotteurism* often occurs in public places with an unsuspecting victim, but frotteurism involves touching and rubbing against a person without his or her consent. The frotteur usually touches or tries to touch the victim in sexually explicit areas of the body.

One of the most potentially traumatizing forms of victimization is *pedophilia*. This disorder involves sexual fantasies, impulses, or behaviors directed at prepubescent (usually under 13 years of age) children by individuals who are at least 16 years old and who are also at least 5 years older than the child. The target is often a child to whom the pedophile has convenient access, such as a family member, foster child, or a child involved in some form of organization or activity that allows for time alone with the child. Female victimization is more commonly reported than is male victimization, although sex offenders who target boys tend to have more victims than those who target girls (see Cohen & Galynker, 2002, for a review). Pedophiles can be attracted to boys, girls, or both, and they can be exclusively attracted to prepubescent children, postpubescent adolescents, or a combination of adults and children or adolescents. Fantasizing about sexual activities with children and experiencing concomitant distress while not acting on these fantasies still fulfills diagnostic criteria for pedophilia (see also Fagan, Wise, Schmidt, & Berlin, 2002, for a review).

Another form of sexual activity that may involve victimization is *sexual sadism*, which is defined as deriving sexual gratification from making another person suffer physically or psychologically, including acts designed to humiliate. The primary components of the sexual gratification are dominance and control, and specific behaviors vary in degrees of severity, from blindfolding and paddling to cutting, burning, beating, and even killing (APA, 2000; Alison, Santtila, Sandnabba, & Nordling, 2004). The partner may be a nonconsenting victim or a sexual masochist. Sexual masochism involves deriving sexual pleasure from one's own suffering or humiliation. Masochists may have a partner perform the behavior, such as binding them, or they may perform the behavior alone. For example, *autoerotic asphyxiation* (a type of *hypoxyphilia* or *asphyxiophilia*, meaning pleasure derived from suffocation) involves depriving oneself of oxygen via a noose, plastic bag, or other means, usually while masturbating (APA, 2000; Uva, 1995). This behavior can lead to accidental suicide. In addition to the primary categories of paraphilias, the *DSM* also includes a "paraphilia not otherwise specified" category, which encompasses a range of deviant behaviors, including making obscene phone calls (*scatologia*), having sex with animals or corpses, partialism (meaning sexual arousal involving a specific body part, such as feet), and the sexual use of urine, feces, and enemas.

Controversy Over Inclusion and Exclusion of Particular Paraphilias in the DSM   The inclusion of particular paraphilias in the *DSM* is an issue of debate. For example, transvestism may be viewed as an uncommon deviation of normal sexual activities that is not inherently problematic. Distress caused by transvestism likely involves social or interpersonal pressure to not engage in this behavior, rather than reflecting an inherent pathology (Reiersol & Skeid, 2006). Researchers have also argued for the exclusion of mild forms of consensual sadomasochism (McConaghy, 1993; Richters, de Visser, Rissel, Grulich, & Smith, 2008). The inclusion of other paraphilias in the *DSM* has also been questioned, but for different reasons. Some argue that disorders that involve nonconsenting partners, such as pedophilia and sadism with nonconsenting partners, be excluded from the *DSM* because the behaviors leading to a diagnosis are criminal and inclusion of the diagnosis implies that the individual committing the crime has a mental illness that causes or explains his or her behavior. A concern is that labeling these behaviors "disorders" could be akin to excusing these behaviors, which was the argument used against the inclusion in the *DSM* of "paraphilic coercive disorder" or rape (Holden, 1986).

Hypersexual Behavior

Although the *DSM–IV–TR* includes a diagnostic category for individuals who do not want to have sex often enough, wanting to have sex too often is not included in the *DSM–IV–TR* as a specific disorder. Instead, "distress about a pattern of repeated sexual relationships involving a succession of lovers who are experienced by the individual only as things to be used" is provided as an example under the "sexual disorder not otherwise specified" category of the *DSM–IV–TR* (APA, 2000, p. 582). *Excessive sexual drive* is included, however, in the *ICD–10*. Many researchers have suggested that "compulsive sexual behavior" be included in the *DSM* (Bradford, 2001). Excessive sexual drive and behavior has been given a variety of names with varied meanings, including sexual addiction, sexual impulsivity disorder, and hypersexual desire disorder or simply hypersexual disorder.

Although this problem is not clearly defined and encompasses a wide range of thoughts and behaviors, most definitions include characteristics such as the lack of control over sexual thoughts or activities, the repetitive, time-consuming nature of these thoughts and activities, and the experience of personal distress, impairment, or other negative consequences that do not deter the behavior (Black, Kehrberg, Flumerfelt, & Schlosser, 1997; Kafka, 2003a; Wiederman, 2004). The use of the term *sexual addiction* is controversial in that it may be perceived as using a disease model, as in drug addiction. Nevertheless, when compared to existing disorders in the *DSM*, hypersexual behavior shares similar criteria with substance dependence and impulse control disorders (e.g., pathological gambling), in which the behavior causes negative outcomes or distress, but there is repeated failure to minimize or cease to engage in the behavior after repeated attempts (Giugliano, 2009). Although somewhat more commonly used, the term *compulsive sexual behavior* may also be problematic. Hypersexual behavior may include unwanted, intrusive thoughts, as in obsessions, but given that the sexual behavior is likely to be pleasurable and may or may not be used to decrease anxiety, the repetitive compulsions performed to mitigate the obsessions found in obsessive-compulsive disorder do not necessarily fit with hypersexual behavior. A consensus on the diagnostic label for hypersexual behavior has yet to be reached (Giugliano, 2009).

The problematic behavior of hypersexuality may be paraphilic in terms of the sexual activities involved, or the behavior may be common sexual practice that is excessive and that causes distress or negative outcomes (Kafka, 1997a). The sexual activity or preoccupations may include excessively high rates of masturbation, excessive use of pornography or telephone sex, or excessive sex with multiple partners, with prostitutes, with nonconsenting partners, or with one consenting partner that results in relationship difficulties (Kafka, 2003a; Raymond, Coleman, & Miner, 2003). A rare, high-risk subpopulation that has recently been identified as having high rates of hypersexual behavior is men who have sex with men without using condoms with the intent to contract HIV, self-identified as *bug chasers* (Moskowitz & Roloff, 2007). These individuals are more likely than other men who have sex with men (who also do not use condoms) to participate in sexual activities involving submission to a partner and humiliation, and it has been proposed that the idea of contracting HIV is viewed as a sexually arousing act of submission for these individuals (Moskowitz & Roloff, 2007).

Operational definitions of hypersexuality have included Kinsey et al.'s (Kinsey, Pomeroy, & Martin, 1948, , as cited in Kafka, 1997a) recommendation of at least seven orgasms a week, through any and all means, for several consecutive months, termed "total sexual outlet." An additional criterion is the average amount of time spent per week devoted to real or imagined sexual activity (Kafka, 1997a). Other researchers suggest that "impersonal sex" be used as a criterion, meaning that the person disregards the other person (if present) in favor of focus on the sex act itself. This criterion is supported by the finding that high rates of impersonal sexual behavior and interests are linked to less satisfaction with life; further, women who previously experienced sexual abuse or assault are more likely to report excessive impersonal sexual activities (Langstrom & Hanson, 2006).

About 5% of the U.S. population engages in hypersexual behavior, according to some estimates (Coleman, Raymond, & McBean, 2003), although individuals may be reluctant to report this problem, and few studies have addressed its prevalence. Among Germans seeking treatment for hypersexual behaviors, their most prevalent symptoms, according to their therapists, were pornography dependence (40%), compulsive masturbation (31%), and ongoing promiscuity (24%), with males being more highly represented in the first two symptom categories and females being more highly represented in the third (Briken, Habermann, Berner, & Hill, 2007). Hypersexual behavior is believed to be an anxiety-mitigating strategy, an impulse control or self-regulation difficulty, or some combination of these (Raymond et al., 2003; Stinson, Becker, & Sales, 2008). Although there may be an initial reduction in tension after the sexual act, individuals often feel guilty about engaging in the behavior (Black et al., 1997; Wiederman, 2004).

Treatment of compulsive sexual behavior depends on the nature of the behavior (e.g., whether it is compulsive masturbation, exhibitionism, or indiscriminate sex with others). As previously noted, hypersexual behavior can include high-risk sexual behavior, such as repeated sexual behavior with multiple partners without condom use. This behavior is a serious health risk and warrants intervention (Coleman, 2002). Regardless of the types of behaviors involved, however, treatment generally includes cognitive and behavioral techniques to increase alternative behaviors and diminish sexual thoughts and activities. In therapy, individuals are encouraged to develop coping strategies to regulate stress and mood (Coleman et al., 2003). Couples therapy may be useful in some cases, as well as a group therapy format modeled after other addictions treatment (such as 12-step programs); however, the goal is usually to reduce the behavior, such as with overeating, and not necessarily to eliminate the sexual behavior, unless it is harmful (Schneider, 1989). Medications used to treat impulse-control disorders and antidepressants with sexual side effects have been indicated as treatments for hypersexual behavior (Raymond, Grant, Kim, & Coleman, 2002). Naltrexone, which blocks opioid receptors and is used primarily to treat substance abuse, has been shown to be beneficial in treating hypersexual behavior (Raymond, Grant, & Coleman, 2010; Ryback, 2004). However, more research is needed to better understand and treat the wide range of hypersexual behaviors.

Epidemiology of Paraphilias

Researchers have had difficulty obtaining accurate estimates of the prevalence of the paraphilias, as some of these behaviors are illegal, are often viewed by society with disgust, disdain, or disapproval, and are relatively rarely seen in clinical settings as the predominant reason for treatment. Further, many areas of the world are unwilling to undertake this research (Bhugra, Popelyuk, & McMullen, 2010). Nevertheless, a large-scale, nationally representative Swedish study reported prevalence rates of at least one occurrence of exhibitionistic behavior at 3%, and voyeuristic behavior at 8% among 18- to 60-year-olds (Langstrom & Seto, 2006). Approximately 68% of those who engaged in exhibitionistic behaviors and 76% of those who engaged in voyeuristic behaviors were male. Lifetime experience of at least one occurrence of transvestic fetishism was reported at rates of approximately 3% for men and less than 1% for women (Langstrom & Zucker, 2005). One-year incidence rates for sexual behaviors involving bondage, discipline, sadomasochism, or dominance and submission were approximately 2%, with higher rates for males than for females (Richters et al., 2008). The paraphilias tend to occur together, as individuals who engage in exhibitionism or voyeurism also have higher rates of sadomasochistic behavior and cross-dressing (Langstrom & Seto, 2006). One potential explanation for the comorbidity of the paraphilias is that individuals with paraphilias tend to report being more easily sexually aroused and engage in higher rates of masturbation (Langstrom & Seto, 2006; Langstrom & Zucker, 2005); therefore, a greater potential for arousal to a larger variety of situations, fantasies, or objects may be possible for these individuals.

Etiology of Paraphilias

Behavioral Factors   Classical or Pavlovian conditioning has been widely used to explain the development of the paraphilias (see Akins, 2004, for a review). The development of a sexual fetish, for example, might be traced to a prior sexual experience that involved simultaneous arousal and presence of a particular object. This experience may occur during adolescence, which is the age at which most paraphilias begin. Once the association is acquired, the individual touches or smells the object to experience or enhance arousal, and repeated pairings of the object with masturbation and orgasm strengthen the association. In addition to the development of sexual fetishes, the pairing of sexual arousal with a particular object, situation, or type of person will likely be involved in the development of the other paraphilias. Operant conditioning may also reinforce the behavior, as people who expose themselves, make obscene phone calls, or rub up against unsuspecting victims may be rewarded by the strong reaction of the victim (such as disgust, anger, or surprise) or by the satisfaction of the act itself and the evasion of punishment if they are not caught. The types of sexual stimuli that elicit arousal are also likely to be learned to some extent through social and cultural norms. For example, shoes are more likely to be a fetish object than are tables. Important role models, such as parents, may also teach the deviant behavior through varying degrees of subtle or blatant modeling of the behavior (Stoller, 1985).

Psychosocial Factors and Comorbid Disorders or Difficulties   In addition to behavioral conditioning and modeling, many other factors, including one's psychosocial history and comorbid problems and disorders, are likely to play a role in the paraphilias. For example, a history of sexual abuse may be an etiological factor. A substantial portion of individuals who develop pedophilia, for example, report a history of sexual abuse (Cohen & Galynker, 2002). After controlling for gender, a history of sexual abuse was significantly more likely among individuals who engaged in voyeuristic behavior, particularly men (Langstrom & Seto, 2006). Substance abuse is often a comorbid condition, and being under the influence of a substance may lower sexual inhibitions or impulses (Kafka & Hennen, 2002; Raymond, Coleman, Ohlerking, Christenson, & Miner, 1999). Individuals with paraphilias or a history of sexual offenses are also more likely to have substance-abusing parents compared to the general population (Langevin, Langevin, Curnoe, & Bain, 2006). The paraphilias have been associated with a variety of additional difficulties, including a higher rate of psychological difficulties and dissatisfaction with life (Langstrom & Seto, 2006), as well as mood disorders, social anxiety, attention-deficit/hyperactivity disorder, and impulse-control difficulties (Kafka & Hennen, 2002). For example, sexual offenders' impaired social skills and social anxiety have been implicated in their disorder (Hoyer, Kunst, & Schmidt, 2001), to the extent that they may have difficulty recognizing social cues and may target vulnerable individuals, such as children, perhaps partly due to their difficulty forming relationships with adults (Emmers-Sommer et al., 2004). Among adolescent sex offenders, including pedophiles, the majority had one or more comorbid psychological disorder, with the most prevalent being conduct disorder, developmental disorders, and personality disorders (Van Wijk, Blokland, Duits, Vermeiren, & Harkink, 2007).

Biological Factors in the Paraphilias   The neurotransmitters that are believed to be involved in impulse control, mood, and sexual functioning, namely, the monoamines (including norepinephrine, dopamine, and serotonin), are implicated in the paraphilias and hypersexual behavior (Bradford, 2001; Kafka, 2003b). Further, multiple sclerosis, temporal lobe epilepsy, as well as brain lesions and brain tumors in various areas have been associated with the paraphilias and hypersexual behavior. For example, the frontal lobe (which is involved in impulse control) and the temporal lobe (believed to be involved in sexual arousal) have both been implicated in these sexual disorders (Bradford, 2001; Cohen & Galynker, 2002; see also Fedoroff, 2008, and Joyal, Black, & Dassylva, 2007, for reviews). However, frontotemporal pathways have also been linked to criminal activity in general and may not be specific to the paraphilias or sexual offending (Joyal et al., 2007). Additionally, the paraphilias reflect a wide range of behaviors and varying degrees of violence and impulsivity, and as such, research that groups different individuals together may find conflicting results (Joyal et al., 2007).

Levels of sex hormones, particularly androgens, are likely to play a role in sexual desire and activity (Bradford, 2001), which has been used as one explanation as to why the paraphilias are more common among males than among females (Arndt, 1991; Fagan et al., 2002; Langstrom & Zucker, 2005). Gender differences in the paraphilias have also been explained by socially prescribed gender roles. For example, cross-dressing among men is more likely to be noticed and pathologized than is cross-dressing among women; further, cases of women who derive sexual pleasure from wearing men's clothing may be underreported or may not be as interpersonally distressing (Devor, 1996). Exposure to media and cultural norms that sexualize women and their clothing and undergarments (compared to that of men) may also play a role in the predominance of males versus females with paraphilias (Bhugra et al., 2010). In addition, sexual scripts in many cultures specify that (in heterosexual relationships) men should be the pursuers and women should be pursued. Taken a step further, some men may sexually harass women or violate their rights, as in frotteurism, voyeurism, exhibitionism, scatologia, and the like, not for sexual gratification but in an attempt to exert dominance and control. Paraphilic behaviors among women, however, can have different motivations and outcomes than the same behaviors among men, as females tend to be more sexualized than males. For example, female exhibitionists report exposing themselves to men for positive attention and to experience the excitement of the situation (Hugh-Jones, Gough, & Littlewood, 2005).

Psychological Treatments of the Paraphilias

Individuals with paraphilias are often reluctant to seek treatment, either because (a) they do not believe their behavior is problematic, (b) they are embarrassed about their unusual sexual activities, or (c) their sexual activities are illegal. Accordingly, much of the research on the treatment of paraphilias includes samples of individuals who have been arrested and found guilty of sexual crimes and are mandated to receive therapy. These individuals are usually highly motivated to report that the treatment has worked but may not necessarily be motivated to change. Individuals whose paraphilic behaviors have caused relationship discord—such as transvestic fetishism with a disapproving partner—may be more motivated to change their behaviors to preserve their relationships. Most of the research on treatment of the paraphilias, however, involves treatment of sexual offenders.

A predominant model in the treatment of sexual offenders (and criminal offenders in general) is the risk-need-responsivity (RNR) treatment model (Andrews, Bonta, & Hoge, 1990; see also Andrews & Bonta, 2010, for a recent review). Assessment of risk of reoffending is the first step, with higher-risk individuals assigned to more intensive treatment than those who are considered lower risk. The second component of the model is to identify and match the "criminogenic needs" of the individual (meaning behavioral problems or characteristics that are related to offending) to appropriate treatment to address target difficulties or behaviors, such as social skills training. Cognitive-behavioral and social cognitive approaches are often used in this model. The third component, responsivity, involves tailoring the treatment to the skills, background, motivation, and abilities of the individual so that the treatment modality will likely have the greatest impact; in other words, so that the individual will respond well to the treatment. Treatment providers consider whether individual or group therapy (or both) would be most helpful, for example, or whether more or less structure in treatment would be useful for a given individual. Research has generally shown favorable outcomes of the RNR approach in terms of reducing recidivism (Andrews & Bonta, 2010). This model has been criticized, however, for potentially leading treatment providers to view the person from a deficit perspective, as a series of risk factors and areas of insufficient development, rather than promoting the view of the offender as a whole person, with personal strengths and positive life goals (Ward & Marshall, 2004; Whitehead, Ward, & Collie, 2007).

An alternative model, termed the *good lives model* (GLM) of rehabilitation, has been developed more recently not only to identify risk factors for sexual offenders' relapse, but also to emphasize the individual's personal goals and strengths and to use these factors in treatment to motivate positive change (Ward & Marshall, 2004). The emphasis of this model on self-regulation, sociocultural and social learning considerations, and positive mastery experiences makes it consistent with the social cognitive approach to psychotherapy. Additionally, research shows that when a sexual offender is being released from prison, community reintegration planning is important so that these individuals can develop healthy, stable lives without reoffending (Willis & Grace, 2008). Although the GLM shows promise based on initial findings (Whitehead et al., 2007), large-scale studies are needed to confirm its efficacy.

Both the RNR model and the GLM apply cognitive-behavioral therapy (CBT) techniques as part of their treatment, and CBT has been used to treat the paraphilias in general, including those involving sexual offenses (see Schaffer, Jeglic, Moster, & Wnuk, 2010, for a review). Behavioral techniques may include extinguishing the arousal response that is triggered by the conditioned stimulus, such as a pair of shoes or a picture of a child. Aversion therapy or aversive conditioning includes the presentation of an aversive stimulus with imagined or real presentation of the paraphilic stimulus. For example, the individual may become aroused by a pedophilic scenario and is then presented with a noxious odor or receives an electric shock or nausea-inducing substance (Marshall, 1974). Covert sensitization involves creating an imagined scene involving the deviant behavior that results in a negative experience or consequence, such as embarrassment or apprehension (Akins, 2004). Reconditioning the individual to become aroused to acceptable sexual stimuli, such as consenting adults, may also be used (Johnston, Hudson, & Marshall, 1992). Treatment may additionally include techniques such as role playing to facilitate improved anger management and emotional regulation, increase empathy for others, enhance communication skills, and improve identification and interpretation of social cues. Relapse prevention involves assisting the client in identifying patterns of behavior, as well as cues and situations, that may increase the risk for reoffending (Emmers-Sommer et al., 2004; Saleh & Guidry, 2003).

Cognitive strategies are also an important component of CBT for individuals with paraphilias (Schaffer et al., 2010). Psychoeducation is used to help clients better understand their problems, how these problems have developed over time, and how to develop strategies to control their behaviors. Clinicians also refute sexual myths and schemas that the client may hold, such as the concept that "no means yes," that all women are manipulative, that children should be taught about sex through experience, or that a victim who is frozen with fear is providing consent. Clinicians may also facilitate imagery that involves a new sequence of events, such as a scenario involving control of the unwanted impulses (Akins, 2004). In addition to cognitive and behavioral techniques, group therapy may be used. For disorders involving nonconsenting partners, such as pedophilia, the group format can be too confrontational in order to address clients' defensiveness, denial, and minimization of the harm they have caused others (Cohen & Galynker, 2002; Fagan et al., 2002). Although more research on the efficacy of CBT for all of the paraphilias is needed, research has generally demonstrated that CBT for sexual offenders is a preferred psychotherapeutic treatment method (Losel & Schmucker, 2005; O'Reilly, Carr, Murphy, & Cotter, 2010).

Medical Treatments for the Paraphilias

Researchers have reported some success in treating the paraphilias with antidepressants that influence serotonergic pathways (see Kafka, 1997b, for a review), as well as medications that reduce the effects of androgens, which are hormones believed to influence sexual desire and activity. Antiandrogens are medications that reduce the effects of androgens by competing with them at their receptor sites. One type of antiandrogen, cyproterone acetate (CPA), blocks androgen receptors and affects hormones that influence the release of testosterone. Medroxyprogesterone acetate (MPA; Depo-Provera) also results in a decrease in testosterone levels, although through a different mechanism of action. These medications have demonstrated success in treating paraphilias, particularly those involving nonconsenting partners, although they can also have serious side effects (Bradford, 2001; Maletzky, Tolan, & McFarland, 2006; Saleh & Guidry, 2003).

Newer medications with fewer side effects have recently been tested, such as the gonadotropin-releasing hormone (GnRH) agonists and the luteinizing hormone-releasing hormone (LHRH) agonists (Greenfield, 2006). These agonists reduce the effect of the hormones that signal the release of androgens by paradoxically stimulating the hypothalamus to release more hormones, until the down-regulation of receptors occurs. In many patients, an initial boost in sexual desire is followed by a steady decrease in desire as feedback mechanisms adjust to this overstimulation of the hypothalamus. For example, the GnRH agonist triptorelin successfully decreased hypersexual behavior in adult men without paraphilias (Safarinejad, 2008), and one type of LHRH agonist, leuprolide acetate, has shown promising results at reducing sexual thoughts and activities among sexual offending paraphiliacs (Saleh & Guidry, 2003). The term *chemical castration* has been used to describe medications that reduce the effects of androgens, particularly the drug MPA; however, these medications do not necessarily cause impotence and their effects are often reversible, depending on the type of medication used. Mandatory treatment with these medications, however, has been an issue of serious debate (Miller, 1998).

Gender Identity Disorder

Defining and Describing Gender Identity Disorder

One's sex refers to anatomical indicators of being male or female. One's gender refers to the sense that one is male or female—in other words, the gender with which one identifies (Lips, 2006). Gender identity disorder is the experience of an inconsistency between one's sex and one's gender. Individuals who take steps toward changing their gender or appearing as the opposite sex may be referred to as *transsexuals*, often specified as male-to-female transsexuals and female-to-male transsexuals (Stoller, 1985). The term *transgender* is used as a broader term to include individuals who opt not to have sex reassignment surgery, but who live as the opposite gender, although the terms transsexual and transgender are often used inconsistently (see Carroll, Gilroy, & Ryan, 2002, for a comprehensive list of terms). According to the *DSM–IV–TR*, gender identity disorder refers to strong and persistent cross-gender identification, such that the person with this disorder feels persistent discomfort with his or her sex and has a strong desire to be the opposite sex. The person asserts that he or she is "in the wrong body," and the experience is significantly distressing or results in impairment in functioning. Gender identity (one's subjective sense of being male or female) is not to be confused with sexual orientation (to whom one is attracted).

In children, gender identity disorder typically involves preference for opposite-sex dress, play behaviors, playmates, and urinary position, as well as the persistent assertion that the child is the opposite sex. Although more boys than girls are generally diagnosed with this disorder, this may be due to greater parental disapproval of stereotypically feminine behaviors in boys than for stereotypically masculine behavior in girls (Devor, 1996; Zucker & Bradley, 1995). The majority of children with gender identity disorder do not continue to have this disorder into adolescence or adulthood, although most individuals with gender identity disorder in adulthood recall having the disorder as children. The majority of boys with this disorder identify as bisexual or homosexual as they mature (Zucker & Bradley, 1995). Since gender identity disorder tends not to persist into adulthood, some researchers argue that this disorder should not be diagnosed among children (Lev, 2005).

Among adolescents and adults with gender identity disorder, behaviors may include cross-dressing, as well as breast binding in women to reduce the appearance of their breasts. Unlike transvestic fetishism, however, the aim of cross-dressing in gender identity disorder is usually to appear to be the opposite gender, which is consistent with the person's sense of self, rather than cross-dressing for the purpose of sexual arousal, although a person might have both aims (Buhrich & McConaghy, 1978). *Autogynephilia* refers to sexual arousal as a result of the mental or physical image of oneself as a woman, and researchers have highly conflicting views about the extent to which autogynephilia is related to gender identity disorder (Blanchard, 2010; Moser, 2010). Many contend that sexual arousal or sexual preferences and gender identity are distinct phenomena and that researchers tend to pathologize transgendered individuals and their sexual functioning (Moser, 2010). For example, if the primary impetus for a man to become a woman were for purposes of sexual arousal (which would be going to extreme lengths just for arousal), then he would not want to proceed with hormone medications that decrease sexual arousal as part of the process of becoming female, but the majority of male-to-female transsexuals do proceed with these medications. Additionally, women who are biologically born female may feel sexy in lingerie, just as women who are male-to-female transgendered may feel sexy in lingerie (Moser, 2010).

Researchers are beginning to discover that individuals with gender identity disorder are a more heterogeneous group than was previously thought. These individuals vary with respect to their sexual orientation, the presence of paraphilias (such as transvestic fetishism), and age of onset of their gender dysphoria. Lev (2005) reviewed several categories of experiences that seem to be missing from the transgender nomenclature, including individuals who do not want medical intervention but who do want to appear as the opposite gender, those who desire hormones but not surgery, those who have more than one gender identity and have or would like to have both male and female genitalia, those who want to appear more masculine or feminine with surgery that does not involve sex reassignment, and those who view their gender as nonstatic and do not wish to identify as one gender or the other.

Epidemiology and Etiology of Gender Identity Disorder

Gender identity disorder is relatively rare. Research conducted in the Netherlands estimates that transsexualism occurs in 1 in 11,900 males and 1 in 30,400 females, although this estimate may be high compared to countries that are less accepting of transsexualism (Bakker, van Kesteren, Gooren, & Bezemer, 1993). The etiology of gender identity disorder is complex and not fully understood, and theories about the development of this disorder are areas of serious debate.

Biological Factors in Gender Identity Disorder   Some evidence points to biological factors in the development of gender identity disorder. Neuroimaging research has studied whether brain activation patterns in transsexual individuals is different from their biologically male or female counterparts. These studies are often limited, however, by small sample sizes and the confounding effect of the hormone treatments that the transsexual patients are receiving. Nevertheless, research supports that male-to-female transsexuals may have different brain activation compared to heterosexual, nongender-dysphoric males during mental rotation tasks (Schoning et al., 2010) and in response to sexual stimuli (Gizewski et al., 2009).

One biological hypothesis of the origin of gender identity disorder is that prenatal exposure to varying levels of sex hormones influences subsequent gender identity development. Although measuring prenatal hormone levels usually is not feasible or practical, comparative finger length on one's hand—particularly between the index and ring fingers—is believed to be related to androgen exposure in the womb (Manning, Scutt, Wilson, & Lewis-Jones, 1998). Among male-to-female transsexuals, there is evidence of a difference in the ratio of length of the second to fourth fingers that is more similar to females than it is to nontranssexual males (Schneider, Pickel, & Stalla, 2006). Although digit ratios are now a popular measure, the validity of this measure as an indicator of prenatal androgen exposure is still being confirmed. Handedness has also been studied, with results showing that both types of transsexuals (male-to-female and female-to-male), as well as boys with gender identity disorder, are significantly more likely to be left handed than are people in the general population (Orlebeke, Boomsma, Gooren, Verschoor, & van den Bree, 1992; Zucker, Beaulieu, Bradley, Grimshaw, & Wilcox, 2001).

Other research has examined chromosomal and gonadal or hormonal anomalies that blur the line between the male and female sexes. For example, infants born with congenital adrenal hyperplasia (CAH) may have female chromosomes, but their bodies produce excessive amounts of androgens (masculinizing hormones) due to adrenal gland dysfunction. At birth, these infants may have large clitorises or even appear male. Regardless of whether they are assigned to the female or male gender, most grow up without developing gender identity disorder, although they do have higher rates of gender identity disorder when compared to the very low rates in the general population. Individuals with CAH who are assigned to the male gender, particularly those whose gender is reassigned later in childhood, tend to have higher rates of gender identity issues (Dessens, Slijper, & Drop, 2005).

In addition to CAH, a number of other physiological and chromosomal anomalies can occur that result in ambiguous genitalia. One abnormality (5-alpha-reductase-2 deficiency), which has been studied among individuals in villages in the Dominican Republic, occurred in genetically male children who had ambiguous genitalia, but appeared female, most of whom were reared as girls (Imperato-McGinley, Guerrero, Gautier, & Peterson, 1974). These children then developed masculine secondary sex characteristics at puberty, their testes descended, and their ambiguous genitalia developed into penises. They were known in the community as "*machihembra*," meaning "half man, half woman," or "*guevedoces*," meaning "penis at age 12." Most of these individuals adopted male gender roles as adults, although follow-up research shows that one of them in particular expressed the desire for sex reassignment surgery in adulthood to become a woman (Sobel & Imperato-McGinley, 2004). Finally, in separate research, the famous case of the boy (John/Joan) with the botched circumcision who was unsuccessfully reared as a girl also points to the role that biology plays in gender identity (Diamond & Sigmundson, 1997). Like any other psychological process, however, gender identity development is likely to be influenced by both biological and environmental factors, which interact with each other in a bidirectional manner.

Psychosocial Factors in Gender Identity Disorder   The concepts of gender and anatomical sex are socially constructed. For example, in most societies, there are two sex categories: male and female. In some societies, however, such as India and Thailand, there is a third category for individuals who wear women's clothing but have male (or sometimes intersex or ambiguous) genitalia and do not try to pass as female (Marecek et al., 2004). Even in societies with two sexes, research suggests that gender identity occurs along a continuum rather than being dichotomous. In other words, most people have varying degrees of identification with their own gender and with the opposite gender (Dunne, Bailey, Kirk, & Martin, 2000; McConaghy, 1993).

From a social cognitive perspective, gender identity development involves learning gender roles through *observational learning* (learning by viewing a model), experiencing others' evaluative reactions to one's behavior, and being rewarded and punished for gender-typical or gender-atypical behavior (Bussey & Bandura, 2004). These environmental forces typically exert pressure on children to conform to gender norms. Despite this pressure to conform, individuals with gender identity disorder may persist in their sex-atypical behavior or their assertion that they are the opposite sex. Many explanations have been provided for this unexpected result. In terms of psychosocial factors, researchers have proposed that children with gender identity disorder have identified with and imitated a person of the opposite gender or that they have been reinforced for gender-atypical behaviors (Halle, Schmidt, & Meyer, 1980; King, 1996).

Treatment for Gender Identity Disorder

Unlike treatments for most disorders, which involve helping individuals to change their thoughts, feelings, and behaviors, successful treatment of gender identity disorder often involves helping individuals change their gender or sex. This transition may include hormone treatments, electrolysis for men to remove unwanted hair, and varying degrees of surgery. The primary focus of psychotherapy may be preparing the client for changes in his or her relationships with others and with the broader society. Addressing emotional wounds from prejudice and discrimination may also be a central part of therapy (Carroll et al., 2002).

The treatment of gender dysphoria in children and adolescents has become a controversial issue. Psychotherapeutic approaches may involve teaching the child or adolescent to develop more gender-consistent behaviors. Opponents argue that this treatment is unethical and that it involves imposing narrowly defined social expectations for gender roles onto children and adolescents (Isay, 1999; Lev, 2005). Although some clinicians argue that retraining children to act in a more gender-role consistent manner will reduce peer and other interpersonal problems, Lev (2005) noted:

> in other areas where children are routinely bullied, for example racial or ethnic discrimination and physical or mental disabilities, the focus of intervention has been policy directed towards changing the social conditions that maintain abuse, not on changing children to better fit in to oppressive circumstances. (p. 49)

Researchers further assert that children with gender-atypical behavior may simply be gay, lesbian, or bisexual, and thus psychotherapy for these children should follow the American Psychological Association's (2000) *Guidelines for Psychotherapy with Lesbian, Gay, and Bisexual Clients*, which involves support and acceptance of feelings and behaviors that vary from socially prescribed gender roles.

Others argue that detection of gender identity disorder in children can be useful to assist them to make a transition to the opposite sex during adolescence. This early transition allows the individual to avoid the continued stress of living life in the gender that is inconsistent with the sense of self. Additionally, secondary sex characteristics become evident during adolescence and can be problematic for adolescents with gender identity disorder. In cases involving extreme, unwavering gender dysphoria since childhood and a clear desire for sex reassignment surgery, hormone therapy and surgery for both male-to-female and female-to-male adolescent transsexuals have resulted in a positive outcome. It is noteworthy, however, that most of these adolescents did not undergo full genital surgery because of their desire to wait for advances in surgical techniques (Cohen-Kettenis & van Goozen, 1997). Not all researchers agree, however, that adolescents are developmentally ready to make such a consequential decision as a transsexual transformation, and the standard practice guidelines for gender identity disorder state that irreversible procedures should not be performed on individuals under the age of 18 (World Professional Association for Transgender Health, 2001).

Since sex reassignment surgery is such a serious, irreversible, and life-changing transformation, surgeons are cautious about accepting patients for this surgery. The current treatment practice for transsexuals is based on the *Standards of Care for Gender Identity Disorders* (2001) guidelines, provided by the World Professional Association for Transgender Health. These guidelines specify that certain conditions must be met before sex reassignment surgery may be performed, including a gender identity disorder diagnosis, recommendation from one or more psychotherapists (depending on the type of surgery requested), and living as the opposite gender for 1 year while receiving hormone injections. Some researchers have expressed concern that individuals who want sex reassignment surgery have learned to report certain expected case histories, including that they are homosexual, that they have been gender dysphoric since childhood, and that they do not have transvestic fetishism because they believe it will increase their chances of being accepted for surgery (see Lev, 2005, for a review). Some argue that transsexualism is not a disorder and that the requirements for sex reassignment surgery are expensive, demeaning, and invalid (Denny, 2004). Moreover, research suggests that patients who do not comply with the 1-year transgender experience guideline prior to surgery have postoperative outcomes that are no different from patients who do comply (Lawrence, 2003). In most cases, sex reassignment surgery results in positive mental and physical health outcomes (De Cuypere et al., 2005; Smith, Van Goozen, Kuiper, & Cohen-Kettenis, 2005), as well as satisfaction with sexual functioning (see Klein & Gorzalka, 2009, for a review). Negative outcomes often involve dissatisfaction or problems with the surgical procedure, which usually cannot be predicted (Lawrence, 2003). For liability reasons, physicians and surgeons will likely continue to screen their patients for sex reassignment surgery and continue to deny some individuals who are not viewed to be "good candidates" for the surgery.

Summary, Current Issues, and Future Directions

Sexual dysfunctions, the paraphilias, and gender identity disorder reflect a vast array of behaviors, all of which lie along a continuum and have varying degrees of concomitant distress, ranging from no distress to severe distress. Biological, social, and psychological factors play a role in each of these disorders, and one cannot separate the influence of these factors for a given individual. The sexual dysfunction literature, which used to emphasize Masters and Johnson's behavioral techniques, is now dominated by medical research that assesses and treats these problems from a biological perspective. Erectile dysfunction has been a predominant area of research, and successful treatment with medications has made this problem profitable to drug manufacturers and relatively easily solved by the consumer (Levine, 2010). Medical interest in female sexual dysfunction, while historically ignored, is now increasing, largely as a result of the potential for a finding a popular drug that could be the female counterpart to drugs such as sildenafil (Hartley, 2006). Nevertheless, conceptualizations and treatments of sexual functioning that consider interpersonal, psychological, and social factors are still recommended (Hatzichristou et al., 2004).

The paraphilias include a variety of behaviors, some of which may simply reflect unusual sexual preferences, while other behaviors involve harmful and illegal activities, such as acting on pedophilic impulses. Behavioral explanations of how deviant sexual behavior is learned are prevalent in this area of research. Much of the research emphasis, however, is devoted to pedophiles and sexual offenders and their treatment, which is a much needed line of research, although more research is needed to address the other paraphilias as well. Behavioral techniques involving punishment or changing learned associations may be used to treat these problems, although particularly for sexual offenders, medications to lower sexual desire are likely to be more prevalent in the future (Saleh & Guidry, 2003).

Gender identity disorder involves a conviction that one is or should have been the opposite sex. This problem reflects a wider range of beliefs about one's gender and desired physical changes than was originally thought, including individuals who want to live as the opposite gender with or without hormone therapy and with or without sex reassignment surgery (Lev, 2005). Individuals may also be intersexed or have ambiguous genitalia at birth. A wide variety of biological and psychosocial factors have been proposed to explain gender identity disorder, although the etiology of gender identity disorder is complicated and not clearly understood. For those individuals who opt for sex reassignment surgery, there are commonly used guidelines that typically must be met before the surgery can be performed, but most transsexuals make a successful transition postoperatively and are relieved of their gender dysphoria (Smith et al., 2005).

The DSM and Future Potential Diagnostic Categories

If the past is a guide to the future, the number of sexual dysfunctions and disorders listed in the *DSM* is likely to increase, which may lead to pathologizing behavior that may otherwise be considered normal, on the one hand, as well as developing more successful treatments for a wider range of sexual difficulties, on the other hand. Recommendations from the Committee on the Definitions, Classifications and Epidemiology of Sexual Dysfunction include the addition of *persistent sexual arousal disorder* (recurrent, unwanted genital arousal), as well as the addition of *anejaculation*, meaning orgasm in men that occurs without ejaculation (Lewis et al., 2004). The third International Consultation on Sexual Medicine (ICSM) resulted in several similar proposals and recommendations for the upcoming DSM–5, including persistent genital arousal disorder and the stratification of sexual arousal disorders into physiological or psychological arousal subtypes (Basson, Wierman, van Lankveld, & Brotto, 2010). Other committees have discussed the possible addition of sexual satisfaction disorder, defined as not being sexually satisfied, despite satisfactory reports of desire, arousal, and orgasm (Basson et al., 2000). Another proposed potential disorder is noncoital sexual pain disorder (Basson et al., 2000). Researchers have also noted an absence of disorders that are specifically relevant to sexual behaviors beyond heterosexual coitus; thus, anodyspareunia, or pain during receptive anal sex, has been proposed as a possible diagnostic category (Hollows, 2007). Further, defining premature ejaculation in terms of vaginal intercourse excludes men who have sex with men.

Research has consistently shown that women can experience a discrepancy between their psychological experience of sexual arousal and their physiological sexual arousal response (Basson et al., 2010). Researchers thus propose that female sexual arousal be divided into three disorders: one indicating the lack of genital arousal (genital sexual arousal disorder), the second including lack of the subjective feeling of sexual arousal and pleasure (subjective arousal disorder), and the third including both the first and second symptoms (combined genital and subjective arousal disorder; Basson et al., 2004, 2010; Lewis et al., 2004; Segraves, Balon, & Clayton, 2007). Further, women may experience sexual desire during, rather than prior to sex, and women may not necessarily be sexually motivated by fantasies and sexual thoughts, which suggests that sexual desire disorder should be revised (Basson, 2005). In line with the acknowledgment of the importance of both psychological and neurobiological factors in sexual dysfunction in men as well, researchers have recommended that premature ejaculation be divided into four categories: (1) lifelong premature ejaculation, (2) acquired premature ejaculation, (3) natural variable premature ejaculation (a subclinical variant of this problem), and (4) premature-like ejaculatory dysfunction (in which the person subjectively ejaculates earlier than he feels he should, but ejaculatory time is within a normal range; Waldinger, 2008). To address the difficulty defining premature ejaculation, the International Society for Sexual Medicine has proposed that for lifelong premature ejaculation, the general guideline of ejaculation at approximately 1 min after vaginal penetration or the inability to delay ejaculation when so desired should be used (McMahon et al., 2008). Further, they noted that social cognitive constructs, such as self-efficacy and interpersonal consequences, should be integrated into the definition of premature ejaculation.

An additional proposal is to move sexual aversion disorder to the category of anxiety disorders in the *DSM*, as one of the types of specific phobias (Brotto, 2010). The rationale for this proposal is that this disorder is often comorbid with anxiety disorders, and its presentation is much more similar to the avoidance seen in individuals with anxiety disorders. In addition, women who avoid sex due to genital pain may be more accurately grouped with individuals with vaginsmus or dyspareunia (Brotto, 2010). Other researchers (e.g., Segraves et al., 2007) have proposed combining existing diagnostic categories that tend to be comorbid or are difficult to differentiate, although these proposals have been met with some criticism ("Responses to the Proposed DSM-V Changes," 2010). The proposals include the grouping of vaginismus and dyspareunia into one disorder: genito-pelvic pain disorder, and the combining of desire and arousal disorders into sexual interest arousal disorder, or perhaps delineating desire disorders, arousal disorders, and combined disorders.

Another potential revision to the *DSM* is the addition of compulsive sexual disorder or hypersexual disorder, which several researchers have recommended (Bradford, 2001; Kafka, 2010). The proposed diagnostic criteria of hypersexual disorder, according to Kafka (2010), would include excessive time devoted to sexual thoughts or activities that interfere with daily life, engaging in sexual thoughts or behaviors as a means to cope with negative mood or stress, repeatedly failing to decrease or restrain these thoughts or behaviors, repeatedly engaging in the sexual behaviors without regard for negative consequences or harm, and experiencing clinically significant distress or impairment from the thoughts or activities. The disorder would not be primarily substance induced and would include one of the following specifiers as the focus of sexual thoughts or activities: masturbation, pornography, sexual behavior with consenting adults, cybersex, telephone sex, strip clubs, or "other."

Some researchers advocate a complete reconceptualization of the categorization of sexual dysfunctions, particularly as they apply to women. Based on qualitative data, researchers have proposed eliminating the current categories and replacing them with the following four categories (which each include individual subcategories): (1) sexual problems resulting from sociocultural, political, or economic factors (such as body image issues or lack of gynecological health care or sexual education); (2) sexual problems relating to one's partner or relationship; (3) sexual problems resulting from psychological factors (such as depression and anxiety); and (4) sexual problems resulting from medical factors (Nicholls, 2008). This framework is termed the "new view" approach to classification. Additional research is needed to determine if this conceptualization is also applicable to men and their sexual experience.

Substantial debate has also continued regarding the diagnostic category of the paraphilias. Researchers have argued that paraphilic behaviors should be stratified into nonclinical paraphilias, which do not result in significant impairment or distress, and paraphilic disorders, which do result in significant impairment or distress (Blanchard, 2010). For example, transvestic behavior could be classified as a lifestyle choice, while transvestic disorder (in place of transvestic fetishism) would involve clinically significant distress or dysfunction. Further, transvestic disorder would include the specifiers "with fetishism" and "with autogynephilia" in place of the existing specifier "with gender dysphoria" (Blanchard, 2010). The specifier "with gender dysphoria" would be removed because an individual who met the criteria for both disorders would have a dual diagnosis of gender identity disorder and transvestic disorder (Blanchard, 2010). However, these recommended changes are not universally agreed upon, as once an individual becomes a male-to-female transsexual, it is unclear how autogynephilia or transvestic disorder would be applicable, particularly since autogynephilia, by definition, does not apply to women (Moser, 2010). Research also indicates that gender identity disorder may be subcategorized into a variety of components that reflect the wide range of gender variant identification, behaviors, and desires for treatment (Lev, 2005).

Internet Sexuality

Although sexual activities were taboo discussion topics in the past, in many cultures, these topics are now receiving more attention. Sexual behavior and sexual function and dysfunction are pervasive in daily society, as books, magazine articles, television shows and commercials, and other forms of media promote ideas about what it means to have a fulfilling sex life. With the advent of the Internet, much more information is readily accessible to people than ever before. At the same time, the Internet can also be a place where pedophilia, sexual addictions, and a host of sexually deviant fantasies can flourish (see Durkin, Forsyth, & Quinn, 2006, for a review). Sexual behaviors that may be rare or considered deviant in one's immediate community are commonplace in online communities that bring together individuals who may be thousands of miles apart (Rosenmann & Safir, 2006). The 24-hour availability, low cost, relative anonymity, and lack of risk for disease on the Internet, combined with the lack of accessibility to the same types of sexual experiences in one's daily interpersonal life, may facilitate excessive Internet sexual activity (termed *Internet sexual compulsivity*; Rosenmann & Safir, 2006). This problematic behavior can take the form of either viewing sexual material or sexual computer-mediated relating (CMR; Cooper, McLoughlin, & Campbell, 2004). *Cybersex* is a term recently applied to sexual online correspondence. A large-scale Swedish study found that 30% of men and 34% of women reported having engaged in this online sexual correspondence (Daneback, Cooper, & Mansson, 2005). When online sexual viewing or correspondence becomes excessive, it can damage relationships and result in diminished work productivity and job loss (Cooper, Safir, & Rosenmann, 2006; Orzack, Voluse, Wolf, & Hennen, 2006). Attempting to control Internet-mediated sexual activity is a major issue for corporations, families, and educational institutions. Yet, online sexual activity can also add excitement to a committed relationship and can provide a "safe" space to discuss sexual fantasies or sexual issues (Cooper et al., 2004). The sense of anonymity of the Internet may also facilitate online sex therapy, as preliminary research suggests (van Diest, van Lankveld, Leusink, Slob, & Gijs, 2007).

The Medicalization of Sexual Dysfunction

Researchers who support the view that sexual dysfunction has been socially constructed argue that any sexual experience, activity, or level of desire that does not fit nicely into the restricted definition of "normal sex" becomes medicalized as a disorder (Bancroft, 2002; Lavie-Ajayi, 2005; Pacey, 2008). A highly lucrative industry (pharmaceuticals) has profited from this perspective, as diagnostic categories lend themselves to treatment with medical interventions. Psychotherapy, which may or may not be covered by an individual's health insurance plan, may take longer to work than a pill, and generally is not promoted through television and other advertisements, is therefore at a disadvantage when compared to pharmaceutical treatments, which have enjoyed increasing popularity. As Tiefer (2006) explained:

> The trend of looking towards biology for the "most basic" explanations of complex human behavior, sidelined during the socially conscious 1970s and revived by sociobiology in the 1980s, escalated in the 1990s along with the mania for genetics and molecular biology and their magical promises. (p. 282)

Proponents of the sexual dysfunction categories assert, however, that these categories allow researchers and treatment professionals to more effectively identify, study, and treat these difficulties. Individuals receiving treatment can also be assured that their problems are valid concerns that warrant attention and treatment, particularly if the problem is framed as a medical one. Further, a serious consequence of sexual difficulties or dysfunctions is the inability to conceive among couples who wish to have a child (Tulla, Dunn, Antilus, & Muneyyirci-Delale, 2006). As such, these couples may wish to explore both psychotherapeutic and medical options to address this difficulty. Moreover, for all couples with sexual difficulties, treatment does not have to be either medical or psychotherapeutic, as a combined, multidisciplinary approach to assessment and treatment is recommended to address the multifaceted etiology of these difficulties (Basson et al., 2010). The majority of treatment outcome studies, however, promote one medication compared to another or to a placebo, rather than using a biopsychosocial approach (Pacey, 2008).

Major demographic trends include increased longevity in the population in general and the "Baby Boomer" generation now embarking upon their 50s and 60s. This trend has important implications for the marketing and selling of medications to treat sexual dysfunctions to this large potential market of consumers, particularly since sexual problems, such as erectile dysfunction, tend to increase with age (Prins et al., 2002). Although sexual functioning clearly has a biological component, many argue that the explanation of sexual dysfunction as purely biological in origin oversimplifies the problem, disregards interpersonal and psychosocial factors, and blames the individual (Tiefer, 2001). Moreover, the use of medication to encourage people who are otherwise satisfied to want to have sex may be viewed as a symptom of a youth-obsessed and sex-obsessed society, rather than a symptom of a medical condition (Potts, Grace, Gavey, & Vares, 2004), particularly since research shows that sexual desire naturally decreases over time as individuals get older (Bitzer et al., 2008; Eplov et al., 2007; Stanworth & Jones, 2008). Nevertheless, diagnostic categories that determine "appropriate" sexual behavior will likely continue to be used, for better or for worse.

References

Akins, C. K. (2004). The role of Pavlovian conditioning in sexual behavior: A comparative analysis of human and nonhuman animals. *International Journal of Comparative Psychology, 17*, 241–262.

Alison, L., Santtila, P., Sandnabba, N. K., & Nordling, N. (2004). Sadomasochistically oriented behavior. In M. S. Kimmel & R. F. Plante (Eds.), *Sexualities: Identities, behaviors, and society* (pp. 258–265). New York: Oxford.

Althof, S. E., Leiblum, S. R., Chevret-Measson, M., Hartmann, U., Levine, S. B., McCabe, M., … Wylie, K. (2005). Psychological and interpersonal dimensions of sexual function and dysfunction. *Journal of Sexual Medicine, 2*(6), 793–800.

American Psychiatric Association. (1980). *Diagnostic and statistical manual of mental disorders* (3rd. ed.). Washington, DC: Author.

American Psychiatric Association. (1987). *Diagnostic and statistical manual of mental disorders* (3rd rev. ed.). Washington, DC: Author.

American Psychiatric Association. (2000). *Diagnostic and statistical manual of mental disorders* (4th ed., text rev.). Washington, DC: Author.

American Psychological Association. (2000). *Guidelines for psychotherapy with lesbian, gay, and bisexual clients*. Retrieved October 31, 2006, from http://www.apa.org/pi/lgbt/resources/guidelines.aspx

Andrews, D. A., & Bonta, J. (2010). Rehabilitating criminal justice policy and practice. *Psychology, Public Policy, and Law, 16*(1), 39–55.

Andrews, D. A., Bonta, J., Hoge, R. D. (1990). Classification for effective rehabilitation: Rediscovering psychology. *Criminal Justice and Behavior, 17*(1), 19–52.

Araujo, A. B., Durante, R., Feldman, H. A., Goldstein, I., & McKinlay, J. B. (1998). The relationship between depressive symptoms and male erectile dysfunction: Cross-sectional results from the Massachusetts Male Aging study. *Psychosomatic Medicine, 60*, 458–465.

Archer, S. L., Gragasin, F. S., Webster, L., Bochinski, D., & Michelakis, E. D. (2005). Aetiology and management of male erectile dysfunction and female sexual dysfunction in patients with cardiovascular disease. *Drugs and Aging, 22*(10), 823–844.

Arndt, W. B. Jr. (1991). *Gender disorders and the paraphilias.* Madison, CT: International Universities Press.

Asboe, D., Catalan, J., Mandalia, S., Dedes, N., Florence, E., Schrooten, W., … Colebunders, R. (2007). Sexual dysfunction in HIV positive men is multi-factorial: A study of prevalence and associated factors. *AIDS Care, 19*(8), 955–965.

Aubrey, J. S. (2007). The impact of sexually objectifying media exposure on negative body emotions and sexual self-perceptions: Investigating the mediating role of body self-consciousness. *Mass Communication and Society, 10*(1), 1–23.

Backman, H., Widenbrant, M., Bohm-Starke, N., & Dahlof, L. G. (2008). Combined physical and psychosexual therapy for provoked vestibulodynia—an evaluation of a multidisciplinary treatment model. *Journal of Sex Research, 45*(4), 378–385.

Bakker, A., van Kesteren, P. J., Gooren, L. J., & Bezemer, P. D. (1993). The prevalence of transsexualism in the Netherlands. *Acta Psychiatrica Scandinavica, 87*(4), 237–238.

Baldwin, D., Moreno, R. A., & Briley, M. (2008). Resolution of sexual dysfunction during acute treatment of major depression with milnacipran. *Human Psychopharmacology, 23*(6), 527–532.

Balon, R., & Segraves, R. T. (2008). Survey of treatment practices for sexual dysfunction(s) associated with anti-depressants. *Journal of Sex and Marital Therapy, 34*(4), 353–365.

Bancroft, J. (2002). The medicalization of female sexual dysfunction: The need for caution. *Archives of Sexual Behavior, 31*(5), 451–455.

Bancroft, J., Loftus, J., & Long, J. S. (2003). Distress about sex: A national survey of women in heterosexual relationships. *Archives of Sexual Behavior, 32*(3), 193–208.

Barlow, D. H. (1986). Causes of sexual dysfunction: The role of anxiety and cognitive interference. *Journal of Consulting and Clinical Psychology, 54*(2), 140–148.

Barnes, T., & Eardley, I. (2007). Premature ejaculation: The scope of the problem. *Journal of Sex and Marital Therapy, 33*(2), 151–170.

Basson, R. (2002). Women's sexual desire—disordered or misunderstood? *Journal of Sex and Marital Therapy, 28*(Suppl.), 17–28.

Basson, R. (2005). Women's sexual dysfunction: Revised and expanded definitions. *Canadian Medical Association Journal, 172*(10), 1327–1333.

Basson, R., Althof, S., Davis, S., Fugl-Meyer, K., Goldstein, I., Leiblum, S., … Wagner, G. (2004). Summary of the recommendations on sexual dysfunctions in women. *Journal of Sexual Medicine, 1*(1), 24–34.

Basson, R., Berman, J., Burnett, A., Derogatis, L., Ferguson, D., Fourcroy, J., … Whipple, B. (2000). Report of the international consensus development conference on female sexual dysfunction: Definitions and classifications. *Journal of Urology, 163*(3), 888–893.

Basson, R., McInnes, R., Smith, M. D., Hodgson, G., & Koppiker, N. (2002). Efficacy and safety of sildenafil citrate in women with sexual dysfunction associated with female sexual arousal disorder. *Journal of Women's Health and Gender-Based Medicine, 11*(4), 367–377.

Basson, R., Wierman, M. E., van Lankveld, J., & Brotto, L. (2010). Summary of the recommendations on sexual dysfunctions in women. *Journal of Sexual Medicine, 7*(1), 314–326.

Baucom, D. H., Shoham, V., Mueser, K. T., Daiuto, A. D., & Stickle, T. R. (1998). Empirically supported couple and family interventions for marital distress and adult mental health problems. *Journal of Consulting and Clinical Psychology, 66*(1), 53–88.

Bayram, G. O., & Beji, N. K. (2010). Psychosexual adaptation and quality of life after hysterectomy. *Sexuality and Disability, 28*(1), 3–13.

Beck, J. G., & Baldwin, L. E. (1994). Instructional control of female sexual responding. *Archives of Sexual Behavior, 23*(6), 665–684.

Beck, J. G., & Barlow, D. H. (1986). The effects of anxiety and attentional focus on sexual responding—II. Cognitive and affective patterns in erectile dysfunction. *Behaviour Research and Therapy, 24*(1), 19–26.

Berman, J. R., & Bassuk, J. (2002). Physiology and pathophysiology of female sexual function and dysfunction. *World Journal of Urology, 20*(2), 111–118.

Berman, J. R., Berman, L., & Goldstein, I. (1999). Female sexual dysfunction: Incidence, pathophysiology, evaluation, and treatment options. *Urology, 54*(3), 385–391.

Betchen, S. J. (2009). Premature ejaculation: An integrative, intersystems approach for couples. *Journal of Family Psychotherapy, 20*(2–3), 241–260.

Bhugra, D., Popelyuk, D., & McMullen, I. (2010). Paraphilias across cultures: Contexts and controversies. *Journal of Sex Research, 47*(2–3), 242–256.

Billups, K. L., Berman, L., Berman, J., Metz, M. E., Glennon, M. E., & Goldstein, I. (2001). A new non-pharmacological vacuum therapy for female sexual dysfunction. *Journal of Sex and Marital Therapy, 27*(5), 435–441.

Bishop, J. R., Ellingrod, V. L., Akroush, M., & Moline, J. (2009). The association of serotonin transporter genotypes and selective serotonin reuptake inhibitor (SSRI)-associated sexual side effects: Possible relationship to oral contraceptives. *Human Psychopharmacology, 24*(3), 207–215.

Bishop, J. R., Moline, J., Ellingrod, V. L., Schultz, S. K., & Clayton, A. H. (2006). Serotonin 2A-1438 G/A and G-protein Beta3 subunit C825T polymorphisms in patients with depression and SSRI-associated sexual side-effects. *Neuropsychopharmacology, 31*(10), 2281–2288.

Bitzer, J., Plantano, G., Tschudin, S., & Alder, J. (2008). Sexual counseling in elderly couples. *Journal of Sexual Medicine, 5*(9), 2027–2043.

Black, D. W., Kehrberg, L. L., Flumerfelt, D. L., & Schlosser, S. S. (1997). Characteristics of 36 subjects reporting compulsive sexual behavior. *American Journal of Psychiatry, 154*(2), 243–249.

Blanchard, R. (2010). The DSM diagnostic criteria for transvestic fetishism. *Archives of Sexual Behavior, 39*(2), 363–372.

Blanker, M. H., Bosch, J. L., Groeneveld, F. P., Bohnen, A. M., Prins, A., Thomas, S., & Hop, W. C. (2001). Erectile and ejaculatory dysfunction in a community-based sample of men 50 to 78 years old: Prevalence, concern, and relation to sexual activity. *Urology, 57*(4), 763–768.

Bodenmann, G., Ledermann, T., Blattner, D., & Galluzzo, C. (2006). Associations among everyday stress, critical life events, and sexual problems. *Journal of Nervous and Mental Disease, 194*(7), 494–501.

Bradford, J. M. (2001). The neurobiology, neuropharmacology, and pharmacological treatment of the paraphilias and compulsive sexual behaviour. *Canadian Journal of Psychiatry, 46*(1), 26–34.

Bradford, A., & Meston, C. M. (2009). Placebo response in the treatment of women's sexual dysfunctions: A review and commentary. *Journal of Sex and Marital Therapy, 35*(3), 164–181.

Braunstein, G. D., Sundwall, D. A., Katz, M., Shifren, J. L., Buster, J. E., Simon, J. A., … Watts, N. B. (2005). Safety and efficacy of a testosterone patch for the treatment of hypoactive sexual desire disorder in surgically menopausal women: a randomized, placebo-controlled trial. *Archives of Internal Medicine, 165*(11), 1582–1589.

Briken, P., Habermann, N., Berner, W., & Hill, A. (2007). Diagnosis and treatment of sexual addiction: A survey among German sex therapists. *Sexual Addiction and Compulsivity, 14*(2), 131–143.

Brotto, L. A. (2010). The DSM diagnostic criteria for sexual aversion disorder. *Archives of Sexual Behavior, 39*(2), 271–277.

Brotto, L. A., Basson, R., & Luria, M. (2008). A mindfulness-based group psychoeducational intervention targeting sexual arousal disorder in women. *Journal of Sexual Medicine, 5*(7), 1646–1659.

Brotto, L. A., Bitzer, J., Laan, E., Leiblum, S., & Luria, M. (2010). Women's sexual desire and arousal disorders. *Journal of Sexual Medicine, 7*(2), 586–614.

Brotto, L. A., Heiman, J. R., Goff, B., Greer, B., Lentz, G. M., Swisher, E., …van Blaricom, A. (2008). A psychoeducational intervention for sexual dysfunction in women with gynecological cancer. *Archives of Sexual Behavior, 37*(2), 317–329.

Buhrich, N., & McConaghy, N. (1978). Two clinically discrete syndromes of transsexualism. *British Journal of Psychiatry, 133*, 73–76.

Bussey, K., & Bandura, A. (2004). Social cognitive theory of gender development and functioning. In A. H. Eagly, A. E. Beall, & R. J. Sternberg (Eds.), *The psychology of gender* (2nd ed., pp. 92–119). New York: Guilford.

Cain, V. S., Johannes, C. B., Avis, N. E., Mohr, B., Schocken, M., Skurnick, J., & Ory, M. (2003). Sexual functioning and practices in a multi-ethnic study of midlife women: Baseline results from SWAN. *Journal of Sex Research, 40*(3), 266–276.

Carbone, D. J., & Seftel, A. D. (2004). Pathophysiology of male erectile dysfunction. In A. D. Seftel, H. Padma-Nathan, C. G. McMahon, F. Giuliano, & S. E. Althof (Eds.), *Male and female sexual dysfunction* (pp. 19–29). New York: Mosby.

Carlson, N. R. (2001). *Physiology of behavior* (7th ed.). Boston: Allyn and Bacon.

Carroll, L., Gilroy, P. J., & Ryan, J. (2002). Counseling transgendered, transsexual, and gender-variant clients. *Journal of Counseling and Development, 80*, 131–139.

Caruso, S., Agnello, C., Intelisano, G., Farina, M., Di Mari, L., & Cianci, A. (2004). Placebo-controlled study on efficacy and safety of daily apomorphine SL intake in premenopausal women affected by hypoactive sexual desire disorder and sexual arousal disorder. *Urology, 63*(5), 955–959.

Carvalho, J., & Nobre, P. (2010). Sexual desire in women: An integrative approach regarding psychological, medical, and relationship dimensions. *Journal of Sexual Medicine, 7*(5), 1807–1815.

Cavender, R. K., & Fairall, M. (2009). Subcutaneous testosterone pellet implant (Testopel) therapy for men with testosterone deficiency syndrome: A single-site retrospective safety analysis. *Journal of Sexual Medicine, 6*(11), 3177–3192.

Christensen, B. S., Gronbaek, M., Osler, M., Pedersen, B. V., Graugaard, C., & Frisch, M. (2011). Sexual dysfunctions and difficulties in Denmark: Prevalence and associated sociodemographic factors. *Archives of Sexual Behavior, 40*(1), 121–132.

Cohen, L. J., & Galynker, I. I. (2002). Clinical features of pedophilia and implications for treatment. *Journal of Psychiatric Practice, 8*(5), 276–289.

Cohen-Kettenis, P. T., & van Goozen, S. H. (1997). Sex reassignment of adolescent transsexuals: A follow-up study. *Journal of the American Academy of Child and Adolescent Psychiatry, 36*(2), 263–271.

Coleman, E. (2002). Promoting sexual health and responsible sexual behavior: An introduction. *Journal of Sex Research, 39*(1), 3–6.

Coleman, E., Raymond, N., & McBean, A. (2003). Assessment and treatment of compulsive sexual behavior. *Minnesota Medicine, 86*(7), 42–47.

Committee on Bioethics. (1998). Female genital mutilation. *Pediatrics, 102*(1), 153–156.

Cooper, A., McLoughlin, I. P., & Campbell, K. M. (2004). Sexuality in cyberspace. In M. S. Kimmel & R. F. Plante (Eds.), *Sexualities: Identities, behaviors, and society* (pp. 285–298). New York: Oxford.

Cooper, A., Safir, M. P., & Rosenmann, A. (2006). Workplace worries: A preliminary look at online sexual activities at the office—emerging issues for clinicians and employers. *CyberPsychology and Behavior, 9*(1), 22–29.

Cyranowski, J. M., Aarestad, S. L., & Andersen, B. L. (1999). The role of sexual self-schema in a diathesis-stress model of sexual dysfunction. *Applied and Preventive Psychology, 8*, 217–228.

Daneback, K., Cooper, A., & Mansson, S. A. (2005). An internet study of cybersex participants. *Archives of Sexual Behavior, 34*(3), 321–328.

Davis, S. R., Davison, S. L., Donath, S., & Bell, R. J. (2005). Circulating androgen levels and self-reported sexual function in women. *Journal of the American Medical Association, 294*(1), 91–96.

De Cuypere, G., T'Sjoen, G., Beerten, R., Selvaggi, G., De Sutter, P., Hoebeke, P., ... Rubens, R. (2005). Sexual and physical health after sex reassignment surgery. *Archives of Sexual Behavior, 34*(6), 679–690.

de Jong, D. C. (2009). The role of attention in sexual arousal: Implications for treatment of sexual dysfunction. *Journal of Sex Research, 46*(2–3), 237–248.

Dennerstein, L., Guthrie, J. R., & Alford, S. (2004). Childhood abuse and its association with mid-aged women's sexual functioning. *Journal of Sex and Marital Therapy, 30*(4), 225–234.

Denny, D. (2004). Changing models of transsexualism. *Journal of Gay and Lesbian Psychotherapy, 8*(1–2), 25–40.

Derogatis, L. R., & Burnett, A. L. (2007). The epidemiology of sexual dysfunctions. *Journal of Sexual Medicine, 5*(2), 289–300.

Derogatis, L. R., Laan, E., Brauer, M., van Lunsen, R. H., Jannini, E. A., Davis, S. R., ... Goldstein, I. (2010). Responses to the proposed DSM-V changes. *Journal of Sexual Medicine, 7*(6), 1998–2014.

Dessens, A. B., Slijper, F. M. E., & Drop, S. L. S. (2005). Gender dysphoria and gender change in chromosomal females with congenital adrenal hyperplasia. *Archives of Sexual Behavior, 34*(4), 389–397.

Devor, H. (1996). Female gender dysphoria in context: Social problem or personal problem. *Annual Review of Sex Research, 7*, 44–89.

Dhillon, S., Yang, L. P. H., & Curran, M. P. (2008). Spotlight on bupropion in major depressive disorder. *CNS Drugs, 22*(7), 613–617.

Diamond, M., & Sigmundson, H. K. (1997). Sex reassignment at birth. Long-term review and clinical implications. *Archives of Pediatrics and Adolescent Medicine, 151*(3), 298–304.

Dominguez, J. M., & Hull, E. M. (2005). Dopamine, the medial preoptic area, and male sexual behavior. *Physiology and Behavior, 86*, 356–368.

Dune, T. M., & Shuttleworth, R. P. (2009). "It's just supposed to happen": The myth of sexual spontaneity and the sexually marginalized. *Sexuality and Disability, 27*(2), 97–108.

Dunn, K. M., Croft, P. R., & Hackett, G. I. (1999). Association of sexual problems with social, psychological, and physical problems in men and women: A cross sectional population survey. *Journal of Epidemiology and Community Health, 53(3)*, 144–148.

Dunne, M. P., Bailey, J. M., Kirk, K. M., & Martin, N. G. (2000). The subtlety of sex-atypicality. *Archives of Sexual Behavior, 29*(6), 549–565.

Durkin, K., Forsyth, C. J., & Quinn, J. F. (2006). Pathological internet communities: A new direction for sexual deviance research in a post modern era. *Sociological spectrum, 26*(6), 595–606.

Elgaali, M., Strevens, H., & Mardh, P. A. (2005). Female genital mutilation—an exported medical hazard. *European Journal of Contraception and Reproductive Health Care, 10*(2), 93–97.

Emmers-Sommer, T. M., Allen, M., Bourhis, J., Sahlstein, E., Laskowski, K., Falato, W. L., … Cashman, L. (2004). A meta-analysis of the relationship between social skills and sexual offenders. *Communication Reports, 17*(1), 1–10.

Eplov, L., Giraldi, A., Davidsen, M., Garde, K., & Kamper-Jorgensen, F. (2007). Sexual desire in a nationally representative Danish population. *Journal of Sexual Medicine, 4*(1), 47–56.

Fagan, P. J. (2004). *Sexual disorders: Perspectives on diagnosis and treatment.* Baltimore: Johns Hopkins University Press.

Fagan, P. J., Wise, T. N., Schmidt, C. W. Jr., & Berlin, F. S. (2002). Pedophilia. *Journal of the American Medical Association, 288*(19), 2458–2465.

Fedoroff, J. P. (2008). Sadism, sadomasochism, sex, and violence. *Canadian Journal of Psychiatry, 53*(10), 637–646.

Feldman, H. A., Goldstein, I., Hatzichristou, D. G., Krane, R. J., & McKinlay, J. B. (1994). Impotence and its medical and psychosocial correlates: Results of the Massachusetts Male Aging Study. *Journal of Urology, 151*(1), 54–61.

Ferenidou, F., Kapoteli, V., Moisidis, K., Koutsogiannis, I., Giakoumelos, A., & Hatzichristou, D. (2008). Presence of a sexual problem may not affect women's satisfaction from their sexual function. *Journal of Sexual Medicine, 5*(3), 631–639.

Fisher, W., Boroditsky, R., & Morris, B. (2004). The 2002 Canadian Contraception Study: Part 2. *Journal of Obstetrics and Gynaecology Canada, 26*(7), 646–656.

Foley, S. M. (1994). Contemporary sex therapy. In R. Lechtenberg & D. A. Ohl (Eds.), *Sexual dysfunction: Neurologic, urologic, and gynecologic aspects* (pp. 259–274). Baltimore: Lea and Febiger.

Frank, E., Anderson, C., & Rubinstein, D. (1978). Frequency of sexual dysfunction in "normal" couples. *New England Journal of Medicine, 299*(3), 111–115.

Fugl-Meyer, K., & Fugl-Meyer, A. R. (2002). Sexual disabilities are not singularities. *International Journal of Impotence Research, 14*(6), 487–493.

Gagnon, J. H., Rosen, R. C., & Leiblum, S. R. (1982). Cognitive and social aspects of sexual dysfunction: Sexual scripts in sex therapy. *Journal of Sex and Marital Therapy, 8*(1), 44–56.

Gambescia, N., Sendak, S. K., & Weeks, G. (2009). The treatment of erectile dysfunction. *Journal of Family Psychotherapy, 20*(2–3), 221–240.

Gambescia, N., & Weeks, G. (2006). Sexual dysfunction. In N. Kazantzis & L. L'Abate (Eds.), *Handbook of homework assignments in psychotherapy* (pp. 351–368). New York: Springer.

Garrusi, B., & Faezee, H. (2008). How do Iranian women with breast cancer conceptualize sex and body image? *Sexuality and Disability, 26(3)*, 159–165.

Gehring, D. (2003). Couple therapy for low sexual desire: A systematic approach. *Journal of Sex and Marital Therapy, 29*(1), 25–38.

Giugliano, J. R. (2009). Sex addiction: Diagnostic problems. *International Journal of Mental Health and Addiction, 7*(2), 283–294.

Gizewski, E. R., Krause, E., Schlamann, M., Happich, F., Ladd, M. E., Forsting, M., & Senf, W. (2009). Specific cerebral activation due to visual erotic stimuli in male-to-female transsexuals compared with male and female controls: An fMRI study. *Journal of Sexual Medicine, 6*(2), 440–448.

Goldstein, I. (2004). Androgen physiology in sexual medicine. *Sexuality and Disability, 22*(2), 165–169.

Gonzalez, M., Viafara, G., Caba, F., & Molina, E. (2004). Sexual function, menopause and hormone replacement therapy (HRT). *Maturitas, 48*(4), 411–420.

Grant, J. E. (2005). Clinical characteristics and psychiatric comorbidity in males with exhibitionism. *Journal of Clinical Psychiatry, 66*(11), 1367–1371.

Greenfield, D. P. (2006). Organic approaches to the treatment of paraphilics and sex offenders. *Journal of Psychiatry and Law, 34*(4), 437–454.

Greenstein, A., Abramov, L., Matzkin, H., & Chen, J. (2006). Sexual dysfunction in women partners of men with erectile dysfunction. *International Journal of Impotence Research, 18*(1), 44–46.

Grover, S. A., Lowensteyn, I., Kaouache, M., Marchand, S., Coupal, L., DeCarolis, E., … Defoy, I. (2006). The prevalence of erectile dysfunction in the primary care setting: Importance of risk factors for diabetes and vascular disease. *Archives of Internal Medicine, 166*(2), 213–219.

Gruszecki, L., Forchuk, C., & Fisher, W. A. (2005). Factors associated with common sexual concerns in women: New findings from the Canadian contraception study. *Canadian Journal of Human Sexuality, 14*(1–2), 1–13.

Halle, E., Schmidt, C. W. Jr., & Meyer, J. K. (1980). The role of grandmothers in transsexualism. *American Journal of Psychiatry, 137*(4), 497–498.

Hartley, H. (2006). The "pinking" of Viagra culture: Drug industry efforts to create and repackage sex drugs for women. *Sexualities, 9*(3), 363–378.

Hatzichristou, D., Rosen, R. C., Broderick, G., Clayton, A., Cuzin, B., Derogatis, L., ... Seftel, A. (2004). Clinical evaluation and management strategy for sexual dysfunction in men and women. *Journal of Sexual Medicine, 1*(1), 49–57.

Heiman, J. R. (2002). Sexual dysfunction: Overview of prevalence, etiological factors, and treatments. *Journal of Sex Research, 39*(1), 73–78.

Heiman, J. R., Gittelman, M., Costabile, R., Guay, A., Friedman, A., Heard-Davison, A., ... Stephens, D. (2006). Topical alprostadil (PGE1) for the treatment of female sexual arousal disorder: in-clinic evaluation of safety and efficacy. *Journal of Psychosomatic Obstetrics and Gynecology, 27*(1), 31–41.

Heiman, J. R., & Meston, C. M. (1997). Empirically validated treatment for sexual dysfunction. *Annual Review of Sexual Research, 8,* 148–194.

Helgason, A. R., Adolfsson, J., Dickman, P., Arver, S., Fredrikson, M., Göthberg, M., & Steineck, G. (1996). Sexual desire, erection, orgasm and ejaculatory functions and their importance to elderly Swedish men: A population-based study. *Age and Ageing, 25*(4), 285–291.

Holden, C. (1986). Proposed new psychiatric diagnoses raise charges of gender bias. *Science, 231*(4736), 327–328.

Hollows, K. (2007). Anodyparuenia: A novel sexual dysfunction? An exploration into anal sexuality. *Sexual and Relationship Therapy, 22*(4), 429–443.

Hoyer, J., Kunst, H., & Schmidt, A. (2001). Social phobia as a comorbid condition in sex offenders with paraphilia or impulse control disorder. *Journal of Nervous and Mental Disease, 189*(7), 463–470.

Hugh-Jones, S., Gough, B., & Littlewood, A. (2005). Sexual exhibitionism as "sexuality and individuality": A critique of psycho-medical discourse from the perspectives of women who exhibit. *Sexualities, 8*(3), 259–281.

Imperato-McGinley, J., Guerrero, L., Gautier, T., & Peterson, R. E. (1974). Steroid 5alpha-reductase deficiency in man: An inherited form of male pseudohermaphroditism. *Science, 186*(4170), 1213–1215.

Irvine, J. M. (1990). *Disorders of desire: Sex and gender in modern American sexology.* Philadelphia: Temple University Press.

Isay, R. A. (1999). Gender in homosexual boys: Some developmental and clinical considerations. *Psychiatry: Interpersonal and Biological Processes, 62*(2), 187–194.

Janata, J. W., & Kingsberg, S. A. (2005). Sexual aversion disorder. In R. Balon & R. T. Segraves (Eds.), *Handbook of sexual dysfunction* (pp. 111–121). New York: Taylor and Francis.

Janssen, P. K. C., Bakker, S. C., Rethelyi, J., Zwinderman, A. H., Touw, D. J., Olivier, B., & Waldinger, M. D. (2009). Serotonin transporter promoter region (5-HTTLPR) polymorphism is associated with the intravaginal ejaculation latency time in Dutch men with lifelong premature ejaculation. *Journal of Sexual Medicine, 6*(1), 276–284.

Johnston, P., Hudson, S. M., & Marshall, W. L. (1992). The effects of masturbatory reconditioning with nonfamilial child molesters. *Behaviour Research and Therapy, 30*(5), 559–561.

Joyal, C. C., Black, D. N., & Dassylva, B. (2007). The neuropsychology and neurology of sexual deviance: A review and pilot study. *Sexual Abuse: A Journal of Research and Treatment, 19*(2), 155–173.

Kadri, N., Alami, K. H. M., & Tahiri, S. M. (2002). Sexual dysfunction in women: Population based epidemiological study. *Archives of Women's Mental Health, 5*(2), 59–63.

Kafka, M. P. (1997a). Hypersexual desire in males: An operational definition and clinical implications for males with paraphilias and paraphilia-related disorders. *Archives of Sexual Behavior, 26*(5), 505–526.

Kafka, M. P. (1997b). A monoamine hypothesis for the pathophysiology of paraphilic disorders. *Archives of Sexual Behavior, 26*(4), 343–358.

Kafka, M. P. (2003a). Sex offending and sexual appetite: The clinical and theoretical relevance of hypersexual desire. *International Journal of Offender Therapy and Comparative Criminology, 47*(4), 439–451.

Kafka, M. P. (2003b). The monoamine hypothesis for the pathophysiology of paraphilic disorders: An update. *Annals of the New York Academy of Sciences, 989,* 144–153.

Kafka, M. P. (2010). Hypersexual disorder: A proposed diagnosis for DSM-V. *Archives of Sexual Behavior, 39*(2), 377–400.

Kafka, M. P., & Hennen, J. (2002). A DSM-IV Axis I comorbidity study of males (n = 120) with paraphilias and paraphilia-related disorders. *Sexual Abuse: A Journal of Research and Treatment, 14*(4), 349–366.

Kao, J., Mantz, C., Garofalo, M., Milano, M. T., Vijayakumar, S., & Jani, A. (2003). Treatment-related sexual dysfunction in male nonprostate pelvic malignancies. *Sexuality and Disability, 21*(1), 3–20.

Kaplan, H. S. (1979). *Disorders of sexual desire.* New York: Brunner/Mazel.

Kennedy, S. H., Dickens, S. E., Eisfeld, B. S., & Bagby, R. M. (1999). Sexual dysfunction before antidepressant therapy in major depression. *Journal of Affective Disorders, 56*(2–3), 201–208.

Kimmel, M. S., & Plante, R. F. (2004). *Sexualities: Identities, behaviors, and society.* New York: Oxford.

King, B. M. (1996). *Human sexuality today* (2nd ed.). Upper Saddle River, NJ: Prentice-Hall.

King, M., Holt, V., & Nazareth, I. (2007). Women's views of their sexual difficulties: Agreement and disagreement with clinical diagnoses. *Archives of Sexual Behavior, 36*(2), 281–288.

Klein, C., & Gorzalka, B. B. (2009). Sexual functioning in transsexuals following hormone therapy and genital surgery: A review. *Journal of Sexual Medicine, 6*(11), 2922–2939.

Knegtering, H., van der Moolen, A. E. G. M., Castelein, S., Kluiter, H., & van den Bosch, R. J. (2003). What are the effects of antipsychotics on sexual dysfunctions and endocrine functioning? *Psychoneuroendocrinology, 28*, 109–123.

Koukounas, E., & Over, R. (2001). Habituation of male sexual arousal: Effects of attentional focus. *Biological Psychology, 58*(1), 49–64.

Kriston, L., Gunzler, C., Agyemang, A., Bengel, J., & Berner, M. M. (2010). Effect of sexual function on health-related quality of life mediated by depressive symptoms in cardiac rehabilitation. Findings of the SPARK project in 493 patients. *Journal of Sexual Medicine, 7*, 2044–2055.

Langevin, R., Langevin, M., Curnoe, S., & Bain, J. (2006). Generational substance abuse among male sexual offenders and paraphilics. *Victims and Offenders, 1*(4), 395–409.

Langstrom, N., & Hanson, R. K. (2006). High rates of sexual behavior in the general population: Correlates and predictors. *Archives of Sexual Behavior, 35*(4), 37–52.

Langstrom, N., & Seto, M. C. (2006). Exhibitionistic and voyeuristic behavior in a Swedish national population survey. *Archives of Sexual Behavior, 35*(1), 427–435.

Langstrom, N., & Zucker, K. J. (2005). Transvestic fetishism in the general population: Prevalence and correlates. *Journal of Sex and Marital Therapy, 31*(2), 87–95.

Larsen, S. H., Wagner, G., & Heitmann, B. L. (2007). Sexual function and obesity. *International Journal of Obesity, 31*(8), 1189–1198.

Laumann, E. O., Glasser, D. B., Neves, R. C. S., & Moreira, E. D. (2009). A population-based survey of sexual activity, sexual problems and associated help-seeking behavior patterns in mature adults in the United States of America. *International Journal of Impotence Research, 21*(3), 171–178.

Laumann, E. O., Paik, A., Glasser, D. B., Kang, J. H., Wang, T., Levinson, B., ... Gingell, C. (2006). A cross-national study of subjective sexual well-being among older women and men: Findings from the Global Study of Sexual Attitudes and Behaviors. *Archives of Sexual Behavior, 35*(2), 145–161.

Laumann, E. O., Paik, A., & Rosen, R. C. (1999). Sexual dysfunction in the United States: Prevalence and predictors. *Journal of the American Medical Association, 281*(6), 537–544.

Lavie-Ajayi, M. (2005). "Because all real women do": The construction and deconstruction of "female orgasmic disorder." *Sexualities, Evolution, and Gender, 7*(1), 57–72.

Lawrence, A. A. (2003). Factors associated with satisfaction or regret following male-to-female sex reassignment surgery. *Archives of Sexual Behavior, 32*(4), 299–315.

Lechtenberg, R., & Ohl, D. A. (1994). *Sexual dysfunction: Neurologic, urologic, and gynecologic aspects.* Philadelphia: Lea and Febiger.

Lev, A. I. (2005). Disordering gender identity: Gender identity disorder in the *DSM-IV-TR. Journal of Psychology and Human Sexuality, 17*(3–4), 35–69.

Levine, S. B. (2010). Commentary on consideration of diagnostic criteria for erectile dysfunction in DSM-V. *Journal of Sexual Medicine, 7*(7), 2388–2390.

Lewis, R. W., Fugl-Meyer, K. S., Bosch, R., Fugl-Meyer, A. R., Laumann, E. O., Lizza, E., & Martin-Morales, A. (2004). Epidemiology/risk factors of sexual dysfunction. *Journal of Sexual Medicine, 1*(1), 35–39.

Lewis, R. W., Fugl-Meyer, K. S., Corona, G., Hayes, R. D., Laumann, E. O., & Moreira, E. D. (2010). Definitions/epidemiology/risk factors for sexual dysfunction. *Journal of Sexual Medicine, 7*, 1598–1607.

Lips, H. M. (2006). *A new psychology of women: Gender, culture, and ethnicity* (3rd ed.). New York: McGraw Hill.

LoPiccolo, J., & Lobitz, W. C. (1972). The role of masturbation in the treatment of orgasmic dysfunction. *Archives of Sexual Behavior, 2*(2), 163–171.

Losel, F., & Schmucker, M. (2005). The effectiveness of treatment for sexual offenders: A comprehensive meta-analysis. *Journal of Experimental Criminology, 1*(1), 117–146.

Lutfey, K. E., Link, C. L., Rosen, R. C., Wiegel, M., & McKinlay, J. B. (2009). Prevalence and correlates of sexual activity and function in women: Results from the Boston Area Community Health (BACH) survey. *Archives of Sexual Behavior, 38*(4), 514–527.

Maletzky, B. M., Tolan, A., & McFarland, B. (2006). The Oregon depo-Provera program: A five-year follow-up. *Sexual Abuse: A Journal of Research and Treatment, 18*(3), 303–316.

Manning, J. T., Scutt, D., Wilson, J., & Lewis-Jones, D. I. (1998). The ratio of 2nd to 4th digit length: A predictor of sperm numbers and concentrations of testosterone, luteinizing hormone and oestrogen. *Human Reproduction, 13*(11), 3000–3004.

Marecek, J., Crawford, M., & Popp, D. (2004). On the construction of gender, sex, and sexualities. In A. H. Eagly, A. E. Beall, & R. J. Sternberg (Eds.), *The psychology of gender* (pp. 192–216). New York: Guilford.

Marshall, W. L. (1974). A combined treatment approach to the reduction of multiple fetish-related behaviors. *Journal of Consulting and Clinical Psychology, 42*(4), 613–616.

Masters, W. H., & Johnson, V. E. (1966). *Human sexual response*. Boston: Little, Brown.

Masters, W. H., & Johnson, V. E. (1970). *Human sexual inadequacy*. Boston: Little, Brown.

Masters, W. H., Johnson, V. E., & Kolodny, R. C. (1985). *Masters and Johnson on sex and human loving*. Boston: Little, Brown.

Matlin, M. W. (2000). *The psychology of women* (4th ed.). New York: Harcourt.

McCabe, M. P. (2001). Evaluation of a cognitive behavior therapy program for people with sexual dysfunction. *Journal of Sex and Marital Therapy, 27*(3), 259–271.

McCarthy, B. W., & McDonald, D. O. (2009). Psychobiosocial versus biomedical models of treatment: Semantics or substance. *Sexual and Relationship Therapy, 24*(1), 30–37.

McConaghy, N. (1993). *Sexual behavior: Problems and management*. New York: Plenum.

McCormick, N. B. (1987). Sexual scripts: Social and therapeutic implications. *Sexual and Marital Therapy, 2*(1), 3–27.

McMahon, C. G. (2004). The ejaculatory response. In A. D. Seftel, H. Padma-Nathan, C. G. McMahon, F. Giuliano, & S. E. Althof (Eds.), *Male and female sexual dysfunction* (pp. 43–57). New York: Mosby.

McMahon, C. G., Althof, S., Waldinger, M. D., Porst, H., Dean, J., Sharlip, I., ... Segraves, R. (2008). An evidence-based definition of lifelong premature ejaculation: Report of the International Society for Sexual Medicine Ad Hoc Committee for the definition of premature ejaculation. *BJU International, 102*(3), 338–350.

Meston, C. M. (2004). The effects of hysterectomy on sexual arousal in women with a history of benign uterine fibroids. *Archives of Sexual Behavior, 33*(1), 31–42.

Meston, C. M., & Ahrold, T. (2010). Ethnic, gender, and acculturation influences on sexual behaviors. *Archives of Sexual Behavior, 39*(1), 179–189.

Meyer III, W., Bockting, W., Cohen-Kettenis, P., Coleman, E., DiCeglie, D., Devor, H., et al. (February, 2001). The standards of care for gender identity disorders (sixth version). *The International Journal of Transgenderism, 5*(1), Retrieved from: http://www.symposion.com/ijt/soc_2001/index.htm

Miclutia, I. V., Popescu, C. A., & Macrea, R. S. (2008). Sexual dysfunctions of chronic schizophrenic female patients. *Sexual and Relationship Therapy, 23*(2), 119–129.

Miller, R. D. (1998). Forced administration of sex-drive reducing medications to sex offenders: Treatment or punishment? *Psychology, Public Policy, and Law, 4*(1–2), 175–199.

Montgomery, S. A., Baldwin, D. S., & Riley, A. (2002). Antidepressant medications: A review of the evidence for drug-induced sexual dysfunction. *Journal of Affective Disorders, 69*(1–3), 119–140.

Moore, C. K. (2010). The impact of urinary incontinence and its treatment on female sexual function. *Current Urology Reports, 11*(5), 299–303.

Moser, C. (2010). Blanchard's autogynephilia theory: A critique. *Journal of Homosexuality, 57*(6), 790–809.

Moskowitz, D. A., & Roloff, M. E. (2007). The ultimate high: Sexual addiction and the bug chasing phenomenon. *Sexual Addiction and Compulsivity, 14*(1), 21–40.

Murthy, S., & Wylie, K. R. (2007). Sexual problems in patients on antipsychotic medication. *Sexual and Relationship Therapy, 22*(1), 97–107.

Nicholls, L. (2008). Putting the new classification scheme to an empirical test. *Feminism and Psychology, 18*(4), 515–526.

Nicolosi, A., Laumann, E. O., Glasser, D. B., Brock, G., King, R., & Gingell, C. (2006). Sexual activity, sexual disorders and associated help-seeking behavior among mature adults in five Anglophone countries from the Global Survey of Sexual Attitudes and Behaviors (GSSAB). *Journal of Sex and Marital Therapy, 32*(4), 331–342.

Nicolosi, A., Laumann, E. O., Glasser, D. B., Moreira, E. D. Jr., Paik, A., & Gingell, C. (2004). Sexual behavior and sexual dysfunctions after age 40: The global study of sexual attitudes and behaviors. *Urology, 64*(5), 991–997.

Nicolosi, A., Moreira, E. D. Jr., Shirai, M., Bin Mohd Tambi, M. I., & Glasser, D. B. (2003). Epidemiology of erectile dysfunction in four countries: Cross-national study of the prevalence and correlates of erectile dysfunction. *Urology, 61*(1), 201–206.

Nijland, E. A., Weijmar Schultz, W. C. M., Nathorst-Boos, J., Helmond, F. A., Van Lunsen, R. H. W., Palacios, S., ... LISA Study Investigators. (2008). Tibolone and transdermal E₂/NETA for the treatment of female sexual dysfunction in naturally menopausal women: Results of a randomized active-controlled trial. *Journal of Sexual Medicine, 5*(3), 646–656.

Nobre, P. J., & Pinto-Gouveia, J. (2006). Dysfunctional sexual beliefs as vulnerability factors to sexual dysfunction. *Journal of Sex Research, 43*(1), 68–75.

Nobre, P. J., & Pinto-Gouveia, J. (2009). Questionnaire of cognitive schema activation in sexual context: A measure to assess cognitive schemas activated in unsuccessful sexual situations. *Journal of Sex Research, 46*(5), 425–437.

Nyunt, A., Stephen, G., Gibbin, J., Durgan, L., Fielding, A. M., Wheeler, M., & Price D. E. (2005). Androgen status in healthy premenopausal women with loss of libido. *Journal of Sex and Marital Therapy, 31*(1), 73–80.

Oberg, K., Fugl-Meyer, K. S., & Fugl-Meyer, A. R. (2002). On sexual well-being in sexually abused Swedish women: Epidemiological aspects. *Sexual and Relationship Therapy, 17*(4), 329–341.

O'Reilly, G., Carr, A., Murphy, P., & Cotter, A. (2010). A controlled evaluation of a prison-based sexual offender intervention program. *Sexual Abuse: A Journal of Research and Treatment, 22*(1), 95–111.

Orlebeke, J. F., Boomsma, D. I., Gooren, L. J. G., Verschoor, A. M., & van den Bree, M. J. M. (1992). Elevated sinistrality in transsexuals. *Neuropsychology, 6*(4), 351–355.

Orzack, M. H., Voluse, A. C., Wolf, D., & Hennen, J. (2006). An ongoing study of group treatment for men involved in problematic Internet-enabled sexual behavior. *CyberPsychology and Behavior, 9*(3), 348–360.

Osvath, P., Fekete, S., Voros, V., & Almasi, J. (2007). Mirtazapine treatment and sexual functions: Results of a Hungarian, multi-centre, prospective study in depressed out-patients. *International Journal of Psychiatry in Clinical Practice, 11*(3), 242–245.

Pacey, S. (2008). The medicalisation of sex: A barrier to intercourse? *Sexual and Relationship Therapy, 23*(3), 183–187.

Pfaus, J. G. (2009). Pathways of sexual desire. *Journal of Sexual Medicine, 6*(6), 1506–1533.

Pinel, J. P. J. (2003). *Biopsychology* (5th ed.). New York: Allyn and Bacon.

Plante, R. F. (2006). *Sexualities in context: A social perspective.* Boulder, CO: Westview.

Potts, A., Grace, V., Gavey, N., & Vares, T. (2004). "Viagra stories": Challenging "erectile dysfunction." *Social Science and Medicine, 59*(3), 489–499.

Potts, A., Grace, V. M., Vares, T., & Gavey, N. (2006). "Sex for life"? Men's counter-stories on "erectile dysfunction," male sexuality and aging. *Sociolology of Health and Illness, 28*(3), 306–329.

Prins, J., Blanker, M. H., Bohnen, A. M., Thomas, S., & Bosch, J. L. (2002). Prevalence of erectile dysfunction: A systematic review of population-based studies. *International Journal of Impotence Research, 14*(6), 422–432.

Pujols, Y., Seal, B. N., & Meston, C. M. (2010). The association between sexual satisfaction and body image in women. *Journal of Sexual Medicine, 7*(2), 905–916.

Raymond, N. C., Coleman, E., & Miner, M. H. (2003). Psychiatric comorbidity and compulsive/impulsive traits in compulsive sexual behavior. *Comprehensive Psychiatry, 44*(5), 370–380.

Raymond, N. C., Coleman, E., Ohlerking, F., Christenson, G. A., & Miner, M. (1999). Psychiatric comorbidity in pedophilic sex offenders. *American Journal of Psychiatry, 156*(5), 786–788.

Raymond, N. C., Grant, J. E., & Coleman, E. (2010). Augmentation with naltrexone to treat compulsive sexual behavior: A case series. *Annals of Clinical Psychiatry, 22*(1), 56–62.

Raymond, N. C., Grant, J. E., Kim, S. W., & Coleman, E. (2002). Treatment of compulsive sexual behaviour with naltrexone and serotonin reuptake inhibitors: Two case studies. *International Clinical Psychopharmacology, 17*(4), 201–205.

Reffelmann, T., & Kloner, R. A. (2010). Erectile dysfunction. In P. P. Toth & C. P. Cannon (Eds.), *Contemporary cardiology: Comprehensive cardiovascular medicine in the primary care setting* (pp. 411–422). New York: Springer.

Reiersol, O., & Skeid, S. (2006). The ICD diagnoses of fetishism and sadomasochism. *Journal of Homosexuality, 50*(2–3), 243–262.

Reissing, E. D., Binik, Y. M., Khalife, S., Cohen, D., & Amsel, R. (2003). Etiological correlates of vaginismus: Sexual and physical abuse, sexual knowledge, sexual self-schema, and relationship adjustment. *Journal of Sex and Marital Therapy, 29*(1), 47–59.

Reissing, E. D., Laliberte, G. M., & Davis, H. J. (2005). Young women's sexual adjustment: The role of sexual self-schema, sexual self-efficacy, sexual aversion and body attitudes. *Canadian Journal of Human Sexuality, 14*(3–4), 77–85.

Richters, J., de Visser, R. O., Rissel, C. E., Grulich, A. E., & Smith, A. M. A. (2008). Demographic and psycho-social features of participants in bondage and discipline, "sadomasochism" or dominance and submission (BDSM): Data from a national survey. *Journal of Sexual Medicine, 5*(7), 1660–1668.

Rosen, R. C., & Laumann, E. O. (2003). The prevalence of sexual problems in women: How valid are comparisons across studies? Commentary on Bancroft, Loftus, and Long's (2003) "Distress about sex: A national survey of women in heterosexual relationships." *Archives of Sexual Behavior, 32*(3), 209–211.

Rosenmann, A., & Safir, M. P. (2006). Forced online: Push factors of internet sexuality: A preliminary study of online paraphilic empowerment. *Journal of Homosexuality, 51*(3), 71–92.

Rowland, D. L. (2006). Neurobiology of sexual response in men and women. *CNS Spectrums, 11*(8, Suppl. 9), 6–12.

Ryback, R. S. (2004). Naltrexone in the treatment of adolescent sexual offenders. *Journal of Clinical Psychiatry, 65*(7), 982–986.

Sadeghi-Nejad, H., & Seftel, A. D. (2004). Vacuum devices and penile implants. In A. D. Seftel, H. Padma-Nathan, C. G. McMahon, F. Giuliano, & S. E. Althof (Eds.), *Male and female sexual dysfunction* (pp. 129–143). New York: Mosby.

Safarinejad, M. R. (2008). Treatment of nonparaphilic hypersexuality in men with a long-acting analog of gonadotropin-releasing hormone. *Journal of Sexual Medicine, 6*(4), 1151–1164.

Saigal, C. S., Wessells, H., Pace, J., Schonlau, M., & Wilt, T. J. (2006). Predictors and prevalence of erectile dysfunction in a racially diverse population. *Archives of Internal Medicine, 166*(2), 207–212.

Saleh, F. M., & Guidry, L. L. (2003). Psychosocial and biological treatment considerations for the paraphilic and nonparaphilic sex offender. *Journal of the American Academy of Psychiatry and the Law, 31*(4), 486–493.

Salonia, A., Zanni, G., Nappi, R. E., Briganti, A., Deho, F., Fabbri, F., … Montorsi, F. (2004). Sexual dysfunction is common in women with lower urinary tract symptoms and urinary incontinence: Results of a cross-sectional study. *European Urology, 45*(5), 642–648.

Sanjuan, P. M., Langenbucher, J. W., & Labouvie, E. (2009). The role of sexual assault and sexual dysfunction in alcohol/other drug use disorders. *Alcoholism Treatment Quarterly, 27*(2), 150–163.

Scepkowski, L. A., Wiegel, M., Bach, A. K., Weisberg, R. B., Brown, T. A., & Barlow, D. H. (2004). Attributions for sexual situations in men with and without erectile disorder: Evidence from a sex-specific attributional style measure. *Archives of Sexual Behavior, 33*(6), 559–569.

Schaffer, M., Jeglic, E. L., Moster, A., & Wnuk, D. (2010). Cognitive-behavioral therapy in the treatment and management of sex offenders. *Journal of Cognitive Psychotherapy: An International Quarterly, 24*(2), 92–103.

Schneider, H. J., Pickel, J., & Stalla, G. K. (2006). Typical female 2nd-4th finger length (2D:4D) ratios in male-to-female transsexuals—possible implications for prenatal androgen exposure. *Psychoneuroendocrinology, 31*(2), 265–269.

Schneider, J. P. (1989). Rebuilding the marriage during recovery from compulsive sexual behavior. *Family Relations, 38*(3), 288–294.

Schoning, S., Engelien, A., Bauer, C., Kugel, H., Kersting, A., Roestel, C., … Konrad, C. (2010). Neuroimaging differences in spatial cognition between men and male-to-female transsexuals before and during hormone therapy. *Journal of Sexual Medicine, 7*(5), 1858–1867.

Segraves, R. T. (2002). Female sexual disorders: Psychiatric aspects. *Canadian Journal of Psychiatry, 47*(5), 419–425.

Segraves, R. T., Balon, R., & Clayton, A. (2007). Proposal for changes in diagnostic criteria for sexual dysfunctions. *Journal of Sexual Medicine, 4*(3), 567–580.

Segraves, R., Clayton, A., Croft, H., Wolf, A., & Warnock, J. (2004). Bupropion sustained release for the treatment of hypoactive sexual desire disorder in premenopausal women. *Journal of Clinical Psychopharmacology, 24*(3), 339–342.

Serati, M., Salvatore, S., Uccella, S., Nappi, R. E., & Bolis, P. (2009). Female urinary incontinence during intercourse: A review on an understudied problem for women's sexuality. *Journal of Sexual Medicine, 6*(1), 40–48.

Serretti, A., & Chiesa, A. (2009). Treatment-emergent sexual dysfunction related to antidepressants: A meta-analysis. *Journal of Clinical Psychopharmacology, 29*(3), 259–266.

Shifren, J. L. (2004). The role of androgens in female sexual dysfunction. *Mayo Clinic Proceedings, 79*(4 Suppl.), S19–S24.

Shifren, J. L., Braunstein, G. D., Simon, J. A., Casson, P. R., Buster, J. E., Redmond, G. P., … Mazer, N. A. (2000). Transdermal testosterone treatment in women with impaired sexual function after oophorectomy. *New England Journal of Medicine, 343*(10), 682–688.

Shifren, J. L., Davis, S. R., Moreau, M., Waldbaum, A., Bouchard, C., Derogatis, L., ... Kroll, R. (2006). Testosterone patch for the treatment of hypoactive sexual desire disorder in naturally menopausal women: Results from the INTIMATE NM1 study. *Menopause, 13*(5), 770–779.

Shiri, R., Koskimaki, J., Hakama, M., Hakkinen, J., Tammela, T. L., Huhtala, H., & Auvinen, A. (2003). Prevalence and severity of erectile dysfunction in 50- to 75-year-old Finnish men. *Journal of Urology, 170*(6), 2342–2344.

Simons, J. S., & Carey, M. P. (2001). Prevalence of sexual dysfunctions: Results from a decade of research. *Archives of Sexual Behavior, 30*(2), 177–219.

Sipski, M. L. (2002). Central nervous system based neurogenic female sexual dysfunction: Current status and future trends. *Archives of Sexual Behavior, 31*(5), 421–424.

Smith, K. B., Pukall, C. F., Tripp, D. A., & Nickel, J. C. (2007). Sexual and relationship functioning in men with chronic prostatitis/chronic pelvic pain syndrome and their partners. *Archives of Sexual Behavior, 36*(2), 301–311.

Smith, Y. L., Van Goozen, S. H., Kuiper, A. J., & Cohen-Kettenis, P. T. (2005). Sex reassignment: Outcomes and predictors of treatment for adolescent and adult transsexuals. *Psychological Medicine, 35*(1), 89–99.

Sobel, V., & Imperato-McGinley, J. (2004). Gender identity in XY intersexuality. *Child and Adolescent Psychiatric Clinics of North America, 13*(3), 609–622.

Sommer, F., Goldstein, I., & Korda, J. B. (2010). Bicycle riding and erectile dysfunction: A review. *Journal of Sexual Medicine, 7*(7), 2346–2358.

Stanworth, R. D., & Jones, T. H. (2008). Testosterone for the aging male; current evidence and recommended practice. *Clinical Interventions in Aging, 3*(1), 25–44.

Stinson, R. D. (2009). The behavioral and cognitive-behavioral treatment of female sexual dysfunction: How far we have come and the path left to go. *Sexual and Relationship Therapy, 24*(3–4), 271–285.

Stinson, J. D., Becker, J. V., & Sales, B. D. (2008). Self-regulation and the etiology of sexual deviance: Evaluating causal theory. *Violence and Victims, 23*(1), 35–51.

Stoller, R. J. (1985). *Presentations of gender.* New Haven, CT: Yale University Press.

Stulberg, D., & Ewigman, B. (2008). Antidepressants causing sexual problems? Give her Viagra. *The Journal of Family Practice, 57*(12), 793–796.

ter Kuile, M. M., Both, S., & van Lankveld, J. J. D. M. (2010). Cognitive behavioral therapy for sexual dysfunctions in women. *Psychiatric Clinics of North America, 33*(3), 595–610.

Tiefer, L. (1991). Historical, scientific, clinical and feminist criticisms of "The Human Sexual Response Cycle" model. *Annual Review of Sex Research, 2,* 1–23.

Tiefer, L. (2001). A new view of women's sexual problems: Why new? Why now? *Journal of Sex Research, 38*(2), 89–96.

Tiefer, L. (2006). The Viagra phenomenon. *Sexualities, 9*(3), 273–294.

Trotta, M. P., Ammassari, A., Murri, R., Marconi, P., Zaccarelli, M., Cozzi-Lepri, A., ... AdICoNA and AdeSpall Study Group. (2008). Self-reported sexual dysfunction is frequent among HIV-infected persons and is associated with suboptimal adherence to antiretrovirals. *AIDS Patient Care and STDs, 22*(4), 291–299.

Trussell, J. C., Anastasiadis, A. G., Padma-Nathan, H., & Shabsigh, R. (2004). Oral type 5 phosphodiesterase therapy for male and female sexual dysfunction. In A. D. Seftel, H. Padma-Nathan, C. G. McMahon, F. Giuliano, & S. E. Althof (Eds.), *Male and female sexual dysfunction* (pp. 107–119). New York: Mosby.

Tulla, M. E., Dunn, M. E., Antilus, R., & Muneyyirci-Delale, O. (2006). Vaginismus and failed in vitro fertilization. *Sexual and Relationship Therapy, 21*(4), 439–443.

Turkistani, I. Y. A. (2004). Sexual dysfunction in Saudi depressed male patients. *International Journal of Psychiatry in Clinical Practice, 8,* 101–107.

Utian, W. H., MacLean, D. B., Symonds, T., Symons, J., Somayaji, V., & Sisson, M. (2005). A methodology study to validate a structured diagnostic method used to diagnose female sexual dysfunction and its subtypes in postmenopausal women. *Journal of Sex and Marital Therapy, 31*(4), 271–283.

Uva, J. L. (1995). Review: Autoerotic asphyxiation in the United States. *Journal of Forensic Sciences, 40*(4), 574–581.

Van Diest, S. L., van Lankveld, J. J. D. M., Leusink, P. M., Slob, A. K., & Gijs, L. (2007). Sex therapy through the internet for men with sexual dysfunctions: A pilot study. *Journal of Sex and Marital Therapy, 33*(2), 115–133.

van Lankveld, J. J., & Grotjohann, Y. (2000). Psychiatric comorbidity in heterosexual couples with sexual dysfunction assessed with the composite international diagnostic interview. *Archives of Sexual Behavior, 29*(5), 479–498.

Van Wijk, A. P., Blokland, A. A. J., Duits, N., Vermeiren, R., & Harkink, J. (2007). Relating psychiatric disorders, offender and offence characteristics in a sample of adolescent sex offenders and non-sex offenders. *Criminal Behaviour and Mental Health, 17*(1), 15–30.

Waldinger, M. D. (2008). Premature ejaculation: Different pathophysiologies and etiologies determine its treatment. *Journal of Sex and Marital Therapy, 34*(1), 1–13.

Waldinger, M. D., Zwinderman, A. H., Schweitzer, D. H., & Olivier, B. (2004). Relevance of methodological design for the interpretation of efficacy of drug treatment of premature ejaculation: A systematic review and meta-analysis. *International Journal of Impotence Research, 16*(4), 369–381.

Ward, T., & Marshall, W. L. (2004). Good lives, aetiology and the rehabilitation of sex offenders: A bridging theory. *Journal of Sexual Aggression, 10*(2), 153–169.

Weintraub, D., Koester, J., Potenza, M. N., Siderowf, A. D., Stacy, M., Voon, V., ... Lang, A. E. (2010). Impulse control disorders in Parkinson disease: A cross-sectional study of 3090 patients. *Archives of Neurology, 67*(5), 589–595.

Weisberg, R. B., Brown, T. A., Wincze, J. P., & Barlow, D. H. (2001). Causal attributions and male sexual arousal: the impact of attributions for a bogus erectile difficulty on sexual arousal, cognitions, and affect. *Journal of Abnormal Psychology, 110*(2), 324–334.

West, S. L., Vinikoor, L. C., & Zolnoun, D. (2004). A systematic review of the literature on female sexual dysfunction prevalence and predictors. *Annual Review of Sexual Research, 15*, 40–172.

Whitehead, P. R., Ward, T., & Collie, R. M. (2007). Time for a change: Applying the Good Lives Model of rehabilitation to a high-risk violent offender. *International Journal of Offender Therapy and Comparative Criminology, 51*(5), 578–598.

Wiederman, M. W. (2004). Self-control and sexual behavior. In R. F. Baumeister & K. D. Vohs (Eds.), *Handbook of self-regulation: Research, theory, and applications* (pp. 525–536). New York: Guilford.

Wiggins, D. L., Wood, R., Granai, C. O., & Dizon, D. S. (2007). Sex, intimacy, and the gynecologic oncologists: Survey results of the New England Association of Gynecologic Oncologists (NEAGO). *Journal of Psychosocial Oncology, 25*(4), 61–70.

Willis, G. M., & Grace, R. C. (2008). The quality of community reintegration planning for child molesters: Effects on sexual recidivism. *Sexual Abuse: A Journal of Research and Treatment, 20*(2), 218–240.

Wolpe, J. (1958). *Psychotherapy by reciprocal inhibition*. Stanford, CA: Stanford University Press.

World Health Organization. (2006). *International classification of diseases* (10th ed., Section F52). Retrieved from http://www.who.int/classifications/apps/icd/icd10online/

Wylie, K., & MacInnes, I. (2005). Erectile dysfunction. In R. Balon & R. T. Segraves (Eds.), *Handbook of sexual dysfunction* (pp. 155–191). New York: Taylor and Francis.

Zisook, S., Rush, A. J., Haight, B. R., Clines, D. C., & Rockett, C. B. (2006). Use of bupropion in combination with serotonin reuptake inhibitors. *Biological Psychiatry, 59*(3), 203–210.

Zucker, K. J., Beaulieu, N., Bradley, S. J., Grimshaw, G. M., & Wilcox, A. (2001). Handedness in boys with gender identity disorder. *Journal of Child Psychology and Psychiatry, 42*(6), 767–776.

Zucker, K. J., & Bradley, S. J. (1995). *Gender identity disorder and psychosexual problems in children and adolescents*. New York: Guilford.

13
Somatoform and Dissociative Disorders

GEORG H. EIFERT and ELLEN MCCORMACK

Schmid College of Science and Technology
Chapman University, Orange, California

MICHAEL J. ZVOLENSKY

Department of Psychology
University of Houston, Texas

Individuals who exhibit multiple somatic symptoms often present to medical practitioners believing that they are physically ill, yet upon evaluation, they are informed that there is no known physiological source underlying their reports of distress. Although many of these patients will be satisfied with negative medical examination results, a significant subgroup will anxiously continue to worry about the possibility of suffering from a yet undiagnosed physical disease—a phenomenon known as *somatization*. Somatization denotes the presence of physical symptoms (e.g., chest pain) for which no demonstrable disease process or bodily oriented pathology can be identified as the cause. These individuals are likely to continue to seek help for their physical symptoms, demand more physical examinations and specialist referrals, undergo costly laboratory tests, and in rare cases, even end up on an operating table (Harth & Hermes, 2007; Warwick & Salkovskis, 1990). At the extreme, such somatization behavior can interfere with life activities and goals, resulting in clinically significant impairment—a phenomenon typically classified as *somatization disorder*. Yet, somatization processes frequently occur in other "somatic disorders," including hypochondriasis, pain disorder, conversion disorder, and body dysmorphic disorder, as well as many other psychiatric conditions (e.g., panic disorder, major depressive disorder).

Somatization is a relatively common occurrence in the general medical system. For instance, several studies suggest that approximately 30% of somatic symptoms in primary care and related clinic settings are medically unexplained (Khan, Khan, & Kroenke, 2000; Kroenke & Price, 1993; Marple, Kroenke, Lucey, Wilder, & Lucas, 1997; Narrow, Rae, Robins, & Regier, 2002; Smith et al., 2003). Moreover, somatization appears to maintain cross-cultural and cross-national applicability (Zvolensky, Feldner, Eifert, Vujanovic, & Solomon, 2008).

Somatization is associated with a high degree of personal suffering measured in both financial and human terms. For example, Katon, Sullivan, and Walker (2001) analyzed several studies with community, primary care, and medical specialty samples and determined that individuals with unexplained somatic symptoms experienced severe personal distress and corresponding life impairment. Somatizing individuals have higher rates of inpatient and outpatient health care utilization and incur correspondingly higher inpatient and outpatient medical costs (Barsky, Orav, & Bates, 2005; Hansen, Fink, Frydenberg, & Oxhoj, 2002). In the United States, some estimates suggest the cost associated with treating somatization at approximately $256 billion a year (Barsky et al., 2005).

Importantly, somatization does not necessarily rule out the possibility of a true physical illness. In fact, many physical health care problems, typically quite mild, can be found among individuals with somatization problems (e.g., hypertension). Thus, somatization denotes an excess degree of worry about physical health and overuse of medical services, relative to the severity of *identifiable* illness. Perhaps not surprisingly, those individuals without a medical explanation for their suffering seem to experience more anxiety and depression than others with similar illness experiences that do have diagnoses (Katon et al., 2001). This difference even held in one study that examined individuals who sacrificed extensive amounts of energy and time to their care (individuals in the top 10% of frequent primary care visitors); those without an identifiable illness reported a higher degree of physical, social, and mental impairments compared to their "diagnosable" counterparts (Vedsted, Fink, Sørensen, & Olesen, 2004). Typically, these impairments are longstanding (occur across most phases of life) and tend to be exacerbated by concurrent stressors in everyday life. Although somatization is indeed a vexing health care problem, this domain represents an exciting opportunity for researchers from diverse disciplines to work together in a collaborative manner to better understand the relations between "body and mind" and health and disease.

The main goal of this chapter is to provide a contemporary overview of the process of somatization as it applies to somatoform disorders. To some extent, our discussion is necessarily organized around the categories and classification of somatoform disorders in the American Psychiatric Association' s (APA) *Diagnostic and Statistical Manual of Mental Disorders* (fourth edition; *DSM–IV*; APA, 1994). However, we attempt to move beyond *DSM* categories toward a more function-based dimensional perspective of somatization problems. We believe such an approach is potentially useful because it targets analyses at fundamental biobehavioral processes and thereby provides information that is likely to be directly useful for the design of clinical interventions.

The first section of this chapter briefly reviews somatoform disorders from a traditional *DSM–IV* perspective, highlighting the prevalence, nature, and the diagnostic validity of such diagnoses. We then outline how a *dimensional perspective* that focuses on key biobehavioral processes may be a more useful approach for understanding somatoform disorders than the *DSM*'s categorical approach. We then address some key vulnerability processes for somatoform disorders. Finally, we address how a dimensional perspective and focus on dysfunctional processes related to illness behavior can be translated into treatments for somatoform disorders.

Classification, Prevalence, and Course of Somatoform Disorders

According to *DSM–IV*, the common feature of the somatoform disorders is the presence of physical symptoms that suggest a general medical condition (hence, the term somatoform) but are not fully (currently) explained by a general medical condition, the direct effects of substance, or by another mental disorder. The physical symptoms must result in substantial personal, social, and occupational impairment and are not feigned or voluntarily produced, as in malingering or factitious disorder. Although symptoms are not feigned, the fact that no medical explanation can be found for patient complaints makes it difficult at times to differentiate somatoform disorders from malingering.

Although the exact prevalence of specific somatoform disorders is not exactly known, most estimates place these problems collectively at under 1% of the general population. *DSM–IV* distinguishes between five somatoform disorders: somatization disorder, hypochondriasis, pain disorder, conversion disorder, and body dysmorphic disorder. By way of background, we begin our discussion with a brief overview of these categories. It should be noted, however, that the DSM–5 work group (APA, 2010) is proposing to rename the somatoform disorder category: "Since somatization disorder, hypochondriasis, undifferentiated somatoform disorder, and pain disorder share certain common features, namely somatic symptoms and cognitive distortions, the work group is proposing that these disorders be grouped under a common rubric called complex somatic symptom disorder" (p. 1). The APA work group notes further that the current terminology for somatoform disorders is confusing and that these disorders all involve presentation of physical symptoms or concern about medical illness. "In addition, because of the implicit mind-body dualism and the unreliability of assessments of 'medically unexplained symptoms,' these symptoms are no longer emphasized as core features of many of these disorders" (APA, 2010, p. 1).

Somatization disorder is characterized by many physical complaints without clear or known physical causes. The condition may last for many years and, in some cases, extend over the entire adult lifespan. To meet the *DSM–IV* diagnostic criteria, an individual needs to present with a history of pain related to at least four different sites or functions (e.g., head, back, abdomen, joints), two gastrointestinal symptoms (e.g., diarrhea, food intolerance), one sexual symptom (e.g., irregular menses, indifference to sex), and one pseudoneurological symptom (e.g., poor balance, numbness, paralysis). These symptoms lead to frequent and multiple medical consultations, complex medical history, and to alterations of the person's lifestyle. Physical and laboratory findings cannot detect a plausible medical condition as the cause of the symptoms. Somatization disorder is a relatively rare phenomenon with recent community and epidemiological studies citing prevalence rates between 0.4 and 0.7% (4–7 per 1,000; Bass & Murphy, 1990; Robins et al., 1984). Its onset is in early adulthood, the course is often chronic, and the prognosis is generally regarded as poor.

Perhaps the most well-known somatoform disorder is *hypochondriasis*, defined as fears, suspicions, or convictions that one has a serious and often fatal illness such as heart disease, cancer, or AIDS. Patients frequently seek reassurance, check their bodies, and avoid illness-related situations. Merely informing patients of the absence of a disease process, or explaining the benign nature of the symptoms, only results in temporary reassurance, which is followed by renewed worry over symptoms and continuing overuse of medical services (Salkovskis & Warwick, 2001). The onset of hypochondriasis is frequently in early adulthood. The course of hypochondriasis is typically chronic, and the condition frequently takes on a dominant role in the person's life and relationships.

Pain disorder is characterized by acute or chronic pain in one or more body parts that is not easily understood or cannot be fully accounted for by a known medical condition. Pain is considered acute when it exists for less than 6 months and chronic when it persists beyond 6 months. Chronic pain, in particular, is often associated with depression and major changes in behavior, such as decreased activity and job loss or change (Breivik, Collett, Ventafridda, Cohen, & Gallacher, 2006). Pain disorder is relatively common and may occur in adults of all ages (Breivik et al., 2006). White, McMullan, and Doyle's (2009) study of palliative clinics found that pain was the most common symptom, at 72% of patients. The proliferation of special pain clinics could be seen as another indication of the high number of pain patients seeking professional help.

Conversion disorder is characterized by symptoms suggesting a neurological disorder with medical investigations that fail to identify a neurological or general medical disorder. At times, the particular symptoms may even be inconsistent with general neurological knowledge. Patients may present with any one or a combination of motor symptoms (e.g., paralysis), seizures or convulsions, and sensory deficits (e.g., blindness, anesthesia, and aphonia). An important requirement for the diagnosis is the temporal relation between conversion symptoms and a psychological stressor, such as acute grief or victimization. Patients are typically unaware of any psychological basis for their symptoms and report being unable to control them. The diagnosis of conversion disorder is rare and difficult to establish, with estimates ranging between 0.001

and 0.3% (1–300 per 100,000; APA, 1994). Although conversion disorder may occur at any age, onset is typically in late childhood or early adulthood. Onset is often sudden and in response to conflicts or stressful situations, such as unresolved grief and sexual trauma (Sar, Islam, & Öztürk, 2009).

Body dysmorphic disorder (BDD) is characterized by a preoccupation with an imagined or exaggerated body disfigurement or an excessive concern that there is something wrong with the shape or appearance of body parts. The perceived defect or abnormality is generally not or barely noticeable to others. Objects of concern typically refer to the face (e.g., shape or size of nose), head (e.g., hearing loss), sexual characteristics (size of penis, breasts), or general body appearance (tallness or shortness). Other concerns may involve scars, wrinkles, or body odor. Cognitive features are excessive preoccupation, intrusive thoughts, and sometimes ideas of reference. For instance, an individual may persist in the belief that he or she is physically ill due to blemishes on the skin or somewhat atypical marks on the skin. Behavioral features include avoidance (e.g., of body exposure, direct social contact, talking about the problem, looking in the mirror), camouflaging or concealing imagined deformities (wearing a hat or glasses), excessive grooming and checking, and reassurance seeking. Because of these obsessive-compulsive features, the DSM–5 work group is recommending that BDD be reclassified from somatoform disorders to a new category of anxiety and obsessive-compulsive spectrum disorders (APA, 2010).

Rief et al. (2006) estimated the prevalence of BDD at 1 to 2% of the population. Individuals with BDD had higher somatization scores and higher rates of suicidal ideation, and they made more suicide attempts than those not meeting the criteria for BDD. BDD was also found to be associated with higher rates of unemployment, lower financial income, and lower rates of living with a significant other. There are no firmly established gender differences in prevalence rates of BDD since research has been inconclusive. Onset of BDD may be gradual or sudden, and its course is generally continuous and chronic, though fluctuating in intensity. BDD is thought to start in adolescence when preoccupation with physical appearance is very common. Sociocultural factors that influence people's attitudes toward and dissatisfaction with their bodies seem to play a role in determining the extent to which a real or imagined physical abnormality becomes a cause for concern and preoccupation.

A preoccupation with physical appearance and distorted body image can also be found in individuals with eating disorders. The difference is that those with eating disorders also exhibit abnormal patterns of eating (binging, purging, extreme dieting), whereas such abnormal eating patterns are not typical for those with BDD.

Although not classified among the somatization disorders, pathological dissociation and the dissociative disorders are worth mentioning here because of the developmental similarities and diagnostic overlap they share with somatization disorders. The potential link between the two disorders has been discussed since the onset of late 19th-century theories of female hysteria, but actual empirical evidence has been mixed (Brown, Schrag, & Trimble, 2005). Dissociation and somatization are both strongly linked with childhood trauma (Brown et al., 2005; Nijenhuis, Spinhoven, van Dyck, van der Hart, & Vanderlinden, 1998; Webster, 2001), which suggests potentially common mechanisms.

The dissociative disorders are: (a) *dissociative amnesia*, where there is no awareness of critical personal information, usually of a traumatic nature, not due to a medical injury or condition; (b) *dissociative fugue*, an extremely rare disorder where an individual abruptly and unexpectedly takes leave of his or her surroundings and travels for days, months, or even years, remaining unaware or confused about his or her identity; (c) *dissociative identity disorder*, formerly known as multiple personality disorder, where an individual has more than one distinct personality that repeatedly surfaces and about whose activities the dominant personality often remains unaware; and (d) *depersonalization disorder*, where an individual recurrently feels detached from his or her own body, sense of self, or experience, which happens severely and frequently enough to impair functioning. Pathological dissociation is thought to occur in about 1 to 3% of the general population, with no significant gender differences (Maaranen et al., 2006; Martínez-Taboas, Canino, Wang, García, & Bravo, 2006). Several strong comorbid factors have emerged from the research, with dissociation occurring almost 9 times more among depressed individuals, 4 times more among suicidal individuals, and 7 times more among those with alexithymia (i.e., deficiency in understanding or describing emotions; Maaranen et al., 2006).

Dissociation occurs most frequently in individuals who have experienced trauma and abuse, particularly sexual abuse, in infancy or early childhood. One community study found that of 44 young adults experiencing dissociative symptoms, 43 had also experienced victimization of some kind (Martínez-Taboas et al., 2006). The experience of trauma often resurfaces for these individuals in the form of recurrent nightmares and frequent intrusive memories (Agargun et al., 2003). The relationship of dissociative behavior and trauma has been related to attachment theory, which views insecure or anxious interpersonal attachment patterns as one of the root causes of dissociative behavior (Ainsworth & Bowlby, 1991). For these poorly attached individuals, the world cannot be relied upon to meet their needs or keep them safe. Securely attached individuals, or those with strong, flexible, and fulfilling interpersonal attachments, were less likely to develop dissociative disorders following traumatic experiences (Dimitrova et al., 2010; Pasquini, Liotti, Mazzotti, Fassone, & Picardi, 2002).

Diagnostic Validity of DSM-Defined Somatoform Disorders

The diagnostic validity of somatoform disorders in relation to one another as well as to other clinical syndromes is problematic and continues to be the focus of intense debates (Löwe et al., 2008; Mayou, Kirmayer, Simon, & Sharpe, 2005). Scholars have frequently observed that these conditions do not necessarily represent distinct conditions, and difficulties distinguishing between symptoms of somatoform disorders and physical health problems abound (Mayou et al., 2005). These disorders are often highly influenced by contextual factors (e.g., cultural influences).

The distinctiveness of the somatoform disorders has been questioned repeatedly. As a category, somatoform disorders continue to lack conceptual coherence and clearly defined diagnostic criteria. The only common feature to all the somatoform disorders is that they cannot be explained by a general medical condition. Starcevic (2006) criticized the current group of somatoform disorders as simply too heterogeneous. For example, BDD shares few features with the rest of the group other than people's focus on bodily changes. In fact, BDD shares more conceptual and functional features with mood and anxiety disorders—particularly obsessive-compulsive disorder and social anxiety (Castle, Rossell, & Kyrios, 2006).

Also, the diagnostic criteria overlap greatly with other psychiatric disorders that have associated somatic symptoms, leading to high rates of multiple diagnoses. Depression and somatization, for instance, are 4 times more likely to co-occur than not (Leiknes, Finset, Moum, & Sandanger, 2008). Löwe et al. (2008) reviewed several studies and concluded that overlap with depressive or anxiety disorders occurred in as many as 26 to 59% of cases. Even the authors of the *DSM–IV* concede that the grouping of these disorders in a single section is based on clinical utility rather than on assumptions regarding shared etiology (APA, 1994). Mayou et al. (2005) pointed out that the subcategories have been found to be unreliable and arbitrary. Many of the subcategories have failed to achieve acceptable standards of reliability, which can negatively affect patient's rights to medical, legal, and insurance entitlements.

For example, pain may occur in any of the somatoform disorders. Ambiguous criteria such as "the person's concern is grossly in excess of what would be expected," and "slight physical abnormality" further hamper clear differentiation of these problems. The distinction between BDD and normal concerns about appearance is as difficult to make as the distinction between BDD and delusional disorder (somatic subtype). Bass and Murphy (1995) questioned the distinction between somatoform disorders and personality disorders, given the high rates of comorbidity between the two. More recent research by Garcia-Campayo, Alda, Sobradiel, Olivan, and Pascual (2007) showed that individuals with somatization disorders were 2.2 times more likely to have a personality disorder than other individuals with psychiatric diagnoses. Chaturvedi, Desai, and Shaligram (2006) noted that somatization and *abnormal illness behavior* are intricately related. Perhaps new diagnostic standards should pay greater attention to an individual's actions, but then again, abnormal illness behavior can develop anywhere, irrespective of a person's psychiatric diagnosis.

Cultural influences on somatization processes are well documented (Ryder et al., 2008; Zvolensky et al., 2008). Based on a review of data from cross-cultural studies, Escobar, Allen, Nervi, and Gara (2001) initially concluded that there is "considerable cultural variation in the expression of somatizing syndromes" (p. 226). Kirmayer and Sartorious (2009, p. 23) explained this variation as a function of different "symptom schemas" that reflect cultural conceptions of suffering and distress and are rooted in cultural causal explanations (e.g., cellular biology in Western medicine; the balance of the body's basic constituents—fire, earth, metal, water, wood— in traditional Korean culture; preservation of vital energy in Native American culture, etc.). Thus, the specific symptoms of certain disorders often appear to be more a function of the individual's culture than of some underlying (distinct) biologically based disease process. Acknowledging that the types and frequency of somatic symptoms differ across cultures, the *DSM–IV* even suggests that symptom lists should be adjusted to the culture. For example, it would be helpful for clinicians to know that for some individuals of Native American descent, the experience of semen in the urine (*dhat*) is frequently not a delusion but a somatization related to fatigue and depression, a representation of feeling zapped of "vital energy"; likewise, it would also be helpful to know that epigastric burning among individuals of Korean descent may not be heartburn but a somatic experience of intense, culturally inappropriate emotion (*hwa-byong* or "fire illness"; Kirmayer & Sartorious, 2009). Symptom lists for Europe and North America would, by contrast, focus on the most frequent areas of concern in these locations: heart disease and cancer.

Mayou et al. (2005) noted that the terms *somatoform* and *somatization* are often unacceptable to patients because they imply that the patients' symptoms are in their minds and "not real." Patients doubt that clinicians appreciate the reality and authenticity of their symptoms. At a more fundamental level, Mayou et al. (2005) criticized the distinction between somatic and psychological problems as inherently dualistic, which does not translate well into other cultures that have a less dualistic view of mind and body (e.g., Asia and China) than Western culture. The notion that problems can be neatly divided into those that can and cannot be explained by disease is indeed unlikely at best. Several authors also point to potential pathophysiological mechanisms that may underlie unexplained physical symptoms such as chest pain (Pilgrim & Wyss, 2008; Sharpe & Bass, 1992; Yilmaz et al., 2008). We often just do not understand them very well—and that is what we should tell patients rather than using terms such as nonorganic when describing their symptoms. We also need to recognize is that there is frequently a reciprocal relation or "looping effect" between health anxiety and somatic symptoms, in which attending to sensations increases their salience and intensity (Kirmayer & Sartorious, 2009). This could occur either indirectly, through psychological processes, or directly, involving the behaviors designed to reduce anxiety over physical symptoms paradoxically increasing physical symptoms (e.g., constantly checking/scratching a lump, increasing its size and irritation).

Toward a Dimensional Framework for Understanding Pathogenic Processes

In light of the current diagnostic problems with the somatoform disorder category in *DSM–IV*, Mayou et al. (2005) suggested abolishing this category in DSM–5 because the concept and category has consistently failed clinicians and patients alike. They suggest redistributing the current somatoform disorders to other diagnostic categories, specifically, BDD should be redefined as a form of obsessive-compulsive disorder and hypochondriasis should be placed with the anxiety disorders and renamed *health anxiety disorder* because it is conceptually and functionally closer to the anxiety disorders than to any of the other somatoform disorders. Clinicians could use new language, referring to *somatic symptoms* as aspects of other diagnoses, and distinguishing between *functional* somatizations—those that lack association with a general medical condition—and nonfunctional somatizations. Löwe et al. (2008), on the other hand, argued against a complete abolition of the somatoform disorder category on the basis that, faulty or no, it has come to have huge personal, clinical, and societal importance, and abolishing the category would effectively abandon a large group of patients and exclude them from treatment. They argued for revisions that would integrate somatoform disorders into the greater medical field, so that mental and physical health workers have identical, interdisciplinary diagnostic and treatment standards. Furthermore, these diagnoses should not be solely based on the absence of organic disease, but also on the presence of the psychosocial features of dysfunctional cognitions, excessive health care use, selective attention to bodily signals, persistent attribution of symptoms to undiagnosed conditions, avoidance and decreased activity, and functional impairments due to somatization (Löwe et al., 2008, p. 7).

Eifert and colleagues have argued (Eifert, Lejuez, & Bouman, 1998; Eifert, Zvolensky, & Lejuez, 2000) that overlap between related categories is not a problem of "comorbidity" or inaccurate definitions but rather a result of similar psychological processes involved in these conditions. Accordingly, we suggested adopting a dimensional approach to understanding illness-related concerns that can identify key biobehavioral processes. To illustrate this approach, we discuss focal dimensions of health anxiety, a psychological process that characterizes, in part, many somatoform disorders as well as related conditions (e.g., panic disorder). We view health anxiety as a psychological process where individuals present with problems that fall on a continuum along four dimensions:

1. Preoccupation with the body and its functioning. Such bodily preoccupation, especially when coupled with somatic complaints, may produce a state of somatic uncertainty and form the basis for the other three dimensions of the disorder.
2. Disease suspicion or conviction. The person has the suspicion or is convinced of having a serious physical disease; suspicion and conviction are on a continuum of strength, and in rare cases the conviction may reach delusional intensity.
3. Disease fear. The person fears having a serious physical disease.
4. Safety-seeking behavior such as repeated requests for medical examinations and tests, bodily checking, verbal complaints, and seeking reassurance. The function of such behavior is to reduce worry and anxiety over physical illness (Eifert et al., 2000; Salkovskis & Warwick, 2001).

A person could obtain a high score on any one or all four dimensions of health anxiety. For example, disease suspicion or conviction may or may not be accompanied by a strong fear of the suspected disease. Clinically, this feature is most apparent in the patient's resistance to medical reassurance that nothing is wrong. This is particularly evident in a study by Rief, Heitmüller, Reisberg, and Rüddel (2006) who found that when patients with medically unexplained symptoms were asked to recall meetings with their doctor, the patients remembered a higher likelihood of medical explanations than their doctors actually gave. Accordingly, a dimensional classification system could help overcome some challenges inherent to a traditional diagnostic perspective of somatoform disorders. Moreover, identifying dimensions that allow a classification of illness behavior based on the function that such behavior serves, rather than just its topography, might lead to a better understanding and improved treatments of those with somatoform problems (Eifert & Lau, 2001).

General Vulnerability Processes for Abnormal Illness Behavior

Given our previous discussion as to prototypical characteristics of health anxiety, the next logical question pertains to the types of processes that increase or decrease the risk for developing abnormal illness behavior. As discussed at the onset of this chapter, just about everyone experiences distressing physical sensations at some point in his or her life. Moreover, a substantial percentage will even experience robust internal physical (interoceptive) reactions in the form of panic attacks, limited symptom panic attacks, gastrointestinal distress, respiratory infections, strained muscles, and so on. In fact, such bodily distress is so common to the human experience that it seems almost inconceivable to imagine a person going through life without experiencing at least some significant somatic disturbance. These normal experiences of physical symptoms become problematic when they begin to interfere with a person's life due to obsessive preoccupation with them and excessive rigid behaviors designed to control, reduce, or escape from them. Such pervasive experiential avoidance behavior seems to be at the core of many anxiety-related clinical problems (Forsyth, Eifert, & Barrios, 2006; Walker & Furer, 2008)—in fact, maladaptive avoidance behavior is a core feature of *all* anxiety disorders (Eifert & Forsyth, 2005).

Although systematic knowledge about causes is lacking, factors such as parental modeling, stressful life events, biological or genetic components, and greater cultural acceptance of physical versus mental illness appear to be related to the development of somatoform disorders (Heinrich, 2004). One finding, that there is a decreased likelihood of somatoform diagnoses when primary care physicians have a more personal and long-term relationship with patients, also suggests that open, honest doctor–patient relationships protect against somatization diagnoses (Gureje, 2004). Difficulty tolerating emotions (experiential avoidance) has also been shown to be associated with the development of somatization symptoms (Chawla & Ostafin, 2007). Difficulty expressing emotions (alexithymia) and negative affect or neuroticism are associated with symptom increase and persistence (De Gucht, 2002).

As these studies indicate, there are a number of biopsychosocial processes that increase vulnerability for the development of somatoform pathology or abnormal illness behavior generally. The processes that we will focus on in this section include (a) an inherited risk for emotional responsivity to physical sensations, (b) deficits in emotion regulatory skills, and (c) language-based and observational learning.

Before this discussion, however, we need to briefly define what we mean by the term *abnormal illness behavior*. Pilowsky (1993, p. 62) defined abnormal illness behavior as the "persistence of a maladaptive mode of experiencing, perceiving, evaluating, and responding to one's own health status," despite the fact that a doctor has conducted a comprehensive assessment of relevant biological, psychological, and social and cultural factors and provided the patient with feedback about the results of these assessments and opportunities for discussion and clarification of the results. Thus, abnormal illness behavior essentially refers to the disagreement between the doctor and patient about the sick role to which the patient feels entitled. The concept of abnormal illness behavior is valuable for understanding not only patients with functional somatic symptoms but also the behavioral aspects of all illness (Chaturvedi et al., 2006).

Inherited Risk for Emotional Responsivity to Physical Sensations

There is consistent empirical evidence that there is a strong inherited component or substrate for negative emotionality. Researchers have referred to this inherited disposition by a number of different terms, including *negative affectivity*, *trait anxiety*, and *neuroticism* (Barlow, 2001; Lau, Ely, & Stevenson, 2006). These synonymous labels are intended to capture a general predisposition to experience negative affect (e.g., anxiety) and perhaps abrupt emotional reactivity (e.g., panic) to challenging or stressful life events.

Although the characteristics of negative affectivity vary across specific negative emotional experiences (e.g., panic versus anger), they all posit that high degrees of negative emotionality are associated with a lower threshold of initial affective response, slower recovery to baseline, and greater reactivation of arousal with repeated exposure to stressful events. High reactivity is generally associated with inhibited temperament, whereas low reactivity is associated with uninhibited temperament (Kagan, 1989; Letcher, Smart, Sanson, & Toumbourou, 2009). Thus, individual differences in temperament are often related to the experience and regulation of affect because they constrain or facilitate certain types of responding. For example, the temperamental characteristic of neuroticism was found to relate to tendencies to experience low levels of self-esteem in situations of interpersonal conflict, and global and day-to-day perceptions of relationships were more dependent on self-esteem in highly neurotic individuals than in others (Denissen & Penke, 2008).

As behavioral genetic research continues to make important strides in our understanding of emotional functioning, we may eventually have specific models to articulate the extent to which a specific gene or combination of genes contributes to a specific anxiety disorder or health disorder. At this stage, however, it appears that a general disposition for negative affectivity is inherited. The contribution of this inherited component is estimated to be at approximately 30% in the development of somatoform-related disorders (Kendler, Walters, Truett, & Heath, 1995). No research has documented the exact proportion of explained variance for the development of a specific disorder, although there is some evidence that there are both shared and specific genetic vulnerabilities across anxiety-related disorders (Smoller, Block, & Young, 2009). It is likely that a genetic predisposition creates the biological conditions that make people prone to respond with anxiety and panic reactions to certain bodily changes and processes (Walker & Furer, 2008, p. 369). One research challenge in this domain will be to specify *how* genetic vulnerabilities (once they are identified) might influence the pathogenesis of a specific disorder.

Development of Emotion Self-Regulatory Skills

Research has shown that early in life humans develop a repertoire of regulatory-oriented skills to deal with elevated levels of bodily arousal and concomitant emotional distress. For example, parents often distract distressed infants by orienting them to other stimuli, and children eventually learn to reorient and soothe themselves (Rueda & Rothbart, 2009, p. 26). Thus, the effective management of bodily states, particularly negative emotional experiences, is a critical early step in psychological development. As children mature, they learn to approach and avoid salient environmental stimuli, and the members of society increasingly expect them to gain better emotion regulatory skills (e.g., suppression of crying in school). By adulthood, the individual is expected to have sophisticated emotional control skills and the ability to learn new regulatory skills for a variety of changing sociocultural contexts. For example, adults are not supposed to demonstrate signs of emotional distress in social, performance, or work settings. Adults without emotion regulation skills often suffer in modern society. An interesting series of studies by Kantor-Martynuska (2009) provides some insights why this may be the case. She found that highly emotionally reactive individuals were more likely to prefer music at low volumes and to recall music as having been played loudly. This suggests that reactive individuals may have an increased sensitivity to arousing stimuli (music) and a tendency to experience it as aversive.

The preceding discussion highlights the notion that emotion regulation skills are expected to increase consistently across the lifespan and are an integral component of mental health (Stewart, Zvolensky, & Eifert, 2002). When individuals lack the ability to effectively alter their emotional experiences, they are more susceptible to physical discomfort, negative affect, and anxiety (Rothbart, Ziaie, & O'Boyle, 1992). An important way in which children learn emotional regulation skills is through exercising their capacity to explore their world, both literally and metaphorically. Developmental researchers originally referred to these experiences as *mastery learning opportunities* (Rothbart, 1989). Impoverished environments, where parents or caregivers (e.g., teachers) respond to children in a noncontingent manner, produce more emotional distress than do environments characterized by contingent outcomes. For example, van der Bruggen, Stams, Bögels, and Paulussen-Hoogeboom (2010) found that maternal rejection mediated a relationship between parent perceptions of children's negative emotionality and the children's anxiety or depression. The researchers hypothesized that maternal rejection instills a sense of helplessness in children, making them less likely to experience mastery of their negative feelings, and thereby increasing the likelihood that negative emotions eventually lead to symptoms of anxiety and depression. Similar findings have been observed in studies of animals raised in environments with little control over important outcomes (e.g., availability of food; Mineka, Gunnar, & Champoux, 1986; Roma, Champoux, & Suomi, 2006). Such findings are important to understanding somatoform disorders because greater degrees of perceived uncontrollability are predictive of the tendency to view ambiguous internal stimuli as threatening (NASA STI Office, 2004; Zvolensky, Eifert, Lejuez, & McNeil, 1999).

Coping with emotional distress is, of course, a multidimensional process. Recent work indicates that coping responses are best viewed from a hierarchical model that includes first-order and higher-order dimensions (Compas et al., 2001). Indeed, researchers increasingly suggest that coping with emotional distress involves strategic (voluntary) and automatic (involuntary) responses. Additionally, Compas et al. (2001) have categorized these coping responses along the dimensions of engagement and disengagement. *Engagement* responding includes active, primary control oriented responding aimed at altering the immediate situation in some sort of direct manner (e.g., leaving a situation that one finds uncomfortable because of cardiac-related distress and tension). *Disengagement* responding includes secondary control-oriented responding aimed at adapting to an uncontrollable situation by purposively altering one's cognitive-affective response to that situation (indirect responding). For instance, an individual might adapt to pain or other aversive bodily sensations by altering his or her cognitive response to such events (e.g., acceptance, distraction, reframing). Overall, it is likely that individuals will develop a variety of emotion regulatory skills across the lifespan, and these skills are likely to be a product of early learning experiences.

Language-Based Learning

Aside from direct forms of learning, individuals also will experience affective responses to body-related events and sensations through the utilization of language. Language serves important symbolic functions by providing humans with emotional experiences without exposure to the actual physical stimuli or events that ordinarily elicit those responses (Luoma, Hayes, & Walser, 2007; Staats & Eifert, 1990). For instance, both "knowing what to do" and "knowing what to feel" involve verbal understanding of the relation between them. Thus, the meaning of health-related anxiety in a psychological sense represents a complex act of relating largely arbitrary verbal-symbolic events with other events and psychological functions within a particular context. For instance, words such as anxiety and fear either implicitly or explicitly establish relations with other events, such as "I am anxious or afraid of … something, some event, or someone."

The relational quality of terms denoting emotions, in turn, must be tied to descriptions of behavior and events with a variety of stimulus functions (e.g., eliciting, evoking, reinforcing, and punishing) and meanings (e.g., good, bad, pleasant, unpleasant, painful). In turn, people often describe their emotional experiences metaphorically in ways that others can understand (e.g., "When I feel anxious it's like a knife going through my chest"). These metaphorical extensions have no real counterpart inside the person. Instead, they function to communicate the meaning of emotional experience (feeling threatened to the point of fearing death) by identifying and relating events with known stimulus functions (a sharp knife can cut into a chest and cause death).

Society determines what kind of stimuli and events are placed in relation to one another and the nature of that relation (Hayes & Wilson, 1994). These arbitrary relations are learned and function in a variety of ways (Sidman, 1994; Staats & Eifert, 1990). Individuals become anxious about particular health-related experiences or "symptoms" because they read and hear about them in the specific cultural context in which they live. This may be one of the main reasons why cultural variations in somatoform disorders are widespread and can be observed with such great regularity (Escobar et al., 2001). For instance, people in Western societies become anxious when they notice a fast or irregular heartbeat because they have seen or heard many times that this event may be a sign of a heart attack. In Southeast Asian and African cultures it is quite common to observe a phenomenon that has been labeled "*koro*," which describes an individual overcome with the belief that his penis—or, in females, her nipples—is retracting or shrinking, with fear that the organ will disappear (Barlow, 2002). In contrast, this phenomenon is quite rare in Western culture. Thus, the overwhelming finding from cross-cultural studies is that the somatic manifestation and expression of emotional distress is universal, but the focus of somatic concern may vary in different cultures.

The most important point is that those with somatoform disorders have likely developed complex repertoires of verbal and other symbolic responses that elicit negative affect and serve as discriminative stimuli for escape or avoidance behavior (Staats & Eifert, 1990). Thus, for otherwise healthy people, the sensations of a beating heart or chest pain may lead to a sequence of verbal and autonomic events that result in the belief that they are having a heart attack (Eifert, 1992). In this instance, a fast or irregular heartbeat is not just a felt beating heart. Instead, it is an acquired and verbally mediated formulation of what it *means* to have a fast or irregular heartbeat or chest pain (e.g., "I have heart disease" or "I am suffering from a heart attack"). Not only may the person respond to such sensations by rushing to an emergency room, but also any other public or private stimulus events associated with this response may now acquire similar negative functions (e.g., physical exercise, smoking, working hard). In this way, a variety of behaviors and events can come to elicit the physiological event that the person then misconstrues as dangerous.

Observational Learning

It is also likely that individuals who develop somatoform disorders have been exposed to negative health-related events to a greater degree than those who do not develop these disorders. For example, some studies indicate that a significant number of individuals with cardiophobia, defined as someone who has an irrational fear of heart disease, have observed heart disease and its potentially lethal effects (e.g., death) in relatives and close friends (Eifert et al., 2000). These individuals had been exposed directly to the physical and emotionally painful consequences of heart disease. As a result, they may also have had more exposure to heart-focused perceptions and interpretations of physical symptoms and physiological processes.

Observational learning is strongly involved in learning pain tolerance, pain ratings, and nonverbal expressions of pain (Flor, Birbaumer, & Turk, 1990). Such observational learning may increase the likelihood of expressing and interpreting arousal and pain in later life as a heart problem because socially acquired perceptions and interpretations of symptoms largely determine how people deal with illness. For instance, if one or both parents have heart disease, children might observe their parent's response to a heart problem. If the behavior that is modeled is maladaptive (e.g., excessive illness behavior), these children will not only be more likely to respond to stress with increased cardiovascular activity, but they will have also learned maladaptive labeling and interpretation of such symptoms and have fewer adaptive coping skills.

Taken together, research suggests a variety of general factors that may promote the development of the type of abnormal illness behavior found in somatoform disorders. These processes are likely nonspecific in the sense that they increase the chance of negative emotional responding and poor affect regulatory strategies. Exposure to specific illnesses or to those who model the potential dangers of certain physical disorders may increase an individual's general vulnerability. Continued research in each of these general domains will improve our ability to predict who will develop a specific type of somatoform disorder.

General Treatment Strategies for Somatoform Disorders

Cognitive-behavioral theories and research have been helpful in providing a fledgling basis for a better understanding and treatment of those with somatization problems. Important progress has been made, in particular for those with health anxiety (Eifert & Lau, 2001; Salkovskis & Warwick, 2001) and chronic pain (Flor et al. 1990; Kerns, Thorn, & Dixon, 2006; Schermelleh, Eifert, Moosbrugger, & Frank, 1997). This section will overview these treatment strategies at a general level and how they can be applied to specific types of somatoform disorders.

Psychologically distressed patients who present with unexplained somatic symptoms are high users of medical care, and their doctors regard them as frustrating and difficult to treat (Mayou, 2009). There is often a mismatch between the expectations of these patients and their doctors' abilities and communication skills. For instance, terms such as *functional heart problem*, *nervous heart*, *atypical chest pain*, and *pseudoangina*, when used to "diagnose" unexplained chest pain, can easily be misinterpreted by a patient who is determined to believe that some significant cardiac disease is being described (Eifert et al., 2000). Health care providers often feel frustrated and emotionally drained because these patients obviously need psychological support but resent being referred to a psychologist or psychiatrist.

Patients often perceive the use of diagnostic labels such as hypochondriasis as an insult because these labels seem to imply that the patients' problems are not real and "just in their head." Wainwright, Calnan, O'Neil, Winterbottom, and Watkins (2006) attributed this effect to modern society's moral "hierarchy of illness," in which observable, stoically born physical pathology is elevated and legitimized, and somatization is denigrated and thought of as "faking it" or malingering (p. 79). They therefore argued that accepting and understanding, rather than refuting or arguing with the patient's symptoms, is the more important strategy for engaging the patient in a therapeutic working relationship. Lipsitt and Starcevic (2006) similarly stated that it is extremely important for health care providers to treat the somatizing patient in a warm, respectful manner, without prejudice based on previous assessments from other clinicians. Health care professionals can help make the patient feel listened to and let him or her know they regard the patient's symptoms as "real" and do not view the patient as "crazy." They can also ease the patient's anxieties and enhance the relationship with the patient by telling the patient that worrying about his or her symptoms is reasonable and legitimate. A solid and trusting working relationship is essential for optimal help. In the engagement stage of treatment, patients can also be told that there may be alternative explanations for the difficulties they are experiencing (e.g., pathophysiological pathways; Pilgrim & Wyss, 2008; Yilmaz et al., 2008). The general treatment strategy is to test such alternative or benign medical explanations for symptoms and to conduct therapy in the context of an experiment that provides an opportunity for testing alternative hypotheses (Eifert & Lau, 2001; Salkovskis, 1996).

Rather than merely telling patients there is no "organic" reason for their chest pain, an explanation of symptoms that overcomes the nonorganic–organic dualism provides the patient with a more acceptable rationale and reassurance (Eifert, Hodson, Tracey, Seville, & Gunawardane,

1996). For instance, to provide a patient with a credible explanation of how anxiety and chest wall muscle tension can result in chest pain, patients may be given a chest-focused relaxation with electromyogram feedback that literally shows them how they can change their chest tension levels. Salkovskis and Warwick (2001) found that reassurance that only informs the patients there is nothing organically wrong with their bodies will actually increase future reassurance-seeking rather than decrease it. Appropriate reassurance and feedback that provides the patient with new and alternative explanations is the key to successful treatment and may help prevent the development of chronic somatization problems. In a controlled case study, Eifert and Lau (2001) found that behavioral experiments were not only useful in developing alternative symptom explanations but also in teaching the patient to reassure him- or herself rather than seeking therapist reassurance. The treatment strategies and techniques targeting the dimensions of abnormal illness behavior related to heart-focused anxiety are summarized in Table 13.1.

Medical professionals need to be trained to provide alternative explanations rather than vague pseudo-medical labels and to acknowledge rather than dismiss patients' concerns. At the same time, withholding unnecessary medication and medical examinations (response prevention for safety-seeking behavior) is a crucial part of treatment. For instance, in their interviews with British physicians, Wainwright et al. (2006) described how some doctors have adopted patient-centered philosophies and view diagnosis as a negotiated process that can approach psychosocial causality covertly over several sessions, thereby balancing a doctor's ethical commitment to scientifically rigorous standards of practice while accommodating a patient's resistance to psychological explanations. The researchers also found, however, that many physicians still struggle when dealing with these issues, so the focus should remain on developing programs for health care providers that help them communicate more effectively with their patients. Early work focused on arming physicians with basic psychological intervention skills, such as empathic listening to complaints and symptoms (Goldberg, Gask, & O'Dowd, 1989;

Table 13.1 Key Treatment Components Targeting Various Dimensions and Symptoms of Heart-Focused Anxiety

Dimensions	Treatment Strategies and Techniques
Preoccupation with heart	Demonstrate that chest pain/heart sensations are not dangerous • *Reduce avoidance/expose to cardiac-related stimuli*
Disease fear	Extinction of fear and exposure to avoided activities • *Exposure to interoceptive (particularly cardioceptive) cues* • *Reinforce "dangerous" behavior (e.g., strenuous exercise)*
Disease conviction	Testing alternative symptom explanations • *Explain impact of anxiety and tension on body (chest pain)* • *Conduct behavioral experiments to test hypotheses* • *Review evidence for/against heart disease* • *Review evidence for cardiac versus tension chest pain*
Safety/reassurance seeking	Extinction of help and reassurance seeking • *Review results of previous tests* • *Withhold reassurance* • *Refuse further tests* • *Do physical exercise while preventing pulse checking*
Physical (panic) symptoms	Reduce chronic tension and overbreathing • *Chest muscle relaxation* • *Teach slow diaphragmatic versus thoracic breathing*

Note: Although this example deals with heart-focused anxiety, the process dimensions are adaptable and applicable to other somatization problems. (Adopted from Eifert and Lau, 2001.)

Rost, Kashner, & Smith, 1995; Smith, Rost, & Kashner, 1995). Physicians were also taught not to reinforce patients' abnormal illness behavior by providing expensive diagnostic procedures, surgeries, and hospitalizations (Rost et al., 1995; Smith et al., 1995). Withholding such procedures also prevents iatrogenic diseases and counteracts patients' disease convictions. Mayou (2009) recommended the use of a stepped care approach, which involves mixing therapeutic intervention with medical reassessment at various set intervals. This should also help counteract patients' disease convictions while still moving them forward in their treatment. The results of these physician-focused interventions suggest that this balanced approach to patient care can reduce health care costs and at the same time increase the psychological adjustment of patients.

Finally, it is essential that we move patients from an almost exclusive focus on symptoms, which may or may not be changeable or controllable, to goals and behaviors that are controllable and changeable. After an initial empathic discussion of symptoms, treatment needs to shift toward more changeable behavioral targets, such as occupational problem solving, social skills training, and quality of life enhancement (Mayou, 2009; Rief, Hiller, Geissner, & Fichter, 1995). Behavioral activation treatment programs (Lejuez, Hopko, & Hopko, 2001) appear to be valuable therapist tools to help move patients in their "valued direction" (Hayes, Strosahl, & Wilson, 2000) and at the same time reduce negative affect.

Acceptance and commitment therapy (ACT), a new acceptance-based behavior therapy, has shown great promise in the treatment of chronic pain (Vowles, Wetherell, & Sorrell, 2009) and anxiety disorders (Eifert & Forsyth, 2005). In the future, this approach could easily be extended to people suffering from all types of health-related anxiety and concerns because it directly targets the experiential avoidance behavior that tends to interfere with people's daily functioning. ACT helps people refocus their efforts on areas in their lives where they can affect change and where they are in control, rather than wasting their time with fruitless attempts to control or change bodily sensations and their evaluations of them, which are very difficult, if not impossible, to change. ACT provides very useful therapeutic tools for helping people reorient their lives away from managing symptoms, pain, and disability to moving forward and living a life guided by their values—what truly matters to them (McKay, Forsyth, & Eifert, 2010).

Specific Treatment Recommendations

Somatization Disorder

It may be most useful to think of somatic problems as requiring management rather than treatment (Bass & Benjamin, 1993). Early diagnosis and the prevention of unnecessary medical and surgical investigation are of primary importance. For instance, a study by Hoyer et al. (2008) showed that the specific assessment of heart-focused anxiety (HFA) may help identify individuals with elevated levels of HFA who might benefit from interventions and help them adjust to the effects of surgery and lingering cardiac problems. Most somatization patients have specific expectations regarding treatment goals and procedures and try to persuade their doctors to follow their wishes for further medical investigations and treatments. Bass and Murphy (1990) stated that treatment often involves long-term supportive psychotherapy and must be directed toward controlling the demands on medical care as well as the treatment of symptoms and social disability. They recommended the following four steps:

1. Encourage a long-term supportive relationship with only one understanding primary care physician to prevent doctor shopping and to coordinate all actions;
2. See patients at regular appointments rather than on demand to prevent reinforcement of illness behavior;

3. View patient's physical complaints as a form of communication rather than as evidence of disease; and

4. Minimize the use of psychotropic drugs or analgesic medication.

In general, adaptive behavior is encouraged and promoted, whereas sick role behavior is ignored as much as possible. Kashner, Rost, Cohen, Anderson, and Smith (1995) focused on coping with the nature and consequences of the physical symptoms, general problem solving, and helping patients take more control of their lives. These authors found that eight sessions of brief group therapy improved physical and mental health at 1-year follow-up.

A randomized controlled trial examining a comprehensive cognitive-behavioral approach for dealing with medically unexplained physical symptoms was conducted by Speckens et al. (1996). A cognitive-behavioral intervention group of 39 general medical outpatients was compared with a control group of 40 patients receiving optimized medical care. Treatment included imaginary exposure and distraction techniques to break the vicious circles of cognitive avoidance and preoccupation; activity scheduling, exposure in vivo, and response prevention to decrease avoidance behavior; relaxation training, breathing exercises, and physical exercises; and problem-solving or social skills training to overcome any problems in interpersonal relationships. At both 6- and 12-month follow-ups, the intervention group reported lower intensity and frequency of symptoms, reduced illness behavior, less sleep impairment, and fewer limitations in social and leisure activities than did the control group.

Hypochondriasis

Traditionally, individuals with hypochondriasis have been considered difficult to treat and their prognosis has been regarded as poor. For instance, early studies assessing the effectiveness of a variety of psychological interventions available at that time (e.g., Kenyon, 1964) found 40% of patients with primary hypochondriasis to be unchanged or worse following treatment. Although patients with unexplained physical symptoms or health anxiety still pose a considerable challenge for therapists, cognitive-behavioral interventions have yielded encouraging results.

The first comprehensive cognitive-behavioral treatment formulations were provided by Warwick and Salkovskis (1990). Patients were instructed to self-monitor during hypochondriacal episodes, paying careful attention to environmental events, physical symptoms, associated cognitions, and their resulting hypochondriacal behavior. As indicated, their treatment was directed at evaluating alternative, nonthreatening explanations of body-related observations that the patient misinterprets as signs of serious disease. Two possible explanations for the patient's problem are considered together rather than as mutually exclusive alternatives (Salkovskis, 1996). Patients were then asked to engage in a variety of behavioral experiments to test these new explanations, and therapy proceeds as an evaluation of the relative merits of the alternative views. Salkovskis (1996) emphasized that the inappropriate safety seeking of hypochondriacal individuals prevents them from discovering that their fears are groundless. Hence, the key function of exposure exercises and response prevention is to bring patients into contact with the actual rather than expected consequences of their symptoms (Eifert & Lau, 2001). By allowing patients to repeatedly experience feared bodily sensations without the dreaded consequences, they learn that what they are afraid of does not actually happen. Using a similar approach, Martinez and Botella (2005) found that cognitive-behavioral treatment resulted in significant statistical and clinical improvement in hypochondriacal patients, which was maintained at 6-month follow-up with 75% of patients reporting noticeable improvement.

A system of differential reinforcement may need to be added for individuals who gain sympathy or interest for their physical complaints but little attention otherwise. In those cases, family members and other individuals the patient has contact with (including the therapist) should reinforce patient initiation of conversation on any topic other than symptoms (healthy conversation). This reinforcement could consist of praise or increased attention. As the patient engages in more healthy conversation, the natural contingencies (e.g., reduced medical bills, more pleasant interactions with others) should begin to maintain behavior and the frequency and magnitude of artificial reinforcement can be slowly reduced.

In an early study, Visser and Bouman (1992) found that patients with hypochondriasis improved significantly following in vivo exposure, response suppression, and cognitive therapy. In this study exposure and response suppression (behavioral components) appeared to have accounted for more of the improvement than the cognitive component (i.e., attempting to change directly the patient's misconceptions about symptoms). The positive results of this series of single case studies were supported in a first controlled trial that showed cognitive-behavioral therapy to be superior to a wait-list control condition (Warwick, Clark, Cobb, & Salkovskis, 1996).

For patients whose main concern is fear of a specific disease, without significant conviction of having the disease, a more focused program of tension reduction (e.g., through relaxation) is important. Lidbeck's (2003) cognitive-behavioral intervention was particularly successful with hypochondriacal participants (decreases in medication usage, anxiety, and hypochondriasis scores maintained at 18-month follow-up), perhaps because of its focus on relaxation training, which accounted for roughly 56% of the program time and two thirds of participants rated to be of "great help" (p. 451). Exposure to the feared stimuli and prevention of checking and safety seeking are also important intervention tools (Eifert, 1992). Walker and Furer (2008), for instance, used repeated interoceptive exposure in therapy using in vivo exercises (e.g., spinning to experience feared dizziness) and in vitro exercises (e.g., vividly imagining terrible leg pain). Psychoeducation has also shown some success in reducing hypochondrical beliefs and fears. For instance, Lidbeck's (2003) program included a weekly group psychoeducation component, and Bouman (2002) found that group psychoeducation was an effective intervention, with a mean 40% reduction in the frequency of medical service utilization.

Overall, cognitive-behavioral treatments are the most promising interventions for patients with hypochondriasis. Also, the prognosis for patients who are treated with cognitive-behavioral interventions seems more favorable than previously thought. In general, patients with mild, short-lived hypochondriasis that is not associated with any complicating factors have the best prognosis for recovery (Taylor, 2005). There are preliminary data to suggest that high trait anxiety and older age are associated with fewer therapeutic gains, but more extensive and controlled studies are needed to determine the most crucial treatment components and the mechanisms that explain their success (Buwalda & Bouman, 2008).

Pain Disorder

Earlier approaches for pain management were based on psychodynamic principles and used hypnotic suggestions to help people deal with pain. A review by Turk, Meichenbaum, and Genest (1983) found that these techniques are ineffective when used alone, and that treatment effects are due to the unwitting inclusion of behavioral and cognitive treatment components.

Early researchers realized that pain behavior is not an expression or side effect of a pain problem, instead it is *the* problem (Rachlin, 1985). Therefore, the goal of treatment is to extinguish maladaptive pain behavior and teach and reinforce the use of more adaptive pain coping strategies (Nicholas, Wilson, & Goyen, 1991). Treatment begins with a thorough functional analysis of current pain behavior and the environmental contingencies associated with that behavior. Once the consequences of maintaining the maladaptive pain behavior are determined, attempts are made to reduce reinforcement for that behavior and increase reinforcement for adaptive pain coping behavior (cf. Fordyce, Roberts, & Sternbach, 1985; Nicholas et al., 1991; Thorn & Kuhajda,

2006). In addition to changing a patient's maladaptive pain behavior, cognitive-behavioral therapy also attempts to alter associated thought patterns and the patient's perceived competence in dealing with pain (Schermelleh-Engel et al., 1997; Thorn & Kuhajda, 2006). Pain management programs typically require active patient participation and include fostering a patient's real and perceived competence to deal with pain, teaching skills and adaptive responses to problems (including self-attribution for change and success), and planning maintenance.

Based on the assumption that pain is mediated by thoughts and images, cognitive methods involving imagery and distraction have often been added to pain management programs (Buenaver, McGuire, & Haythornthwaite, 2006). Patients are encouraged to create and focus on those thoughts and images that alleviate pain, while ignoring those that exacerbate pain. Particularly for patients who engage in few activities, a *behavioral* activation program is beneficial in more than one way (Lejuez et al., 2001). Such programs encourage and reinforce patients engaging in a host of activities. As patients continue with these activities, they frequently recognize the intrinsically reinforcing value of the activities and their mood enhancing effects.

Although the cognitive-behavioral approach to pain management has been identified as an empirically validated treatment by the Task Force on Promotion and Dissemination of Psychological Procedures (Chambless, 1995), patients are often reluctant to get involved in such programs. Acceptance-based behavior therapy, or ACT, is focused on motivating people to change what they can change and accept what they cannot change. Specifically, ACT teaches people how to bring compassion and acceptance to the pain they cannot control while engaging in life-goal–related actions that they can control (Dahl & Lundgren, 2006; Vowles et al., 2009). This intriguing new approach has been successful in reducing long-term disability resulting from chronic pain (Dahl, Wilson, & Nilsson, 2004)

Conversion Disorder

An important first step in the treatment of conversion symptoms is their early recognition, for which a physical examination plays a crucial role. In many cases, a positive diagnosis can be made on the basis of the rather untypical or bizarre symptoms. Since conversion symptoms vary widely across patients, treatment needs to be individualized. Identifying precipitating stressors is crucial so that patients can be taught more adaptive ways of coping with these stressors. Occasionally, manipulation of the patient's social environmental is necessary to reduce the influence of secondary gain, such as attention from family and friends. Partners and significant others may have to learn how to reinforce the patient's nonsymptomatic behavior.

Behavior therapy has shown some efficacy in the treatment of conversion disorder, particularly for patients who primarily exhibit motor symptoms and gait disturbances (Lipsitt & Starcevic, 2006; Speed, 1996). The program consisted of providing or withholding reinforcement depending on the patient's attempt at normalizing gait and increasing motor movement through specific exercises.

Body Dysmorphic Disorder

Behavioral interventions for BDD aim toward changing avoidance behavior, reassurance seeking, checking, and excessive grooming. Exposure in vivo is used to counter avoidance of social situations (meeting people, having a conversation, being in the spotlight) and prevent individuals from attempting to cover their ostensible blemishes (e.g., by wearing camouflaging clothing such as baggy pants, long hair, sun glasses). Patients are encouraged to expose themselves to social situations rather than avoid them and to observe the reactions of other people to their imagined deformity. Rosen (1995) suggested exposure assignments such as wearing trendy clothes, using makeup to accentuate features, standing closer to people, and undressing in front of one's spouse. Response prevention may involve refraining from looking in the mirror for excessive periods of time, the use of makeup, and inspecting skin blemishes.

A few treatment studies for BDD have examined the use of exposure and response prevention (Neziroglu & Yaryura-Tobias, 1993) and social skills training (Braddock, 1982). Geremia and Neziroglu (2001) described several successful cognitive-behavioral therapy cases in which participants reported statistically significant reductions in depression, anxiety, and dissatisfaction with body parts. Half of their small subject pool also demonstrated decreases in body dysmorphic obsessions and compulsions, like checking and grooming, and reduction in overvalued ideas, like "beauty is the most important attribute."

To date the largest controlled outcome study of the treatment of BDD (Rosen, Reiter, & Orosan, 1995) compared the effectiveness of cognitive-behavioral therapy with a wait-list control condition in 54 females. Treatment involved eight 2-hour small group sessions and was aimed at modifying dysfunctional thoughts about the patients' body image, reducing checking of their appearance, and increasing exposure to avoided situations. Results at posttest and 4-months follow-up showed improvement in the active treatment condition on several measures of body image, whereas no such changes occurred in the control condition. The results of this study are promising, but more controlled studies are needed to corroborate existing data and to examine the role of the various treatment components.

Dissociative Disorders

Dissociation is thought to be a coping mechanism for trauma—individuals literally dissociate themselves from an experience that is presumably too traumatic for the conscious self to acknowledge or experience. Since dissociation often is associated with trauma or abuse, treatment focuses on reprocessing these experiences through exposure, and ultimately, seeking to reintegrate these memories with the conscious self. Therapists have used a variety of therapeutic approaches, including exposure, cognitive restructuring, hypnosis, and metaphorical imagery, to help facilitate gaining access to personally relevant memories (van der Hart, van der Kolk, & Boon, 1999). In this domain, hypnosis is often considered a suggestive therapeutic tool. However, therapists must beware of creating false memories (Loftus & Davis, 2006). Clients who are successful in integrating memories of real trauma and dissociated self states experience decreased levels of dissociation, depression, posttraumatic stress disorder, distress, and suicidality (Brand, Classen, McNary, & Zaveri, 2009). Since dissociative experiences can reoccur even after successful treatment, it has been suggested that treatments should incorporate long-term self-management techniques. Pharmacological interventions are also always an option, but long-term studies suggest they do not produce better results than psychotherapy, which is more conducive to the long-term goal of "total integration" (Maldonado & Spiegel, 2009).

Conclusions

Unexplained and unexplainable somatic symptoms, complaints, and concerns are very common in the general population. These problems are costly to the individuals concerned in terms of distress and financial expense as well as to society in terms of lost productivity and health care costs. Compared to other common psychological dysfunctions (e.g., anxiety and depression), our present conceptual understanding of somatoform disorders is poor, and comprehensive integrative models are still lacking.

One factor that has impeded a better understanding of the somatoform disorders is the unsatisfactory and somewhat arbitrary nature of their current *DSM* classification. In view of the existing conceptual and diagnostic confusion, vagueness, and imprecision, we question the utility of the current criteria for and distinctions among somatoform disorders and the wisdom of keeping hypochondriasis in particular separate from the anxiety disorders. "Comorbidity" of somatoform disorders with anxiety disorders and depression is not a diagnostic problem but an indication that there are similarities in the underlying psychopathological processes (Aikens, Zvolensky, & Eifert, 2001). We have outlined some commonalities in emotional dysregulation processes, particularly in relation to anxiety. A practical consequence for researchers and clinicians is to give up their focus on the individual disorders and increase their efforts at identifying the common functions of symptoms in those with different somatoform problems (Eifert, 1996; Kirmayer & Sartorious, 2009).

The complex relation between the physical and psychological aspects of somatoform disorders has led to much confusion. We caution against an overreliance on medical diagnostic procedures and medical theory. At the same time, research and service delivery would benefit from a more balanced approach. This approach should focus not just on finding or excluding somatic abnormalities, but also on combining current medical knowledge and diagnostic techniques with the psychological assessments of a patient's behavior, cognitive processes, and social relationships (cf. Fink, 1996; Löwe et al., 2008). In our work with cardiac patients we have observed how a simple reliance on one source of information (medical or psychological) was inadequate for many patients. Instead, it was the combination of sophisticated medical tests and psychological information that yielded the type of knowledge that was most useful for recommending and designing the most appropriate treatment for the individual patient.

Hence, perhaps one of the most compelling conclusions arising from this chapter is that somatoform disorders cannot be adequately understood, assessed, and treated from a single perspective. Both the classification and research could be improved by adopting a multidisciplinary approach and an integrated biopsychosocial perspective. For example, Mayou, Bass, and Sharpe (1995) proposed a multidimensional classification of patients with functional somatic symptoms along five dimensions: (1) number and type of somatic symptoms; (2) mental state (mood and psychiatric disorder); (3) cognitions (e.g., symptom misinterpretations, disease conviction); (4) behavioral and functional impairment (illness behavior, avoidance, use of health services); and (5) pathophysiological disturbance (organic diseases, physiological mechanisms such as hyperventilation). As described in the section on health anxiety, Löwe et al. (2008) presented an alternate diagnostic system that focused on the presence of behaviors, some of which are classified *abnormal illness behaviors*. Individuals should be assessed for (1) dysfunctional cognitions; (2) excessive health care use; (3) selective attention to bodily signals; (4) persistent attribution of symptoms to undiagnosed conditions; (5) avoidance and decreased activity; and (6) functional impairments due to somatization. These criteria are behavioral and would be of more immediate relevance for treatment than diagnosing according to physiological phenomena we cannot observe or measure. Rather than attempting to find the "correct diagnosis," we recommend assessment along the crucial dimensions involved in the regulation of maladaptive illness behavior and devising treatment programs based on such assessments. This may be more valuable than diagnosing according to the number and type of physical complaints.

A multicausal perspective suggests several potentially fruitful lines for future psychological research into somatoform disorders, such as an increased focus on information-processing behavior (attribution, attention, and memory) and environmental contingencies for illness behavior (e.g., social, occupational, medical). Psychoneuroimmunological studies may help clarify particular aspects of the nature of the interface between pathophysiological changes and individual responses to such changes, as exemplified in some chronic pain research (Flor et al., 1990). Although the past emphasis on the problems of patients with no demonstrable physical pathology was worthwhile and deserves continued attention, the gray area of those with some organic pathology, bodily symptoms, and psychological distress deserves greater recognition and needs to be investigated more carefully.

Treatment programs and outcomes are likely to be enhanced by an improved conceptual understanding of these problems. The need for better theories and treatments is even more pressing for those somatoform problems that have been particularly neglected in the past, such as BDD and conversion problems. The relative success of recent cognitive-behavioral treatment programs for those with unexplained physical symptoms, health anxiety, or chronic pain is promising. These treatment successes may help change the common perception of health care providers that people with such problems are just a "pain in the neck" and invariably difficult, or even impossible, to treat.

References

Agargun, M. Y., Kara, H., Özer, Ö. A., Selvi, Y., Kiran, Ü., & Özer, B. (2003). Clinical importance of nightmare disorder in patients with dissociative disorders. *Psychiatry and Clinical Neurosciences, 57*(6), 575–579.

Aikens, J. E., Zvolensky, M. J., & Eifert, G. H. (2001). Fear of cardiopulmonary sensations in emergency room noncardiac chest pain patients. *Journal of Behavioral Medicine, 24,* 155–167.

Ainsworth, M. D. S., & Bowlby, J. (1991). An ethological approach to personality development. *American Psychologist, 46,* 333–341.

American Psychiatric Association. (1994). *Diagnostic and statistical manual of mental disorders* (4th ed.). Washington, DC: Author.

American Psychiatric Association. (2010, May 28). *Somatoform disorders.* Online forum on proposed revisions to DSM disorders and criteria. Retrieved from http://www.dsm5.org/ProposedRevisions/Pages/SomatoformDisorders.aspx

Barlow, D. H. (2001). *Anxiety and its disorders: The nature and treatment of anxiety and panic* (2nd ed.). New York: Guilford.

Barsky, A., Orav, E., & Bates, D. (2005). Somatization increases medical utilization and costs independent of psychiatric and medical comorbidity. *Archives of General Psychiatry, 62*(8), 903–910.

Bass, C. M., & Benjamin, S. (1993). The management of the chronic somatizer. *British Journal of Psychiatry, 162,* 472–480.

Bass, C. M., & Murphy, M. R. (1990). Somatization disorder: Critique of the concept and suggestions for future research. In C. M. Bass (Ed.), *Somatization: Physical symptoms and psychological illness* (pp. 301–332). Oxford: Blackwell.

Bass, C. M., & Murphy, M. R. (1995). Somatoform and personality disorders: Syndromal comorbidity and overlapping developmental pathways. *Journal of Psychosomatic Research, 39,* 403–427.

Bouman, T. K. (2002). A community-based psychoeducational group approach to hypochondriasis. *Psychotherapy and Psychosomatics, 71,* 326–332.

Braddock, L. E. (1982). Dysmorphophophobia in adolescence: A case report. *British Journal of Psychiatry, 140,* 199–201.

Brand, B., Classen, C. C., McNary, S. W., & Zaveri, P. (2009). A review of dissociative disorders treatment studies. *Journal of Nervous and Mental Disease, 197*(9), 646–654.

Breivik, H., Collett, B., Ventafridda, V., Cohen, R., & Gallacher, D. (2006). Survey of chronic pain in Europe: Prevalence, impact on daily life, and treatment. *European Journal of Pain, 10*(4), 287–333.

Brown, R. J., Schrag, A., & Trimble, M. R. (2005). Dissociation, childhood interpersonal trauma, and family functioning in patients with somatization disorder. *American Journal of Psychiatry, 162,* 899–905.

Buenaver, L., McGuire, L., & Haythornthwaite, J. (2006). Cognitive-behavioral self-help for chronic pain. *Journal of Clinical Psychology, 62,* 1389–1396.

Buwalda, F., & Bouman, T. (2008). Predicting the effect of psychoeducational group treatment for hypochondriasis. *Clinical Psychology and Psychotherapy, 15*(6), 396–403.

Castle, D. J., Rossell, S., & Kyrios, M. (2006). Body dysmorphic disorder. *Psychiatric Clinics of North America, 29,* 521–538.

Chambless, D. L. (1995). Training in and dissemination of empirically validated psychological treatments: Report and recommendations by the Task Force on Psychological Procedures. *Clinical Psychologist, 48,* 3–23.

Chaturvedi, S., Desai, G., & Shaligram, D. (2006). Somatoform disorders, somatization and abnormal illness behavior. *International Review of Psychiatry, 18*(1), 75–80.

Chawla, N., & Ostafin, B. (2007). Experiential avoidance as a functional dimensional approach to psychopathology: An empirical view. *Journal of Clinical Psychology, 63*(9), 871–890.

Compas, B. E., Conner-Smith, J. K., Saltzman, H., Thomsen, A. H., & Wadsworth, M. E. (2001). Coping with stress during childhood and adolescent: Problems, progress, and potential in theory and research. *Psychological Bulletin, 127*, 87–127.

Dahl, J., & Lundgren, T. (2006). *Living beyond your pain.* Oakland, CA: New Harbinger.

Dahl, J., Wilson, K. G., & Nilsson, A. (2004). Acceptance and commitment therapy and the treatment of persons at risk for long-term disability resulting from stress and pain symptoms: A preliminary randomized trial. *Behavior Therapy, 35*, 785–802.

De Gucht, V. (2002). Neuroticism, alexithymia, negative affect and positive affect as predictors of medically unexplained symptoms in primary care. *Acta Neuropsychiatrica, 14*(4), 181–185.

Denissen, J., & Penke, L. (2008). Neuroticism predicts reactions to cues of social inclusion. *European Journal of Personality, 22*, 497–517.

Dimitrova, N., Pierrehumbert, B., Glatz, N., Torrisi, R., Heinrichs, M., Halfon, O., & Chouchena, O. (2010). Closeness in relationships as a mediator between sexual abuse in childhood or adolescence and psychopathological outcome in adulthood. *Clinical Psychology and Psychotherapy, 17*(3), 183–195.

Eifert, G. H. (1992). Cardiophobia: A paradigmatic behavioral model of heart-focused anxiety and non-anginal chest pain. *Behaviour Research and Therapy, 30*, 329–345.

Eifert, G. H. (1996). More theory-driven and less diagnosis-based behavior therapy. *Journal of Behavior Therapy and Experimental Psychiatry, 27*, 75–86.

Eifert, G. H., & Forsyth, J. P. (2005). *Acceptance and commitment therapy for anxiety disorders.* Oakland, CA: New Harbinger.

Eifert, G. H., Hodson, S. E., Tracey, D. R., Seville, J. L., & Gunawardane, K. (1996). Heart-focused anxiety, illness beliefs, and behavioral impairment: Comparing healthy heart-anxious patients with cardiac and surgical inpatients. *Journal of Behavioral Medicine, 19*, 385–399.

Eifert, G. H., & Lau, A. (2001). Using behavioral experiments in the treatment of cardiophobia: A case study. *Cognitive and Behavioral Practice, 8*, 305–317.

Eifert, G. H., Lejuez, C. W., & Bouman, T. K. (1998). Somatoform disorders. In A. S. Bellack & M. Hersen (Series Eds.), *Comprehensive clinical psychology* (Vol. 6, pp. 543–565). Oxford: Pergamon.

Eifert, G. H., Zvolensky, M. J., & Lejuez, C. W. (2000). Heart-focused anxiety and chest pain: A conceptual and clinical review. *Clinical Psychology: Science and Practice, 7*, 403–417.

Escobar, J. I., Allen, L. A., Nervi, C. H., & Gara, M. A. (2001). General and cross-cultural considerations in a medical setting for patients presenting with medically unexplained symptoms. In G. J. G. Asmundson, S. Taylor, & B. Cox (Eds.), *Health anxiety: Clinical research perspectives on hypochondriasis and related disorders* (pp. 220–245). New York: Wiley.

Fink, P. (1996). Somatization: Beyond symptom count. *Journal of Psychosomatic Research, 40*, 7–10.

Flor, F., Birbaumer, N., & Turk, D. C. (1990). The psychobiology of chronic pain. *Advances in Behaviour Research and Therapy, 12*, 47–84.

Fordyce, W. E., Roberts, A. H., & Sternbach, R. A. (1985). The behavioural management of chronic pain: A response to critics. *Pain, 22*, 113–125.

Forsyth, J. P., Eifert, G. H., & Barrios, V. (2006). Fear conditioning research as a clinical analog: What makes fear learning disordered? In M. G. Craske, D. Hermans, & D. Vansteenwegen (Eds.), *Fear and learning: Basic science to clinical application* (pp. 133–153). Washington, DC: American Psychological Association.

Garcia-Campayo, J., Alda, M., Sobradiel, N., Olivan, B., & Pascual, A. (2007). Personality disorders in somatization disorder patients: A controlled study in Spain. *Journal of Psychosomatic Research, 62*(6), 675–680.

Geremia, G., & Neziroglu, F. (2001). Cognitive therapy in the treatment of body dysmorphic disorder. *Clinical Psychology and Psychotherapy, 8*, 243–251

Goldberg, D., Gask, L., & O'Dowd, T. (1989). The treatment of somatization: Teaching techniques of reattribution. *Journal of Psychosomatic Research, 33*, 689–695.

Gureje, O. (2004). What can we learn from a cross-national study of somatic distress? *Journal of Psychosomatic Research, 56*, 409–412.

Hansen, M., Fink, P., Frydenberg, M., & Oxhoj, M. (2002). Use of health services, mental illness, and self-rated disability and health in medical inpatients. *Psychosomatic Medicine, 64*, 668–675.

Harth, W., & Hermes, B. (2007). Psychosomatic disturbances and cosmetic surgery. *Journal der Deutschen Dermatologischen Gesellschaft, 5*(9), 736–743.

Hayes, S. C., Strosahl, K., & Wilson, K. (2000). *Acceptance and commitment therapy: Understanding and treating human suffering.* New York: Guilford.

Hayes, S. C., & Wilson, K. G. (1994). Acceptance and commitment therapy: Altering the verbal support for experiential avoidance. *Behavior Analyst, 17*, 289–303.

Heinrich, T. (2004). Medically unexplained symptoms and the concept of somatization. *Wisconsin Medical Journal, 103*(6), 83–87.

Hoyer, J., Eifert, G. H., Einsle, F., Zimmermann, K., Krauss, S., Knaut, M., … Köllner, V. (2008). Heart-focused anxiety before and after cardiac surgery. *Journal of Psychosomatic Research, 64*, 291–297.

Kagan, J. (1989). Temperamental contributions to social behavior. *American Psychologist, 44*, 668–674.

Kantor-Martynuska, J. (2009) The listener's temperament and perceived tempo and loudness of music. *European Journal of Personality, 23*, 655–673.

Kashner, T. M., Rost, K., Cohen, B., Anderson, M., & Smith, G. R. (1995). Enhancing the health of somatization disorder patients. Effectiveness of short-term group therapy. *Psychosomatics, 36*, 462–470.

Katon, W., Sullivan, M., & Walker, E. (2001). Medical symptoms without identified pathology: Relationship to psychiatric disorders, childhood and adult trauma, and personality traits. *Annals of Internal Medicine, 134*(9.2), 917–925.

Kendler, K. S., Walters, E. E., Truett, K. R., & Heath, A. C. (1995). A twin-family study of self-report symptoms of panic, phobia, and somatization. *Behavior Genetics, 25*, 499–515.

Kenyon, F. E. (1964). Hypochondriasis: A clinical study. *British Journal of Psychiatry, 110*, 478–488.

Kerns, R., Thorn, B., & Dixon, K. (2006). Psychological treatments for persistent pain: An introduction. *Journal of Clinical Psychology, 62*(11), 1327–1331.

Khan, A. A., Khan, A., & Kroenke, K. (2000). Symptoms in primary care: Etiology and outcome. *Journal of General Internal Medicine, 15*, 76–77.

Kirmayer, L., & Sartorious, N. (2009). Cultural models and somatic syndromes. In J. Dimsdale, Y. Xin, A. Kleinman, V. Patel, W. Narrow, P. Sirovatka, & D. Regier (Eds.), *Somatic presentations of mental disorders: Refining the research agenda for DSM-V* (pp. 19–40). Arlington, VA: American Psychiatric Association.

Kroenke, K., & Price, R. (1993). Symptoms in the community: Prevalence, classification, and psychiatric comorbidity. *Archives of Internal Medicine, 153*, 2474–2480.

Lau, J., Ely, T., & Stevenson, J. (2006). Examining the state-trait anxiety relationship: A behavioural genetic approach. *Journal of Abnormal Child Psychology, 34*(1), 19–27.

Leiknes, K., Finset, A., Moum, T., & Sandanger, I. (2008). Overlap, comorbidity, and stability of somatoform disorders and the use of current versus lifetime criteria. *Psychosomatics, 49*(2), 152–162.

Lejuez, C. W., Hopko, D. R., & Hopko, S. D. (2001). A brief behavioral activation treatment for depression. *Behavior Modification, 25*, 255–286.

Letcher, P., Smart, D., Sanson, A., & Toumbourou, J. (2009). Psychosocial precursors and correlates of differing internalizing trajectories from 3 to 15 years. *Social Development, 18*(3), 618–646.

Lidbeck, J. (2003). Group therapy for somatization disorders in primary care: Maintenance of treatment goals of short cognitive-behavioural treatment one-and-a-half-year follow-up. *Acta Psychiatrica Scandinavica, 107*, 449–456.

Lipsitt, D. R., & Starcevic, V. (2006). Psychotherapy and pharmacotherapy in the treatment of somatoform disorders. *Psychiatric Annals, 36*, 341–350.

Loftus, E. F., & Davis, S. (2006). Recovered memories. *Annual Review of Clinical Psychology, 2*, 469–498.

Löwe, B., Mundt, C., Herzog, W., Brunner, R., Backenstrass, M., Kronmüller, K., & Henningsen, P. (2008). Validity of current somatoform disorder diagnoses: Perspectives for classification in DSM-V and ICD-11. *Psychopathology, 41*, 4–9.

Luoma, J., Hayes, S., & Walser, R. (2007). *Learning ACT: An acceptance and commitment therapy skills-training manual for therapists.* Oakland, CA: New Harbinger.

Maaranen, P., Tanskanen, A., Honkalampi, K., Haatainen, K., Hintikka, J., & Vinamäki, H. (2006). Factors associated with pathological dissociation in the general population. *Australian and New Zealand Journal of Psychiatry, 39*(5), 387–394.

Maldonado, J. R., & Spiegel, D. (2009). Dissociative disorders. In J. A. Bourgeois, R. E. Hales, J. S. Young, & S. C. Yudofsky (Eds.), *The American Psychiatric Publishing board review guide for psychiatry* (pp. 413–424). Arlington, VA: American Psychiatric Publishing.

Marple, R., Kroenke, K., Lucey, C., Wilder, J., & Lucas, C. (1997). Concerns and expectations in patients presenting with physical complaints: Frequency, physician perceptions and actions, and two-week outcomes. *Archives of Internal Medicine, 157*, 1482–1488.

Martinez, M. P., & Botella, C. (2005). An exploratory study of the efficacy of a cognitive-behavioral treatment for *hypochondriasis* using different measures of change. *Psychotherapy Research, 15*, 392–408.

Martínez-Taboas, A., Canino, G., Want, M. Q., García, P., & Bravo, M. (2006). Prevalence and victimization correlates of pathological dissociation in a community sample of youths. *Journal of Traumatic Stress, 19*(4), 439–448.

Mayou, R. (2009). Are treatments for common mental disorders also effective for functional symptoms and disorders? In J. Dimsdale, Y. Xin, A. Kleinman, V. Patel, W. Narrow, P. Sirovatka, & D. Regier (Eds.), *Somatic presentations of mental disorders: Refining the research agenda for DSM-V* (pp. 131–142). Arlington, VA: American Psychiatric Association.

Mayou, R., Bass, C. M., & Sharpe, M. (Eds.). (1995). *Treatment of functional somatic symptoms.* Oxford: Oxford University Press.

Mayou, R., Kirmayer, L., Simon, G., & Sharpe, M. (2005). Somatoform disorders: Time for a new approach in DSM-V. *American Journal of Psychiatry, 162*, 847–855.

McKay, M., Forsyth, J. P., & Eifert, G. H. (2010). *Your life on purpose: How to find what matters and create the life you want.* Oakland, CA: New Harbinger.

Mineka, S., Gunnar, M., & Champoux, M. (1986). Control and early socioemotional development: Infant rhesus monkeys reared in controllable versus uncontrollable environments. *Child Development, 57*, 1241–1256.

Narrow, W., Rae, D., Robins, L., & Regier, D. (2002). Revised prevalence estimates of mental disorders in the United States: Using a clinical significance criterion to reconcile 2 surveys' estimates. *Archives of General Psychiatry, 59*, 115–123.

NASA Scientific and Technical Information Program Office. (2004). *Stress, cognition, and human performance: Literature review and conceptual framework.* (Pub. No. 2004–212824). Hanover, MD: NASA Center for AeroSpace Information.

Neziroglu, F. A., & Yaryura-Tobias, J. A. (1993). Exposure, response prevention, and cognitive therapy in the treatment of body dysmorphic disorder. *Behavior Therapy, 24*(3), 431–438.

Nicholas, M. K., Wilson, P. H., & Goyen, J. (1991). Operant-behavioural and cognitive-behavioural treatment of chronic low back pain. *Behaviour Research and Therapy, 29*, 225–238.

Nijenhuis, E. R. S., Spinhoven, P., van Dyck, R., van der Hart, O., & Vanderlinden, J. (1998). Degree of somatoform and psychological dissociation in dissociative disorder is correlated with reported trauma. *Journal of Traumatic Stress, 11*(4), 711–730.

Pasquini, P., Liotti, G., Mazzotti, E., Fassone, G., & Picardi, A. (2008). Risk factors in the early family life of patients suffering from dissociative disorders. *Acta Psychiatrica Scandinavica, 105*(2), 110–116.

Pilgrim, T., & Wyss, T. (2008). Takotsubo cardiomyopathy or transient left ventricular apical ballooning syndrome: A systematic review. *International Journal of Cardiology, 124*(3), 283–292.

Pilowsky, I. (1993). Aspects of abnormal illness behaviour. *Psychotherapy and Psychosomatics, 60*, 62–74.

Rachlin, H. C. (1985). Pain and behavior. *Behavioral and Brain Sciences, 8*, 43–83.

Rief, W., Buhlmann, U., Wilhelm, S., Borkenhagen, A., & Brahler, E. (2006). The prevalence of body dysmorphic disorder: A population-based survey. *Psychological Medicine, 36*, 877–885.

Rief, W., Heitmüller, A., Reisberg, K., & Rüddel, H. (2006). Why reassurance fails in patients with unexplained symptoms—an experimental investigation of remembered probabilities. *PLOS Medicine, 3*(8): e269. doi:10.1371/journal.pmed.0030269.

Rief, W., Hiller, W., Geissner, E., & Fichter, M. M. (1995). A two-year follow-up study of patients with somatoform disorders. *Psychosomatics, 36*, 376–386.

Robins, L. N., Helzer, J. E., Weissman, M. M., Orvaschel, H., Gruenberg, E., Burke, J. D., & Regier, D. A. (1984). Lifetime prevalence of specific psychiatric disorders in three sites. *Archives of General Psychiatry, 41*(10), 949–958.

Roma, P., Champoux, M., & Suomi, S. (2006). Environmental control, social context, and individual differences in behavioral and cortisol responses to novelty in infant rhesus monkeys. *Child Development, 77*(1), 118–131.

Rosen, J. C. (1995). The nature of body dysmorphic disorder and treatment with cognitive behavior therapy. *Cognitive and Behavioral Practice, 2*, 143–166.

Rosen, J. C., Reiter, J., & Orosan, P. (1995). Cognitive-behavioral therapy for negative body image in body dysmorphic disorder. *Journal of Consulting and Clinical Psychology, 63*, 263–269.

Rost, K., & Kashner, T. M., & Smith, G. R. (1995). Effectiveness of psychiatric intervention with somatization disorder patients. *General Hospital Psychiatry, 16*, 381–387.

Rothbart, M. K. (1989). Temperament and development. In G. Kohnstamm, J. Bates, & M. K. Rothbart (Eds.), *Temperament in childhood* (pp. 187–248). Chichester: Wiley.

Rothbart, M. K., Ziaie, H., & O'Boyle, C. G. (1992). Self-regulation and emotion in infancy. In N. Eisenberg & R. A. Fabes (Eds.), *Emotion and its regulation in early development* (pp. 7–24). San Francisco: Jossey-Bass.

Rueda, M., & Rothbart, M. (2009). The influence of temperament on the development of coping: The role of maturation and experience. In E. Skinner & M. Zimmer-Gembeck (Eds.), *Coping and the development of regulation* (pp. 19–31). San Francisco: Jossey-Bass.

Ryder, A., Yang, J., Xiongzhao, Z., Shugiao, Y., Yi, J., Heine, J., & Bagby, R. (2008). The cultural shaping of depression: Somatic symptoms in China, psychological symptoms in North America? *Journal of Abnormal Psychology, 117*(2), 300–313.

Salkovskis, P. M. (1996). The cognitive approach to anxiety: Threat beliefs, safety seeking behavior, and the special case of health anxiety and obsessions. In P. M. Salkovskis (Ed.), *Frontiers of cognitive therapy* (pp. 49–74). New York: Guilford.

Salkovskis, P. M., & Warwick, H. M. C. (2001). Making sense of hypochondriasis: A cognitive model of health anxiety. In G. J. G. Asmundson, S. Taylor, & B. Cox (Eds.), *Health anxiety: Clinical research perspectives on hypochondriasis and related disorders* (pp. 46–64). New York: Wiley.

Sar, V., Islam, S., & Öztürk, E. (2009). Childhood emotional abuse and dissociation in patients with conversion symptoms. *Psychiatry and Clinical Neuroscience, 63*(5), 670–677.

Schermelleh-Engel, K., Eifert, G. H., Moosbrugger, H., & Frank, D. (1997). Perceived competence and anxiety as determinants of maladaptive and adaptive coping strategies of chronic pain patients. *Personality and Individual Differences, 22*, 1–10.

Sharpe, M., & Bass, C. M. (1992). Pathophysiological mechanisms in somatization. *International Review of Psychiatry, 4*, 81–97.

Sidman, M. (1994). *Equivalence relations and behavior: A research story*. Boston: Authors Cooperative.

Smith, R. C., Lein, C., Collins, C., Lyles, J. S., Given, B., Dwamena, F. C., … Given, C. W. (2003). Treating patients with medically unexplained symptoms in primary care. *Journal of General Internal Medicine, 18*(6), 478–489.

Smith, G. R., Rost, K., & Kashner, T. M. (1995). A trial of the effect of a standardized psychiatric consultation of health outcomes and cost in somatizing patients. *Archives of General Psychiatry, 52*, 238–243.

Smoller, J., Block, S., & Young, M. (2009). Genetics of anxiety disorders: The complex road from DSM to DNA. *Depression and Anxiety, 26*(11), 965–975.

Speckens, A. E. M., van Hemert, A. M., Spinhoven, P., Hawton, K. E., Bolk, J. H., & Rooijmans, H. G. M. (1996). Cognitive behavioral therapy for medically unexplained physical symptoms: A randomised controlled trial. *British Medical Journal, 311*, 1328–1332.

Speed, J. (1996). Behavioral management of conversion disorder: Retrospective study. *Archives of Physical Medicine and Rehabilitation, 77*, 147–154.

Staats, A. W., & Eifert, G. H. (1990). A paradigmatic behaviorism theory of emotion: Basis for unification. *Clinical Psychology Review, 10*, 539–566.

Starcevic, V. (2006). Somatoform disorders and DSM-V: Conceptual and political issues in the debate. *Psychosomatics, 47*, 277–281.

Stewart, S. H., Zvolensky, M. J., & Eifert, G. H. (2002). The relations of anxiety sensitivity, experiential avoidance, and alexithymic coping to young adults' motivations for drinking. *Behavior Modification, 26*, 274–296.

Taylor, S. (2004). Understanding and treating health anxiety: A cognitive-behavioral approach. *Cognitive and Behavioral Practice, 11*(1), 112–123.

Thorn, B., & Kuhajda, M. (2006). Group cognitive therapy for chronic pain. *Journal of Clinical Psychology, 62*, 1355–1366.

Turk, D. C., Meichenbaum, D., & Genest, M. (1983). *Pain and behavioral medicine: A cognitive-behavioral perspective*. New York: Guilford.

van der Bruggen, C., Stams, G., Bögels, S., & Paulussen-Hoogeboom, M. (2010). Parenting behaviour as a mediator between young children's negative emotionality and their anxiety/depression. *Infant and Child Development, 19*(4), 354–365.

van der Hart, O., van der Kolk, B., & Boon, S. (1999). Treatment of dissociative disorders. In J. Douglas & M. D. Bremner (Eds.), *Trauma, memory, and dissociation. Progress in psychiatry* (pp. 253–284). Arlington, VA: American Psychiatric Publishing.

Vedsted, P., Fink, P., Sørensen, H., & Olesen, F. (2004). Physical, mental and social factors associated with frequent attendance in Danish general practice. A population-based cross-sectional study. *Social Science Medicine, 59*(4), 813–823.

Visser, S., & Bouman, T. (1992). Cognitive-behavioural approaches in the treatment of hypochondriasis: Six single case cross-over studies. *Behaviour Research and Therapy, 30*, 301–306.

Vowles, K. E., Wetherell, J. L., & Sorrell, J. T. (2009). Targeting acceptance, mindfulness, and values-based action in chronic pain: Findings of two preliminary trials of an outpatient group-based intervention. *Cognitive and Behavioral Practice, 16*, 49–58.

Wainwright, D., Calnan, M., O'Neil, C., Winterbottom, A., & Watkins, C. (2006). When pain in the arm is "all in the head": The management of medically unexplained suffering in primary care. *Health, Risk and Society, 8*(1), 71–88.

Walker, J., & Furer, P. (2008). Interoceptive exposure in the treatment of health anxiety and hypochondriasis. *Journal of Cognitive Psychotherapy: An International Quarterly, 22*(4), 366–378.

Warwick, H. M. C., Clark, D. M., Cobb, A. M., & Salkovskis, P. M. (1996). A controlled trial of cognitive-behavioural treatment of hypochondriasis. *British Journal of Psychiatry, 169*, 189–195.

Warwick, H. M. C., & Salkovskis, P. M. (1990). Hypochondriasis. *Behaviour Research and Therapy, 28*, 105–117.

Webster, R. E. (2001). Symptoms and long-term outcomes for children who have been sexually assaulted. *Psychology in the Schools, 38*(6), 533–547.

White, C., McMullan, D., & Doyle, J. (2009). "Now that you mention it, doctor …": Symptom reporting and the need for systematic questioning in a specialist palliative care unit. *Journal of Palliative Medicine, 12*(5), 447–450.

Yilmaz, A., Mahrholdt, H., Athanasiadis, A., Vogelsberg, H., Meinhardt, G., Voehringer, M., … Sechtem, U. (2008). Coronary vasospasm as the underlying cause for chest pain in patients with PVB19 myocarditis. *Heart, 94*(11), 1456–1463.

Zvolensky, M. J., Feldner, M. T., Eifert, G. H., Vujanovic, A. A., & Solomon, S. E. (2008). Cardiophobia: A critical analysis. *Transcultural Psychiatry, 45*, 231–252.

14
Substance Use Disorders[1]

KEITH KLOSTERMANN and MICHELLE L. KELLEY

Old Dominion University
Norfolk, Virginia

Of the major public health concerns of the 21st century, alcoholism and drug addiction are among the most pervasive, with devastating social, legal, and economic consequences for individuals and families not only in the United States but around the world. The World Health Organization (WHO) estimates that 76.3 million individuals have an alcohol use disorder and 5.3 million individuals have drug use disorders (WHO, 2010). The *National Survey on Drug Use and Health* reports more than half of the U.S. population, aged 12 and older, uses alcohol. Of these, 23.3% engage in binge drinking (i.e., drinking five or more drinks on the same occasion at least once in the past month), and nearly 7% are heavy drinkers (Office of Applied Studies, 2009). Along these lines, approximately 25% of children under the age of 18 are exposed to familial alcohol abuse or alcohol dependence (Grant et al., 2006). Although the prevalence rates of other drug use disorders are much lower than for alcohol, they are sizable by nearly any standard. For illicit psychoactive substances, the lifetime prevalence of drug abuse or dependence is roughly 6% in the United States, with lifetime cannabis abuse (i.e., 4.6%) being the most common after alcohol (Haynes, 2002). Substance use in the United States claims 600,000 lives annually, including 440,000 attributable to nicotine use, 125,000 from alcohol use, and 10,000 from heroin and cocaine use (exclusive of deaths from HIV; McCrady & Epstein, 1999). Alcoholism is the third major cause of death in the United States (behind coronary heart disease and cancer), with the lifespan of individuals with alcoholism being about 12 years shorter than their nonalcoholic counterparts (Mokdad, Marks, Stroup, & Gerberding, 2004). In addition to the serious problems individuals with alcohol or drug problems create for themselves, victims of family violence, accidents, and violent crime add to the numbers of those adversely affected. On days when alcohol is used, intimate partner violence increases (Mignone, Klostermann, & Chen, 2009). Parental substance use is associated with a host of emotional, behavioral, and social problems for children (Boris, 2009; Osborne & Berger, 2009), which may evolve into problems with alcohol and drugs as these children progress through adolescence and into adulthood. Thus, the effects of alcoholism and substance abuse can be accurately described as being part of an intractable, multigenerational, vicious cycle.

Aside from the toll in human suffering, estimates of yearly direct and indirect economic and social costs arising from substance abuse are substantial. Individuals who abuse alcohol and other drugs consume a disproportionately large share of social resources from a variety of sources, some of which include specialized drug abuse treatment (Institute of Medicine, 1990), treatment of secondary health effects (Langenbucher, 1994), use of social welfare programs (Plotnick, 1994), and involvement of the criminal justice system (e.g., arrests, incarceration, parole, and probation; Deschenes, Anglin, & Speckart, 1991; Harwood, Hubbard,

---

[1] This research was supported in part by a grant from the National Institute on Drug Abuse (R01DA024740).

Collins, & Rachal, 1988). In the United States, the most recent estimate of the societal cost of drug abuse (focusing on the cost of health care, productivity losses, and criminal justice system and crime victim costs) was $180.9 billion in 2002, with an average annual rise in costs of 5.3% per year since 1992 (Office of National Drug Control Policy, 2004). Similarly, the economic cost of alcoholism (i.e., abuse and dependence) for 1998 (the last year for which figures are available) was $184.6 billion, which translates into approximately $638 for every man, woman, and child in the United States (Grant et al., 2006; Harwood et al., 1988).

The size and scope of substance abuse and dependence in our society have drawn significant and increasing scientific and public attention. Although our understanding of addiction to alcohol and drugs is far from complete, there has been great progress in the understanding of the etiology, course, and treatment of alcoholism and drug abuse. However, progress is not to be confused with consensus. There remains much controversy, not only about the etiology and treatment of substance misuse, but also, on a far more fundamental level, about how to conceptualize and operationalize substance use disorders.

Definition and Description of Substance Use Disorders

For most of U.S. history, chronic and excessive substance use has been viewed either as immoral conduct or as a disease. More recently, with the rising influence of the behavioral sciences in this dialogue, addiction has also been viewed as maladaptive behavior subject to reinforcement contingencies that govern all learned human behavior. In turn, the definition and description of addictive behavior can vary considerably, based on which view (i.e., moral, disease, or behavioral) is emphasized.

Defining Addictive Behavior

The evolution in thinking about what defines addictive behavior is based in large part on the observation that a number of processes are common to excessive behaviors that have been characterized as addictive. Miller (1995) defined addiction as consisting of three primary components: (1) preoccupation; (2) compulsion; and (3) relapse. Using drug addiction as an example, in the *preoccupation* phase, individuals place a great deal of emphasis on acquiring drugs. As such, social relationships and employment are jeopardized in the continuous search for drugs and suffer as a consequence of using drugs. In the *compulsion* phase, the individual continues to use drugs, despite serious negative consequences. During *relapse*, the individual stops using drugs for a period of time, however, eventually resumes using drugs at an abnormal level. To capture the essence of addiction that spans these behaviors, a broad definition has evolved that can be generally applied to all addictive behavior, including addiction to psychoactive substances. From this vantage point, addiction is viewed as a complex, progressive pattern of behavior having biological, psychological, and sociological components. Thus, this pattern of behavior is characterized by the individual's overwhelming pathological involvement in or attachment to substance use, subjective compulsion to continue use, and inability to exert control over it. Moreover, this behavior pattern continues despite its negative impact on the physical, psychological, and social functioning of the individual.

Although this depiction provides an overarching description of addictive behavior, it provides little insight into how to discern when use of drugs or alcohol crosses the normal threshold into problematic use, and similarly, from problematic use to disorder. More specifically, because of widely divergent social attitudes toward and prejudices about alcohol and drug use, there have been few generally accepted and agreed-on operational criteria for what level of use constitutes social use, abuse, and dependence. Substance use can follow one of several patterns; addiction "is not an all-or-nothing" phenomenon, but a continuum from recreational use to severe compulsion (Peele, Brodsky, & Arnold, 1991, p. 133).

Labels and Diagnostic Systems

Throughout history, a number of value-laden terminologies have been used to describe individuals who use alcohol and other drugs, as well as the problems such use can create (Carroll & Miller, 2006). Labels assigned to behaviors may have tremendous implications for the way the individual and problem are conceptualized; names used to describe a given phenomenon greatly influence the way one thinks about a problem and how one addresses it. Individuals with alcohol problems have been called, at various times, drunks, dipsomaniacs, alcoholics, alcohol abusers, and so on. Those who use illicit drugs have been called addicts, dope fiends, freaks, and criminals. Of course, these labels have important implications for how we think about people who have these problems and what can be done about the problems. In response to these issues, more formal diagnostic systems have come to the fore in recognition of the importance of labels and to bring order to the labeling system.

Although *use*, *abuse*, and *addiction* are best viewed as a continuum of behavior, much effort has been put forth to delineate boundaries between critical points on this continuum. There are several different definitional frameworks used to categorize various levels of addictive behavior that are widely referenced in the scientific and lay press. The most widely used framework is the psychiatric diagnostic approach, exemplified in the current *Diagnostic and Statistical Manual of Mental Disorders* (*DSM-IV-TR*; American Psychiatric Association, 2000) and the *International Classification of Diseases* (*ICD-10*; WHO, 1992). Using the *DSM-IV* system as an example, the diagnosis of alcohol or psychoactive substance use disorders includes two general subcategories—abuse and dependence—collectively considered substance use disorders. *Substance dependence* is marked by a cluster of cognitive, behavioral, and physiological symptoms, indicating that the individual continues to use a given psychoactive substance despite significant substance-related problems. To meet diagnostic criteria for dependence on a psychoactive substance, an individual must display at least three of the following seven symptoms:

1. Physical tolerance
2. Withdrawal
3. Unsuccessful attempts to stop or control substance use
4. Use of larger amounts of the substance than intended
5. Loss of or reduction in important recreational, social, or occupational activities
6. Continued use of the substance despite knowledge of physical or psychological problems that are likely to have been caused or exacerbated by the substance
7. Excessive time spent using the substance or recovering from its effects

In contrast, the essential feature of *substance abuse* is a maladaptive pattern of problem use leading to significant adverse consequences. This includes one or more of the following:

1. Failure to fulfill major social obligations in the context of work, school, or home
2. Recurrent substance use in situations that create the potential for harm (e.g., drinking and driving)
3. Recurrent substance-related legal problems
4. Continued substance use despite having persistent social or interpersonal problems caused or exacerbated by the effects of the substance

However, given the complexity of addictive behavior, it appears that a binary, either–or view implicit in the psychiatric diagnostic approach is too simplistic and provides little understanding of the complexities of the addictive process and how to change it. As noted by Shaffer and Neuhaus (1985), addictive behavior is not easily categorized and, as such, is not easily defined by a set of consensually agreed-on criteria. Indeed, different diagnostic systems often place greater emphases on different aspects of behavioral and physiological functioning in their definitions. In turn, these differences lead to fairly divergent estimates about the prevalence of alcohol and drug use disorders in the general population (for a review of this issue, see Grant & Dawson, 1999). Moreover, O'Brien, Volkow, and Li (2006) argued that dependence is often confused with physical dependence, which may occur with therapeutic applications of a variety of medications and, as a result, may create apprehension among clinicians to prescribe medications (e.g., pain) out of fear of creating addiction (Kranzler & Li, 2010). In response to this concern, given its emphasis on behavioral aspects of substance use, these authors advocate a return to using the term *addiction* in the upcoming DSM–5 because it seems to accurately capture the chronic, relapsing, and compulsive nature of substance use that often occurs despite negative consequences. Accordingly, as noted on the American Psychiatric Association (2010) DSM–5 development website, the word dependence will be limited to physiological dependence, which is a normal response to repeated doses of many medications, including beta-blockers, antidepressants, opioids, antianxiety agents, and other drugs. Tolerance and withdrawal symptoms are not considered for the diagnosis of a substance abuse disorder when occurring in the course of appropriate medical treatment with prescribed medications.

A Biopsychosocial Perspective

Behavioral scientists have proposed an alternative biopsychosocial approach to defining alcoholism and drug abuse. According to this framework, alcohol and drug use disorders are not defined as unitary diseases, nor is it implicitly assumed that the observed substance use symptoms are the manifestation of a disease state. Instead, symptoms are viewed as acquired habits that emerge from a combination of genetic, social, pharmacological, and behavioral factors. Addiction is viewed as involving physiological changes in individuals (many of whom may be genetically or psychologically predisposed) and the complex interaction of environmental stressors and individual aspects of the person (including his or her experiential history) that produce and maintain addictive behaviors.

A comprehensive understanding of the synergistic relationship among these factors is essential not only to understand the degree and severity of substance use, but also to recognize when use becomes abuse. This approach largely deemphasizes labels and places greater emphasis on understanding the interplay between multiple factors that have led to and maintained the observed behavior.

Cultural and Social Issues

Definitions of substance abuse do not develop in isolation; the point at which substance use is said to move from recreational to disordered is determined by the social and cultural context in which the behavior occurs (Thombs, 2006). Thus, societal norms and definitions of substance use and abuse are inextricably intertwined. How we determine what qualifies as an alcohol or drug problem is derived from the boundaries implicitly (e.g., social stigma associated with being labeled an alcoholic or drug addict) or explicitly (e.g., laws prohibiting use of certain substances) drawn by the society in which the behavior takes place. In many respects, the norms for acceptable drinking and other drug use are delineated and communicated (implicitly or explicitly) to members of the society by the way the culture defines addiction.

A Sociocultural View of Alcoholism and Drug Abuse

From a sociological perspective, clinical diagnostic criteria for alcoholism and other drug abuse are derived from societal norms and thus vary depending on when and where the diagnosis is made. More specifically, drinking or drug-taking behaviors that are considered disordered are those that deviate from socially accepted standards. Perhaps the cultural foundations of alcoholism, which can also be applied to other addictive behaviors, are best captured by Vaillant (1990), who stated: "Normal drinking merges imperceptibly with pathological drinking. Culture and idiosyncratic viewpoints will always determine where the line is drawn" (p. 6).

Moreover, problems with alcoholism and drug abuse have become increasingly medicalized, and certain factions appear to have an agenda in viewing these behaviors as symptoms of a disease state and convincing others to view them in a similar manner. If addictive behavior is defined as a disease, the label itself gives credibility to physicians' efforts to control, manage, and supervise the care provided to individuals seeking treatment. Thus, the medical community may have a strong, vested interest in defining addictive behavior as a disease. At its core, treatment of substance abuse is a business; as with all businesses, economics play a critical role (Carlson, 2006). The label serves to make legitimate such financially lucrative efforts as hospital admissions, insurance billing, expansion of the pool of patients available for hospital admission, consulting fees, and so forth.

However, it would be short sighted to assume that societal norms alone shape the parameters for defining alcoholism and drug addiction. In some respects, the process of labeling what constitutes substance abuse or dependence restricts drinking and drug using behavior by members of a given culture. In our culture, public intoxication, drinking early in the morning, drinking while at work, and drinking and driving are considered signs of problem drinking, which are included as indicators in many of our widely used diagnostic instruments (e.g., Michigan Alcoholism Screening Test [MAST], Selzer, 1971; Alcohol Use Disorders Identification Test [AUDIT], Babor, Higgins-Biddle, Saunders, & Monteiro, 2001). Clearly, these "symptoms" are culturally derived and are based on a commonly held set of beliefs about acceptable substance use; the nature of the symptoms would likely be different in another culture that holds a different set of social norms. Thus, understanding the cultural beliefs and practices of individuals from diverse backgrounds and how they relate to substance use will be critical in the development of successful prevention and intervention programs (Grant et al., 2006).

The Disease–Moral Model of Addictive Behavior

The disease model of alcoholism and abuse of other drugs is not the only theoretical conceptualization of these disorders and, in some contexts, not the predominant one. From a social policy perspective, the idea that addictive behavior is deviant and immoral is on at least an equal footing with the disease model. This disease–moral model is summed up by a passage from a turn-of-the-century temperance lecturer, John B. Gough (1881), who wrote that he considered "drunkenness as a sin, but I consider it also a disease. It is a physical as well as moral evil" (p. 443). The disease and moral models of substance abuse are, in many respects, strange bedfellows. These models hold divergent and, at times, inconsistent views about the etiology and maintenance of addictive behavior. Although the moral view holds that drinking and drug use are freely chosen acts for which individuals are responsible, the disease model, in many respects, espouses the opposite position. Thus, the conclusions and outcomes of the disease–moral model are, at times, rife with contradiction. For example, it is difficult to reconcile the inherent contradiction in treating the "illness" of psychoactive substance abuse with punishment (e.g., incarceration). How many other illnesses are routinely punished?

At a social policy level, much energy and effort is expended in veering between these two models. Yet, it is the disease–moral model that is the guiding hand that drives alcohol and drug policies today, with neither perspective completely displacing the other. For instance, judges sentence those convicted of driving while intoxicated (DWI) to attend Alcoholics

Anonymous (AA) meetings or face jail. As noted by Peele (1996), the synthesis of disease and law enforcement models is perhaps manifested most clearly in the debate between those who believe drug abusers should be treated and those who believe they should be incarcerated.

Gender Issues

Although social norms provide a context in which to understand addictive behavior, it is also important to understand that science does not stand above or outside of its social context, but is immersed in and highly influenced by it (Kuhn, 1962). As with all areas of inquiry, social and cultural factors influence the way scientists study alcoholism and drug abuse. The relationship between addictive behavior and gender is an important case in point. Alcoholism and other addictions have traditionally been considered problems of men; as such, it has been the study of addictive behavior among men that has shaped our understanding of the nature and course of these disorders. Two of the most widely known and influential investigations of alcoholism, Jellinek's (1952) on the phases of alcoholism and Vaillant's (1995) 45-year prospective longitudinal study of alcohol abuse in inner-city and college cohorts, were limited to male participants. Treatment methods and programs were also initially designed to treat male substance abuse; it was not unusual for women who needed treatment for addictive disorders to be placed in psychiatric wards, whereas men were treated in specialized alcoholism or drug abuse treatment programs (Blume, 1998).

Because the majority of research conducted in the area of substance abuse has been based largely on studies with male participants, a significant concern is that conclusions drawn from these studies may not generalize to women with substance use disorders (Straussner & Zelvin, 1997). More recently, women have become the focus of increased attention by the research and treatment communities. Comparisons of substance use by men and women have revealed several important differences in epidemiology, development, and treatment. Wilsnack and Wilsnack (2002) identified two important public health policy implications of women's drinking: (1) women with drinking problems may be reluctant to seek treatment or may be prevented by embarrassed family members, and (2) prevalence rates of women's drinking may be underestimated, which makes it difficult to accurately determine the amount of harm caused by female drinking.

Epidemiological and Etiological Comparisons

Data from the 2008 National Survey on Drug Use and Health (Substance Abuse and Mental Health Services Administration, 2009) reveal that the rate of substance abuse or dependence for males 12 and older were nearly twice as high as for females. However, important changes in use patterns have taken place as a function of gender. In 2008, for males, the rate of abuse or dependence dropped to 11.5% from 12.5% in 2007, while among females, the rate was 6.4%, which signified an increase from the 5.7% reported in 2007. The change in use patterns is especially notable in younger cohorts. Among youth aged 12 to 17, the rate of substance abuse or dependence was higher for females than for males (8.2 vs. 7.0%). Moreover, a cross-national epidemiological study from 17 countries participating in the WHO's Mental Health Survey Initiative concluded that there was consistent evidence across countries suggesting a general shift may be occurring with respect to traditional gender differences in drug use (Degenhardt et al., 2008).

Another area of difference between men and women are the factors that appear associated with drinking and drug use. For example, Winfield, George, Swartz, and Blazer (1990) found that the lifetime prevalence of alcohol abuse or dependence was 3 times higher and abuse of other drugs was 4 times higher among women who reported a history of sexual assault. In a study of women recruited from community violence agencies, women with recent incidents of intimate partner violence were more likely to report using alcohol as a coping behavior (Kaysen et al., 2007). Moreover, sexual assault during adulthood appears associated with substance use. In a sample of women applying for a protection order from a domestic violence unit, those who experienced more than one sexual assault from a partner, as compared to just one, were 3.5 times as likely to start or escalate substance use (McFarlane et al., 2005). These predictors (e.g., sexual and intimate partner violence) are important in that they are experiences women typically have more often than men.

In addition, female substance abusers have higher rates of comorbid (i.e., co-occurring) psychiatric disorders, especially depressive and anxiety disorders, than do men (Brady & Randall, 1999). It also appears that male significant others who use drugs strongly influence women's patterns of substance use. In comparison to women, men are more likely to introduce their partners to the use of drugs and to supply drugs to them (Amaro & Hardy-Fosta, 1995). Moreover, women frequently report using or discontinuing substance use for the sake of their partners (Sun, 2007); and having a partner who abuses alcohol or drugs is more strongly related to relapse for women than for men (Grella, Scott, Foss, Joshi, & Hser, 2003). Taken together, these findings suggest that women may be more likely to rely on substance use as a form of self-medication for mood disturbances and interpersonal problems, which has been termed *effortful avoidance* (Feuer, Nishith, & Riseck, 2005). Moreover, their partners' substance use may be more likely to affect women than men.

The Stigma of Addiction for Women

Sociocultural factors also play important roles in the substance use patterns of men and women. In nearly all societies in which alcohol or other drugs are consumed, the cultural norms, attitudes, stereotypes, and legal sanctions often differ for men versus women. Most cultures expect that women will drink less alcohol than men. These expectations may serve as a protective factor, reducing the incidence of alcohol use disorders among women (Kubicka, Csemy, & Kozeny, 1995).

However, the intense stigma associated with drinking and drug use by women can also create serious social problems. Society tolerates some behaviors exhibited by intoxicated men, but views the same behavior as scandalous and morally objectionable if exhibited by intoxicated women. As Blume (1991) argued, women who are intoxicated are often subjected to unwanted sexual overtures, and men believe that intoxicated women who say "No" to these advances really mean "Yes." In a study of beliefs about rape, participants viewed rapists who were intoxicated as less responsible for their crimes than sober rapists and viewed rape victims who had been drinking as more to blame for the rape than victims who had not been drinking (Richardson & Campbell, 1982). Thus, it is not surprising that alcoholic women are much more likely to be victims of violent crime, including rape, than their nonalcoholic counterparts (McClelland & Teplin, 2001). Some contend that society at large views women who abuse alcohol or other drugs as partially or fully responsible for sexual advances made by men, thus making these women acceptable targets for physical and sexual aggression (Stormo, Lang, & Stritzke, 1997).

An important result of the stigma associated with women's alcohol and drug use is denial by the person, the family, and society. These various forms of denial, in turn, are barriers that may prevent women from seeking treatment. As noted by Schober and Annis (1996), women often are reluctant to acknowledge a substance use problem publicly by seeking treatment because of intense fear of being stigmatized as a substance abuser. In comparison to their male counterparts, fears about the stigma associated with the label of *alcoholic* or *substance abuser* may be a more powerful disincentive for women to seek treatment than denial of having a problem or accessibility and cost of treatment (Marlatt, Tucker, Donovan, & Vuchinich, 1997).

Along with personal denial, family denial is also a significant barrier to women entering treatment for substance abuse. In fact, the response by family members to women entering treatment appears to be more negative than it is for men. For example, Beckman and Amaro (1986) found that nearly 25% of women in a treatment sample reported opposition from family or friends compared to only 2% of men. In addition, child care and child custody issues influence the decision to seek treatment.

Women often fear that entering treatment will lead to the perception that they are unfit as mothers and may be deprived of custody of their children. These fears are not unfounded. Women who use alcohol and other drugs during pregnancy have been prosecuted on charges of prenatal child abuse or delivery of a controlled substance to a minor (via the umbilical cord). Such practices have not prevented substance use during pregnancy but have discouraged pregnant substance users from seeking prenatal or addiction treatment (Blume, 1997).

In addition to these personal and familial barriers, several factors related to the type and process of treatment have increased women's reluctance to seek help. Less than 14% of all women who need treatment for substance abuse receive it; less than 12% of pregnant women receive help (Center on Addiction and Substance Abuse, 1996). Dawson, Grant, Stinson, and Chou (2006) found that individuals who seek treatment differ in many ways, with men being more likely to seek help than women. Unfortunately, these findings are not surprising; most treatments for addictive behaviors have been developed largely to meet the needs of men and thus may not be as effective for women (Ramlow, White, Watson, & Luekefeld, 1997). A major obstacle to more women engaging in treatment is that most programs fail to provide services (e.g., child care, obstetrician services) that make it easier for women to enter treatment (Nelson-Zlupko, Dore, Kauffman, & Kaltenbach, 1996; Stewart, Gossop, & Trakada, 2007). Some studies do, in fact, suggest that treatment programs designed specifically to meet the treatment needs of substance-abusing women have higher retention rates and better outcomes than standard outpatient or residential treatment programs (Dahlgren & Willander, 1989; Roberts & Nishimoto, 1996). Yet, gender specific treatment programs are not widely available. In a review of the Alcohol and Drug Services Study (ADSS) conducted by the U.S. Department of Health and Human Services, Brady and Ashley (2005) found that women-only treatment availability ranged from about 2% of outpatient nonmethadone facilities to 21% of nonhospital residential facilities.

Sexual Orientation and Alcohol and Drug Use Disorders

Sexual Minority Women

For three decades, researchers have demonstrated that lesbian and bisexual women are at greater risk for substance use and substance use disorders than are heterosexual women (Brandsma & Pattison, 1982; McCabe, Hughes, Bostwick, West, & Boyd, 2009; McKirnan & Peterson, 1989; Parson, Kelly, & Wells, 2006; Wilsnack, Hughes, & Johnson, 2008). Using data from a large-scale national survey, McCabe et al. (2009) estimated past year prevalence rates for lesbians and bisexual women were 20% and 25% for heavy drinking and 13% and 16% for alcohol dependence. In a convenience sample of lesbian participants, Amadio, Adam, and Buletza (2006) found 24% were categorized as alcoholic on the MAST (Selzer, 1971). Gilman et al. (2001) found the 12-month prevalence rates for sexual minority women were 19.5% for any substance abuse, 13.3% for alcohol abuse, and 15.3% for substance dependence compared to 7.8%, 5.2%, and 6.2 %, respectively, for heterosexual women.

In addition, a growing body of research suggests that young sexual minority teenage girls have higher rates of initial substance use and experience steeper substance use trajectories than do heterosexual youth (Marshal, Friedman, Stall, & Thompson, 2009), which may continue into adulthood (Hughes et al., 2006). In their recent meta-analysis, Marshal et al. (2008) found that the odds of substance use for young, nonheterosexual women were, on average, 400 times higher than for heterosexual youth. In a study of 1,514 high school students, Orenstein (2001) found gay or lesbian youth were approximately twice as likely as heterosexual students to have ever used marijuana; however, for "hard drug" use, differences were more substantial. For instance, 2% of heterosexual students have at some point used cocaine or crack, whereas 27% of gay and lesbian students reported cocaine or crack use. Similarly, 1% of heterosexual adolescents surveyed indicated that they had used an intravenous drug, whereas 9% of gay or lesbian adolescents indicated they had injected a drug. Findings from previous research lead Marshal et al. (2009) to conclude that a significant proportion of lesbian, gay, and bisexual (LGB) youth are on high-risk substance use trajectories that had begun in young adulthood.

The growing awareness of substance use disparities between heterosexual and sexual minority women has led to an increasing search to understand the causal mechanisms associated with these differences. "Syndemics" are defined by the Centers for Disease Control and Prevention's Syndemics Prevention Network as "two or more afflictions, interacting synergistically, contributing to excess burden of disease in a population" (Centers for Disease Control and Prevention, n.d., para.1). In early life the pressure to conform may result in stress. Children who are viewed as different may experience greater peer rejection and bullying. In turn, this stress may lead to initial alcohol or drug use. However, in young adulthood, sexual minorities may begin to socialize in bars and clubs in an attempt to seek social support and community identification, thereby increasing their exposure to environments where alcohol and drugs are widespread (Marshal et al., 2009). In addition, sexual minority stress, a multifaceted construct that includes stress related to identity concealment and confusion, experienced and anticipated rejections and discrimination, and internalized homophobia, may also contribute to substance use and misuse (Lewis, Derlega, Berndt, Morris, & Rose, 2001; Meyer, 2003).

Etiology of Alcohol and Other Drug Use Disorders

Research on the etiology of substance use disorders is a multidimensional, multidisciplinary effort, and findings that have appeared in the literature are truly voluminous; this is a consequence of the multiple theoretical conceptualizations of the development and maintenance of these disorders. For instance, investigators who view alcoholism and drug abuse as diseases are often most interested in examining genetic and biological contributions. Behavior-oriented researchers are more apt to explore antecedent and consequent events that may serve to initiate and reinforce substance use. Sociologists examine macrolevel variables, such as peer and societal influences that contribute to the onset and maintenance of addictive behavior. To be clear, development of an addiction to alcohol or other drugs is a complex process involving many factors; however, the exact role of each of these ingredients has not been fully determined and operates differently for each individual. Genetics, biology, environment, sociocultural factors, and the biochemical properties of the psychoactive substances themselves appear to contribute substantially to the process (Sandbak, Murison, Sarviharju, & Hyytiae, 1998).

Neurobiology of Addiction

Neurobiological research on addiction tends to focus on identifying neuroadaptive mechanisms within specific brain circuits that mediate the transition from infrequent and controlled substance use to chronic addiction (Cruz, Bajo, Schweitzer, & Roberto, 2008). Central to the neurochemical process underlying addiction is the manner by which alcohol or other drugs become reinforcing. Most neurobiological studies of addiction have focused on the dopamine system, which is considered to be the neurotransmitter system through which most drugs of abuse exert their reinforcing effects (Koob & Bloom, 1988). A *reinforcer* is operationally defined as an event that increases the likelihood of a subsequent response; drugs of abuse, which appear to have substantial effects on the dopamine system, are much stronger reinforcers than natural reinforcers, such as food and sex (Wightman & Robinson, 2002).

A network of four circuits may be largely responsible for drug abuse and addiction: (1) reward, located in the nucleus accumbens and the ventral pallidum; (2) motivation or drive, located in the orbitofrontal cortex and the subcallosal cortex; (3) memory and learning, located in the amygdala and the hippocampus; and (4) control, located in the prefrontal cortex and the anterior cingulate gyrus (Volkow, Fowler, & Wang, 2003). These four circuits receive innervations (i.e., are stimulated into action) from dopaminergic neurons but are also connected to one another through direct and indirect pathways. The circuits work together and can be changed with experience. Thus, during the development and maintenance of addiction to a psychoactive substance, the enhanced value of the substance in the reward, motivation, and memory circuits eventually overcomes any inhibitory control exerted by other parts of the brain (e.g., the prefrontal cortex). This, in turn, creates a positive feedback loop that is initiated by the ingestion of the psychoactive substance and then perpetuated by the activation of the motivation or drive and memory circuits. For individuals addicted to drugs, the value of the drug of abuse is enhanced in the reward and motivation or drive circuits; increases in dopamine induced by drugs are 3 to 5 times higher than those of natural reinforcers (Wise, 2002).

Genetic Propensity

Many studies have examined the genetic predisposition to substance abuse and addiction, and a substantial literature suggests addiction problems and disorders have a genetic component (Dick, & Agrawal, 2008). The familial nature of alcoholism has long been recognized and is well documented (Merikangas et al., 1998; Nurnberger et al., 2004). Although alcoholism appears to run in families, it is difficult to disentangle genetic factors from environmental influences because members of nuclear families typically share both genetic and environmental factors. As an example, a number of genes are believed to contribute to an individual's susceptibility to substance dependence; thus, there may be many idiographic combinations of these genes resulting in different combinations for different people. Environmental influences, in particular the environment–gene interaction, may also impact alcohol and drug use (Heath et al., 2002). With this caveat in mind, studies of twins also support the role of genetic factors in the development of alcoholism. The level of twin-pair concordance for a disorder or trait can be compared between identical (monozygotic, or MZ) and fraternal (dizygotic, or DZ) twins. A higher concordance for MZ than DZ twins is an indication of genetic heritability; 100% heritability indicates a disorder is entirely genetic, 50% heritability means there is a substantial contribution from genetic and environmental factors, and 0% indicates genetic factors do not play a role. In general, adult twin studies of alcohol dependence show a heritability of 50 to 60% (Hasin, Hatzenbuehler, & Waxman, 2006).

Only a few studies have sought to determine a familial influence in the development of substance use disorders other than alcohol. Compton, Thomas, Conway, and Colliver (2005) estimated that 40–60% of variability in the risk of addiction is accounted for by genetic factors (including genetic–environmental interactions). Similarly, a recent population-based twin study of abuse or dependence found that the median heritability estimate was 53% for males and 55% for females, respectively (Kalaydjian & Merikangas, 2008). In addition, a preference for specific types of drugs may occur among family members of drug abusers; MZ twins appear to display a greater similarity than DZ twin pairs in their preference for, and response to, certain types of drugs (Schuckit, 1987).

Examining the genetic link for the abuse of drugs other than alcohol is often far more difficult than for alcohol because individuals must be exposed to the psychoactive substance for the behavioral manifestation of the genetic propensity toward a certain behavior to appear. Most individuals have had exposure to alcohol; this is not the case for many other drugs of abuse (e.g., heroin, cocaine).

Family Environment Influences

Not only do individuals who abuse alcohol and other drugs often develop physiological dependence, they can also develop a strong psychological dependence. Essentially, they become dependent on the drug to help them cope with negative emotional states and stressful social situations. Because substance abuse often leads to significant problems for people across multiple domains of functioning, we must ask, "How is psychological dependence on alcohol or other drugs learned?"

As has been argued by many investigators, the family is an extremely important molding influence for children across a variety of domains. Although the misuse of alcohol and other psychoactive substances by adults often has serious physical, emotional, behavioral, and economic consequences, the ancillary short- and long-term negative effects on those who live with these adults are often no less destructive. In particular, children who live with parents who abuse alcohol and other drugs may be victimized by the deleterious environments these caregivers frequently create. Generally, there is an inverse relationship between parental monitoring and youth behavior problems (Snyder, 2002). However, in comparison to matched controls, alcohol- and drug-abusing parents are less able to monitor their children's behavior (Fals-Stewart, Kelley, Fincham, Golden, & Logsdon, 2004). Robertson, Baird-Thomas, and Stein (2008) found alcohol use disorders were associated with lower levels of parental monitoring, which seemed to impact significantly youth alcohol and marijuana use, hard drug use (e.g., cocaine), sexual risk behavior, and delinquency. Stress and negative affect, which are comparatively high in families with an alcoholic family member, are associated with alcohol use in adolescents (Chassin, Curran, Hussong, & Colder, 1996).

Personality and Psychiatric Factors

Several psychoanalytic explanations for the development and maintenance of alcoholism and drug abuse have been proposed. For example, Wurmser (1984) viewed substance abusers as having overly harsh superegos and proposed that these individuals use alcohol and other drugs to escape intense feelings of anger and fear. Khantzian, Halliday, and McAuliffe (1990) theorized that inadequacies of the ego underlie substance misuse and argued that a person's drug of choice has particular self-medicating properties for his or her particular type of ego deficit. Other psychoanalytic formulations also have been put forth (for a review, see Leeds & Morgenstern, 1995); however, because they are difficult to test scientifically, these models have not been widely accepted in the research community.

A related theory that is often used to explain substance abuse (most often in the popular press) is the idea of an *alcoholic personality*—a type of character organization that predisposes a person to use alcohol rather than some other strategy for coping with emotional and social stress. Some investigators have found that individuals at high risk for developing alcoholism are significantly more impulsive and aggressive than those at low risk for abusing alcohol (Morey, Skinner, & Blashfield, 1984). However, results of studies regarding a predisposition to drinking or other drug use have been mixed, and most alcoholism and drug abuse investigators have largely dismissed the traditional notion of the existence of an alcoholic personality. Yet, there is strong evidence that certain disorders and substance abuse are linked. For example, roughly half of individuals diagnosed with schizophrenia are also either alcohol or drug dependent (Kosten, 1997). The relationship between antisocial personality and substance use is strong (Harford & Parker, 1994; Kwapil, 1996), although the direction of the causal link (if there is one at all) is unclear (Carroll, Ball, & Rounsaville, 1993). Some investigators have suggested that there is a strong relationship between depressive disorders and alcoholism (Kranzler, Del Boca, & Rounsaville, 1997) and that this relationship may be stronger among women than among men (Moscato et al., 1997).

Although the nature of the relationship between substance abuse and other mental disorders is unclear, comorbidity is important to consider in treatment planning. Providing the best possible treatment for substance-abusing clients who have co-occurring psychological disorders requires (a) more cross-disciplinary collaboration, (b) greater integration of substance abuse and mental health treatments, and (c) more comprehensive training to treatment providers in the assessment of and intervention with common co-occurring conditions.

Behavior-Oriented Explanations

Early learning explanations for substance abuse were based on two fundamental assumptions: (1) substance use is a learned behavior, and (2) substance use is reinforced because it reduces anxiety and tension. To test these assumptions, Masserman, Yum, Nicholson, and Lee (1944) induced an experimental neurosis in cats. After the cats were trained to eat food at a food box, they were given an aversive stimulus (e.g., an air blast to the face or an electric shock) whenever they approached the food. In turn, the cats stopped eating and displayed various symptoms, including anxiety, psychophysiological disturbances, and peculiar behaviors. When the cats were given alcohol, however, their symptoms were alleviated and they were able to eat again. Based on these findings, it was concluded that the anxiety-reducing properties of the alcohol are reinforcing and are thus responsible for maintaining drinking behavior.

In general, however, the tension reduction model of substance use is difficult to test, and research with alcoholic participants has produced conflicting findings. Paradoxically, in some individuals, prolonged drinking is associated with increased anxiety and depression (McNamee, Mello, & Mendelson, 1968). Along these lines, if tension reduction alone explained the development of substance use disorders, anyone who finds drugs or alcohol tension reducing would be in danger of becoming a substance abuser. We would expect alcoholism and drug abuse to be far more common than it is because psychoactive substances tend to reduce tension for most people who use them.

Several investigators have concluded that expectancies play a central role in the initiation and maintenance of alcohol and drug use disorders (Marlatt et al., 1998; Mendelson & Mello, 1995; Read & Curtin, 2007). Expectancies of the positive effects of substance use develop from repeated pairings of alcohol or other drugs with their reinforcing effects. Thus, expectancies can be conceptualized as conditioned cognitions, which can themselves be associated with positive experiences, or positive subjective responses, to alcohol or other drugs. Positive expectancies can facilitate more frequent use and thus contribute to the development of dependence (Rotgers, 1996). Expectancy theory has been supported by research. For example, expectancies of social benefit can influence adolescents' decisions to start drinking and predict their consumption of alcohol (Christiansen, Smith, Roehling, & Goldman, 1989) and alcohol-related problems (Moulton, Moulton, Whittington, & Cosio, 2000).

Sociocultural Factors in the Etiology of Substance Abuse

What is ultimately labeled alcoholism or drug addiction varies based on the temporal, geographic, and religious context. In the mid-1800s, the average American consumed roughly 3 times more alcohol than the average person consumes today. Thus, what would be considered alcoholic drinking then would differ substantially from our present-day definition. During the 1600s and much of the 1700s, alcohol was not even seen as an addictive substance, and habitual drunkenness was not, by and large, seen as problematic (Levine, 1978).

Additionally, the effect of cultural attitudes toward drinking is well illustrated by Mormons and Muslims, whose religious values prohibit the use of alcohol. As such, the prevalence of alcoholism, using standard diagnostic systems, is extremely low in these groups. Any drinking is considered problematic use by members of these religious groups. This is not dissimilar from many cultures that consider any use of "hard drugs" (e.g., heroin, cocaine) to be problematic use.

Although alcohol plays a significant role in some Jewish family rituals (Lawson & Lawson, 1998), excessive consumption is viewed as inexcusable behavior. Thus, within the Jewish culture, norms are for frequent drinking of alcohol, but in small amounts. These cultural norms serve to protect Jewish people from developing problems with alcohol (Glassner & Berg, 1980). In general, among cultures where drinking is integrated into religious rites and social customs and where self-control, sociability, and "knowing how to hold one's liquor" are important, alcoholism is rare (Blum & Blum, 1969).

In comparison, the prevalence of alcoholism is high in Europe and those countries that have been highly influenced by European culture (i.e., Argentina, Canada, Chile, Japan, the United States, and New Zealand). Although these countries make up less than 20% of the world's population, they consume 80% of the alcohol (Barry, 1982). In particular, the French have the highest rate of alcoholism in the world (i.e., roughly 15% of the population); France is also marked by the highest per capita alcohol consumption and the highest death rate from cirrhosis of the liver (Alcohol Abuse Essentials, n.d.).

It is also generally accepted that Irish Catholics have a comparatively high rate of alcoholism (Lawson & Lawson, 1998). Vaillant (1983) found that Irish participants in his study on the longitudinal course of alcoholism were more likely to develop alcohol problems than were those from other ethnic groups. Interestingly, Irish participants were also more likely to abstain as a way of controlling drinking. As noted by Vaillant (1983), "It is consistent with Irish culture to view alcohol in terms of black or white, good or evil, drunkenness or complete abstinence" (p. 226). Viewing drinking behavior dichotomously, as either good or sinful, may serve to eliminate models of social drinking. In the Irish culture, there appears to be a shared norm that drinking is an acceptable method to deal with personal distress (Bales, 1980).

Studies have found consistent differences between cultures that generally engage in moderate drinking and those where a disproportionately large percentage of its members appear to have drinking problems (Maloff, Becker, Fonaroff, & Rodin, 1982; Peele & Brodsky, 1996). Cultural groups with comparatively low rates of alcoholism share four characteristics regarding alcohol use. First, drinking is accepted and is governed by social custom; thus, individuals in these cultures learn constructive norms for drinking. Second, differences between "good" and "bad" patterns of drinking are explicitly taught. Third, skills for drinking responsibly are taught. Fourth, drunkenness and misbehavior under the influence of alcohol are disapproved. In cultures where alcohol consumption is more problematic, agreed-on social standards for alcohol use have not been established, so drinkers must rely on an internal standard or their peer group's standards. Drinking is disapproved by members of the culture and, moreover, abstinence is encouraged; thus, norms of social drinking are not available. Finally, people in these cultures expect that alcohol will overpower the individual's capacity for self-management.

Social customs and cultural norms have an enormous influence on substance use. In addition, the behavior that is displayed while under the influence of psychoactive substances also appears to be affected by cultural factors. For example, Lindman and Lang (1994) studied alcohol-related behavior in eight countries and found that although participants generally believed aggression would follow consumption of many alcoholic drinks, there were significant national differences in the expectancy that excessive alcohol consumption leads to aggression. These differences were unrelated to self-reported alcoholic beverage preference, frequency of drinking to intoxication, or rates of personal involvement in episodes of alcohol-related aggression. Thus, the expectation that drinking leads to aggression is determined to a significant extent by contextual factors and cultural traditions related to alcohol use. Previous studies using real and mock alcoholic beverages have shown that individuals who believed they had consumed alcohol began to act more aggressively, regardless of the beverage they had actually consumed (Bushman, 1997).

Thus, how we learn to drink alcohol and consume other drugs is determined largely by the drinking and drug use we observe and by the people with whom we engage in these behaviors. There is a strong interdependence between the drinking and drug use patterns of those who associate with one another regularly in the same social circle. Indeed, in the broadest sense, each individual is linked, to a greater or lesser extent, to all other members of his or her culture. It is within this social fabric that patterns of belief and behaviors about alcohol and other drug use are modeled through a combination of examples, reinforcements, punishments, encouragement, and the many other means that societies use to communicate norms, attitudes, and values (Heath, 1982).

It is important to note that alcohol and drug abuse are not mutually exclusive (Hasin, Stinson, Ogburn, & Grant, 2007). As noted by the National Epidemiological Survey of Alcohol and Related Conditions, 5.6% of adults in the U.S. population reported both alcohol and drug use in the past year. Moreover, findings also revealed that co-use of alcohol and drugs was highest among the 18- to 24-year-old age group.

Treatment

Given that conceptualizations of addiction have varied throughout history, different treatment approaches have predominated based largely on the theoretical model holding sway. At present, the range of treatment possibilities is fairly extensive, varying greatly in terms of philosophy and general treatment goals. Consequently, those seeking help now have a broad variety of choices in their attempts to resolve substance abuse problems.

Pharmacotherapy

Intuitively, a reasonable solution to drug or alcohol addiction is to identify molecules that oppose the actions of these substances. Much scientific effort has been put forth based on this idea, and the results are manifested in the large variety of pharmacotherapies now available to treat addictive behavior. These include medications to reduce cravings to use drugs, to reduce the reinforcing effects of the psychoactive substances, to make taking drugs aversive, and to treat co-occurring mental disorders that may potentially underlie the drinking or drug use (Romach & Sellers, 1998).

Several pharmacotherapies have been developed for the treatment of alcoholism. Disulfiram (Antabuse) produces a sensitivity to alcohol that results in a highly unpleasant reaction when the patient ingests even small amounts of alcohol. Disulfiram blocks the oxidation of alcohol at the acetaldehyde stage. Accumulation of acetaldehyde in the blood produces a complex of highly unpleasant reactions, such as flushing, throbbing in head and neck, throbbing headache, respiratory difficulty, nausea, copious vomiting, sweating, thirst, chest pain, and so forth.

However, the effectiveness of disulfiram has been mixed, particularly if used as the sole intervention. Because it is generally self-administered, the alcoholic client can simply cease taking the disulfiram, wait for the drug to leave his or her system (roughly 2 weeks), and resume drinking. In fact, controlled clinical trials indicate that, unless its administration is supervised (e.g., by a family member or treatment provider), disulfiram does not significantly improve abstinence rates compared to placebo (Hughes & Cook, 1997). In general, patients who seem to respond well to disulfiram treatment are characterized as being older, possessing longer drinking histories, having social stability, and as motivated for recovery (Fuller & Gordis, 2004; Suh, Pettinati, Kampman, & O'Brien, 2006). Given the potential serious adverse response resulting when the medication is combined with alcohol, some have suggested that disulfiram be used only in abstinence-based programs (Arias & Kranzler, 2008).

Another medication used to treat alcoholism is naltrexone, which helps to reduce craving for alcohol by blocking the pleasure-producing effects of ethanol. O'Malley et al. (1996) have shown that use of naltrexone reduced alcohol intake and lowered the incentive to drink for alcoholics compared to those given a placebo. Naltrexone has been most consistently found to be effective in reducing heavy drinking, with less support for reductions in percentage of drinking days or in increasing the likelihood of abstinence (Bouza, Angeles, Munoz, & Amate, 2004; Srisurapanont & Jarusuraisin, 2005). Although some studies have found naltrexone to be ineffective (Krystal, Cramer, Krol, Kirk, & Rosenheck, 2001), the majority of trials to date support its efficacy and safety (Bouza et al., 2004).

Acamprosate has also demonstrated effectiveness in treating alcohol addiction. In a recent meta-analytic review of 17 studies, 6-month continuous abstinence rates were significantly higher for those taking acamprosate compared to a placebo (Mann, Chabac, Lehert, Potgieter, & Henning, 2004). Acamprosate appears to reduce craving for alcohol, but the mechanism underlying acamprosate's action remains unknown, although some evidence suggests that it blocks the glutamate receptor (Harris et al., 2002).

Finally, antidepressant medications have been used to treat alcohol-dependent individuals with co-occurring depression. Mason, Kocsis, Ritvo, and Cutler (1996) reported that tricyclic antidepressants reduced depressive symptoms, and, to a certain extent, drinking behavior. Others have found that selective serotonin reuptake inhibitors, such as fluoxetine (Prozac), reduce the frequency of drinking among alcohol-dependent patients with major depression (Cornelius et al., 1997).

Significant progress also has been made in the pharmacotherapy of opiate addiction. The most effective and commonly used pharmacotherapies for opiate addiction involve the use of agonists (i.e., drugs that occupy and activate the same receptors as opiates). The approach involves administration of drugs with similar action to those of the abuse drug, but with different pharmacotherapeutic effects (e.g., longer acting, less reinforcing, decreased euphoria).

Two widely used agonists, methadone and L-alpha-acetylmethadol (LAAM), have been approved in the United States to treat opiate dependence and are only available through licensed programs that closely monitor the patient's substance use and may also provide psychiatric help as needed (Arias & Kranzler, 2008). Methadone and LAAM reduce the subjective effects of heroin and other opiates through cross-tolerance. The usefulness of these two agonists lies in the fact that they satisfy the craving for heroin or other opiate-based illicit drugs; however, it is important to note that they are equally physiologically addictive. Thus, the advantage of methadone and LAAM over heroin is that methadone and LAAM are administered in a controlled environment as part of treatment. Methadone and LAAM are often combined with other psychosocial treatments to be fully effective (Fals-Stewart, O'Farrell, & Birchler, 2001; McLellan, Arndt, Metzger, Woody, & O'Brien, 1993). LAAM is similar to methadone, but it is administered every 3 days rather than daily. The main difficulty with LAAM, however, is that it takes time to achieve initial stabilization, thus increasing relapse risk (Jaffe, 1995).

Both LAAM and methadone also reduce such concomitant negative behaviors as crime and needle sharing and seem to enable those dependent on opiates to function well enough to maintain employment and other social obligations. Many who are involved in LAAM or methadone maintenance programs are also able to function in their communities and within their families. The quality and dosing of LAAM and methadone is strictly controlled via well-monitored government standards compared to that of street heroin and other illegal opiate-based substances. Yet, the practice of weaning drug abusers from heroin only to addict them to a government-controlled substance is considered by many to be morally and ethically questionable. Moreover,

LAAM and methadone maintenance treatments are often difficult for participants to manage because they may require secrecy from employers, friends, and family members due to concerns about the stigma associated with being maintained on these drugs. It can also be difficult for participants to develop a drug-free social network—a task that many see as a crucial part of successful recovery.

Buprenorphine, an opioid agonist approved in 2002 by the U.S. Food and Drug Administration (FDA) for the treatment of opiate addiction, blocks the subjective effects of heroin and other opiates and has been shown to reduce heroin use and increase compliance with psychosocial treatment (Strain, Stitzer, Liebson, & Bigelow, 1994). Compared to methadone, an advantage of buprenorphine is that it has less abuse potential and overdose risk. In addition, it can be obtained by prescription from a psychiatrist or primary care physician who has completed approved training, rather than through attendance at a specialized methadone clinic (O'Malley & Kosten, 2006).

Naltrexone is another approved treatment for opiate addiction. Naltrexone is a competitive antagonist (i.e., it binds to receptors), but instead of activating these receptors as agonists do, it blocks them. Thus, naltrexone works by preventing receptors from being activated by heroin and other opiates. Yet, unlike its use in alcohol treatment, naltrexone has not been very successful in treating opiate dependence, largely because of poor patient compliance (O'Brien & McLellan, 1996). Naltrexone appears to be effective with individuals highly motivated to quit, particularly those in high-level professional positions (attorneys, physicians, etc.; Meandzija & Kosten, 1994), and as part of other psychosocial treatments that include patient monitoring (Fals-Stewart & O'Farrell, 2003).

Although over 50 different medications have been tried as treatments for cocaine and amphetamine addiction, none are presently FDA approved and none have been demonstrated to be effective (Mendelson & Mello, 1996). No medications are yet available to treat clients suffering from abuse of other drugs, such as cannabis, phencyclidine, and inhalants (Wilkins & Gorelick, 1994).

Psychosocial Interventions

Although medications are an important part of the treatment armamentarium of clinicians working with clients suffering from psychoactive substance use disorders, most experts agree that the mainstay of treatment for addiction is some form of peer support or psychosocial therapy. AA and other 12-step peer support groups (e.g., Narcotics Anonymous, Cocaine Anonymous) are the largest and most widely known self-help support groups for treating those with alcohol and other drug problems. These programs operate primarily as self-help counseling programs in which both person-to-person and group relationships are emphasized. Meetings consist mainly of discussions of participants' problems with alcohol and other drugs, with testimonials from those who have recovered. Participants are encouraged to "work" the 12 steps of AA, which include admitting powerlessness over alcohol, believing a higher power can restore sanity, and developing a searching and fearless moral inventory of oneself (Alcoholics Anonymous, 1976). AA promotes total abstinence from alcohol and drugs. Although widely used, evidence for the effectiveness of AA and the related peer support groups is mostly anecdotal rather than based on well-controlled studies, largely because AA does not endorse participation in research. However, Fiorentine (1999) reported that affiliation with AA after outpatient treatment was associated with better outcomes than non-AA involvement.

A commonly used formal treatment approach derived from AA and the disease model is twelve-step facilitation (TSF). In TSF, substance dependence is viewed not as symptomatic of another illness, but as a primary problem with biological, emotional, and spiritual underpinnings and presenting features. Alcoholism and drug abuse are seen as progressive illnesses, marked largely by denial. The primary goals of treatment are to encourage clients to work through their denial and work the 12 steps of AA. This is typically done in the context of individual and group therapy and involves strong encouragement to attend 12-step self-help groups on a regular basis. Along with individual and group counseling, medical and religious services are also considered important parts of treatment because the disease of alcoholism and other drug use is viewed as affecting the biological and spiritual realms, as well as psychosocial functioning. Despite being the most common form of treatment in the United States, relatively little research has been conducted on the efficacy of TSF as compared to other forms of treatment. In a review of TSF as compared to other psychosocial interventions, Ferri, Amato, and Davoli (2006) found limited support that AA is more effective than alternative treatments.

One of the strongest predictors of success of treatment for alcoholism has been motivation to change. A treatment intervention that has grown out of this observation is motivational enhancement therapy (MET), which attempts to engage clients who are resistant to behavior change and is considered the most acceptable approach for new patients (Arias & Kranzler, 2008). A central technique of MET is motivational interviewing (Gray & Zide, 2006), which is defined as a directive, client-centered therapy style designed to elicit change by assisting clients with exploring and resolving ambivalence. Several studies have now demonstrated that MET is an effective treatment for alcoholism and other drug abuse (Vasilaki, Hosier, & Cox, 2006).

Cognitive and behavioral treatments have been among the most widely used and investigated psychosocial treatments for substance dependence. Cognitive-behavioral therapy (CBT) teaches clients coping skills to reduce or eliminate drinking or substance use. Techniques that characterize CBT include identifying high-risk situations for relapse, instruction and rehearsal strategies for coping with those situations, self-monitoring and behavioral analysis of substance use, strategies for recognizing and coping with cravings, coping with lapses, and instruction on problem solving (Carroll & Onken, 2005).

It has long been maintained by providers and researchers alike that treatment for substance use disorders would be more effective if important patient characteristics were taken into account in selecting treatments (Mattson et al., 1994). This hypothesis was tested in the most comprehensive study of patient–treatment matching for alcoholism, Project MATCH. In this investigation, the efficacy of TSF, MET, and CBT were compared. Overall, the study involved 1,726 participants who were treated in 26 alcohol treatment programs in the United States by 80 different therapists. The investigators evaluated patients on 10 characteristics shown to predict treatment outcome (Project MATCH Group, 1997): diagnosis, cognitive impairment, conceptual ability level, gender, desire to seek meaning in life, motivation, psychiatric severity, severity of alcohol involvement, social support for drinking versus abstinence, and the presence of antisocial personality disorder. The results of the study were somewhat surprising to many in the treatment and research communities—matching the patients to particular treatments did not appear to influence treatment effectiveness. TSF, MET, and CBT were shown to be equally effective across multiple domains of functioning. One conclusion drawn from these findings was that clients who received interventions in competently run programs will do equally well with any of the three treatments (Cooney, Babor, DiClemente, & Del Boca, 2003).

Relapse Prevention

Without question, one of the most vexing problems facing substance abuse treatment providers is relapse. Polich, Armor, and Braiker (1981) found that, over a 4-year posttreatment period, only 7% of their total sample (922 males) abstained from alcohol during the entire follow-up interval. Given that the goal of treatment was abstinence, 7% is a disturbingly low rate of success. Equally disturbing, 54% continued to show alcohol-related problems. Thus, increasing the long-term benefits made during any primary intervention has become a major part of overall treatment planning. A cognitive-behavioral approach to preventing relapse that has been widely used is described in the classic work by Marlatt and Gordon (1985), in which relapse is viewed as a key behavior in substance abuse treatment. The behaviors underlying relapse are seen as indulgent behaviors based on an individual's learning history. When a person is abstinent, he or she gains a greater sense of personal control over the indulgent behaviors. The longer the person stays abstinent, the greater his or her sense of self-efficacy. In this model, relapse is a process that begins with a series of small, seemingly irrelevant decisions, even while maintaining abstinence. These decisions make relapse inevitable. For example, an alcoholic who buys beer to keep in his house to be prepared for visits by friends who drink has made a decision that may ultimately lead to relapse.

Another relapse behavior that is also often observed involves the abstinence violation effect, in which any use of drugs or alcohol is viewed by the substance abuser as complete failure. In many respects, this notion is advocated by a large number of treatment programs and grows from an axiom often heard at AA meetings: "One drink, one drunk." Thus, when a substance user who has been abstinent for an extended period drinks or uses drugs, because the goal of complete abstinence has been violated, the individual's self-efficacy for abstinence plummets, and he or she may assume that a return to regular use of the drug is inevitable and then behave in a way that fulfills this prophecy.

As part of the relapse prevention program, clients are taught to recognize the apparently irrelevant decisions that serve as warning signals of the possibility of relapse. High-risk situations are identified and targeted, and the individuals learn to assess their own vulnerability to relapse. To counter the abstinence violation effect, clients are also taught not to become excessively discouraged if they do relapse. In this respect, clients are taught that relapse is part of the recovery process and are encouraged to develop plans to address relapse when it happens.

Controlled Drinking: A Controversial Outcome

Some interventions for drug and alcohol abuse are based on the hypothesis that some individuals need not give up drinking or drug use, but they can learn to use it moderately (Lang & Kidorf, 1990; Sobell & Sobell, 1995). Several approaches have been used to teach controlled drinking, and some research has suggested that certain alcohol-dependent individuals can control their drinking. For example, self-control training techniques (e.g., behavioral self-control training; BSCT), in which the goal of treatment is to have alcohol-dependent clients reduce their drinking without necessarily abstaining from alcohol, has much appeal for some clients (Harris & Miller, 1990). A computer program is now available that provides instruction on self-control training and has been shown in a well-controlled study to reduce problem drinking (Hester & Delaney, 1997). In general, the best candidates for this type of intervention are young, motivated clients with no biomedical impairment from alcohol abuse (Thombs, 2006).

In the United States, the vast majority of treatment professionals have rejected the idea that substance abusers can control their drinking or drug use and thus insist on a total abstinence approach. However, controlled drinking interventions are less controversial in other parts of the world (e.g., the Netherlands, Australia) and have been used effectively in other countries (Dawe & Richmond, 1997). The debate regarding controlled drinking as an acceptable treatment goal has raged for over 25 years. Some investigators have noted that controlled drinking can be efficacious (Heather, 1995; Kahler, 1995), whereas others have argued that alcohol-dependent individuals cannot maintain control over drinking and, as such, controlled drinking is not an acceptable treatment objective (Glatt, 1995).

Conclusion

Substance use disorders are among the most pressing and intransigent mental health problems facing society today. Concerns about abuse of alcohol, tobacco, and other psychoactive substances date as far back as biblical times: "He shall separate himself from wine and strong drink, and shall drink no vinegar of wine, or vinegar of strong drink, neither shall he drink any liquor of grapes, nor eat moist grapes, or dried" (Num. 6:3). Despite such a long history, scientific scrutiny of these problems is a fairly recent phenomenon. However, a large and evolving body of literature about the epidemiology, etiology, neurobiology, and treatment of addictive behavior has accumulated. These and other aspects of addictive behavior continue to be the focus of extensive clinical and experimental research.

The study of substance use and misuse has been marked by extensive controversy and heated debate. These conflicts have been fueled by a fundamental disagreement among scientists, clinicians, social policymakers, and the public about whether to view addiction as a disease in need of medical treatment, as sin in need of punishment and containment, or as learned behaviors that can be modified by contingencies. The debate has important implications for research, treatment, and social policy. For example, interventions shown to be effective in research settings are often ignored in the treatment community because they are viewed as philosophically opposed to a conventional wisdom about what works best. Unfortunately, the beliefs about what constitutes effective treatment are often not supported by the empirical research. Those who view alcoholism and other drug use as diseases are ethically and, in some instances, morally opposed to the use of controlled use treatments, which they view as irresponsible. Drug users fill our criminal justice system, while treatment providers lament the criminalization of these "diseases." Yet, proponents of legalization of drugs, who are in the minority, note that legalization will help contain many of the social ills associated with substance use. Others see such a stance as irresponsible and immoral because it would increase the exposure of those with a genetic propensity for addiction to the substances that would activate the addictive process. In turn, they believe that such policies would contribute to greater social decay. Because the emotional, legal, and economic stakes in the debate are so high, no end to the debate is in sight.

Acknowledgment

The authors wish to acknowledge William Fals-Stewart for his contributions to earlier versions of this chapter.

References

Alcohol Abuse Essentials. (n.d.). *Alcohol abuse and world statistics*. Retrieved from http://www.alcohol-abuse-essentials.com/Alcohol_Abuse_and_World_Statistics.html

Alcoholics Anonymous. (1976). *Living sober: Some methods A.A. members have used for not drinking*. New York: Alcoholics Anonymous World Services.

Amadio, D. M., Adam, T., & Buletza, K. (2008). Gender differences in alcohol use and alcohol-related problems: Do they hold for lesbians and gay men? *Journal of Gay and Lesbian Social Services, 20*, 315–327.

Amaro, H., & Hardy-Fosta, C. (1995). Gender relations in addiction and recovery. *Journal of Psychoactive Drugs, 27*, 325–333.

American Psychiatric Association. (2000). *Diagnostic and statistical manual of mental disorders* (4th ed., text rev.). Washington, DC: Author.

American Psychiatric Association DSM-5 Development. (2010). *Substance-related disorders*. Retrieved from http://www.dsm5.org/proposedrevisions/pages/substance-relateddisorders.aspx

Arias, A. J., & Kranzler, H. R. (2008). Treatment of co-occurring alcohol and other drug use disorders. *Alcohol, Research, and Health, 31*, 155–167.

Babor, T. F., Higgins-Biddle, J. C., Saunders, J. B., & Monteiro, M. G. (2001). *The alcohol use disorders identification test: Guidelines for use in primary health care* (2nd ed.). WHO/MSD/MSB/01.6a. Retrieved from http://whqlibdoc.who.int/hq/2001/who_msd_msb_01.6a.pdf

Bales, F. (1980). Cultural differences in roles of alcoholism. In D. Ward (Ed.), *Alcoholism: Introduction to theory and treatment* (pp.). Dubuque, IA: Kendall/Hunt.

Barry, H. III. (1982). Cultural variations in alcohol abuse. In I. Al-Issa (Ed.), *Culture and psychopathology* (pp. 309–338). Baltimore: University Park Press.

Beckman, L. J., & Amaro, H. (1986). Personal and social difficulties faced by women and men entering alcoholism treatment. *Journal of Studies on Alcohol, 47,* 135–145.

Blum, R. H., & Blum, E. M. (1969). A cultural case study. In R. H. Blum (Ed.), *Drugs I: Society and drugs* (pp. 226–227). San Francisco: Jossey-Bass.

Blume, S. B. (1991). Sexuality and stigma: The alcoholic woman. *Alcohol Health and Research World, 15*(2), 139–146.

Blume, S. B. (1997). Women and alcohol: Issues in social policy. In R. Wilsnack & S. Wilsnack (Eds.), *Gender and alcohol: Individual and social perspectives* (pp. 462–489). New Brunswick, NJ: Rutgers Center of Alcohol Studies.

Blume, S. B. (1998). Addictive disorders in women. In R. J. Frances & S. I. Miller (Eds.), *Clinical textbook of addictive disorders* (2nd ed., pp. 413–429). New York: Guilford.

Boris, N. W. (2009). Parental substance abuse. In C. H. Zeanah, Jr. (Ed.), *Handbook of infant health* (3rd ed., pp. 171–179). New York: Guilford.

Bouza, C., Angeles, M., Munoz, A., & Amate, J. M. (2004). Efficacy and safety of naltrexone and acamprosate in the treatment of alcohol dependence: A systematic review. *Addiction, 99,* 811–828.

Brady, T. M., & Ashley, O. S. (2005). *Women in substance abuse treatment: Results from the Alcohol and Drug Services Study (ADSS).* (DHHS Publication No. SMA 04-3968, Analytic Series A-26). Rockville, MD: Substance Abuse and Mental Health Services Administration, Office of Applied Studies.

Brady, K. T., & Randall, C. L. (1999). Gender differences in substance use disorders. *Psychiatric Clinics of North America, 22,* 241–252.

Brandsma, J. M., & Pattison, E. M. (1982). Homosexuality and alcohol. In J. M. Pattison & E. Kaufman (Eds.), *Encyclopedia handbook of alcoholism* (pp. 736–741). New York: Gardner.

Bushman, B. J. (1997). Effects of alcohol on human aggression: Validity of proposed explanations. In M. Galanter (Ed.), *Recent developments in alcoholism* (pp. 227–243). New York: Plenum.

Carlson, R. G. (2006). Ethnography and applied substance misuse research: Anthropologic and cross-cultural factors. In K. M. Carroll & W. R. Miller (Eds.), *Rethinking substance abuse: What the science shows, and what we should do about it* (pp. 201–222). New York: Guilford.

Carroll, K. M., Ball, S. A., & Rounsaville, B. J. (1993). A comparison of alternate systems for diagnosing antisocial personality disorder in cocaine abusers. *Journal of Nervous and Mental Diseases, 181,* 436–443.

Carroll, K. M., & Miller, W. R. (2006). Defining and addressing the problem. In K. M. Carroll & W. R. Miller (Eds.), *Rethinking substance abuse: What the science shows, and what we should do about it* (pp. 3–7). New York: Guilford.

Carroll, K. M., & Onken, L. S. (2005). Behavioral therapies for drug abuse. *American Journal of Psychiatry, 162*(8), 1452–1460.

Centers for Disease Control and Prevention. (n.d.). Syndemics Prevention Network. *Definitions.* Retrieved from http://www.cdc.gov/syndemics/definition.htm

Center on Addiction and Substance Abuse. (1996). *Substance abuse and American women.* New York: Author.

Chassin, L., Curran, P. J., Hussong, A. M., & Colder, C. R. (1996). The relation of parent alcoholism to adolescent substance use: A longitudinal follow-up. *Journal of Abnormal Psychology, 105*(1), 70–80.

Christiansen, B. A., Smith, G. T., Roehling, P. V., & Goldman, M. S. (1989). Using alcohol expectancies to predict adolescent drinking behavior after one year. *Journal of Consulting and Clinical Psychology, 57,* 93–99.

Compton, W. M., Thomas, Y. F., Conway, K. P., & Colliver, J. D. (2005). Developments in the epidemiology of drug use and drug use disorders. *American Journal of Psychiatry, 162,* 1494–1502.

Cooney, N. L., Babor, T. F., DiClemente, C. C., & Del Boca, F. K. (2003). Clinical and scientific implications of Project MATCH. In T. F. Babor & F. K. Del Boca (Eds.), *Treatment matching in alcoholism* (pp. 222–237). New York: Cambridge University Press.

Cornelius, J. R., Salloum, I. M., Ehler, J. G., Jarrett, P. J., Cornelius, M. D., Perel, J. M., … Black, A. (1997). Fluoxetine in depressed alcoholics: A double-blind placebo-controlled trial. *Archives of General Psychiatry, 54,* 700–705.

Cruz, M. T., Bajo, M., Schweitzer, P., & Roberto, M. (2008). Shared mechanisms of alcohol and other drugs. *Alcohol, Research, and Health, 31,* 137–147.

Dahlgren, L., & Willander, A. (1989). Are special treatment facilities for female alcoholics needed? A controlled 2-year follow-up study from a specialized female unit (EWA) versus a mixed male/female treatment facility. *Alcoholism: Clinical and Experimental Research, 13*, 499–504.

Dawe, S., & Richmond, R. (1997). Controlled drinking as a treatment goal in Australian alcohol treatment agencies. *Journal of Substance Abuse, 14*, 81–86.

Dawson, D. A., Grant, B. F., Stinson, F. S., & Chou, P. S. (2006). Estimating the effect of help-seeking on achieving recovery from alcohol dependence. *Addiction, 101*, 824–834.

Degenhardt, L., Chiu, W.-T., Sampson, N., Kessler, R. C., Anthony, J. C., de Girolamo, G, … Wells, J. E. (2008). Toward a global view of alcohol, tobacco, cannabis, and cocaine use: Findings from the WHO World Mental Health Surveys. *PLoS Med, 5*(7), e141.

Deschenes, E. P., Anglin, M. D., & Speckart, G. (1991). Narcotics addiction: Related criminal careers, social and economic costs. *Journal of Drug Issues, 21*, 383–411.

Dick, D. D., & Agrawal, A. (2008). The genetics of alcohol and other drug dependence. *Alcohol, Research, and Health, 2*, 111–117.

Fals-Stewart, W., Kelley, M. L., Fincham, F. D., Golden, J., & Logsdon, T. (2004). Emotional and behavioral problems of children living with drug-abusing fathers: Comparison with children living with alcoholic fathers and nonsubstance-abusing fathers. *Journal of Family Psychology, 18*, 319–330.

Fals-Stewart, W., & O'Farrell, T. J. (2003). Behavioral family counseling and naltrexone for male opioid–dependent patients. *Journal of Consulting and Clinical Psychology, 71*, 432–442.

Fals-Stewart, W., O'Farrell, T. J., & Birchler, G. R. (2001). Behavioral couples therapy for male methadone maintenance patients: Effects on drug-using behavior and relationship adjustment. *Behavior Therapy, 32*, 391–411.

Fiorentine, R. (1999). After drug treatment: Are 12-step programs effective in maintaining abstinence? *American Journal of Drug and Alcohol Abuse, 25*(1), 93–116.

Ferri, M., Amato, L., & Davoli, M. (2006). Alcoholics Anonymous and other 12-step programmes for alcohol dependence. Cochrane Database of Systematic Reviews, Issue 3. Art.No.: CD005032. DOI: 10.1002/14651858.CD005032.pub2.

Feuer, C. A., Nishith, P., & Resick, P. (2005). Prediction of numbing and effortful avoidance in female rape survivors with chronic PTSD. *Journal of Traumatic Stress, 18*, 165–170.

Fuller, R. K., & Gordis, E. (2004). Does disulfiram have a role in alcohol treatment today? *Addiction, 99*, 21–24.

Gilman, S. E., Cochran, S. D., Mays, V., Hughes, M., Ostrow, D., & Kessler, R. C. (2001). Risk of psychiatric disorders among individuals reporting same-sex sexual partners in the National Comorbidity Survey. *American Journal of Public Health, 91*, 933–939.

Glassner, B., & Berg, B. (1980). How Jews avoid drinking problems. *American Sociological Review, 45*, 647–664.

Glatt, M. M. (1995). Controlled drinking after a third of a century. *Addiction, 90*, 1157–1160.

Gough, J. B. (1881). *Sunlight and shadow*. Hartford, CT: Worthington.

Grant, B. F., & Dawson, D. A. (1999). Alcohol and drug use, abuse, and dependence: Classification, prevalence, and comorbidity. In B. S. McCrady & E. E. Epstein (Eds.), *Addiction: A comprehensive textbook* (pp. 9–29). New York: Oxford University Press.

Grant, B. F., Dawson, D. A., Stinson, F. S., Chou, S. P., Dufour, M. C., & Pickering, R. P. (2006). The 12-month prevalence and trends in DSM-IV alcohol abuse and dependence. *Alcohol, Research, and Health, 29*, 79–91.

Grant, B. F., Stinson, F. S., Dawson, D. A., Chou, S. P., Ruan, W. J., & Pickering, R. P. (2005). Co-occurrence of 12-month alcohol and drug use disorders and personality disorders in the United States: Results from the National Epidemiologic Survey on Alcohol and Related Conditions. *Archives of General Psychiatry.39*,1–9.

Gray, S. W., & Zide, M. R. (2006). *Psychopathology: A competency-based treatment model for social workers*. Belmont, CA: Thomson.

Grella, C. E., Scott, C. K., Foss, M. A., Joshi, V., & Hser, Y. I. (2003). Gender differences in drug treatment outcomes among participants in the Chicago Target Cities Study. *Evaluation and Program Planning, 26*, 297–310.

Harford, T. C., & Parker, D. A. (1994). Antisocial behavior, family history, and alcohol dependence symptoms. *Alcoholism, 18*, 265–268.

Harris, K. B., & Miller, W. R. (1990). Behavioral self-control training for problem drinkers: Components of efficacy. *Psychology of Addictive Behaviors, 4*, 82–90.

Harris, B. R., Prendergast, M. A., Gibson, D. A., Rogers, D. T., Blanchard, J. A., Holley, R. C., ... Littleton, J. M. (2002). Acamprosate inhibits the binding and neurotoxic effects of trans-ACPD, suggesting a novel site of action at metabotropic glutamate receptors. *Alcoholism: Clinical and Experimental Research, 26,* 1779–1793.

Harwood, H. J., Hubbard, R. L., Collins, J. J., & Rachal, J. V. (1988). The costs of crime and the benefits of drug abuse treatment: A cost-benefit analysis using TOPS data. In C. G. Luekefeld & F. M. Tims (Eds.), *Compulsory treatment of drug abuse: Research and clinical practice* (Research Monograph Series 86, pp. 209–235). Rockville, MD: National Institute on Drug Abuse.

Hasin, D., Hatzenbuehler, M., & Waxman, R. (2006). Genetics of substance use disorders. In K. M. Carroll & W. R. Miller (Eds.), *Rethinking substance abuse: What the science shows, and what we should do about it* (pp. 61–80). New York: Guilford.

Hasin, D. S., Stinson, F. S., Ogburn, E., & Grant, B. F. (2007). Prevalence, correlates, disability and co-morbidity of DSM-IV alcohol abuse and dependence in the United States: Results from the National Epidemiologic Survey on Alcohol and Related Conditions. Survey on alcohol and related conditions. *Archives of General Psychiatry, 64,* 830–842.

Haynes, V. D. (2002, August 9). Nevada blazes trail for legal marijuana. *Chicago Tribune, 1,* 14.

Heath, A. C., Todorov, A. A., Nelson, E. C., Madden, P. A., Bucholz, K. K., & Martin, N. G. (2002). Gene environment interaction effects on behavioral variation and risk of complex disorders: The example of alcoholism and other psychiatric disorders. *Twin Research, 5*(1), 30–37.

Heath, D. B. (1982). Sociocultural variants in alcoholism. In E. M. Pattison & E. Kaufman (Eds.), *Encyclopedic handbook of alcoholism* (pp. 426–440). New York: Gardner.

Heather, J. (1995). The great controlled drinking consensus. Is it premature? *Addiction, 90,* 1160–1163.

Hester, R. K., & Delaney, H. D. (1997). Behavioral self-control program for Windows: Results of a controlled clinical trial. *Journal of Consulting and Clinical Psychology, 65,* 686–693.

Hughes, J. C., & Cook, C. C. (1997). The efficacy of disulfiram: A review of outcome studies. *Addiction, 92,* 381–395.

Hughes, T. L., Wilsnack, S. C., Szalacha, L. A., Johnson, T., Bostwick, W. B., Seymour, R., ... Kinnison, K. E. (2006). Age and racial/ethnic differences in drinking and drinking-related problems in a community sample of lesbians. *Journal of Studies on Alcohol, 67,* 579–590.

Institute of Medicine. (1990). *Treating drug problems.* Washington, DC: National Academy Press.

Jaffe, J. H. (1995). Pharmacological treatment of opioid dependence: Current techniques and new findings. *Psychiatric Annals, 25,* 369–375.

Jellinek, E. M. (1952). Phases of alcohol addiction. *Quarterly Journal of Studies on Alcohol, 13,* 673–684.

Kahler, C. W. (1995). Current challenges and an old debate. *Addiction, 90,* 1169–1171.

Kalaydjian, A., & Merikangas, K. (2008). Physical and mental comorbidity of headache in a nationally representative sample of US adults. *Psychosomatic Medicine, 70,* 773–780.

Kaysen, D., Dillworth, T. M., Simpson, T., Waldrop, A., Larimer, M. E., & Resick P. A. (2007). Domestic violence and alcohol use: Trauma-related symptoms and motives for drinking. *Addictive Behaviors, 32,* 1272–1283.

Khantzian, E. J., Halliday, K. S., & McAuliffe, W. E. (1990). *Addiction and the vulnerable self: Modified dynamic group therapy for substance abusers.* New York: Guilford.

Kosten, T. R. (1997). Substance abuse and schizophrenia. *Schizophrenia Bulletin, 23,* 181–186.

Koob, G. F., & Bloom, F. E. (1988). Cellular and molecular mechanisms of drug dependence. *Science, 242,* 715–723.

Kranzler, H. R., & Li, T. (2010). *What is addiction?* National Institute on Alcohol Abuse and Alcoholism. Retrieved from http://pubs.niaaa.nih.gov/publications/arh312/93-95.htm

Kranzler, H. R., Del Boca, F. K., & Rounsaville, B. (1997). Comorbid psychiatric diagnosis predicts three-year outcomes in alcoholics: A posttreatment natural history study. *Journal of Studies on Alcohol, 57,* 619–626.

Krystal, J. H., Cramer, J. A., Krol, W. F., Kirk, G. F., & Rosenheck, R. A. (2001). Naltrexone in the treatment of alcohol dependence. *New England Journal of Medicine, 345,* 1734–1739.

Kubicka, L., Csemy, L., & Kozeny, J. (1995). Prague women's drinking before and after the "velvet revolution" of 1989: A longitudinal study. *Addiction, 90,* 1471–1478.

Kuhn, T. (1962). *The structure of scientific revolutions.* Chicago: University of Chicago Press.

Kwapil, T. R. (1996). A longitudinal study of drug and alcohol use by psychosis-prone and impulsive-non-conforming individuals. *Journal of Abnormal Psychology, 105*(1), 114–123.

Lang, A. R., & Kidorf, M. (1990). Problem drinking: Cognitive behavioral strategies for self control. In M. E. Thase, B. A. Edelstein, & M. Hersen (Eds.), *Handbook of outpatient treatment of adults* (pp. 413–442). New York: Plenum.

Langenbucher, J. (1994). Offsets are not add-ons: The place of addictions treatment in American health care reform. *Journal of Substance Abuse, 6,* 117–122.

Lawson, A., & Lawson, G. (1998). *Alcoholism and the family: A guide to treatment and prevention* (2nd ed.). Gaithersburg, MD: Aspen.

Leeds, J., & Morgenstern, J. (1995). Psychoanalytic theories of substance abuse. In F. Rotgers, D. S. Keller, & J. Morgenstern (Eds.), *Treating substance abuse: Theory and technique* (pp. 68–83). New York: Guilford.

Levine, H. G. (1978). The discovery of addiction: Changing conceptions of habitual drunkenness in America. *Journal of Studies on Alcohol, 39,* 143–174.

Lewis, R. J., Derlega, V. J., Berndt, A., Morris, L. M., & Rose, S. (2001). An empirical analysis of stressors for gay men and lesbians. *Journal of Homosexuality, 42,* 63–88.

Lindman, R. E., & Lang, A. R. (1994). The alcohol-aggression stereotype: A cross-cultural comparison of beliefs. *International Journal of Addictions, 29,* 1–13.

Maloff, D., Becker, H. S., Fonaroff, A., & Rodin, J. (1982). Informal social controls and their influence on substance use. In N. E. Zinberg & W. M. Harding (Eds.), *Control over intoxicant use* (pp. 53–76). New York: Human Sciences Press.

Mann, K., Chabac, S., Lehert, P., Potgieter, A., & Henning, S. (2004, December). *Acamprosate improves treatment outcome in alcoholics: A polled analysis of 11 randomized placebo controlled trials in 3338 patients.* Poster presented at the annual conference of the American College of Neuropsychopharmacology, Puerto Rico.

Marlatt, G. A., Baer, J. S., Kivahan, D. R., Dimeoff, L. A., Larimer, M. E., Quigley, L. A., … Williams, E. (1998). Screening and brief intervention for high-risk college student drinkers: Results from a 2-year follow up assessment. *Journal of Consulting and Clinical Psychology, 66,* 604–615.

Marlatt, G. A., & Gordon, J. R. (1985). *Relapse prevention: Maintenance strategies in the treatment of addictive behaviors.* New York: Guilford.

Marlatt, G. A., Tucker, J. A., Donovan, D. M., & Vuchinich, R. E. (1997). Help-seeking by substance abusers: The role of harm reduction and behavioral-economic approaches to facilitate treatment entry and retention. In L. S. Onken, J. D. Blaine, & J. J. Boren (Eds.), *Beyond the therapeutic alliance: Keeping the drug-dependent individual in treatment* (pp. 44–84). Rockville, MD: National Institute on Drug Abuse.

Marshal, M. P., Friedman, M. S., Stall, R., & Thompson, A. L. (2009). Individual trajectories of substance use in lesbian, gay, and bisexual youth and heterosexual youth. *Addiction, 104,* 974–981.

Mason, B. J., Kocsis, J. H., Ritvo, E. C., & Cutler, R. B. (1996). A double-blind placebo-controlled trial of desipramine in primary alcoholics stratified on the presence or absence of major depression. *Journal of the American Medical Association, 275,* 1–7.

Masserman, J., Yum, K., Nicholson, J., & Lee, S. (1944). Neurosis and alcohol: An experimental study. *American Journal of Psychiatry, 101,* 389–395.

Mattson, M. E., Allen, J. P., Longabaugh, R., Nickless, C. J., Connors, G. J., & Kadden, R. M. (1994). A chronological review of empirical studies matching alcoholic clients to treatment. *Journal of Studies on Alcohol, 12,* 16–29.

McCabe, S. E., Hughes, T. L., Bostwick, W. B., West, B. T., & Boyd, C. J. (2009). Sexual orientation, substance use behaviors, and substance use dependence in America. *Addiction, 104,* 1333–1345.

McClelland, G. M., & Teplin, L. A. (2001). Alcohol intoxication and violent crime: Implications for public health policy. *American Journal for Addictions, 10*(Suppl.), 70–85.

McCrady, B. S., & Epstein, E. E. (1999). Introduction. In B. S. McCrady & E. E. Epstein (Eds.), *Addiction: A comprehensive textbook* (pp. 3–8). New York: Oxford University Press.

McFarlane, J., Maleha, A., Gist, J., Watson, K., Batten, E., Hall, I., & Smith, S. (2005). Intimate partner sexual assault against women and associated victim substance use, suicidality, and risk factors for femicide. *Issues in Mental Health Nursing, 26,* 953–967.

McKirnan, D. J., & Peterson, P. L. (1989). Alcohol and drug use among homosexual men and women: Epidemiology and population characteristics. *Addictive Behaviors, 14,* 545–553.

McLellan, A. T., Arndt, I. O., Metzger, D. S., Woody, G. E., & O'Brien, C. P. (1993). The effects of psycho-social services in substance abuse treatment. *Journal of the American Medical Association, 260,* 1953–1959.

McNamee, H. B., Mello, N. K., & Mendelson, J. H. (1968). Experimental analysis of drinking patterns of alcoholics: Concurrent psychiatric observations. *American Journal of Psychiatry, 124,* 1063–1069.

Meandzija, B., & Kosten, T. R. (1994). Pharmacologic therapies for opioid addiction. In N. S. Miller (Ed.), *Principles of addiction medicine* (sect. XII, chap. 4, pp. 1–5). Chevy Chase, MD: American Society of Addiction Medicine.

Mendelson, J. H., & Mello, N. K. (1995). Alcohol, sex, and aggression. In J. A. Inciardi & K. McElrath (Eds.), *The American drug scene: An anthology* (pp. 50–56). Los Angeles: Roxbury.

Mendelson, J. H., & Mello, N. K. (1996). Management of cocaine abuse and dependence. *New England Journal of Medicine, 334,* 965–972.

Merikangas, K. R., Stolar, M., Stevens, D. E., Goulet, J., Preisig, M. A., Fenton, B., … Rounsaville, B. J. (1998). Familial transmission of substance use disorders. *Archives of General Psychiatry, 55,* 973–979.

Meyer, I. H. (2003). Prejudice, social stress, and mental health in lesbian, gay, and bisexual populations: Conceptual issues and research evidence. *Psychological Bulletin, 129,* 674–697.

Mignone, T., Klostermann, K., & Chen, R. (2009). The relationship between relapse to alcohol and relapse to violence. *Journal of Family Violence, 24,* 497–506.

Miller, N. S. (1995). *Addiction psychiatry: Current diagnosis and treatment.* New York: Wiley.

Mokdad, A. H., Marks, J. S., Stroup, D. S., & Gerberding, G. L. (2004). Actual causes of death in the United States, 2000. *Journal of the American Medical Association, 291,* 1238–1245.

Morey, L. C., Skinner, H. A., & Blashfield, R. K. (1984). A typology of alcohol abusers: Correlates and implications. *Journal of Abnormal Psychology, 93,* 403–417.

Moscato, B. S., Russell, M., Zielezny, M., Bromet, E., Egri, G., Mudar, P., & Marshall, J. R. (1997). Gender differences in the relation between depressive symptoms and alcohol problems: A longitudinal perspective. *American Journal of Epidemiology, 146,* 966–974.

Moulton, M., Moulton, P., Whittington, A. N., & Cosio, D. (2000). The relationship between negative consequence drinking, gender, athletic participation, and social expectancies among adolescents. *Journal of Alcohol and Drug Education, 45*(2), 12–22.

Nelson-Zlupko, L., Dore, M. M., Kauffman, E., & Kaltenbach, K. (1996). Women in recovery: Their perceptions of treatment effectiveness. *Journal of Substance Abuse Treatment, 13,* 51–59.

Nurnberger, J. I. Jr., Wiegand, R., Bucholz, K., O'Connor, S., Meyer, E. T., Reich, T., … Porjesc, B. (2004). A family study of alcohol dependence: Coaggregation of multiple disorders in relatives of alcohol-dependent probands. *Archives of General Psychiatry, 61,* 1246–1256.

O'Brien, C. P., & McLellan, A. T. (1996). Myths about the treatment of addiction. *Lancet, 347,* 237–240.

O'Brien, C. P., Volkow, N., & Li, T. K. (2006). Addiction versus dependence for DSM-V. *American Journal of Psychiatry, 163,* 764–775.

Office of Applied Studies. (2009). *Results from the 2008 National Survey of Drug Use and Health: National findings.* Rockville, MD: Substance Abuse Services and Mental Health Services Administration.

Office of National Drug Control Policy. (2004). *The economic costs of drug abuse in the United States: 1992– 2002.* Washington, DC: Executive Office of the President.

O'Malley, S. S., Jaffe, A. J., Chang, G., Rode, S., Schottenfeld, R., Meyer, R. E., & Rounsaville, B. (1996). Six month follow-up of naltrexone and psychotherapy for alcohol dependence. *Archives of General Psychiatry, 53,* 217–224.

O'Malley, S. S., & Kosten, T. R. (2006). Pharmacotherapy of addictive disorders. In K. M. Carroll & W. R. Miller (Eds.), *Rethinking substance abuse: What the science shows, and what we should do about it* (pp. 240–256). New York: Guilford.

Orenstein, A. (2001). Substance use among gay and lesbian adolescents. *Journal of Homosexuality, 41,* 1–15.

Osborne, C., & Berger, L. M. (2009). Parental substance abuse and child well-being: A consideration of parents' gender and coresidence. *Journal of Family Issues, 30,* 341–370.

Parson, J. T., Kelly, B. C., & Wells, B. E. (2006). Difference in club drug use between heterosexual and lesbian/bisexual females. *Addictive Behavior, 12,* 2344–2349.

Peele, S. (1996). Assumptions about drugs and the marketing of drug policies. In W. K. Bickel & R. J. DeGrandpre (Eds.), *Drug policy and human nature: Psychological perspectives on the prevention, management, and treatment of illicit drug abuse* (pp. 199–220). New York: Plenum.

Peele, S., & Brodsky, A. (1996). The antidote to alcohol abuse: Sensible drinking messages. In S. Peele (Ed.), *Wine in context: Nutrition, physiology, and policy* (pp. 66–70). Davis, CA: American Society for Enology and Viticulture.

Peele, S., Brodsky, A., & Arnold, M. (1991). *The truth about addiction and recovery.* New York: Simon and Schuster.

Plotnick, R. D. (1994). Applying benefit-cost to substance use prevention programs. *International Journal of the Addictions, 29,* 339–359.

Polich, J. M., Armor, D. J., & Braiker, H. B. (1981). *The course of alcoholism: Four years after treatment.* New York: Wiley Interscience.

Project MATCH Group. (1997). Project MATCH: Rationale and methods for a multisite clinical trial matching patients to alcoholism treatment. *Alcoholism: Clinical and Experimental Research, 17,* 1130–1145.

Ramlow, B. E., White, A. L., Watson, M. A., & Luekefeld, C. G. (1997). The needs of women with substance use problems: An expanded vision for treatment. *Substance Use and Misuse, 32,* 1395–1404.

Read, J. P., & Curtin, J. J. (2007). Contextual influences on alcohol expectancy processes. *Journal of Studies on Alcohol and Drugs, 68*(5), 759–770.

Richardson, D., & Campbell, J. (1982). The effect of alcohol on attributions of blame for rape. *Personality and Social Psychology Bulletin, 8*, 468–476.

Roberts, A. C., & Nishimoto, R. H. (1996). Predicting treatment retention of women dependent on cocaine. *American Journal of Drug and Alcohol Abuse, 22*, 313–333.

Robertson, A. A., Baird-Thomas, C., & Stein, J. A. (2008). Child victimization and parental monitoring as mediators of youth problem behaviors. *Criminal Justice and Behavior, 35*, 755–771.

Romach, M. K., & Sellers, E. M. (1998). Alcohol dependency: Women, biology, and pharmacotherapy. In E. F. McCance-Katz & T. R. Kosten (Eds.), *New treatments for chemical addictions* (pp. 35–73). Washington, DC: American Psychiatric Press.

Rotgers, F. (1996). Behavioral theory of substance abuse treatment: Bringing science to bear on practice. In F. Rotgers & J. Morgenstern (Eds.), *Treating substance abuse: Theory and technique* (pp. 174–201). New York: Guilford.

Sandbak, T., Murison, R., Sarviharju, M., & Hyytiae, P. (1998). Defensive burying and stress gastricerosions in alcohol-preferring AA and alcohol-avoiding ANA rats. *Alcoholism: Clinical and Experimental Research, 22*, 2050–2054.

Schober, R., & Annis, H. M. (1996). Barriers to help-seeking for change in drinking: A gender-focused review of the literature. *Addictive Behaviors, 21*, 81–92.

Schuckit, M. A. (1987). Biological vulnerability to alcoholism. *Journal of Consulting and Clinical Psychology, 55*, 301–310.

Selzer, M. L. (1971). The Michigan Alcoholism Screening Test: The quest for a new diagnostic instrument. *American Journal of Psychiatry, 127*, 1653–1658.

Shaffer, H. J., & Neuhaus, C. Jr. (1985). Testing hypotheses: An approach for the assessment of addictive behaviors. In H. B. Milkman & H. J. Shaffer (Eds.), *The addictions: Multidisciplinary perspectives and treatments* (pp. 87–103). Lexington, MA: Lexington.

Snyder, J. (2002). Reinforcement and coercion mechanisms in the development of antisocial behavior: Peer processes. In J. R. Reid, G. R. Patterson, & J. Snyder (Eds.), *Antisocial behavior: Prevention, intervention, and basic research* (pp.). Washington, DC: APA Press.

Sobell, M. B., & Sobell, L. C. (1995). Controlled drinking after 25 years: How important was the great debate? *Addiction, 90*, 1149–1153.

Srisurapanont, M., & Jarusuraisin, N. (2005). Opioid antagonists for alcohol dependence. *Cochrane Database of Systematic Reviews, 1*, CD001867.

Stewart, D., Gossop, M., & Trakada, K. (2007). Drug dependent parents: Childcare responsibilities, involvement with treatment services, and treatment outcomes. *Addictive Behaviors, 32*, 1657–1668.

Stormo, K. J., Lang, A. R., & Stritzke, W. G. (1997). Attributions about acquaintance rape: The role of alcohol and individual differences. *Journal of Applied Social Psychology, 27*(4), 279–305.

Strain, E. C., Stitzer, M. L., Liebson, I. A., & Bigelow, G. E. (1994). Comparison of buprenorphine and methadone in the treatment of opioid dependence. *American Journal of Psychiatry, 151*, 1025–1030.

Straussner, S. L. A., & Zelvin, E. (1997). *Gender and addiction: Men and women in treatment.* Northvale, NJ: Aronson.

Substance Abuse and Mental Health Services Administration. (2009). Office of Applied Studies. (2009). *Results from the 2008 National Survey of Drug Use and Health: National Findings. Rockville*, MD: Substance Abuse Services and Mental Health Services Administration.

Suh, J. J., Pettinati, H. M., Kampman, K. M., & O'Brien, C. P. (2006). The status of disulfiram: A half of a century later. *Journal of Clinical Psychopharmacology, 26*, 290–302.

Sun, A. (2007). Relapse among substance-abusing women: Components and processes. *Substance Use and Misuse, 42*, 1–21.

Thombs, D. L. (2006). *Introduction to addictive behavior* (3rd ed.). New York: Guilford.

Vaillant, G. E. (1983). *The natural history of alcoholism.* Cambridge, MA: Harvard University Press.

Vaillant, G. E. (1990). We should retain the disease concept of alcoholism. *Harvard Medical School Mental Health Letter, 6*, 4–6.

Vaillant, G. E. (1995). *The natural history of alcoholism revisited.* Cambridge, MA: Harvard University Press.

Vasilaki, E. I., Hosier, S. G., & Cox, W. M. (2006). The efficacy of motivational interviewing as a brief intervention for excessive drinking: A meta-analytic review. *Alcohol and Alcoholism, 41*(3), 332–335.

Volkow, N. D., Fowler, J. S., & Wang, G. J. (2003). The addicted human brain: Insights from imaging studies. *Journal of Clinical Investigation, 111*, 1444–1451.

Wightman, R. M., & Robinson, D. L. (2002). Transient changes in mesolimbic dopamine and their association with "reward." *Journal of Neurochemistry, 82,* 721–735.

Wilkins, J. N., & Gorelick, D. A. (1994). Pharmacologic therapies for other drugs and multiple drug addiction. In N. S. Miller (Ed.), *Principles of addiction medicine* (sect. XII, chap. 6, pp. 1–6). Chevy Chase, MD: American Society of Addiction Medicine.

Wilsnack, S. C., Hughes, T. L., & Johnson, T. P. (2008). Drinking and drinking-related problems among heterosexual and sexual minority women. *Journal of Studies on Alcohol and Drugs, 69,* 129–139.

Wilsnack, S. C., & Wilsnack, R. W. (2002). International gender and alcohol research: Recent findings and future directions. *Alcohol, Research, and Health, 26,* 245–250.

Winfield, I., George, L. K., Swartz, M., & Blazer, D. G. (1990). Sexual assault and psychiatric disorders among a community sample of women. *American Journal of Psychiatry, 147,* 335–341.

Wise, R. A. (2002). Brain reward circuitry: Insights from unsensed incentives. *Neuron, 36,* 229–240.

World Health Organization. (1992). *ICD-10 classification of mental and behavioural disorders: Clinical descriptions and diagnostic guidelines.* Geneva: Author.

World Health Organization. (2010). Management of substance abuse: Facts and figures. Retrieved from http://www.who.int/substance_abuse/facts/en/index.html

Wurmser, L. (1984). The role of superego conflicts in substance abuse and their treatment. *International Journal of Psychoanalytic Psychotherapy, 10,* 227–258.

15

Mental Health and Aging

AMY FISKE, CAROLINE M. CILIBERTI, CHRISTINE E. GOULD, DANIELLE
K. NADORFF, MICHAEL R. NADORFF, SARRA NAZEM, and SARAH T. STAHL

West Virginia University
Morgantown, West Virginia

MEGAN M. CLEGG-KRAYNOK

Ohio Northern University
Ada, Ohio

The largest cohort in U.S. history is approaching late life, driving unprecedented growth in the older adult population. The leading edge of the Baby Boom generation (born between 1946 and 1964) reached the age of 65 in 2011. By 2030, nearly 20% of the U.S. population will be 65 or older, double the size of the older adult population in 2000 (Federal Interagency Forum on Aging-Related Statistics, 2010). Along with this dramatic population increase, an increase in the number of older adults with mental health problems is anticipated (Jeste et al., 1999), resulting from both larger numbers of older adults in the population and an elevated propensity for psychopathology in the Baby Boom cohort (Hasin, Goodwin, Stinson, & Grant, 2005). Furthermore, it is expected that the coming generation of older adults will seek mental health treatment at higher rates than past generations (Qualls, Segal, Norman, Niederehe, & Gallagher-Thompson, 2002). These changes bring into sharp focus the importance of investigating the presentation, etiology, and treatment of psychopathology in late life.

Psychopathology in late life can best be understood in the context of lifespan development. Developmental psychopathology has been a useful paradigm for studying abnormal behavior situated within a developmental context (Sroufe & Rutter, 1984; see also Chapter 16, this volume), but the work within this field has generally focused on early development (Cicchetti & Toth, 2009). In contrast, a large body of literature within the lifespan developmental psychology tradition offers theoretical and empirical explanations for normal development across the entire lifespan and into old age (e.g., Baltes & Baltes, 1990; Carstensen, Isaacowitz, & Charles, 1999), but less often focuses on psychopathology. This chapter adopts the developmental psychopathology perspective to examine abnormal behavior in late life as a function of development across the lifespan.

Several aspects of the developmental psychopathology perspective have been particularly helpful in organizing our thinking within this chapter. Consistent with this perspective, in which psychopathology is viewed as deviation from normal development (Sroufe & Rutter, 1984; see also Chapter 16, this volume), we begin with an overview of normal cognitive and socioemotional development in late life. In addition, within the developmental psychopathology perspective, emphasis is placed on understanding not only the presence of psychopathology at any point in time, but also the trajectory over time and even the absence of psychopathology in a person at risk. This chapter will differentiate, where possible, between individuals with early onset of disorder that persists into older adulthood and individuals who experience disorder for the first time in late life, referred to as late onset. It should be noted, however, that age of onset is not specified in much of the research on late-life psychopathology. There has been relatively little research examining the absence of psychopathology in late life among individuals at risk, including those with early onset disorder who experienced remission. Future research in this area would make an important contribution to our understanding of lifespan developmental psychopathology. The developmental psychopathology approach also highlights the possibility that psychopathology may manifest itself differently over time, a concept that has been termed *heterotypic continuity* (Cicchetti & Toth, 2009). This issue is especially relevant to the study of late-life psychopathology, since diagnostic rubrics have been based primarily on symptom presentation typically seen earlier in the lifespan. As a result, some forms of psychopathology may be underdetected among older adults. We discuss this issue further in relation to several of the disorders presented below. A final issue to consider is research methodology; both developmental psychopathology and lifespan developmental psychology traditions emphasize the need for longitudinal research before drawing conclusions about age changes. We base our conclusions on longitudinal research wherever possible.

We begin this chapter with a brief overview of biological, cognitive, social, and emotional development in late life. We then examine some of the most prominent forms of psychopathology with respect to epidemiology, presentation, etiology, and treatment. Where the disorder appears to increase or decrease in prevalence compared to earlier points in the lifespan, we evaluate possible explanations for these age-related changes. The disorders we cover include anxiety disorders, mood disorders and suicide, schizophrenia, substance use disorders, personality disorders, sleep disorders, and dementia. For disorders not included in this chapter, the interested reader is referred to Segal, Qualls, and Smyer (2011).

Normal Development in Late Life

Normal development in late life is characterized by both stability and change in biological, cognitive, social, and emotional domains. Biological aging involves changes in the central nervous system and most other organ systems, as well as a concomitant increase in the likelihood of physical illness and disability. Despite these age-related changes, however, most older adults remain independent. Only 4.5% of adults age 65 and older live in skilled nursing facilities (Hetzel & Smith, 2001). Age-related slowing of the central nervous system and other neurological changes are associated with normative declines in cognitive abilities characterized as fluid intelligence (summarized by Zarit & Zarit, 2007, p. 23). In contrast, crystallized intelligence, which involves fund of knowledge, remains stable or even improves into late life (p. 23). Social changes with age include the possibility of bereavement, retirement, caregiving, and other forms of role change. Nevertheless, 75% of older men and 43% of older women are married (p. 13).

An influential meta-theory that purports to explain adaptation to these age-related changes is the Selective Optimization and Compensation model (SOC; Baltes & Baltes, 1990). According to Baltes and Baltes, aging is associated with a narrowing of opportunities, referred to as *selection*. Selection may result from losses, as described above, or may be elective, as when a person chooses to focus on a particular occupation or other objective. Optimization is the process of enhancing existing abilities, such as practicing a skill. Compensation entails use of alternative methods of meeting a goal, such as seeking help or using an assistive device. Individuals age successfully, according to the SOC model, to the extent that they select goals wisely, optimize their preserved abilities, and compensate for their losses. The SOC model provides a framework for understanding some forms of psychopathology in late life, as discussed further below.

Another useful theory for understanding normal development in late life is the socioemotional selectivity theory (SST; Carstensen, Isaacowitz, & Charles, 1999). According to SST, social goals change across the lifespan. In youth (or whenever time is perceived as expansive), individuals pursue more information-oriented social goals, such as learning about social norms or evaluating oneself in relation to others. In contrast, in late life (or whenever the future is perceived to be foreshortened), the focus is on emotion-oriented social goals, such as regulating one's emotional state through contact with others. Consistent with predictions of this theory, older adults typically have smaller social networks than younger adults but are more likely to derive emotional satisfaction from them (Carstensen et al., 1999). Older adults also exhibit improved emotion regulation compared to their younger counterparts (Carstensen et al., 1999; Charles, Reynolds, & Gatz, 2001). These aspects of the theory are particularly relevant for the understanding of psychopathology in late life. Against this backdrop of normal aging, we next consider major types of disorders in late life.

Anxiety

Anxiety disorders involve disturbances in affect, physiology, and cognition and are characterized by avoidance of situations or stimuli that evoke fear or somatic distress when present (Ollendick & Byrd, 2001). Anxiety disorders include generalized anxiety disorder (GAD), simple phobia, social phobia, panic disorder, agoraphobia without panic disorder, obsessive-compulsive disorder (OCD), and posttraumatic stress disorder (PTSD; see also Chapter 8, this volume).

Anxiety disorders tend to be chronic, sometimes lasting years or decades (Barlow, 2002). Nonetheless, both the lifetime and 12-month prevalence of all anxiety disorders drops after age 65 (Gum, King-Kallimanis, & Kahn, 2009). According to Gum et al. (2009), the 12-month prevalence of any anxiety disorder is highest among adults aged 18–44 (20.7%), followed by adults aged 45–64 (18.7%), and drops to 7.0% among adults aged 65 and older.

According to Gum et al. (2009), the most common anxiety disorder among people aged 65 and up is specific phobia, with a lifetime prevalence of 6.8%, followed by social phobia (6.3%), GAD (3.3%), panic disorder and PTSD (2.1% each), and agoraphobia without panic disorder (1.6%). Other researchers have found that GAD is the most common anxiety disorder among older adults (e.g., Beekman et al., 1998). Since anxiety disorders share the common thread of worry, and GAD is characterized by worry, some investigators consider it to be the "basic" anxiety disorder (e.g., Roemer, Orsillo, & Barlow, 2002). Because much of the research on late-life anxiety has focused on GAD, we focus on this disorder in this section.

Description and Course

The American Psychiatric Association's (APA) *Diagnostic and Statistical Manual of Mental Disorder*, fourth edition, text revised (*DSM–IV–TR*; APA, 2000) describes GAD as a disorder characterized by excessive and difficult-to-control worry lasting for a minimum of 6 months, accompanied by at least three of the following six symptoms: fatigue, restlessness or feeling edgy, muscle tension, trouble concentrating or mind going blank, irritability, and disrupted sleep. The proposed set of criteria for GAD in the DSM–5 (APA, 2010) retains the core symptom of worry, but reduces the time frame from 6 to 3 months and shifts the focus away from the six associated symptoms. According to the proposed criteria, one must exhibit excessive and difficult to control worry, along with either restlessness or muscle tension, and one or more behavioral manifestations of worry to meet the new criteria for GAD (APA, 2010). These criteria decrease the focus on somatic symptoms in GAD and may significantly impact the diagnosis of the disorder in late life. Because somatic symptoms of anxiety may overlap with symptoms of physical illness (Palmer, Jeste, & Sheikh, 1997), the proposed DSM–5 diagnostic criteria will likely affect the detection of GAD in older adults. If somatic symptoms simply confound the diagnosis of GAD, then the increased emphasis on nonsomatic symptoms (i.e., worry) will simplify the diagnosis of GAD among older adults. However, the proposed DSM–5 criteria could possibly result in fewer diagnoses of GAD if older adults with anxiety truly present with more physical manifestations of anxiety than their younger counterparts, as some researchers have suggested (e.g., Spar & LaRue, 1990).

Several age-related differences in presentation of GAD are worth noting. The core symptom of GAD is worry. However, worry content may change with age. Wetherell, Le Roux, and Gatz (2003) found that some worries (e.g., worries about family) may be normative among older adults. Other worries are shown to differentiate older adults with GAD from those without GAD, including worries about finances, personal health, small matters, and social matters (Wetherell et al., 2003). Additionally, researchers have examined age-related presentations in the six associated diagnostic symptoms of GAD according to *DSM–IV–TR*. Sleep disturbance and muscle tension seemed to be especially important factors in distinguishing older adults with GAD from those without, while trouble concentrating did not distinguish those with GAD from those with no diagnosis (Wetherell et al., 2003). Though muscle tension is retained as a diagnostic symptom in DSM–5, sleep disturbance is not.

GAD is thought to be a chronic disorder (Roemer et al., 2002). A longitudinal study shows a remission rate of 38% over 5 years (Yonkers, Dyck, Warshaw, & Keller, 2000). However, of those with either fully or partially remitted GAD, many (27% and 39%, respectively) remitted within 3 years. Remission rates are lower when GAD co-occurs with major depression than when GAD is the sole diagnosis (Schoevers, Deeg, van Tilburg, & Beekman, 2005).

Etiology

Researchers have attempted to examine the etiology of GAD and other anxiety disorders. Genetic factors, predictability or control over life events, parenting style, and attributional style may make certain individuals more vulnerable to anxiety disorders (Barlow, 2002). However, much of this research focuses on children and younger adults, and little is known about the etiology of GAD or other anxiety disorders in late life.

Explanation for Age Differences

The reasons for the relatively lower prevalence of GAD in late life compared to earlier in the lifespan are not well understood, but there are several explanations that would be consistent with the empirical evidence. We may observe these decreases in prevalence because older adults are more adept than their younger counterparts at regulating emotions and can reduce the impact of negative emotions (Carstensen et al., 1999). These strategies may allow older adults to successfully manage anxiety symptoms in late life. Further, there is evidence that the probability of treatment contact for anxiety disorders cumulatively increases with age (Wang et al., 2005). Thus, many older adults may have been successfully treated by the time they reach late life.

Certain methodological factors could also account for the lower prevalence of GAD in late life. Measures developed for use with younger adults may miss symptoms of anxiety in older adults. Further, anxiety disorders are often diagnosed with one or more comorbid *DSM* Axis I disorders (Lenze et al., 2000). Physical disorders can also complicate the identification of anxiety disorders in older adults. Older adults with anxiety disorders have more comorbid physical health problems than those without anxiety disorders (Palmer et al., 1997). Anxiety symptoms may mimic the signs of physical illness, and conversely, physical illness may mimic the experience of anxiety (Palmer et al., 1997). Thus, the lower prevalence of GAD in late life may result in part from poor detection of it.

Assessment and Treatment

As noted above, differences in the presentation of GAD in late life compared to earlier in the lifespan should be considered when assessing for the disorder in older adults. There are several evidence-based pharmacologic and psychosocial treatments available to older adults with GAD. Benzodiazepines were historically used to treat anxiety in older adults. However, antidepressants have become a first-line treatment for GAD because of significant risks associated with benzodiazepines (Sheikh & Cassidy, 2000). Of the psychosocial interventions, relaxation training and cognitive-behavior therapy (CBT) have the most support for use with older adults with GAD (Ayers, Sorrell, Thorp, & Wetherell, 2007).

Conclusions

In sum, GAD and other anxiety disorders are relatively common in late life but are less prevalent in this age group than earlier in the lifespan. Older adults may simply experience less anxiety in late life as a result of treatment or more successful emotion regulation strategies. However, prevalence estimates that rely on assessments developed for use with younger adults may underestimate the true number of older adults who meet the criteria for these disorders. Moreover, we know little about the etiology and presentation of anxiety in late life. To answer these questions, there is a need for more longitudinal research on the anxiety disorders.

Mood Disorders

Depression in late life is a relatively common, yet underdiagnosed, disorder, with a wide range of possible physical, emotional, and cognitive consequences (Fiske, Wetherell, & Gatz, 2009). Several types of mood disorders are categorized in the *DSM–IV–TR*, including major depressive disorder, dysthymic disorder, bipolar disorder, and depressive disorder due to general medical condition (see also Chapter 9, this volume). An estimated 1 to 3% of the population aged 65 and older currently meet the criteria for depression (Cole & Dendukuri, 2004). The 12-month prevalence of major depressive disorder is significantly lower among adults aged 65 and older than in any other adult age group (Hasin et al., 2005). Depressive symptoms at a clinically significant level of severity that do not meet the criteria for any diagnosis have also been a focus of much research. It is estimated that as many as 19% of older adults may have clinically significant depressive symptoms (Cole & Dendukuri, 2004). This is of serious concern, as minor depression in older men and major depression in both genders of older adults have demonstrated an increased risk of death that is not fully explained by suicide (Penninx et al., 1999). As most research concerning depression in late life relates to either major depressive disorder or severity of depressive symptoms, these will be the focus in this section. Bipolar disorder is uncommon in late life and will not be discussed in detail in this section. However, the relative absence of a disorder can also be informative from a lifespan developmental psychopathology perspective. Although the reasons for the relatively low prevalence of bipolar disorder in late life are not well understood, there is evidence of midlife remission in a substantial proportion of individuals (Cicero, Epler, & Scher, 2009), and selective mortality from suicide and other causes has been well documented (Angst, Stassen, Clayton, & Angst, 2002; Jamison, 2000).

Description and Course

Major depressive disorder is characterized by pervasive dysphoria or anhedonia and associated symptoms. Depression presents differently in late life than earlier in the lifespan (Christensen et al., 1999; Gallo, Anthony, & Muthén, 1994). Older adults are less likely than younger individuals to endorse cognitive or affective symptoms, including sadness, worthlessness or guilt, and suicidal ideation (Gallo et al., 1994). In contrast, older adults are more likely than younger individuals to endorse somatic symptoms, such as insomnia, fatigue, and psychomotor retardation (Christensen et al., 1999). Cognitive deficits are more often present in depressed older adults, particularly in the case of late-onset disorder.

At least half of older adults with depression developed it for the first time in late life. Brodaty et al. (2001) found that 52% of depressed older adults had their first onset after age 60. Similarly, Bruce et al. (2002) found that 71% of depressed older adult home care patients developed depression for the first time in late life. Depression is a chronic, episodic disorder. A study examining the course of depression in community-dwelling older adults found that after 3 years, 48.3% had remitted, while 51.7% had relapsed (Schoevers et al., 2003).

Etiology

The etiology of depression in late life can be viewed from a developmental diathesis–stress perspective (Gatz, Kasl-Godley, & Karel, 1996). Biological or psychological vulnerabilities to depression, which vary across the lifespan, may interact with stressors characteristic of late life to precipitate a depressive episode. Biological vulnerability may include genetic risk as well as physiological changes related to either aging or disease (e.g., vascular disease; Dent et al., 1999). An example of psychological vulnerability is external locus of control (Beekman et al., 2000). Risk factor research has identified numerous stressors associated with depression or depressive symptoms in late life, including physical limitations (Cui, Lyness, Tang, Tu, & Conwell, 2008; Dent et al., 1999); economic strain (Samuelsson, McCamish-Svensson, Hagberg, Sundström, & Dehlin, 2005); death of a partner or other relatives (Vink et al., 2009); and being a caregiver (reviewed by Fiske et al., 2009). Lowered cognitive functioning has also been associated with late life depression (Cui et al., 2008) and may be a marker of biological change or a psychological stressor. Risk factors may vary based on age of depression onset. Late-onset depression is associated with lower levels of neuroticism but poorer overall physical health than early onset (Nguyen & Zonderman, 2006; Sneed, Kasen, & Cohen, 2007).

Explanation for Age Differences

As with anxiety disorders, the reasons for the relatively low prevalence of depressive disorders in late life are poorly understood. Increased ability to regulate emotions (Carstensen et al., 1999; Charles et al., 2001) may play a part in reducing the likelihood of depression among older adults. The current clinical diagnostic rubric might not detect depression in older adults (Weiss, Nagel, & Aronson, 1986). This may be due to the greater tendency of older adults to endorse somatic symptoms and the reduced likelihood of older adults endorsing dysphoria. Either dysphoria or anhedonia must be present to diagnose major depressive disorder (APA, 2000). Since depression is associated with increased risk of death from suicide and other causes, selective mortality may also partially explain reduced rates of depression in late life.

Assessment and Treatment

Since late-life depression presents differently from depression earlier in the lifespan, often without endorsement of sadness, assessment can be difficult (Fiske & O'Riley, 2008). The Geriatric Depression scale (Yesavage et al., 1983) was developed to measure depressive symptoms in older adults without including somatic symptoms that could be confounded with physical illness, although this strategy risks underdetecting purely somatic presentations of depression, which are more common in late life (for a discussion, see Fiske & O'Riley, 2008).

Both pharmacologic and psychosocial treatments have demonstrated efficacy in treating depression in late life (for a review of pharmacological treatments, see Beyer, 2007). Psychosocial treatments for older adult depression that meet evidence-based criteria include behavioral therapy, CBT, cognitive bibliotherapy, problem-solving therapy, brief psychodynamic therapy, and life review therapy (see Scogin, Welsh, Hanson, Stump, & Coates, 2005, for a review). The outcomes for older adults who are treated for depression are similar to those for younger individuals (Pinquart, Duberstein, & Lyness, 2006). However, effective treatment may take more time, especially for late-onset depression. A study by Driscoll et al. (2005) found that late-onset recurrent depression took longer to respond to treatment than early-onset depression (an average of 12 weeks vs. 8 weeks, respectively), but that those with late onset had similar results for remission (47% for late-onset single, 53% for early-onset recurrent) and relapse (19% for late-onset single,

17% for early-onset recurrent). In addition, older adults may cycle out of recurrent depressive episodes more slowly (Kessler, Foster, Webster, & House, 1992). Treatment of depression in late life may also be improved by integrating mental health treatment into primary care (Bruce et al., 2004; Hunkeler et al., 2006).

Conclusions

Although subsyndromal symptoms are common in late life, major depression and bipolar disorders are less common in late life than in midlife (Fiske et al., 2009). Although direct evidence is lacking, improved ability to regulate emotions may contribute to a true decline in these disorders with age. Mood disorders may also be underdiagnosed in late life due to differences in presentation when compared with presentation earlier in the lifespan. The etiology and risk factors for older adult depression may differ from depression in younger adults, and these differences should be considered when assessing for depression among older adults. Effective pharmacologic and psychosocial treatments are available.

Suicide

Any discussion of mood disorders would be incomplete without consideration of suicide, and this is particularly true when the focus is late-life mood disorders. Suicide among older adults differs in several important ways from suicide earlier in the lifespan. In 2007, the suicide rate in the United States for adults age 65 and older (14.27 per 100,000) was over 30% higher than the suicide rate for individuals age 64 and younger (10.84 per 100,000), primarily due to very high suicide rates in older adult men (Xu, Kochanek, Murphy, & Tejada-Vera, 2010). Gender differences in late life suicide may reflect the fact that older adult men are more likely to use firearms than older adult women (Xu et al., 2010). Additionally, suicide attempts in late life are much more likely to be fatal when compared with attempts by younger adults. It is estimated that there are 100 suicide attempts for every death by suicide among young adults (Jacobziner, 1965), whereas there are four suicide attempts for every death by suicide among older adults (Lawrence, Almeida, Hulse, Jablensky, & Holman, 2000).

Definitions

Suicide is a self-inflicted death in which there is evidence that the individual intended to take his or her life (Silverman, Berman, Sanddal, O'Carroll, & Joiner, 2007). An individual may also have suicidal ideation, which is having thoughts of ending one's life regardless of whether or not the person actually intends to do so (Silverman et al., 2007). A suicide attempt is "a self-inflicted, potentially injurious behavior with a nonfatal outcome for which there is evidence (either explicit or implicit) of intent to die" (Silverman et al., 2007, p. 273). This section will focus on suicide rather than suicidal ideation or attempt.

Etiology

Several theories of suicidal behavior may be informative with respect to late-life suicide. Joiner's (2005) influential "interpersonal theory of suicide" attempts to explain why suicidal thoughts are common but so few individuals die by suicide. Joiner postulates that there are three factors that put an individual at risk of dying by suicide: thwarted belongingness, perceived burdensomeness, and the acquired capability to enact lethal self-harm. According to Joiner, interpersonal factors (thwarted belongingness and perceived burdensomeness) contribute to the desire to die by suicide but are insufficient to enable an individual to enact lethal self-harm. The individual must also have acquired the capability to enact such behaviors through habituation, such as by practicing or working up to the attempt, attempting suicide in the past, or experiencing (personally or vicariously) painful or provocative experiences. As a result of habituation, fear of pain and other normal, protective barriers to suicidal behavior are reduced. This theory provides a compelling argument for why older adults are at greater risk to die by suicide. Older adults face several threats to their belongingness, such as the death of friends and loved ones as well as retirement, and they may also feel like a burden to friends and family if disability forces increased reliance on others. Older adults also have a lifetime of experience with pain, and painful conditions are common in older adults, which may lead to habituation and, therefore, the acquired capability to engage in lethal self-harm behavior, increasing the risk of dying by suicide. In addition, older adults have a longer history of exposure to death and therefore may be less affected by the idea of dying than younger individuals.

Suicidal behavior in older adults may also be understood in the context of the SOC model, discussed earlier (Baltes & Baltes, 1990). Suicidal behavior may result from failures in selection, optimization, or compensation. Failure to reach one's target or goal may lead to helplessness and depression. Further, lack of compensation (including an unwillingness or inability to seek help or to redefine goals) may exacerbate the problem and lead to feelings of hopelessness and suicidal ideation. Therefore, identifying and rectifying failures in selection, optimization, and compensation may be an important step in reducing an older adult's risk of suicide.

Risk factor research suggests that having psychopathology (specifically mood and substance abuse disorders) puts older adults at significantly higher risk of suicide (Beautrais, 2002). Prior suicide attempts are also a risk factor for suicide or serious suicide attempt (Beautrais, 2002). Chronic illnesses also become more prevalent with age, and certain illnesses and physical conditions, such as cancer, vision impairment, and incontinence, may put older adults at greater risk of death by suicide (see review by Fiske, O'Riley, & Widoe, 2008). Mild cognitive impairment is also associated with greater risk of late-life suicide, but there is little evidence of increased risk associated with dementia, Parkinson's disease, or stroke. Evidence suggests that effects may be partially but not fully explained by depression (Fiske et al., 2008).

Assessment and Prevention

Several measures have been created to assess suicidal ideation (Heisel & Flett, 2006) or risk in older adults (Edelstein et al., 2009; Fremouw, McCoy, Tyner, & Musick, 2009). Since late-life depression is treatable, there is hope for reducing suicide risk in late life by treating depression in older adults (Bruce et al., 2004). Since older adult suicide attempts are more likely to be fatal than suicide attempts in younger adults, there are fewer opportunities to intervene following an attempt. Preventing suicide in older adults is further complicated by the fact that older adults do not regularly seek out mental health professionals (Santos & VandenBos, 1982), although there is evidence that the majority of older adults who die by suicide had visited a physician within a month of the death (Luoma, Martin, & Pearson, 2002). Therefore, identifying suicidal risk in settings that older adults frequent, such as primary care or through visiting nurses, is important to treat individuals at risk and reduce the likelihood of death by suicide. Programs that integrate treatment for depression within primary care have demonstrated success in reducing suicidal ideation (Bruce et al., 2004; Hunkeler et al., 2006).

Conclusions

Suicide rates are very high in late life, particularly among older adult men (Xu et al., 2010). Several theories offer possible explanations for these age differences, but they remain to be evaluated empirically. Identifying older adults at risk of suicide is difficult because older adults do not seek out the attention of mental health professionals. However, the primary risk factor for late-life suicide is depression, and suicidal older adults do present to primary care. Therefore, a promising approach may be to develop screening tools specifically for older adults and utilize them in primary care and home care settings, where integrated depression treatment can also be offered. Improving the identification of depression and suicide risk in older adults may increase the number of older adults who receive treatment and reduce the number who die by suicide.

Schizophrenia

Schizophrenia is a lifespan neurodevelopmental disorder. The prevalence is 1.3% in the population aged 18 to 54 and 0.6% among individuals aged 65 and older (Jeste & Nasrallah, 2003; also see Chapter 10, this volume). Schizophrenia with onset in late life has been the focus of recent research and will be discussed specifically below.

Description and Course

DSM–IV–TR diagnostic criteria specify at least two of the following symptoms: delusions; hallucinations; thought disorders manifested in disorganized speech, disorganized or catatonic behavior, or negative symptoms (e.g., blunted affect, loss of motivation, or poverty of speech). Notably, no pathognomic symptom of schizophrenia has been identified, suggesting that the diagnostic category may be heterogeneous, comprising multiple related but distinct disorders.

Several different trajectories characterize the course of schizophrenia across the lifespan. Most commonly, schizophrenia has an onset in late adolescence or early adulthood, but in 25% of older adults with schizophrenia, onset occurred later in life (Jeste & Nasrallah, 2003). Regardless of the age at which the disease is diagnosed, evidence suggests that the disease process begins earlier, as preclinical signs such as cognitive, motor, and social deficits are observed in children, adolescents, and adults who later develop schizophrenia (Walker & Lewine, 1990). The course of schizophrenia is chronic, with continuing symptoms for a minority of patients (25–35%), whereas the course is episodic for more than 50% of patients (Jobe & Harrow, 2010). A subgroup of 20 to 35% of patients functions well after discontinuing antipsychotic medication (Jobe & Harrow, 2010).

Etiology

Leading theories attribute the etiology of schizophrenia to genetic or other biological vulnerability in combination with pre- and perinatal environmental stressors that interfere with normal neurological development (Bearden, Meyer, Loewy, Niendam, & Cannon, 2006). Evidence shows substantial genetic influence (Gottesman & Hanson, 2005). Environmental stressors that have been implicated include birth complications, such as those involving fetal hypoxia (Bearden et al., 2006) and maternal viral infection during the second trimester (Barr, Mednick, & Munk-Jörgensen, 1990).

Explanation for Age Differences

There are several possible explanations for the lower prevalence of schizophrenia in late life compared to early adulthood or middle age. Lower rates of schizophrenia in late life may result, in part, from remission of the disease. Although there are varying estimates of the rate of remission, longitudinal research demonstrates convincingly that remission is possible, even among older adults. In a sample of community-dwelling, middle-aged and older schizophrenia outpatients, 8% met stringent criteria for sustained remission (Auslander & Jeste, 2004). Furthermore, the pattern of symptoms of schizophrenia appears to be characterized by stability or a decline in severity across the lifespan (Folsom et al., 2009; Jeste et al., 2003). Older individuals with schizophrenia appear to have better coping skills than their younger counterparts, and well-being and functioning among older adults with early-onset schizophrenia have been shown to be stable or even reflect an increased level at older ages (Folsom et al., 2009; Jeste et al., 2003). Similarly, in longitudinal research, cognitive performance has been shown to remain stable over time in older adult schizophrenia outpatients (Savla et al., 2006). When compared to age-matched normal controls, however, older adults with schizophrenia show greater symptomatology, poorer functioning, and lower quality of life (Jobe & Harrow, 2010). In addition, stability in symptoms and functioning is only found among non-institutionalized individuals. Institutionalized older adults with early-onset schizophrenia experience more severe symptoms than both younger adults and noninstitutionalized older adults as well as declines in cognitive functioning (Folsom et al., 2009; Savla et al., 2006). An alternative explanation for the lower rates of schizophrenia in late life is selective mortality, that is, an increased likelihood for individuals with schizophrenia of dying before reaching old age (Jobe & Harrow, 2010).

Late- and Very Late-Onset Schizophrenia

Late-onset schizophrenia refers to onset after age 40, and *very late-onset* schizophrenia refers to onset after age 60 (Cohen, 1990; Howard et al., 2000). Given the theorized etiology of schizophrenia as a deviation from normal brain development, onset of the disorder in late life would seem difficult to explain. Some investigators (e.g., Howard et al., 2000) have proposed that late-onset schizophrenia is a disorder distinct from early-onset schizophrenia, with differing epidemiology, presentation, and risk or protective factors. Evidence, however, is mixed.

Cross-sectional research suggests that symptom presentation is similar for early- versus late-onset schizophrenia (see review by Howard et al., 2000), but this finding is mostly restricted to those younger than 60. For older individuals with very late onset, the expression of symptoms is less severe, with more nonspecific symptomatology compared to those with early onset (Häfner et al., 1998). Cognitive impairment is a symptom of schizophrenia for both early and late onset, but for those with late onset, the impairment is milder than for those with early onset (Howard et al., 2000). Some investigators have suggested that late-onset schizophrenia is better understood as a form of dementia, but longitudinal evidence from two studies suggests that this is not the case (Palmer et al., 2003; Rabins, 2003).

Epidemiologic research suggests that risk factors may differ for early- versus late-onset schizophrenia. Individuals with onset of schizophrenia in later life are less likely to have a family history of schizophrenia and more likely to experience sensory impairments than those with early onset (Howard, Almeida, & Raymond, 1994; Howard et al., 2000). Other correlates include being female and being unmarried, but it is unclear whether individuals with late-onset schizophrenia have better or worse social, educational, and occupational functioning compared to those with earlier-onset schizophrenia (Howard et al., 2000). Thus, additional research is needed to better understand whether early-onset and late-onset (or even very late-onset) schizophrenia are the same disorder with different manifestations or if they are distinct disorders.

Assessment and Treatment

Several treatments have demonstrated efficacy in the management of schizophrenia in late life. Antipsychotic medications are effective in controlling positive symptoms, as in younger populations (Auslander & Jeste, 2004). Cognitive-behavioral social skills training is associated with better social functioning, coping skills, and even insight among older adults with schizophrenia (Granholm et al., 2005). Supported employment has demonstrated similar success in improving outcomes in middle-aged and older adults with schizophrenia, as in younger samples (Twamley & Narvaez, 2008).

Conclusions

Based on the findings from the studies reviewed above, the following conclusions can be made. Schizophrenia is rare among older adults, and even rarer is late-onset schizophrenia among older adults. Overall, older adults with late-onset schizophrenia have the same rates of cognitive decline as those with early onset. With some exceptions, either stability in symptomatology and functioning or decreases in deficits or impairments are apparent for noninstitutionalized individuals with schizophrenia. Evidence is inconclusive with respect to whether late-onset schizophrenia represents the same or a different disorder than early-onset schizophrenia, but it does not appear to predict dementia, and individuals with late-onset schizophrenia tend to have a better prognosis and quality of life than those with early onset.

Alcohol Use Disorders

Alcohol use disorders are associated with severe mental and physical health consequences and increased risk of mortality (Thun et al., 1997; see also Chapter 14, this volume). These disorders are less common in late life than earlier in the lifespan, with the prevalence of problematic alcohol use among older adults between 1 and 22% for community populations (Johnson, 2000; Oslin, 2004). However, several methodological, assessment, and etiological factors complicate the study of alcohol use in older age. Despite the fact that excessive drinking declines as individuals enter their 70s and 80s, many older adults still drink more than the suggested consumption guidelines, especially those in the cohort born after 1920, suggesting that cohort effects may be an underlying factor when assessing alcohol use across the lifespan (Moos, Schutte, & Brennan, 2009).

Description and Course

To meet *DSM–IV–TR* criteria for alcohol abuse, an individual must show a maladaptive pattern of substance use, resulting in significant distress or impairment. Alcohol dependence involves continued use despite alcohol-related problems. Diagnostic criteria, which were not developed or validated in older adult populations, may underestimate the prevalence of abuse among older adults (Patterson & Jeste, 1999). For example, diagnostic criteria specify age-dependent consequences (e.g., school or work) that may not be relevant in late life due to age-related role changes (Patterson & Jeste, 1999). An alternative method of studying problematic alcohol use is to measure frequency of drinking behaviors.

Studies suggest that the major risk period for alcohol initiation is over by the age of 20 (DeWit, Adlaf, Offord, & Ogbrone, 2000), and the odds of lifetime alcohol use disorders drop significantly for each increasing year of age at initiation (Grant & Dawson, 1997). However, a majority of this research has relied heavily on adolescent and young adult samples without long-term longitudinal tracking. There is evidence that some older adults start problem drinking after age 50, often referred to as late adult onset or "reactive" drinking (Sattar, Petty, & Burke, 2003). Older adults who begin drinking later in life may do so in response to aging stressors, such as traumatic losses, issues related to retirement, or major illness (Johnson, 2000; Oslin, 2004; Sattar et al., 2003). Regardless of age of onset, alcohol use disorders tend to follow a chronic course (Kerr, Fillmore, & Bostrom, 2002).

Etiology

There are multiple possible causes of problematic alcohol use in late life. Alcohol use disorders arise from an interaction of genetic risk and environmental factors that may vary across the lifespan (Vanyukov & Targer, 2000). Risk factors for late-life drinking include pain, sleep difficulties, and depression (Brennan, Schutte, & Moos, 2005; Sattar et al., 2003; Schonfield & Dupree, 1991). Additionally, lack of social support in late life may lead to the use of alcohol as a negative coping strategy and has been associated with higher chances of relapse (Jason, Davis, Ferrari, & Bishop, 2001; Moos, Finney, & Cronkite, 1990).

Explanations for Age Differences

There are several possible explanations for the reduced prevalence of alcohol use disorders in late life. Longitudinal research shows that excessive drinking behavior declines with age (Moos et al., 2009). Younger alcohol users have been shown to "mature out" of problem drinking well before they reach old age as a consequence of both personality development and role transitions (Littlefield, Sher, & Wood, 2009). Physiological changes may contribute to older adults' increased sensitivity to alcohol, which may be associated with changes in alcohol use behaviors. For example, lean body mass and total body water to fat ratio decreases with age, resulting in increased serum concentrations of alcohol in the body (Oslin, 2004). Although some older adults may reduce consumption of alcohol as a consequence of physiological changes associated with aging, it should be noted that some older adults who continue lifelong drinking patterns unaware of their age-heightened risk may encounter drinking-related problems for the first time in late life (Merrick et al., 2008). An alternative explanation for reduced rates of alcohol use disorders in late life is selective mortality. Individuals with early-onset alcohol abuse or dependence die approximately 10 years earlier than age-matched controls (Fried et al., 1998; Thun et al., 1997), and even in late-onset cases, alcohol abuse has been found to be associated with excess mortality, especially in men (Moore et al., 2006; Moos, Brennan, & Mertens, 1994). In addition, problems with detection may contribute to the low apparent rates of alcohol disorders in late life.

Assessment and Treatment

Accurate assessment of alcohol use disorders is critical for the treatment of these disorders among older adults. Unfortunately, underdetection and underreporting occur in primary care settings, which are often considered the front-line approach to older adult mental health care. D'Amico, Paddock, Burnam, and King (2005) found that problem drinkers were less likely to visit general medical providers than nonproblem drinkers. Additionally, medical professionals were less likely to ask persons aged 50 or older about alcohol use.

Several other barriers have been identified in the detection of older adult alcohol misuse (St. John, Snow, & Tyas, 2010). The symptoms of alcohol use are often the same symptoms portrayed under different older adult disorders. Symptoms like falls, accidental injuries, urinary incontinence, and depression are geriatric problems that share common symptom presentations with those seen in alcohol abusers (Han, Gfroerer, Colliver, & Penne, 2009; Johnson, 2000; Sattar et al., 2003). Furthermore, the harmful effects of drinking also exacerbate problems with physical and mental health functioning. Cognitive impairment, in conjunction with or separate from alcohol disorders, may diminish the likelihood of detection due to self-report difficulties, bias, and symptom misidentification (Blazer & Wu, 2009). In addition, because social patterns change with age (Carstensen, Isaacowitz, & Charles, 1999), many of the social consequences of problem drinking go unnoticed (Sattar et al., 2003). Further complicating this dilemma is the fact that individuals at risk for alcohol problems or binge drinking are less likely to report overt stress (Blazer & Wu, 2009). These factors should be considered when assessing for alcohol use problems in an older adult.

Older adults are amenable to treatment, and outcomes are especially beneficial when elder-specific treatments are used (Blow, Walton, Chermack, Mudd, & Brower, 2000; Oslin, 2004). In fact, most research suggests that late-onset drinkers may be more responsive and receptive to treatment than early-onset drinkers (Oslin, Pettinati, & Volpicelli, 2002), especially since early-onset patients may be more likely than late-onset patients to drop out of treatment (Atkinson, Tolson, & Turner, 1993). Older adults attain several positive outcomes across a range of measures (e.g., alcohol, emotional, social) after receiving and completing substance treatment. Older adults may also respond well to brief interventions (Oslin, 2004). However, few intervention studies use randomized, controlled designs in older adults, making it difficult to suggest which types of treatment interventions are most effective (Oslin, 2004; Sattar et al., 2003).

Conclusions

Cross-sectional and longitudinal research suggests that alcohol use disorders are less prevalent in old age than earlier in the lifespan. Research suggests that these findings may be explained by reduced drinking associated with age-related changes in physiological, personality, and social factors as well as selective mortality. However, the lack of consensus on what is considered problem drinking, as well as difficulty detecting and screening for alcohol use disorders in late life, complicates the picture.

Although alcohol use disorders decrease with age, they still present a significant public health challenge. The number of older adults who will meet criteria for substance use disorder is projected to double from 2.8 million to 5.7 million in 2020 (Han et al., 2009). As the Baby Boom generation gets set to move into old age, researchers will have the unique ability to witness how alcohol use changes in a generation that has historically consumed more alcohol and been more open to psychological treatment than previous generations.

Personality Disorders

Personality disorders (PDs) are defined as pervasive and inflexible patterns of behavior associated with distress or impairment. A more detailed discussion of diagnostic criteria for PDs can be found in Chapter 11, this volume. Although PDs are defined by their longstanding patterns of dysfunctional behavior, some PDs may manifest differently as individuals age. PDs are found among 10% of community-dwelling older adults (Widiger & Seidlitz, 2002), which is slightly lower than the prevalence for younger adults, ranging from 10 to 13% (Weissman, 1993). The *DSM–IV–TR* describes 10 personality disorders, but only 4 with evident age-related differences will be reviewed in detail here. Cross-sectional research suggests that antisocial personality disorder (ASPD) and borderline personality disorder (BPD) are less prevalent in older adults than in younger adults (Segal, Hook, & Coolidge, 2001), whereas schizoid PD and obsessive-compulsive (OC) PD appear to be more prevalent in older compared to younger adults (Engels, Duijsens, Haringsma, & van Putten, 2003; Segal et al., 2001). Among individuals aged 65 to 98 years old, ASPD was diagnosed in 0.2 to 0.3%, schizoid PD in 0.9 to 1.9%, and OCPD in 1.6 to 2.5% of older adults (Balsis, Woods, Gleason, & Oltmanns, 2007).

Description and Course

Schizoid PD is characterized by a lack of interest in interpersonal relationships, ASPD by disregard for and violation of the rights of others, BPD by instability in relationships, affect, and identity, and OCPD by preoccupation with order (APA, 2000).

Age-related differences in presentation of ASPD and BPD are evident. Older adults with ASPD are more likely to endorse lying or deception than younger adults with ASPD (Balsis, Gleason, Woods, & Oltmanns, 2007). This age difference is consistent with the interpretation that violation of the rights of others (e.g., physical fighting and aggression) requires physical strength and agility (Kroessler, 1990), which may diminish as strength declines with age. Several differences in the presentation of BPD are observed as well. Specifically, older adults with BPD may have fewer close relationships, so the pattern of unstable relationships may be less frequently endorsed (Agronin & Maletta, 2000). In addition, older adults are less likely to exhibit impulsive behaviors and are more likely to experience the cognitive symptoms of BPD, such as identity disturbance (Clarkin, Spielman, & Klausner, 1999).

Etiology

Personality disorders can be conceptualized as maladaptive and extreme variants of normal personality traits. As such, they are likely to arise from an interaction of genetic predisposition and early life environment exacerbated by current stressors. The predisposition hypothesis (Sadavoy & Leszcz, 1987, as cited in Zweig & Hillman, 1999) suggests that middle-aged and older adults with PDs are more susceptible to age-related stressors (e.g., loss, physical illness, forced dependency) than their counterparts. Thus, these individuals with PDs may have a higher diathesis prior to encountering stressors. Encountered stressors may lead to poorer prognosis, increased disability, and mortality.

Explanations for Age Differences

There are a few explanations for the age differences in prevalence of specific PDs. The maturation hypothesis posits that certain *immature* personality types (e.g., antisocial, borderline) are more likely to improve with age as impulsivity decreases. On the other hand, *mature* personality disorder types (OCPD, schizoid, and paranoid PDs) are thought to worsen with age as a result of longstanding patterns of behavior, cohort differences (e.g., leading to "miserly" behavior), or mild cognitive impairment (e.g., hoarding in OCPD; Kernberg, 1984; Solomon, 1981, cited in Zweig & Hillman, 1999).

Longitudinal research has yielded findings that are broadly consistent with these explanations. At present, there are several well-constructed and promising longitudinal studies of personality disorders (e.g., McLean Study of Adult Development, Zanarini et al., 2007; Collaborative Longitudinal Personality Disorders Study, Skodol et al., 2005); however, the cohorts are young and yield little information about individuals older than 50 years. Despite this limitation, there is longitudinal evidence of a decrease in impulsive behaviors over time for both ASPD and BPD. The course of ASPD varies with high mortality rates (23.9%), remission of ASPD (17.6%), and continued engagement in antisocial behavior for almost half of the studied individuals (48.5%; Black, Baumgard, & Bell, 1995). In contrast, BPD often remits, with about 75% of patients remitting at 15-year follow-up (Zanarini et al., 2007). Although remission is common, some symptoms of affective instability may still remain (Zanarini, Frankenburg, Hennen, & Silk, 2003). Thus, the distress associated with personality disorders is stable across the lifespan, while the symptom presentation changes (Zanarini et al., 2007).

Age differences may also be reflective of biased diagnostic criteria (Balsis, Gleason et al., 2007) or age differences in the presentation of symptoms. For example, the criteria for schizoid PD may falsely identify as schizoid older adults with social isolation due to disability or decreased functional status. However, an older adult with schizoid PD would have a life-long history of few or no relationships rather than age-related reduction in relationships. Interestingly, some of the criteria for OCPD, which is frequently identified in older adults, may be biased toward younger age groups as the criteria focus on behaviors occurring in a work setting (Agronin & Maletta, 2000). Notwithstanding the potential bias, three other criteria were more frequently endorsed by older adults with OCPD: (1) inflexible about moral, ethical, or values issues, (2) unable to discard worthless objects, and (3) assuming a miserly spending style (Balsis, Gleason et al., 2007).

Additionally, selective mortality may also play a role in the apparent decrease in certain PDs that involve impulsive and potentially harmful behaviors, specifically ASPD and BPD. Individuals with ASPD and BPD are more likely to die from unnatural deaths, such as suicide or other violent deaths, compared to the average population. In a longitudinal study of individuals diagnosed with ASPD, 24% of individuals died after a lengthy follow-up period (16 to 45 years; Black et al., 1995). Individuals with BPD have high rates of completed suicide (about 10%

overall, a rate of 50 times that of the general population) and higher rates of deaths from natural (8%) and premature causes (18.2%; Paris & Zewig-Frank, 2001; see also Lieb, Zanarini, Schmahl, Linehan, & Bohus, 2004).

Assessment and Treatment

Assessment measures used to diagnose personality disorders were created using young adult samples and may be biased when used with older adults (Balsis, Woods, Gleason, & Oltmanns, et al., 2007). In particular, when assessing older adults, it is essential to differentiate behaviors consistent with personality disorders from behavior influenced by medical or neurological disorders (e.g., dementia), role changes (e.g., recently widowed), and other changes in life context (e.g., moving to long-term care facility; Zweig, 2008).

Among older individuals with comorbid PDs and *DSM* Axis I disorders, the course of treatment may be slowed, complicated, and possibly impeded compared to individuals without Axis II disorders (Gradman, Thompson & Gallagher-Thompson, 1999). As there have been few treatment studies, it is not clear whether certain types of psychotherapy are more beneficial than others for individuals with PDs. In recent years, dialectical behavior therapy (DBT) has gained support in treating young adults with BPD (for a brief review, see Lieb et al., 2004), but it has not been widely examined as treatment for personality psychopathology among older adults. DBT was found to be effective in conjunction with medication to treat depression in older adults with comorbid PDs (Lynch et al., 2007).

Conclusions

Personality disorders reflect heterotypic continuity across the lifespan, in that certain symptoms (e.g., impulsivity) vary across the lifespan, while there are some stable, underlying personality characteristics. The stability in the underlying distress of personality disorders is evident as older adults with PDs experience more distress and are more difficult to treat compared to older adults without PDs. Contrary to the assumptions embedded in the diagnostic system, longitudinal studies suggest that BPD is more likely than not to remit across the lifespan. Additionally, individuals with BPD and ASPD may experience selective mortality, which is reflected by some cross-sectional research. Some researchers suggest that schizoid and OCPDs are more prevalent in late life. More longitudinal research is needed to elucidate the course of PDs across the lifespan and into old age.

Insomnia

A third of our life is spent sleeping, yet the important function that sleep plays in our daily lives goes largely unnoticed until our sleep becomes disturbed in some way. Older adults who suffer from sleep difficulties are at greater risk for falling because of fatigue, slower reaction times, and impaired daytime functioning associated with sleep impairment (Ancoli-Israel, Ayalono, & Salzman, 2008). Sleep disturbance has even been linked to elevated risk of mortality (Hardy & Studenski, 2008).

The most common sleep problem clinicians will encounter is insomnia. Insomnia is a diagnostic component of many other psychological and psychiatric disorders; furthermore, diagnoses such as mood and anxiety disorders have been linked to persistent poor sleep quality in longitudinal studies of older adults (Morgan, Healey, & Healey, 1989; Pigeon & Perlis, 2007). Although insomnia can occur at any point in the lifespan, rates increase by 200% around the seven and eighth decades, and insomnia was found to be present in 41% of women age 80 to 89 (Lichstein, Stone, Nau, McCrae, & Payne, 2006). In a large-scale study of adults age 65 and older, up to 34% reported symptoms of insomnia, and half of the women reported such symptomatology (Foley et al., 1995).

Description and Course

The *DSM–IV–TR* criteria for primary insomnia require difficulty sleeping for a minimum of 1 month, with some type of daytime dysfunction not due to drug or medication use or other psychological, medical, or sleep disorder (APA, 2000). In contrast, the *International Classification of Sleep Disorders*, a specialized system for classifying sleep disorders, specifies diagnostic criteria for insomnia that require difficulty sleeping when provided ample opportunity to do so and some type of daytime dysfunction (American Academy of Sleep Medicine, 2005). Subtypes of insomnia are classified according to the time of the night when the problem occurs. Sleep-onset insomnia is broadly defined by difficulty falling asleep, whereas maintenance insomnia is defined by an inability to stay asleep or by waking earlier than desired (Lichstein et al., 2006). Insomnia is often comorbid with other psychological and physical health problems, such as depression, anxiety, diabetes, and heart disease (Ancoli-Israel et al., 2008; Cooke & Ancoli-Israel, 2006; Lichstein et al., 2006).

Etiology

The predominant conceptual model of insomnia is the behavioral model presented by Spielman, Caruso, and Glovinsky (1987). Predisposing factors, which may be biological, psychological, or social, are thought to increase vulnerability to insomnia and interact with precipitating factors, such as acute stressors, in producing the acute phase of insomnia. Behavioral responses, such as extending sleep opportunity and using alcohol to induce sleep, tend to perpetuate the sleep difficulties, leading to chronic insomnia. Predisposing, precipitating, and perpetuating factors may vary in frequency across the lifespan.

Explanations for Age Differences

Changes in sleep continuity that occur with normal aging may predispose older adults to insomnia. Sleep latency, or the time it takes one to fall asleep once in bed, increases with age, becoming most pronounced after the age of 65 (for a meta-analysis, see Ohayon, Carskadon, Guilleminault, & Vitello, 2004). Total sleep time decreases by approximately 10 min for each decade of the lifespan (Ohayon et al., 2004). Additionally, time awake after sleep onset (WASO) also increases approximately 10 min each decade beginning at age 30 (Ohayon et al., 2004).

When examining sleep timing across the lifespan, a normative shift to earlier sleep onset is seen among older adults (Ancoli-Israel, 2005) and demonstrated by examining biochemical markers of sleep (Yoon et al., 2003). This phase shift has been associated with maintenance insomnia, such that older adults often attempt to remain awake until "normal" bedtimes, which are later than their biologically driven sleep-onset times. In tandem, the sleep period is shortened, causing daytime fatigue. Compared to earlier lifespan periods, older adults have more flexible schedules, allowing for "makeup" sleep via daytime naps, which serve to further complicate the advance sleep phase shift–insomnia relation (Yoon et al., 2003).

Assessment and Treatment

Assessment of insomnia often begins with complaints of trouble falling asleep, early awakening, or daytime fatigue at least 3 times per week, which can be documented using a sleep diary. Confirmation of sleep and wake activity levels can be done most cost efficiently by using an actigraph, which is worn on the wrist and measures motion. Effective interventions for insomnia include pharmacologic treatment with hypnotics, which are highly prescribed among older adults and are helpful in the short term, melatonin, and sedating antidepressants, for which evidence is mixed (Lichstein et al., 2006). Though hypnotics are most commonly prescribed for insomnia, there is longitudinal evidence that with long-term use, these drugs are ineffective and can exacerbate insomnia when patients cease taking them (Hohagen et al., 1993). Behavioral techniques that have demonstrated efficacy in treating insomnia, separately or as part of a multicomponent treatment, include stimulus control, which strengthens the association of the bed with sleep, and sleep restriction, which limits time in bed (Perlis, Jungquist, Smith, & Posner, 2005). Recent research has demonstrated that the most efficacious long-term treatment of insomnia is early combined treatment with behavioral and pharmacologic treatment with a phasing-out of pharmacologic aids (Morin et al., 2009).

Conclusions

Older adults are at elevated risk for insomnia (Ancoli-Israel, 2005). Insomnia has been linked to daytime sleepiness, which, if frequent enough, has been linked to serious consequences, including increased mortality rates (Morgan et al., 1989). Because treatment of sleep problems has been related to alleviation of comorbid symptomology, effective sleep treatments, such as behavioral treatments for insomnia, provide hope not only for those suffering from sleep disorders, but also those suffering from other diagnoses.

Dementia

In 2005, approximately 24 million people worldwide were suffering from some form of dementia (Ferri et al., 2005). Prevalence of dementia increases with age; rates for adults in their 60s are approximately 1.5%, with rates increasing to 15–25% for adults in their 80s. Although the underlying mechanisms are not fully understood, dementia is more common in females than in males (Shumaker et al., 2003). Life expectancy decreases with severity of dementia, especially for those older than 85 years, among whom dementia is a predictor of approximately 30% of all deaths in men and 50% of all deaths in women (Aevarsson, Svanborg, & Skoog, 1998). Alzheimer's disease (AD) is the most common type of dementia, accounting for approximately 60 to 80% of all dementia (Alzheimer's Association, 2011). Vascular dementia is the second most common form and has been estimated at 8 to 30% of all dementia cases (DiCarlo et al., 2002). Dementia with Lewy bodies has recently been recognized as a common form of dementia; it is estimated to account for up to 30% of all dementia cases (Williams, Xiong, Morris, & Galvin, 2006). Because AD accounts for the majority of dementia cases, we will focus solely on AD in this section.

Description and Course

According to the *DSM–IV–TR*, the essential features of dementia are memory impairments and progressive cognitive declines in one or more areas of intellectual functioning: aphasia (e.g., language deterioration), apraxia (e.g., impaired ability to complete motor activities), agnosia (e.g., failure to identify objects), or a disturbance in executive functioning (e.g., ability to think abstractly, execute a plan). Such declines in cognitive functioning must be severe enough to interfere with occupational and social functioning. To qualify for a diagnosis of Alzheimer's disease, the deficits cannot be due to any preexisting central nervous system disorder or any other disorder that is known to cause dementia.

Age of onset of AD is typically after age 65 and cognitive deterioration is slow and progressive. Survival time ranges from approximately 3 years (if diagnosed in 80s or 90s) to 7 to 10 years (if diagnosed in 60s and 70s; Cosentino, Scarmeas, Albert, & Stern, 2006). Defining features of AD are the presence of amyloid plaques, neurofibrillary tangles, and brain atrophy.

Etiology

AD involves the progressive deterioration of the cerebral cortex and the hippocampus, which is expressed clinically through impairment in memory and other cognitive abilities. Cognitive reserve capacity, conceptualized as the brain's ability to sustain the effects of injury or disease, varies across individuals and is thought to influence the extent and timing of the clinical expression of AD-related neuropathology (Borenstein, Copenhaver & Mortimer, 2006). As a result, it may be particularly helpful to distinguish between risk factors for neuropathology and risk factors for the clinical expression of AD.

Among risk factors thought to influence AD neuropathology directly, genetic vulnerability is the most prominent (Gatz et al., 2006). The e4 allele of the apolipoprotein (*APOE*) gene is well established as a risk factor for late-onset AD (most cases of AD are late onset; Farrer et al., 1997). *APOE4* is a susceptibility gene; that is, carrying one or two *APOE* e4 alleles does not mean an adult will, without a doubt, develop AD. Other risk factors include head trauma and cardiovascular disease (reviewed by Borenstein et al., 2006).

In contrast, evidence suggests that premorbid intelligence and education may be risk factors associated with the clinical expression of AD (Borenstein et al., 2006). Whalley, Deary, Appleton, and Starr (2004) demonstrated that premorbid childhood IQ acts as a protective factor against cognitive decline. More specifically, children with lower mental ability and fewer years of education tend to show greatest cognitive decline. The association between education level and AD is well established (DiCarlo et al., 2002). Gatz et al. (2007) reported that within adult twin pairs discordant for dementia, the twin with dementia had fewer years of education than the nondemented twin partner, and the effect was independent of genetic influences.

Some investigators suggest the "use it or lose it" hypothesis with respect to cognitive reserve (i.e., neurological resilience), proposing that mental activity and stimulation (e.g., doing crossword puzzles, staying socially engaged) may actually increase synaptic density in the brain and thereby enhance cognitive reserve (Orrell & Sahakian, 1995). The hypothesis is that those with greater cognitive reserves experience fewer cognitive deficits during the aging process (Whalley et al., 2004), but the impact on risk of dementia remains to be fully evaluated.

Explanations for Age Differences

Alzheimer's disease is a progressive neurodegenerative disease. As such, risk increases directly with advancing age. In addition, age-related conditions such as hypertension, high cholesterol, and cardiovascular disease may play a role in AD through causing damage to the vascular system. Furthermore, an overarching theme in the literature is the influence of cognitive reserve on the onset and progression of dementia (Borenstein et al., 2006). Premorbid intelligence is an indicator of cognitive reserve. Cognitive reserve may even have an influence on cognition after a diagnosis of AD has been made (Starr & Lonie, 2008).

Assessment and Treatment

The assessment of AD currently involves neuropsychological testing to evaluate memory and cognitive impairments, as well as a somatic examination and neuroimaging to rule out alternative explanations for the impairment. Autopsy studies validate that this method can be highly accurate (Gatz et al., 2006). Advances in neuroimaging technology, which have recently made it possible to view AD-related neuropathology (amyloid plaques), have made it possible to evaluate factors that affect the clinical expression of AD independent of the neuropathology (Roe et al., 2010). Although this type of neuroimaging may also be helpful in diagnosing AD, diagnostic accuracy is improved by including measures associated with the clinical expression of the disease (Roe et al., 2010).

There are no published interventions for the primary prevention of dementia (Stephan & Brayne, 2008), and there are no available treatments to slow or reverse the progression of brain deterioration in AD. However, the U.S. Food and Drug Administration (FDA) has approved several drugs that can ameliorate symptoms for up to 12 months (Massoud & Gauthier, 2010). The acetyl cholinesterase inhibitors (AChE), such as donepezil (Aricept), have been shown to improve cognition and functioning in mild to moderate AD, whereas the *N*-methyl-d-aspartate receptor antagonist (NMDA) memantine (Namenda) has demonstrated similar outcomes in mild to severely impaired patients (Massoud & Gauthier, 2010). Over 90 clinical trials are investigating experimental therapies on slowing the progression of AD (Alzheimer's Association, 2010).

Although no preventive treatments exist, when examining protective factors, education is consistently found to buffer against age of onset and progression of dementia (DiCarlo et al., 2002). Moreover, clinicians typically focus on preventive treatments of cardiovascular disease, such as controlling modifiable risk factors (e.g., cholesterol levels, blood pressure, and diabetes; Rockwood, 2002). Prevention of such chronic conditions can be achieved through regular exercise, maintaining weight, and lowering blood pressure and cholesterol levels.

Further, because amyloid plaques and neurofibrillary tangles are the hallmark of AD, drug trials aimed at influencing the development of these substances are under way.

Conclusions

Alzheimer's disease is a progressive neurodegenerative disorder that affects almost exclusively older adults. Highly accurate assessment and diagnosis is currently possible, and new methods are on the horizon. Currently available treatments reduce symptom severity and improve functioning.

Psychopathology in Late Life

There is evidence of both similarity and difference in psychopathology in late life relative to earlier ages. Contrary to popular stereotype, late life is associated with lower prevalence of many types of psychopathology, including anxiety disorders, major depressive disorder, bipolar disorder, schizophrenia, alcohol use disorders, and some types of PD. There is longitudinal evidence of attenuation of symptom severity or even remission for most of these disorders. These outcomes are consistent with the improved emotion regulation that has been documented in late life. It is also possible, however, that lower rates of disorder in late life may be a methodological artifact rather than reflecting a true age-related decline. Symptom presentation of many of the disorders differs in older adults compared to younger adults, such that diagnostic rubrics established to describe disorders in younger populations may not capture these disorders when they appear in older populations. In some cases, symptoms may attenuate slightly, such that diagnostic criteria are no longer met, but they remain problematic for the patient. For example, subthreshold depressive and anxiety symptoms are common in late life. Further, selective mortality may explain some of the apparent decline in prevalence of some of these disorders (bipolar, major depressive disorder, substance use disorders, schizophrenia). More research, including longitudinal designs, will be needed to tease apart these alternative explanations.

In contrast to the disorders that appear to decline in prevalence with age, there are several disorders that increase in prevalence with age, including dementia, sleep disorders, select PD, and suicide. Biological changes associated with aging, which are associated with an increased likelihood of executive dysfunction and other cognitive deficits, may explain not only dementia but also other disorders that are linked to cognitive functioning, such as OCPD. Age-related changes in the circadian rhythm have been implicated in increased rates of insomnia. Of note, however, is that biological aging is not always associated with increases in disorder (e.g., changes in metabolism with age can lead to reductions in problem drinking). In addition, behavioral and environmental factors may contribute to increased prevalence of certain disorders in late life. For example, schedule flexibility in old age and sleep-related behaviors may perpetuate insomnia; habituation to painful or provocative experiences may increase risk of highly lethal suicidal behavior; and social role changes may precipitate change in alcohol use.

The assessment of psychopathology in older adults can be challenging due to differences in symptom presentation and comorbid physical illnesses. Age-specific instruments are available for some but not all disorders. Many of the same treatments that have demonstrated efficacy in adult populations have also been shown to work in older adults, and several treatments have been developed specifically for older adults. Nonetheless, outcome research within this age group is scarce.

Increasingly, longitudinal research has begun to reshape our understanding of psychopathology in late life. Additional longitudinal research is needed to elucidate the trajectories of psychopathology across the lifespan. Future research focused on older adults who do not manifest psychopathology in spite of risk factors could be particularly helpful in uncovering protective factors. Finally, assessment and treatment outcome research with a focus on older adults is needed. Considering the impending expansion of the older adult population, this type of research could not be more timely.

References

Aevarson, O., Svanborg, A., & Skoog, I. (1998). Seven-year survival rate after age 85 years: Relation to Alzheimer disease and vascular dementia. *Archival Neurology, 55*, 1226–1232.

Agronin, M., & Maletta, G. (2000). Personality disorders in late life: Understanding the gap in research. *American Journal of Geriatric Psychiatry, 8*, 4–18.

Alzheimer's Association. (2010). Alzheimer's disease facts and figures. *Alzheimer's and Dementia, 6*, 1–74.

Alzheimer's Association. (2011). Alzheimer's disease facts and figures, *Alzheimer's & Dementia, 7*.

American Academy of Sleep Medicine. (2005). *The international classification of sleep disorders: Diagnostic and coding manual* (2nd ed.). Westchester, IL: Author.

American Psychiatric Association. (2000). *Diagnostic and statistical manual of mental disorders* (4th ed., text rev.). Washington, DC: Author.

American Psychiatric Association. (2010). *American Psychiatric Association DSM-5 development*. Retrieved from http://www.dsm5.org/ProposedRevision/Pages/proposedrevision.aspx?rid=167.

Ancoli-Israel, S. (2005). Normal human sleep at different ages: Sleep in the older adult. In M. R. Opp (Ed.), *SRS basics of sleep guide* (pp. 21–26). Westchester, IL: Sleep Research Society.

Ancoli-Israel, S., Ayalon, L., & Salzman, C. (2008). Sleep in the elderly: Normal variations and common sleep disorders. *Harvard Review of Psychiatry, 16*, 279–286.

Angst, F., Stassen, H. H., Clayton, P. J., & Angst, J. (2002). Mortality of patients with mood disorders: Follow-up over 34–38 years. *Journal of Affective Disorders, 68*, 167–181.

Atkinson, R. M., Tolson, R. L., & Turner, J. A. (1993). Factors affecting outpatient treatment compliance of older male problem drinkers. *Journal of Studies on Alcohol, 54*, 102–106.

Auslander, L. A., & Jeste, D. V. (2004). Sustained remission of schizophrenia among community-dwelling older outpatients. *American Journal of Psychiatry, 161*, 1490–1493.

Ayers, C. R., Sorrell, J. T., Thorp, S. R., & Wetherell, J. L. (2007). Evidence-based psychological treatments for late-life anxiety. *Psychology and Aging, 22*, 8–17.

Balsis, S., Gleason, M. E., Woods, C. M., & Oltmanns, T. F. (2007). An item response theory analysis of DSM-IV personality disorder criteria across younger and older age groups. *Psychology and Aging, 22*(1), 171–185.

Balsis, S., Woods, C. M., Gleason, M. E., & Oltmanns, T. F. (2007). Overdiagnosis and underdiagnosis of personality disorders in older adults. *American Journal of Geriatric Psychiatry, 15*, 742–753.

Baltes, P. B., & Baltes, M. M. (1990). Psychological perspectives on successful aging: The model of selective optimization with compensation. In P. B. Baltes & M. M. Baltes (Eds.), *Successful aging: Perspectives from behavioral sciences* (pp. 1–34). Cambridge, MA: Cambridge University Press.

Barlow, D. H. (2002). The experience of anxiety: Shadow of intelligence or specter of death? In D. H. Barlow (Ed.), *Anxiety and its disorders: The nature and treatment of anxiety and panic* (pp. 1–36). New York: Guilford.

Barr, C. E., Mednick, S. A., & Munk-Jörgensen, P. (1990). Exposure to influenza epidemics during gestation and adult schizophrenia: A 40-year study. *Archives of General Psychiatry, 47*, 869–874.

Bearden, C. E., Meyer, S. E., Loewy, R. L., Niendam, T. A., & Cannon, T. (2006). The neurodevelopmental model of schizophrenia: Updated. In D. Cicchetti & D. J. Cohen (Eds.), *Developmental psychopathology* (2nd ed., Vol. 3, pp. 542–569). Hoboken, NJ: Wiley.

Beautrais, A. L. (2002). A case control study of suicide and attempted suicide in older adults. *Suicide and Life-Threatening Behavior, 32*, 1–9.

Beekman, A. T. F., Bremmer, M. A., Deeg, D. J., van Balkom, A. J., Smit, J. H., de Beurs, E., … van Tilburg, W. (1998). Anxiety disorders in later life: a report from the longitudinal aging study Amsterdam. *International Journal of Geriatric Psychiatry, 13*, 717–726.

Beekman, A. T. F., de Beurs, E., van Balkom, A. J. L. M., Deeg, D. J. H., van Dyck, R., & van Tilburg, W. (2000). Anxiety and depression in later life: Co-occurrence and communality of risk factors. *American Journal of Psychiatry, 157*, 89–95.

Beyer, J. L. (2007). Managing depression in geriatric populations. *Annals of Clinical Psychiatry, 19*, 221–228.

Black, D. W., Baumgard, C. H., & Bell, S. E. (1995). A 16- to 45-year follow-up of 71 men with antisocial personality disorder. *Comprehensive Psychiatry, 36*, 130–140.

Blazer, D. G., & Wu, L. (2009). The epidemiology of at-risk and binge drinking among middle-aged and elderly community adults: National survey on drug use and health. *American Journal of Psychiatry, 166*, 1162–1169.

Blow, F. C., Walton, M. A., Chermack, S. T., Mudd, S. A., & Brower, K. J. (2000). Older adult treatment outcome following elder-specific inpatient alcoholism treatment. *Journal of Substance Abuse Treatment, 19*, 67–75.

Borenstein, A. R., Copenhaver, C. I., & Mortimer, J. A. (2006). Early-life risk factors for Alzheimer disease. *Alzheimer Disease and Associated Disorders, 20*, 63–72.

Brennan, P. L., Schutte, K. K., & Moos, R. H. (2005). Pain and use of alcohol to mange pain: Prevalence and 3-year outcomes among older problem and non-problem drinkers. *Addiction, 100*, 777–786.

Brodaty, H., Luscombe, G., Parker, G., Wilhelm, K., Hickie, I., Austin, M. P., & Mitchell, P. (2001). Early and late onset depression in old age: Different aetologies, same phenomenology. *Journal of Affective Disorders, 66*, 225–236.

Bruce, M. L., McAvay, G. J., Raue, P. J., Brown, E. L., Meyers, B. S., Keohane, D. J., … Weber, C. (2002). Major depression in elderly home health care patients. *American Journal of Psychiatry, 159*, 1367–1374.

Bruce, M. L., Ten Have, T. R., Reynolds, C. F. III, Katz, I. R., Schulberg, H. C., Mulsant, B. H., … Alexopoulos, G. S. (2004). Reducing suicidal ideation and depressive symptoms in depressed older primary care patients: A randomized controlled trial. *JAMA, 291*, 1081–1091.

Carstensen, L. L., Isaacowitz, D. M., & Charles, S. T. (1999). Taking time seriously: A theory of socioemotional selectivity. *American Psychologist, 54*, 165–181.

Charles, S. T., Reynolds, C. A., & Gatz, M. (2001). Age-related differences and change in positive and negative affect over 23 years. *Journal of Personality and Social Psychology, 80*, 136–151.

Christensen, H., Jorm, A. F., Mackinnon, A. J., Korten, A. E., Jacomb, P. A., Henderson, A. S., & Rodgers, B. (1999). Age differences in depression and anxiety symptoms: A structural equation modeling analysis of data from a general population sample. *Psychological Medicine, 29*, 325–339.

Cicchetti, D., & Toth, S. L. (2009). The past achievements and future promises of developmental psychopathology: The coming of age of a discipline. *Journal of Child Psychiatry and Psychiatry, 50*, 16–25.

Cicero, D. C., Epler, A. J., & Sher, K. J. (2009). Are there developmentally limited forms of bipolar disorder? *Journal of Abnormal Psychology, 118*, 431–447.

Clarkin, J. F., Spielman, L. A., & Klausner, E. (1999). Conceptual overview of personality disorders in the elderly. In E. Rosowsky, R. C. Abrams, & R. A. Zweig (Eds.), *Personality disorders in older adults: Emerging issues in diagnosis and treatment* (pp. 3–15). Mahwah, NJ: Erlbaum.

Cohen, C. I. (1990). Outcome of schizophrenia into later life: An overview. *Gerontologist, 30*, 790–797.

Cole, M. G., & Dendukuri, N. (2004). The feasibility and effectiveness of brief interventions to prevent depression in older subjects: A systematic review. *Journal of Geriatric Psychiatry, 19*, 1019–1025.

Cooke, J. R., & Ancoli-Israel, S. (2006). Sleep and its disorders in older adults. *Psychiatric Clinics of North America, 29*, 1077–1093.

Cosentino, S., Scarmeas, N., Albert, S., & Stern, Y. (2006). Verbal fluency predicts mortality in Alzheimer disease. *Cognitive Behavioral Neurology, 19*, 123–129.

Cui, X., Lyness, J. M., Tang, W., Tu, X., & Conwell, Y. (2008). Outcomes and predictors of late-life depression trajectories in older primary care patients. *American Journal of Geriatric Psychiatry, 16*, 406–415.

D'Amico, E. J., Paddock, S. M., Burnam, A., & King, F. (2005). Identification of and guidance for problem drinking by general medical providers. *Medical Care, 43*, 229–236.

Dent, O. F., Waite, L. M., Bennett, H. P., Casey, B. J., Grayson, D. A., Cullen, J. S., ... Broe, G. A. (1999). A longitudinal study of chronic disease and depressive symptoms in a community sample of older people. *Aging and Mental Health, 3,* 351–357.

DeWit, D. J., Adlaf, E. M., Offord, D. R., & Ogbrone, A. C. (2000). Age at first alcohol use: A risk factor for the development of alcohol disorders. *American Journal of Psychiatry, 157,* 745–750.

DiCarlo, A., Baldereschi, M., Amaducci, L., Lepore, V., Bracco, L., Maggi, S., ... ILSA Working Group. (2002). Incidence of dementia, Alzheimer disease, and vascular dementia in Italy. The ILSA study. *Journal of the American Geriatrics Society, 50,* 41–48.

Driscoll, H. C., Basinski, J., Mulsant, B. H., Butters, M. A., Dew, M. A., Houck, P. R., ... Reynolds, C. F. (2005). Late-onset major depression: Clinical and treatment-response variability. *International Journal of Geriatric Psychiatry, 20,* 661–667.

Edelstein, B. A., Heisel, M. J., McKee, D. R., Martin, R. R., Koven, L. P., Duberstein, P. R., & Britton, P. C. (2009). Development and psychometric evaluation of the reasons for living—older adults scale: A suicide risk assessment inventory. *Gerontologist, 49,* 736–745.

Engels, G. I., Duijsens, I. J., Haringsma, R., & van Putten, C. M. (2003). Personality disorders in the elderly compared to four younger age groups: A cross-sectional study of community residents and mental health patients. *Journal of Personality Disorders, 17,* 447–459.

Farrer, L. A., Cupples, L. A., Haines, J. L., Hyman, B., Kukull, W. A., Mayeux, R., ... van Duijn, C. M. (1997). Effects of age, sex, and ethnicity on the association between apolipoprotein E genotype and Alzheimer's disease: A meta-analysis. APOE and Alzheimer Disease Meta Analysis Consortium. *JAMA, 278,* 1349–1356.

Federal Interagency Forum on Aging-Related Statistics. (2010, July). *Older Americans 2010: Key indicators of well-being.* Washington, DC: U.S. Government Printing Office.

Ferri, C., Prince, M., Brayne, C., Brodaty, H., Fratiglioni, L., Ganguli, M., ... Alzheimer's Disease International. (2005). Global prevalence of dementia: A Delphi consensus study. *Lancet, 366,* 2112–2117.

Fiske, A., & O'Riley, A. (2008). Late life depression. In J. D. Hunsley & A. J. Mash (Eds.), *A guide to assessments that work* (pp. 138–157). New York: Oxford University Press.

Fiske, A., O'Riley, A. A., & Widoe, R. K. (2008). Physical health and suicide in late life: An evaluative review. *Clinical Geropsychologist, 31*(4), 31–50.

Fiske, A., Wetherell, J. L., & Gatz, M. (2009). Depression in older adults. *Annual Review of Clinical Psychology, 5,* 363–389.

Foley, D. J., Monjan, A. A., Brown, S. L., Simonsick, E. M., Wallace, R. B., & Blazer, D. G. (1995). Sleep complaints among elderly persons: An epidemiologic study of three communities. *Sleep, 18,* 425–432.

Folsom, D. P., Depp, C., Palmer, B.W., Golshan, S., Cardenas, V., Kraemer, H. C., ... Jeste, D. V. (2009). Physical and mental health-related quality of life among older people with schizophrenia. *Schizophrenia Research, 108,* 207–213.

Fremouw, W., McCoy, K., Tyner, E. A., & Musick, R. (2009). Suicidal older adult protocol—SOAP. In J. B. Allen, E. M. Wolf, & L. VandeCreek (Eds.), *Innovations in clinical practice: A 21st century sourcebook* (Vol. 1, pp. 203–212). Sarasota, FL: Professional Resource Press/Professional Resource Exchange.

Fried, L. P., Kronmal, R. A., Newman, A. B., Bild, D. E., Mittelmark, M. B., Polak, J., Robbins, J. A., & Gardin, J. M. (1998). Risk factors for 5-year mortality in older adults: The cardiovascular health study. *Journal of the American Medical Association, 278,* 585–592.

Gallo, J. J., Anthony, J. C., & Muthén, B. O. (1994). Age differences in the symptoms of depression: A latent trait analysis. *Journals of Gerontology, 49,* P251–P264.

Gatz, M., Kasl-Godley, J. E., & Karel, M. J. (1996). Aging and mental disorders. In J. E. Birren & K. W. Schaie (Eds.), *Handbook of the psychology of aging* (4th ed., pp. 365–382). San Diego, CA: Academic Press.

Gatz, M., Mortimer, J. A., Fratiglioni, L., Johansson, B., Berg, S., Andel, R., ... Pedersen, N. L. (2007). Accounting for the relationship between low education and dementia: A twin study. *Physiology and Behavior, 92,* 232–237.

Gatz, M., Reynolds, C. A., Fratiglioni, L., Johansson, B., Mortimer, J. A., Berg, S., ... Pedersen, N. L. (2006). The role of genes and environments for explaining Alzheimer's disease. *Archives of General Psychiatry, 63,* 168–174.

Gottesman, I. I., & Hanson, D. R. (2005). Human development: biological and genetic processes. *Annual Review of Psychology, 56,* 263–286.

Gradman, T. J., Thompson, L. W., & Gallagher-Thompson, D. (1999). Personality disorders and treatment outcome. In E. Rosowsky, R. C. Abrams, & R. A. Zweig (Eds.), *Personality disorders in older adults: Emerging issues in diagnosis and treatment* (pp. 69–94). Mahwah, NJ: Erlbaum.

Granholm, E., McQuaid, J. R., McClure, F. S., Auslander, L. A., Perivoliotis, D., Pedrelli, P., & Jeste, D. V. (2005). A randomized, controlled trial of cognitive behavioral social skills training for middle-aged and older outpatients with chronic schizophrenia. *American Journal of Psychiatry, 162,* 520–529.

Grant, B. F., & Dawson, D. A. (1997). Age at onset of alcohol use and its association with DSM-IV alcohol abuse and dependence: Results from the national longitudinal alcohol epidemiologic survey. *Journal of Substance Abuse, 9,* 103–110.

Gum, A. M., King-Kallimanis, B., & Kohn, R. (2009). Prevalence of mood, anxiety, and substance-abuse disorders for older Americans in the National Comorbidity Survey-Replication. *American Journal of Geriatric Psychiatry, 17,* 769–781.

Häfner, H., Maurer, K., Löffler, W., Heiden, W., Munk-Jørgensen, P., & Hambrecht, M. (1998). The ABC schizophrenia study: A preliminary overview of the results. *Social Psychiatry and Psychiatric Epidemiology, 33,* 380–386.

Han, B., Gfroerer, J. C., Colliver, J. D., & Penne, M. A. (2009). Substance use disorder among older adults in the United States in 2020. *Addiction, 104,* 88–96.

Hardy, S. E., & Studenski, S. A. (2008). Fatigue predicts mortality in older adults. *Journal of the American Geriatric Society, 56,* 1910–1914.

Hasin, D. S., Goodwin, R. D., Stinson, F. S., & Grant, B. F. (2005). Epidemiology of major depressive disorder: Results from the National Epidemiologic Survey on Alcoholism and Related Conditions. *Archives of General Psychiatry, 62,* 1097–1106.

Heisel, M. J., & Flett, G. L. (2006). The development and initial validation of the Geriatric Suicide Ideation scale. *American Journal of Geriatric Psychiatry, 14,* 742–751.

Hetzel, L., & Smith, A. (2001). *The 65 years and over population: 2000–Census 2000 Brief.* Washington, DC: U.S. Census Bureau.

Hohagen, F., Rink, K., Kappler, C., Schramm, E., Riemann, D., Weyerer, S., & Berger, M. (1993). Prevalence and treatment of insomnia in general practice: A longitudinal study. *European Archives of Psychiatry and Clinical Neuroscience, 242,* 329–336.

Howard, R., Almeida, O., & Raymond, L. (1994). Phenomenology, demography and diagnosis in late paraphrenia. *Psychological Medicine, 24,* 97–410.

Howard, R., Rabins, C., Seeman, F. D. Jeste, D. V., & the International Late-Onset Schizophrenia Group. (2000). Late-onset schizophrenia and very-late-onset schizophrenia-like psychosis: An international consensus. *American Journal of Psychiatry, 157,* 172–178.

Hunkeler, E. M., Katon, W., Tang, L., Williams, J. W. Jr, Kroenke, K., Lin, E. H., … Unützer J. (2006). Long term outcomes from the IMPACT randomised trial for depressed elderly patients in primary care. *British Medical Journal (Clinical Research Edition), 332,* 259–263.

Jacobziner, H. (1965). Attempted suicides in adolescence. *Journal of the American Medical Association, 191,* 7–11.

Jamison, K. R. (2000). Suicide and bipolar disorder. *Journal of Clinical Psychiatry, 61,* 47–51.

Jason, L. A., Davis, M. I., Ferrari, J. R., & Bishop, P. D. (2001). Oxford house: A review of research and implications for substance abuse recovery and community research. *Journal of Drug Education, 31,* 1–27.

Jeste, D., Alexopoulos, G. S., Bartels, S. J., Cummings, J. L., Gallo, J. J., Gottlieb, G. L., … Lebowitz, B. D. (1999). Consensus statement on the upcoming crisis in geriatric mental health: Research agenda for the next 2 decades. *Archives of General Psychiatry, 56,* 848–853.

Jeste, D. V., & Nasrallah, H. A. (2003). Schizophrenia and aging: No more dearth of data? *American Journal of Geriatric Psychiatry, 11,* 584–587.

Jeste, D. V., Twamley, E. W., Eyler, B., Zorrilla, L. T., Golshan, S., Patterson, T. L., & Palmer, B. W. (2003). Aging and outcome in schizophrenia. *Acta Psychiatrica Scandinavica,107,* 336–343.

Jobe, T. H., & Harrow, M. (2010). Schizophrenia course, long-term outcome, recovery, and prognosis. *Current Directions in Psychological Science, 19,* 220–225.

Johnson, I. (2000). Alcohol problems in old age: A review of recent epidemiological research. *International Journal of Geriatric Psychiatry, 15,* 575–581.

Joiner, T. (2005). *Why people die by suicide.* Cambridge, MA: Harvard University Press.

Kernberg, O. (1987). *Severe personality disorders: Psychotherapeutic strategies.* New Haven, CT: Yale University Press.

Kerr, W. C., Fillmore, K. M., & Bostrom, A. (2002). Stability of alcohol consumption over time: Evidence from three longitudinal surveys from the United States. *Journal of Studies on Alcohol and Drugs, 63,* 325–333.

Kessler, R. C., Foster, C., Webster, P. S., & House, J. S. (1992). The relationship between age and depressive symptoms in two national surveys. *Psychology and Aging, 7,* 119–126.

Kroessler, D. (1990). Personality disorder in the elderly. *Hospital and Community Psychiatry, 41,* 1325–1329.

Lawrence, D., Almeida, O. P., Hulse, G. K., Jablensky, A. V., & Holman, D. J. (2000). Suicide and attempted suicide among older adults in Western Australia. *Psychological Medicine, 30,* 813–321.

Lenze, E. J., Mulsant, B. H., Shear, M. K., Schulberg, H. C., Dew, M. A., Begley, A., ... Reynolds, C. F. III (2000). Comorbid anxiety disorders in depressed elderly patients. *American Journal of Psychiatry, 157,* 722–728.

Lichstein, K. L., Stone, K. C., Nau, S. D., McCrae, C. S., & Payne, K. L. (2006). Insomnia in the elderly. *Sleep Medicine Clinics, 1,* 221–229.

Lieb, K., Zanarini, M. C., Schmahl, C., Linehan, M. M., & Bohus, M. (2004). Borderline personality disorder. *Lancet, 364*(9432), 453–461.

Littlefield, A. K., Sher, K. J., & Wood, P. K. (2009). Is "maturing out" of problematic alcohol involvement related to personality change? *Journal of Abnormal Psychology, 118,* 360–374.

Luoma, J. B., Martin, C. E., & Pearson, J. L. (2002). Contact with mental health and primary care providers before suicide: A review of the evidence. *American Journal of Psychiatry, 159,* 909–916.

Lynch, T. R., Cheavens, J. S., Cukrowicz, K. C., Thorp, S. R., Bronner, L., & Beyer, J. (2007). Treatment of older adults with co-morbid personality disorder and depression: A dialectical behavior therapy approach. *International Journal of Geriatric Psychiatry, 22,* 131–143.

Massoud, F., & Gauthier, S. (2010). Update on the pharmacological treatment of Alzheimer's disease. *Current Neuropharmacology, 8,* 68–80.

Merrick, E. L., Horgan, C. M., Hodgkin, D., Garnick, D. W., Houghton, S. F. Panas, L., ... Blow, F. C. (2008). Unhealthy drinking patterns in older adults: Prevalence and associated characteristics. *Journal of the American Geriatrics Society, 56,* 214–223.

Moore, A. A., Giuli, L., Gould, R., Hu, P., Zhou, K., Reuben, D., Greendale, G., & Karlamangla, A. (2006). Alcohol use, comorbidity, and mortality. *Journal of American Geriatric Society, 54,* 757–762.

Moos, R. H., Brennan, P. L., & Mertens, J. R. (1994). Mortality rates and predictors of mortality among late-middle-aged and older substance abuse patients. *Clinical and Experimental Research, 18,* 187–195.

Moos, R. H., Finney, J. W., & Cronkite, R. C. (1990). *Alcoholism treatment: Context, process, and outcome.* New York: Oxford University Press.

Moos, R. H., Schutte, K. K., Brennan, P. L., & Moos, B. S. (2009). Older adults' alcohol consumption and late-life drinking problems: A 20-year perspective. *Addiction, 104,* 1293–1302.

Morgan, K., Healey, D. W., & Healey, P. J. (1989). Factors influencing persistent subjective insomnia in old age: A follow-up study of good and poor sleepers aged 65 to 74. *Age and Ageing, 18,* 117–122.

Morin, C. M., Vallieres, A., Guay, B., Ivers, H., Savard, J., Merette, C., ... Baillargeon, L. (2009). Cognitive behavioral therapy, singly and combined with medication, for persistent insomnia: A randomized controlled trial. *Journal of the American Medical Association, 301,* 2005–2015.

Nguyen, H. T., & Zonderman, A. B. (2006). Relationship between age and aspects of depression: Consistency and reliability across two longitudinal studies. *Psychology and Aging, 21,* 119–126.

Ohayon, M. M., Carskadon, M. A., Guilleminault, C., & Vitiello, M. V. (2004). Healthy individuals: Developing normative sleep values across the human lifespan. *Sleep, 27,* 1255–1273.

Ollendick, T. H., & Byrd, D. A. (2001). Anxiety disorders. In M. Hersen & V. B. Van Hasselt (Eds.), *Advanced abnormal psychology* (pp. 223–242). New York: Springer.

Orrell, M., & Sahakian, B. (1995). Education and dementia: Research evidence supports the concept "use it or lose it." *British Medical Journal, 310,* 951–952.

Oslin, D. W. (2004). Late-life alcoholism: Issues relevant to the geriatric psychiatrist. *American Journal of Geriatric Psychiatry, 12,* 571–583.

Oslin, D. W., Pettinati, H., & Volpicelli, J. R. (2002). Alcoholism treatment adherence: Older age predicts better adherence and drinking outcomes. *American Journal of Geriatric Psychiatry, 10,* 740–747.

Palmer, B. W., Bondi, M. W., Twamley, E. W., Thal, L., Shahrokh, G., & Jeste, D. V. (2003). Are late-onset schizophrenia spectrum disorders neurodegenerative conditions? Annual rates of change on two dementia measures. *Journal of Neuropsychiatry and Clinical Neurosciences, 15*(1), 45–52.

Palmer, B. W., Jeste, D. V., & Sheikh, J. I. (1997). Anxiety disorders in the elderly: DSM-IV and other barriers to diagnosis and treatment. *Journal of Affective Disorders, 46*(3), 183–190.

Paris, J., & Zweig-Frank, H. (2001). The 27-year follow-up of patients with borderline personality disorder. *Comprehensive Psychiatry, 42*, 482–487.

Patterson, T. L., & Jeste, D. V. (1999). The potential impact of the baby-boom generation on substance abuse among elderly persons. *Psychiatric Services, 50*, 1184–1188.

Penninx, B. W. J. H., Geerlings, S. W., Deeg, D. J. H., van Eijk, J. T. M., van Tilburg, W., & Beekman, A. T. F. (1999). Minor and major depression and the risk of death in older persons. *Archives of General Psychiatry, 56*, 889–893.

Perlis, M. L., Jungquist, C., Smith, M. T., & Posner, D. (2005). *Cognitive behavioral treatment of insomnia: A session-by-session guide.* New York: Springer.

Pigeon, W. R., & Perlis, M. L. (2007). Insomnia and depression: Birds of a feather? *International Journal of Sleep Disorders, 1*, 82–91.

Pinquart, M., Duberstein, P. R., & Lyness, J. M. (2006). Treatments for later-life depressive conditions: A meta-analytic comparison of pharmacotherapy and psychotherapy. *American Journal of Psychiatry, 163*, 1493–1501.

Qualls, S. H., Segal, D. L., Norman, S., Niederehe, G., & Gallagher-Thompson, D. (2002). Psychologists in practice with older adults: Current patterns, sources of training, and need for continuing education. *Professional Psychology: Research and Practice, 33*, 435–442.

Rabins, P. V. (2003). Long-term follow-up and phenomenologic differences distinguish among late-onset schizophrenia, late-life depression, and progressive dementia. *American Journal of Geriatric Psychiatry, 11*, 589–594.

Rockwood, K. (2002). Vascular cognitive impairment and vascular dementia. *Journal of the Neurological Sciences, 203*, 23–27.

Roe, C. M., Mintun, M. A., Ghoshal, N., Williams, M. M., Grant, E. A., Marcus, D. S., & Morris, J. C. (2010). Alzheimer disease identification using amyloid imaging and reserve variables: Proof of concept. *Neurology, 75*, 42–48.

Roemer, L., Orsille, S. M., & Barlow, D. H. (2002). Generalized anxiety disorder. In D. H. Barlow (Ed.), *Anxiety and its disorders: The nature and treatment of anxiety and panic* (pp. 477–515). New York: Guilford.

Sadavoy, J. (1987). Character disorders in the elderly: An overview. In J. Sadavoy and M. Lesczc (Eds.), *Treating the elderly with psychotherapy: The scope for change in later life* (pp. 175–229). Madison, CT: International Universities Press.

Sattar, S. P., Petty, F., & Burke, W. J. (2003). Diagnosis and treatment of alcohol dependence in older alcoholics. *Clinics in Geriatric Medicine, 19*, 743–761.

Samuelsson, G., McCamish-Svensson, C., Hagberg, B., Sundström, G., & Dehlin, O. (2005). Incidence and risk factors for depression and anxiety disorders: Results from a 34-year longitudinal Swedish cohort study. *Aging and Mental Health, 9*, 571–575.

Santos, J. F., & VandenBos, G. R. (Eds.). (1982). *Psychology and the older adult: Challenges for Training in the 1980's.* Washington, DC: American Psychological Association.

Savla, G., Moore, D. J., Roesch, S. C., Heaton, R. K., Jeste, D. V., & Palmer, B. W. (2006). A evaluation of longitudinal neurocognitive performance among middle-aged and older schizophrenia patients: Use of mixed-model analyses. *Schizophrenia Research, 83*, 215–223.

Schoevers, R. A., Beekman, A. T. F., Deeg, D. J. H., Hooijer, C., Jonker, C., & van Tilburg, W. (2003). The natural history of late-life depression: Results from the Amsterdam Study of the Elderly (AMSTEL). *Journal of Affective Disorders, 76*, 5–14.

Schoevers, R. A., Deeg, D. J., van Tilburg, W., & Beekman, A. T. F. (2005). Depression and generalized anxiety disorder: Co-occurrence and longitudinal patterns in elderly patients, *American Journal of Geriatric Psychiatry, 13*, 31–39.

Schonfield, L., & Dupree, L. W. (1991). Antecedents of drinking for early- and late-onset elderly alcohol abusers. *Journal of Studies on Alcohol and Drugs, 52*, 587–592.

Scogin, F., Welsh, D., Hanson, A., Stump, J., & Coates, A. (2005). Evidence-based psychotherapies for depression in older adults. *Psychological Science and Practice, 12*, 222–237.

Segal, D. L., Hook, J. N., & Coolidge, F. L. (2001). Personality dysfunction, coping styles, and clinical symptoms in younger and older adults. *Journal of Clinical Geropsychology, 7*, 201–212.

Segal, D. L., Qualls, S. H., & Smyer, M. A. (2011). *Aging and mental health* (2nd ed.). Hoboken, NJ: Wiley-Blackwell.

Sheikh, J. I., & Cassidy, E. L. (2000). Treatment of anxiety disorders in the elderly: Issues and strategies. *Journal of Anxiety Disorders, 14*, 173–190.

Shumaker, S., Legault, C., Thal, L., Wallace, R., Ockene, J., Hendrix, S., … WHIMS Investigators. (2003). Estrogen plus progestin and the incidence of dementia and mild cognitive impairment in postmenopausal women. *Journal of the American Medical Association, 289*, 2651–2662.

Silverman, M. M., Berman, A. L., Sanddal, N. D., O'Carroll, P. W., & Joiner, T. E. (2007). Rebuilding the tower of Babel: A revised nomenclature for the study of suicide and suicidal behaviors. Part 2: Suicide-related ideations, communications, and behaviors. *Suicide and Life-Threatening Behavior, 37*, 264–277.

Skodol, A. E., Gunderson, J. G., Shea, M. T., McGlashan, T. H., Morey, L. C., Sanislow, C. A., … Stout, R. L. (2005). The collaborative longitudinal personality disorders study (CLPS): Overview and implications. *Journal of Personality Disorders, 19*, 487–504.

Sneed, J. R., Kasen, S., & Cohen, P. (2007). Early-life risk factors for late-onset depression. *International Journal of Geriatric Psychiatry, 22*, 663–667.

Solomon, K. (1981). Personality disorders in the elderly. In J. R. Lion (Ed.), *Personality disorders, diagnosis, and management* (pp. 310–338). Baltimore, MD: Williams & Wilkins.

Spar, J. E., & LaRue, A. (1990). *Geriatric psychiatry*. Washington, DC: American Psychiatric Press.

Spielman, A., Caruso, L., & Glovinsky, P. (1987). A behavioral perspective on insomnia treatment. *Psychiatric Clinics of North America, 10*, 541–553.

Sroufe, L. A., & Rutter, M. (1984). The domain of developmental psychopathology. *Child development, 55*, 17–29.

Starr, J., & Lonie, J. (2008). Estimated pre-morbid IQ effects on cognitive and functional outcomes in Alzheimer disease: A longitudinal study in a treated cohort. *BMC Psychiatry, 28*, 1–8.

Stephan, B., & Brayne, C. (2008). Vascular factors and prevention of dementia. *International Review of Psychiatry, 20*, 344–356.

St. John, P. D., Snow, W. M., & Tyas, S. L. (2010). Alcohol use among older adults. *Reviews in Clinical Gerontology, 20*, 56–68.

Thun, M. J., Peto, R., Lopez, A. D., Monaco, J. H., Jenley, S. J., Heath, C. W. Jr., & Doll, R. (1997). Alcohol consumption and mortality among middle-aged and elderly US adults. *New England Journal of Medicine, 337*, 1705–1714.

Twamley, E. W., & Narvaez, J. M. (2008). Supported employment for middle-aged and older people with schizophrenia. *American Journal of Psychiatric Rehabilitation, 11*, 76–89.

Vanyukov, M. M., & Targer, R. E. (2000). Genetic studies of substance abuse. *Drug and Alcohol Dependence, 59*, 101–123.

Vink, D., Aartsen, M. J., Comijs, H. C., Heymans, M. W., Penninx, B. W. J. H., Stek, M. L., … Beekman, A. T. F. (2009). Onset of anxiety and depression in the aging population: Comparison of risk factors in a 9-year prospective study. *American Journal of Geriatric Psychiatry, 17*, 642–652.

Walker, E., & Lewine, R. J. (1990). Prediction of adult-onset schizophrenia from childhood home movies of the patients. *American Journal of Psychiatry, 174*, 1052–1056.

Wang, P. S., Lane, M., Olfson, M., Pincus, H. A., Wells, K. B., & Kessler, R. C. (2005). Twelve-month use of mental health services in the United States. *Archives of General Psychiatry, 62*, 629–640.

Weiss, I. K., Nagel, C. L., & Aronson, M. K. (1986). Applicability of depression scales to the old person. *Journal of American Geriatric Sociology, 34*, 215–218.

Weissman, M. (1993). The epidemiology of personality disorders: A 1990 update. *Journal of Personality Disorders, 7*(Suppl.), 44–62.

Wetherell, J. L., Le Roux, H., & Gatz, M. (2003). DSM-IV criteria for generalized anxiety disorder in older adults: Distinguishing the worried from the well. *Psychology and Aging, 18*, 622–627.

Whalley, L., Deary, I., Appleton, C., & Starr, J. (2004). Cognitive reserve and the neurobiology of cognitive aging. *Aging Research Reviews, 3*, 369–382.

Widiger, T. A., & Seidlitz, L. (2002). Personality, psychopathology, and aging. *Journal of Research in Personality, 36*, 335–362.

Williams, M., Xiong, C., Morris, J., & Galvin, J. (2006). Survival and mortality differences between dementia with Lewy bodies vs Alzheimer disease. *Neurology, 67*, 1935–1941.

Xu, J., Kochanek, K. D., Murphy, S. L., & Tejada-Vera, B. (2010). Deaths: Final data for 2007. *National Vital Statistics Reports, 58*(19). Retrieved from http://www.cdc.gov/nchs/data/nvsr/nvsr58/nvsr58_19.pdf

Yesavage, J. A., Brink, T. L., Rose, T. L., Lum, O., Huang, V., Ade, M., & Leirer, V. O. (1983). Development and validation of a geriatric screening scale: A preliminary report. *Journal of Psychiatric Research, 17*, 37–49.

Yonkers, K. A., Dyck, I. R., Warshaw, M., & Keller, M. B. (2000). Factors predicting the clinical course of generalized anxiety disorder. *British Journal of Psychiatry, 176*, 544–549.

Yoon, I., Kripke, D. F., Elliott, J. A., Youngstedt, S. D., Rex, K. M., & Hauger, R. L. (2003). Age-related changes of circadian rhythms and sleep-wake cycles. *Journal of the American Geriatric Society, 51*, 1085–1091.

Zanarini, M. C., Frankenburg, F. R., Hennen, J., & Silk, K. R. (2003). The longitudinal course of borderline psychopathology: 6-year prospective follow-up of the phenomenology of borderline personality disorder. *American Journal of Psychiatry, 160*, 274–283.

Zanarini, M. C., Frankenburg, F. R., Reich, D. B., Silk, K. R., Hudson, J. I., & McSweeney, L. B. (2007). The subsyndromal phenomenology of borderline personality disorder: A 10-year follow-up study. *American Journal of Psychiatry, 164*, 929–935.

Zarit, S. H., & Zarit, J. M. (2007). Normal processes of aging. In *Mental disorders in older adults* (2nd ed., pp. 10–39). New York: Guilford.

Zweig, R. A. (2008). Personality disorder in older adults: Assessment challenges and strategies. *Professional Psychology: Research and Practice, 39*, 298–305.

Zweig, R. A., & Hillman, J. (1999). Personality disorders in adults: A review. In E. Rosowsky, R. C. Abrams, & R. A. Zweig (Eds.), *Personality disorders in older adults: Emerging issues in diagnosis and treatment* (pp. 31–53). Mahwah, NJ: Earlbaum.

Part III
Common Problems of Childhood and Adolescence

16

Developmental Psychopathology
Basic Principles

JANICE ZEMAN

College of William and Mary
Williamsburg, Virginia

CYNTHIA SUVEG

University of Georgia
Athens, Georgia

Researchers and clinicians alike have exerted considerable effort to unravel the intricacies underlying disordered behavior in children and adults. In more recent decades, the foray into charting the precursors and developmental progression of childhood behavioral disturbance has emerged as its own unique subspecialty within clinical and developmental psychology. An exciting advance emanating from this burgeoning interest is the macroparadigm (Achenbach, 1990) of developmental psychopathology (DP). In their seminal article, Sroufe and Rutter (1984) defined DP as "the study of the origins and course of individual patterns of behavioral maladaptation, whatever the age of onset, whatever the causes, whatever the transformations in behavioral manifestation, and however complex the course of the developmental pattern may be" (p. 18). The primary focus of the DP perspective is to study the processes underlying continuity and change in patterns of both adaptive and maladaptive behavior from an interdisciplinary approach. A central tenet is the notion that no single theory can adequately explain all aspects of psychological maladjustment. Instead, psychological functioning is best understood through reliance on and integration of multiple levels of analyses that arise from a variety of disciplines, each with unique theoretical views and methodological approaches. Accordingly, the DP approach draws on diverse scientific fields, such as lifespan developmental psychology, clinical psychology, psychiatry, neuroscience, epidemiology, sociology, neuroendocrinology, genetics, among others, with the goal of providing a comprehensive knowledge base concerning the mutually influencing processes that underlie maladaptation as well as adaptation (Cicchetti & Curtis, 2007).

Although on the surface the DP perspective may seem to be most similar to the subdisciplines of child clinical and developmental psychology, its emphasis differs in important ways. DP is interested in the processes that mediate and moderate the development of disordered behaviors, with a primary focus on the origins of the behaviors and how they manifest themselves in disorder or adaptation over development. Of equal interest are those precursors of maladaptation (e.g., presence of risk factors) that do not lead to disorder. In contrast to clinical psychology, the DP perspective does not focus on differential diagnosis, treatment, or prognosis but rather is interested in the pathways that lead toward and away from disorder. Further, DP researchers are interested in individual differences in patterns of adaptation rather than examining group differences in a particular aspect of a disorder. Relatedly, although DP relies heavily on basic research emanating from lifespan developmental psychologists, it is not as interested in studying the universal processes of normative development as is developmental psychology, but rather examines the complex links between specific normative developmental issues or tasks and the emergence of later disorder (Sroufe & Rutter, 1984). Examining and characterizing the effects of risk and protective factors (e.g., poverty, minority ethnic status, intelligence, socioeconomic status) on developmental processes as they relate to the emergence of disorder is a paradigmatic DP research agenda; it identifies the contextual influences that place children at risk for or buffers and protects them from maladaptation. In sum, psychopathology is viewed as developmental deviation in which specific aspects of the normative developmental trajectory have been derailed and, consequently, maladaptive behaviors manifest (Sroufe & Rutter, 1984). The following sections of this chapter detail the core tenets of the DP perspective, with illustrative examples provided throughout.

Core Tenets

General Principles of Development

To understand the DP perspective more completely, it is important to be familiar with some basic principles of development that underlie most developmental theories (Sroufe & Rutter, 1984). An essential starting point concerns the use of age as a developmental marker. Simply studying a sample of children or adolescents of a particular age does not necessarily constitute a developmental approach in and of itself, nor does it necessarily shed light on a developmental process. Rutter (1989) has suggested that to understand and study the psychological processes that underlie age differences in a particular phenomenon, chronological age should be conceptualized as reflecting four types of influence, including cognitive and biological maturity as well as type and duration of environmental experiences. A developmental approach begins with a topic of interest (e.g., importance of language development in relational aggression) then, based on theory and empirical literature, hypotheses about when differences in development processes may emerge are offered. These hypotheses are then tested by selecting children of differing stages based on cognitive, biological, or experiential factors (e.g., toddler, preschool, early elementary age) or by selected abilities (e.g., expressive language abilities) that theoretically best illuminate important transitions or points of change in the topic of interest. When comparing atypically developing groups of children to a control or comparison group, it is necessary to match these children on constructs of importance to the research question (e.g., reading ability). Thus, although chronological age will continue to be used as a marker of development due to its simplicity and convenience, it is important to consider the effect of its component parts (e.g., biological maturation) on the process under investigation.

Although one theory does not predominate in developmental psychology, there are a number of principles that characterize development (Santostefano, 1978). The principle of *holism* refers to the notion that development consists of a set of interrelated domains that exert transactional effects. Although researchers often refer to physical, social, cognitive, language, or emotional development as if they were separate, independent domains, development in one area influences development in the others. For example, worry is generally considered a normative developmental experience that is more common as children's cognitive abilities become more differentiated and complex (Muris, Merckelbach, Meetsers, & van den Brand, 2002; Vasey, Crnic, & Carter, 1994). For children to experience complex worries (e.g., death concerns), they need the ability to engage in at least rudimentary abstract thought that involves anticipation of the future in which a possible array of potential negative outcomes is considered. Such cognitive skills are most reflective of later stages of cognitive development (i.e., concrete and formal operational periods; Piaget, 1972). Likewise, to manage the affective component of worry successfully, children must have developed emotion regulation skills. The absence, or delay, of these skills might contribute to chronic mismanagement of worry (i.e., avoidance, age-inappropriate clinginess to parents) and result in maladaptive functioning. Undoubtedly, children's emotional, cognitive, and social development are dynamically intertwined (Brown & Dunn, 1992; Denham, 1998).

Directedness refers to the notion that children are active shapers of their environment and not passive recipients of experience (Scarr & McCartney, 1983). Thus, the direction a child's life takes is based on an interaction of genetic influences, a history of experiences, and a series of adaptations to environmental influences that place that child on his or her unique developmental trajectory. *Differentiation of modes and goals* purports that with development, children's behavior becomes more flexible with increased organization and differentiation. These developments, in turn, promote adaptation to the increasingly complex demands present in the environment. Individual differences in flexibility and behavioral organization then lead to different trajectories of psychological adjustment or deviation from developmental norms. Finally, the *mobility of behavioral function* principle states that earlier, more undifferentiated forms of behavior become hierarchically integrated into later forms of behavior. Interestingly, the earlier behavioral forms may lay dormant but can become activated under periods of stress, producing behaviors that appear to be regressed. That is, a child who has mastered toilet training may regress to earlier forms of behavior when stressed by the adjustment to the birth of a sibling.

Overall, development is considered to be the interaction of genetic and environmental influences plus prior adaptation. From within this model, the individual and his or her context is considered to be inseparable because of the mutual and continual interactions between them. The DP perspective is unique in its emphasis on prior experience when investigating the development of adaptation and disorder. That is, each developmental progression is considered to be a series of adaptations or maladaptations that evolve over time to produce a specific outcome. Past experiences are critical in the unfolding of future behaviors because individuals interpret and respond to new situations based on their history. For example, a child who behaves aggressively in preschool with his peers begins to experience mild forms of peer rejection. Although this boy is placed into a new school environment for kindergarten, his history of unpleasant peer relations in preschool and his emergent hostile attribution bias (Dodge, 1980) contribute to his interpretation of ambiguous overtures by peers as provocative and his subsequent selection of a confrontational response to these peers. Thus, this boy adopts an active role in creating his experiences (i.e., niche picking) and in so doing, successive steps toward maladaptation are made. The outcome of these behaviors is not immutable because change remains possible at all steps in development, but the interaction of genes, context, and prior adjustment will guide the direction of the outcome for a certain behavior (Sroufe, 1997).

Mutual Influence of Typical and Atypical Development

Another unique and defining feature of the DP perspective is its emphasis on the study of both typical and atypical development in concert because they are mutually informing and provide a comprehensive understanding of development (Sroufe, 1990). From this perspective, psychopathology is defined as developmental deviation; the implication being that to understand what is considered atypical or abnormal, knowledge of what is normative is of utmost importance. Delineating the pathways to competent functioning when faced with conditions of adversity or other derailing environmental influence (e.g., risk research) is of key importance for constructing a framework to understand fully the complexities of development. Conversely, the study of atypical developmental processes helps to inform and clarify understanding of normative processes. In some instances, when studying normative behavior, the component processes involved in a developmental task are inextricably intertwined and integrated, making it difficult to distinguish each component and its role in the construction of the behavior under examination.

Consider the example of emotion regulation, a construct that has garnered considerable theoretical and empirical discussion (Cole, Martin, & Dennis, 2004). Emotion regulation is "the extrinsic and intrinsic processes responsible for monitoring, evaluating, and modifying emotional reactions, especially their intensive and temporal features, to accomplish one's goals" (Thompson, 1994, pp. 27–28). There are numerous interwoven components that comprise emotion regulation, including emotional reactivity, coping strategies, and emotional understanding, to name just a few. For example, emotional reactivity is one's initial, unmodulated response to an emotion-provoking event, whereas emotion-coping strategies involve the modification of this reactivity through a variety of means (e.g., cognitive interpretation of the arousal, use of distraction, support seeking). To successfully regulate one's emotional experience in response to the demands of the social context, individuals must also employ emotion-understanding skills to identify and label emotions and to understand the causes or consequences of emotional experiences. Thus, emotion regulation is comprised of numerous closely related, interacting processes, and studying each component in isolation from the other may create an incomplete picture of the phenomenon being studied.

Illumination of these component processes can sometimes be achieved through the investigation of atypical development in which functioning in one of the specific facets may have gone awry. For example, empirical research has found that anxious youth exhibit high emotional reactivity (Jacques & Mash, 2004), yet they do not exhibit deficits across all related emotion regulation processes. That is, anxious youth demonstrate less adaptive coping with emotional experiences, poorer understanding of how to dissemble or alter emotional expression, but no differences from nonanxious youth in understanding of emotion cues and multiple emotions (Southam-Gerow & Kendall, 2002; Suveg et al., 2008; Suveg & Zeman, 2004). Taken together, anxious youth seem to have difficulty translating their knowledge of emotion cues into adaptive emotion regulation, suggesting that knowledge of emotion-related skills is a necessary but insufficient condition for adaptive emotion regulation. In sum, by neglecting to study the dynamic interplay between typical and atypical developmental processes, understanding of the pathways to both adaptation and disorder will be incomplete. Each lens or particular emphasis on a developmental process provides important insights into the strengths and vulnerabilities associated with different pathways or trajectories to adjustment or disorder.

The interpretation of a behavior as being adaptive or maladaptive depends on the outcome of that behavior. That is, the adaptive or maladaptive nature of specific behaviors can only be defined with respect to their ultimate end points or outcomes, and these outcomes may differ depending on an individual's unique contextual variables. For example, emotional competence reflects the flexible use of emotional displays that are sensitive to cues in the social context (Saarni, 1999). Children begin to learn these skills in early childhood primarily through parental socialization of emotion (Zeman, Perry-Parrish, & Cassano, 2010). For children living in maltreating environments, however, the normative trajectory for learning these skills is altered. Research indicates that children who are physically maltreated have difficulties displaying their emotions in an adaptive manner throughout childhood, as evidenced in infancy by less flexibility and sensitivity to environmental cues (Gaensbauer, 1982; Shields, Cicchetti, & Ryan, 1994). This pattern continues into middle childhood with less situationally responsive emotional displays in both family and peer contexts (Shipman & Zeman, 2001). Although functional in one context (i.e., the maltreating family), the same method of managing emotion may be maladaptive when utilized in another context (i.e., peers; Jenkins & Oatley, 1998). Thus, it is imperative to consider that particular methods of managing emotional expressions are not in and of themselves maladaptive. The appropriateness of each method is determined by the context in which the emotional experience occurs (Cole & Kaslow, 1988). In summary:

[B]oth positive adaptation and maladaptation can only be defined with respect to outcome, and developmental pathways are only fully defined by considering *both* the normal and abnormal outcomes in which they terminate and the strengths and liabilities of the patterns of adaptation and coping that mark their origins. (Sroufe, 1990, p. 336)

The role of the developmental psychopathologist, then, is to delineate the component parts of the particular developmental process that promote or inhibit optimal functioning by examining the mutual interplay between normative and atypical development.

Developmental Pathways Perspective

When explicating the development of disorder or adaptation from a DP perspective, the concept of *developmental pathways* has been applied. To facilitate understanding of this construct, a commonly used metaphor is that of a tree in which adaptive and optimal development is represented by strong limbs emanating straight and upward from the trunk (Sroufe, 1997; Waddington, 1957). Dysfunction or maladaption is represented by successive growth on weaker branches leading away from the central core of the tree (see Figure 16.1). From this metaphor come four central propositions, as outlined in the sections that follow (Cicchetti & Rogosch, 2002; Sroufe, 1997; Sroufe & Rutter, 1984).

Disorder as Deviation From Normative Development   First is the notion that disorder is considered to arise from a pattern of deviations from normative development that has evolved over time. Understanding what constitutes normative development is essential to determine what represents a deviation from the typical course. Certain pathways or branches represent adaptational failures that will then forecast the probability of later disorder. Repeated difficulty with mastering specific developmental tasks increases the likelihood that future issues with optimal

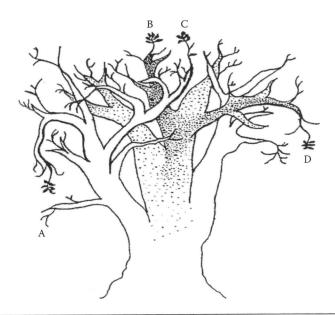

Figure 16.1 A schematic representation of the developmental pathways concept. (A) Continuity of maladaptation, culminating in disorder. (B) Continuous positive adaptation. (C) Initial maladaptation followed by positive change (resilience). (D) Initial positive adaptation followed by negative change toward pathology. From Sroufe, A.L. (2003). Psychopathology as an outcome of development. *Development and Psychopathology, 15*(4), 251–268. Reproduced with permission.

developmental will ensue. From the tree metaphor, each adaptational failure adds an increment of growth on a branch leading away from the core tree growth and strength. One or two small failures likely do not lead far from the core, but an abundance of these maladaptive developmental failures will further the distance from the core and increase the size of the wayward branch. Thus, disorder results when there is a repeated succession of deviations leading away from the blueprint of normative development.

Equifinality   The second key proposition in the pathways framework, *equifinality*, purports that there are multiple pathways to a single outcome. That is, individuals may start on quite distinct points in their developmental origins and then experience varying influences at differing points in their developmental history, yet have phenotypically similar outcomes, including adaptation or disorder despite these differing developmental courses. Thus, effective interventions for these individuals will likely differ despite their common diagnosis or pattern of behavior. For example, the pathways to later depression are quite varied. One adolescent could have a genetic predisposition for depression, whereas another adolescent may have experienced a maltreating home environment, and a third teen may have been raised by a depressed mother (Cicchetti & Rogosch, 2002). Yet the resultant outcome for all three individuals may converge on a depressive disorder, despite their unique preceding sets of biological and environmental influences. Thus, for researchers and clinicians, the principle of equifinality highlights the importance of determining the multitude of prior or predisposing factors that lead to outcomes of both adaptive functioning as well as its converse. Cicchetti and Sroufe (2000) commented that the research agenda with respect to equifinality has progressed from simply determining the antecedents of a behavior to addressing the more complex question, "What are the factors that initiate and maintain individuals on pathways probabilistically associated with X and a family of related outcomes?" (p. 257).

Multifinality   The concept of *multifinality* refers to the notion that even though individuals may begin at a common starting point (e.g., the base of a branch), the unfolding of the outcomes or resultant pathways from that origin may diverge based on the interaction of prior experiences and biological factors that produce different patterns of adaptation or pathology. Even though the outcomes may appear to be quite different from a surface examination (phenotype), it is possible that their underlying causes and etiology (genotype) are more similar than dissimilar (Sroufe, 1997). These differing pathways are thought to arise from the dynamic interplay between risk and protective processes that are unique to each individual and thus produce different pathways. For example, research has indicated that children from low-income, disadvantaged environments who have experienced at least one form of maltreatment do not all exhibit the same types of outcomes but instead show a divergence in maladaptive outcomes. Moreover, a subset of the maltreated children exhibit remarkable resilience and appear to be protected by personal attributes of positive self-esteem, ego resilience, and ego control, whereas the pathway to resilience for nonmaltreated but low-income, disadvantaged children is reliant on relationship factors (i.e., maternal availability, relationship with camp counselor; Cicchetti & Rogosch, 1997). Thus, the interplay between the protective factors in this situation of adversity is crucial to understanding the divergence of pathways. A research agenda with this principle as a guide endeavors to answer the question, "What differentiates those progressing to X from those progressing to Y and those being free from maladaptation or handicapping condition?" (Cicchetti & Sroufe, 2000, p. 257). In sum, classification of disorder based on the principles of multifinality and equifinality necessitates that developmental history be a key factor when describing and understanding adaptation and disorder.

The Nature of Change   Characterizing change and how it relates to the emergence of positive adaptation or disorder is of utmost importance to the DP perspective. As such, despite early adversity, change is thought to be possible at any juncture in development. Pathology is not conceptualized as a stable entity that a child either has or does not have. Rather, altering the course of a maladaptive developmental trajectory remains a viable possibility. When faced with adversity, individuals have a "self-righting" tendency to strive toward adaptive modes of functioning (Waddington, 1957). As described previously, this self-righting, self-organizational tendency has been documented in children who have experienced significant maltreatment within the context of other socioeconomic adversity (Cicchetti & Rogosch, 1997). From this framework, the role of the DP researcher is to investigate the factors that initiate and maintain the processes of self-righting that result in positive adaptation and the underlying mechanisms that interfere with this self-organization process that steers individuals onto a path leading to maladaptive outcomes.

A second corollary to the principle regarding change is that prior adaptation places constraints on the possibility of future change. That is, the longer a child has been on a maladaptive or adaptive pathway, particularly if development has crossed significant developmental milestones or stages (Sroufe, 1997), the more difficult or unlikely the possibility of change. Thus, from the tree metaphor, the farther the branch grows away from the trunk, receiving less support and nutrients from the core of the tree, the more difficult it will be to redirect growth to rejoin the trajectory of positive adaptation. This construct is based on the notion that children are active shapers of their environment, in which they select particular experiences, interpret them according to their biases, and then exert an impact on the environment through their actions; all of these steps interact with one another. A particular type of maladaptation or psychopathology, then, is likely to become stronger over time to the extent that the context facilitates the continuance of the behavior (Steinberg & Avenevoli, 2000). For example, regarding the boy who experienced peer rejection in preschool and continued this pattern in early elementary school, his interpretative frame of social relationships (i.e., hostile attribution bias) will become internalized and solidify with additional experiences that may lead to an escalation of negative, aggressive social relationships, and perhaps ultimately to significant antisocial behavior (Dodge et al., 2003). Research indicates that early intervention is critical to disrupt this dynamic chain of reinforcing behaviors and cognitions and, in essence, help children rejoin the normative, adaptive path to social relationships. The more stable the path to antisocial and aggressive behavior, the more difficult it becomes for enduring change (Conduct Problems Prevention Research, 2011).

In summary, the image of the branching tree provides a helpful metaphor to conceptualize the ways in which pathways to both positive adaptation and maladaptation can occur. As with any metaphor, there are limitations to its applicability. Further, there are a finite number of possible pathways that exist, making the task of characterizing these trajectories a plausible goal rather than a hopeless task (Cicchetti & Rogosch, 2002). We now turn our attention to a few remaining constructs to be discussed from within the DP perspective.

Continuity

One of the core issues of interest to developmental psychopathologists is determining whether the course of development is characterized by continuities or discontinuities across time and, if so, understanding their underlying mechanisms. A central research question concerns the prediction of adult psychopathology based on childhood behavior. That is, does depression at age 10 predict a stable pathway to depression in adulthood, barring any intervention efforts? Research over the past 30 years has made important strides in addressing this type of question.

The course of typical and atypical development is considered to be lawful and coherent (Sroufe & Rutter, 1984), meaning that the way in which an individual develops in any given domain progresses in an orderly fashion that follows developmental principles of growth. This notion is not to be confused with behavioral stability or homotypic continuity in which one would expect to see the same type of behavior exhibited across different developmental stages. This is rarely seen in development (Kagan, 1971). Rather, coherence (meaning congruity, consistency, logical connections) in development is expected regardless of transformations in the observed behavior due to maturation. For example, in the development of locomotor skills in infancy and toddlerhood, there is coherence in development despite the appearance of dramatic transformations in behavior that are exhibited in the progression of motor skills from sitting to crawling or scooting to walking to hopping. Coherence of development refers to the meaning of or the underlying processes involved in the behavior over time, rather than in the outward manifestation of the behavior. Thus, researchers look for heterotypic continuity in processes that involves "persistence of the underlying organization and meaning of behavior despite changing behavioral manifestation" (Cicchetti & Rogosch, 2002, pp. 13–14).

Rutter (1981) has proposed that there are several different ways in which links are established between early development and later disorder. These linkages may be direct in which an early experience (a) leads to or causes the disorder that then endures, (b) leads to a physical changes that then effects subsequent functioning, or (c) results in a change in behavioral patterns that over time leads to maladaptive functioning or disorder. The linkages between early experience and later disorder may also operate in an indirect fashion in which (a) early experiences may change the dynamics and functioning of the family situation, which then produces disordered behavior in the child over time; (b) the experience of early stress affects the development of coping responses, which can either result in increased sensitivity and compromised efforts to respond to stress or can buffer the child against the effects of stress and the development of disorder; (c) through early experiences, the child experiences changes in self-concept, which then influences his or her responses to future situations; and (d) early experiences influence later behavior in terms of the individual's selection of subsequent environments. Thus, the way in which issues and experiences at one developmental period are resolved sets the foundation for subsequent adaptations and issues at later stages. Children's development, then, is characterized by patterns of heterotypic continuities, discontinuities, and dramatic behavioral transformations, all of which make the study of the effect of early experience on later development extraordinarily challenging but also exciting in its potential for discovery.

Comorbidity

Another topic that is viewed differently by developmental psychopathologists than traditional clinical child psychologists is the approach to understanding the nature of overlapping or coexisting diagnostic entities. The term *comorbidity* has arisen from the medical model and implies the existence of two more disorders from the current *Diagnostic and Statistical Manual of Mental Health* diagnostic system (American Psychiatric Association, 2000). Within this diagnostic system, comorbidity appears to be more typical than not (Caron & Rutter, 1991). From a DP perspective, however, comorbidity is viewed as a failure of the categorical system to characterize particular patterns of behavioral disturbance accurately. The focus of research, therefore, is concerned with developing classification systems based on patterns of adaptation and developmental outcomes using the pathways perspective. It may be that the symptom overlap is due to many factors, including (1) presence of shared risk factors, (2) a comorbid association at the level of risk factors, (3) the presence of a unique syndrome, and/or (4) the occurrence of one disorder increasing the risk for the development and occurrence of another disorder (Caron & Rutter, 1991).

Research has attempted to explain common comorbidities in youth by examining variations in symptom patterns or underlying processes in particular developmental domains. For example, anxiety and depression commonly co-occur in children (Brady & Kendall, 1992; Compas & Oppedisano, 2000), but research from a DP perspective has identified emotion-related variables that can differentiate the syndromes (Suveg, Hoffman, Zeman, & Thomassin, 2009). Specifically, poor emotion awareness, emotion dysregulation, poor emotion regulation coping, and high frequency of negative affect are emotion-related variables common to both anxiety and depression symptoms, but low frequency of positive affect is uniquely related to depression symptoms, and frequency of emotion experience and somatic response to emotion activation are specific to anxiety symptoms of youth. Examining overlap in symptoms and syndromes is critical to better understand the underlying pathway(s) to the development of behavioral patterns and illuminates targets for prevention, a primary interest of DP researchers.

Risk and Resilience

A paradigmatic DP research agenda is exemplified by risk and resilience research; namely, what biological or contextual processes influence development either toward or away from adaptation? Risk research examines multiple levels of analysis and considers interactive rather than main effects models. For example, research has recently begun to examine contextual factors that moderate genetic risk for poor socioemotional outcomes. Lesch et al. (1996) have identified the presence of the short allele (homozygous or heterozygous; ss or sl, respectively) of the 5-HTTLPR polymorphism (serotonin transporter gene regulatory region) as a risk factor for poor self-regulation and symptoms of anxiety. Interestingly, a secure attachment relationship was found to protect youth considered at risk by the presence of the 5-HTTLPR polymorphism (Kochanska, Philibert, & Barry, 2009). Other lines of research have examined how contextual variables interact to produce particular outcomes. For example, physiological indicators of child stress reactivity have been associated with poor functioning in the context of family adversity or stress (el-Sheikh, Harger, & Whitson, 2001; Obradović, Stamperdahl, Bush, Adler, & Boyce, 2010). Examining the interaction of multiple factors that span genetic, physiological, behavioral, and environmental domains contributes to a better understanding of the processes underlying adaptation and maladaptation and mediators and moderators of the processes.

Although much debate surrounds the construct of resilience (Luthar, Cicchetti, & Becker, 2000), resilience is generally not viewed as a trait-like quality that the child simply "has" or is endowed with. Rather, resilience is thought to be a dynamic developmental process that operates from within the developmental context such that factors within the environment (e.g., secure attachment history) interact with characteristics of the child (e.g., intelligence) to produce positive outcomes or competence despite exposure to adverse conditions (e.g., living in a high crime neighborhood; Luthar et al., 2000). Thus, simply being intelligent may not produce adaptation when faced with severe adversity, but a history of positive coping efforts in prior stressful situations and the presence of a secure attachment relationship with a primary caregiver may interact with a child's personal attribute of intelligence to yield a specific positive outcome (e.g., academic achievement) in a particular situation. Further, resilience is a multidimensional construct such that some children who are at high risk for maladaptation demonstrate competence in certain domains but not in others. Kaufman, Cook, Arny, Jones, and Pittinsky (1994) examined outcomes in children with a history of maltreatment and found that the majority showed resilience in terms of academic functioning, but only a minority exhibited such resilience within the social domain. Research has also revealed that although some individuals outwardly display resilience and competence in multiple domains, they experience internalizing symptoms (Luthar, 1993) or chronic health-related issues (Werner & Smith, 1992), indicating that resilience does not imply invulnerability.

Although this is an exciting and promising area of research and, in many ways, at the heart of the DP perspective, the current state of the field has been criticized for its definitional ambiguities, the heterogeneity of both the risk and competency factors, the instability of the construct, and the overall utility of the concept of resilience (Luthar et al., 2000). Nevertheless, there remains great potential for gaining an increasingly in-depth, complete understanding of adaptation within this line of inquiry.

Cultural Issues

Considering the DP emphasis on contextual factors, the distinct role that culture plays in children's adaptation is receiving increasing attention. Research and practice must take into account the unique factors of children's cultural norms, socialization practices, and values when considering whether a particular behavior represents a maladaptive response to the dominant culture's demands. Given that the majority of developmental research has been conducted using Western, European American, middle-class samples, it is important to recognize the dominant sociocultural perspective of this society in contrast to others. Mequita and Markus (2004) have identified two distinct, prevalent cultural frameworks. The first model of agency, termed *disjoint*, is reflected in European American cultures with a focus on the self and the notion that the self should be independent, happy, and seek to control and influence the environment. The second model, termed *conjoint*, is reflective of East Asian cultures in which the emphasis is on interdependence, belonging to social groups, and perception of the environment through the perspective of others. Thus, children developing within each of these cultures are likely to display different developmental trajectories and outcomes, and the determination of whether an outcome is adaptive or maladaptive must be considered within the norms of the particular culture. In a comparison of children from Nepal (representing an Asian, collectivistic, conjoint culture) and a rural area in the northeastern section of the United States (representing a Western, individualistic, disjoint culture), Cole, Bruschi, and Tamang (2002) found cultural differences in several aspects of emotional functioning. Specifically, children from the United States were more likely to attempt to change emotion-evoking situations than Nepali youth, who were more likely to accept them. In Western culture, with an emphasis on individual happiness, accepting a situation that caused distress might be less adaptive than in Eastern cultures where group harmony is valued.

Further, from within a specific culture, researchers must consider the role of subcultures that may place importance on values that potentially differ from those of the mainstream culture. For example, within the United States, social acceptance of boys in inner-city, high-crime areas is more likely to be based on aggressive behavior and low academic achievement rather than the typical profile of prosocial, competent behavior valued in middle-class America (Luthar & McMahon, 1996). Thus, examining the dynamic interplay of risk and protective factors in the development of disorder and positive adaptation must take into account the unique role of cultural factors when examining outcomes.

Conclusion

This chapter examined the central tenets of the DP perspective and highlighted its core principles with examples from research. The DP perspective is not a single theory, but rather an approach to the study of the intersection between adaptation and maladaptation that employs multiple levels of analyses to examine interacting and dynamic influences (i.e., genetic, physiological, environmental, contextual) on development. Not concerned with traditional diagnostic classification, the DP approach focuses on identifying processes that underlie pathways to adaptation and disorder and its related mediators and moderators. The role of cultural context in development is considered vitally important because it is essential for understanding the function, value, and appropriateness of a behavior. Further, by taking a process approach to understanding particular pathways to adaptation and disorder, specific targets can be identified for early prevention and intervention. Despite its clear contributions to our understanding of the implications of developmental deviations, challenges to the DP paradigm remain. For instance, because of its emphasis and interest in processes related to stability and change over time, expensive longitudinal methodologies are needed to address these questions adequately. The statistical analyses of multiple interacting factors across different levels of analysis require large sample sizes, which can also be challenging to recruit and sustain over time for a variety of reasons (e.g., resource availability). Further, multiple perspectives from varying fields (e.g., genetics, developmental psychology, sociology) provide the ideal approach to understanding psychosocial adaptation, yet the involvement, coordination, and funding of transdisciplinary teams and the integration of the resultant findings pose unique challenges. Nonetheless, the DP perspective offers a broad understanding and interpretation of development and its deviation that has appeal to a wide array of researchers and is likely to result in a more thorough, complete understanding of such phenomena than adopting simplistic approaches.

References

Achenbach, T. (1990). What is "developmental" about developmental psychopathology? In J. Rolf, A. Masten, D. Cicchetti, K. Nuechterlein, & S. Weintraub (Eds.), *Risk and protective factors in the development of psychopathology* (pp. 29–48). New York: Cambridge University Press.

American Psychiatric Association. (2000). *Diagnostic and statistical manual of mental disorders* (4th rev. ed.). Washington, DC: Author.

Brady, E. U., & Kendall, P. C. (1992). Comorbidity of anxiety and depression in children and adolescents. *Psychological Bulletin, 111*, 244–255.

Brown, J.R., & Dunn, J. (1992). Talk with your mother or your sibling? Developmental changes in early family conversations about feelings. *Child Development, 63*, 336–349.

Caron, D., & Rutter, M. (1991). Comorbidity in child psychopathology: Concepts, issues, and research strategies. *Journal of Child Psychology and Psychiatry, 32*, 1063–1079.

Cicchetti, D., & Curtis, W. J. (2007) Multilevel perspectives on pathways to resilient functioning. *Development and Psychopathology, 19*, 627–629.

Cicchetti, D., & Rogosch, F. A. (1997). The role of self-organization in the promotion of resilience in maltreated children. *Development and Psychopathology, 9*, 799–817.

Cicchetti, D., & Rogosch, F. A. (2002). A developmental psychopathology perspective on adolescence. *Journal of Consulting and Clinical Psychology, 70*, 6–20.

Cicchetti, D., & Sroufe, A. (2000). Editorial: The past as prologue to the future: The times, they've been a-changin'. *Development and Psychopathology, 23*, 255–264.

Cole, P. M., Bruschi, C. J., & Tamang, B. L. (2002). Cultural differences in children's emotional reactions to difficult situations. *Child Development, 73*, 983–996.

Cole, P. M., & Kaslow, N. (1988). Interactional and cognitive strategies for affect regulation: Developmental perspective on childhood depression. In L. B. Alloy (Ed.), *Cognitive processes in depression* (pp. 310–343). New York: Guilford.

Cole, P. M., Martin, S. E., & Dennis, T. A. (2004). Emotion regulation as a scientific construct: Methodological challenges and directions for child development research. *Child Development, 2*, 217–333.

Compas, B. E., & Oppedisano, G. (2000). Mixed anxiety-depression in childhood and adolescence. In A. J. Sameroff, M. Lewis, & S. M. Miller (Eds.), *Handbook of developmental psychopathology* (pp. 531–548). New York: Kluwer Academic/Plenum Publishers.

Conduct Problems Prevention Research Group. (2011). The effects of the Fast Track preventive intervention on the development of conduct disorder across childhood. *Child Development, 82*(1), 331–345.

Denham, S. A. (1998). *Emotional development in young children.* New York: Guilford.

Dodge, K. A. (1980). Social cognition and children's aggressive behavior. *Child Development, 51*, 162–170.

Dodge, K. A., Lansford, J. E., Burks, V. S., Bates, J. E., Pettit, G. S., Fontaine, R., & Price, J. M. (2003). Peer rejection and social information-processing factors in the development of aggressive behavior problems in children. *Child Development, 74,* 374–393.

el-Sheikh, M., Harger, J., & Whitson, S. M. (2001). Exposure to interparental conflict and children's adjustment and physical health: The moderating role of vagal tone. *Child Development, 72,* 1617–1636.

Gaensbauer, T. J. (1982). Regulation of emotional expression in infants from two contrasting caretaking environments. *Journal of the American Academy of Child Psychiatry, 21,* 163–171.

Jacques, H. A. K., & Mash, E. J. (2004). A test of the tripartite model of anxiety and depression in elementary and high school boys and girls. *Journal of Abnormal Child Psychology, 32,* 13–25.

Jenkins, J., & Oatley, K. (1998). The development of emotion schemas in children. In W. F. Flack & J. D. Laird (Eds.). *Emotions in psychopathology: Theory and research* (pp. 45–56). New York: Oxford University Press.

Kagan, J. (1971). *Change and continuity in infancy.* New York: Wiley.

Kaufman, J., Cook, A., Arny, L., Jones, B., & Pittinsky, T. (1994). Problems defining resiliency: Illustrations from the study of maltreated children. *Development and Psychopathology, 6,* 215–229.

Kochanska, G., Philibert, R. A., & Barry, R. A. (2009). Interplay of genes and early mother–child relationship in the development of self-regulation from toddler to preschool age. *Journal of Child Psychology and Psychiatry, 50,* 1331–1338.

Lesch, K., Bengel, D., Hiels, A., Sabol, S., Greenberg, B., Petri, S., ... Murphy, D. (1996). Association of anxiety-related traits with a polymorphism in the serotonin transporter gene regulatory region. *Science, 274,* 1527–1531.

Luthar, S. S. (1993). Annotation: Methodological and conceptual issues in the study of resilience. *Journal of Child Psychology and Psychiatry, 34,* 441–453.

Luthar, S. S., Cicchetti, D., & Becker, B. (2000). The construct of resilience: A critical evaluation and guidelines for future work. *Child Development, 71,* 543–562.

Luthar, S. S., & McMahon, T. (1996). Peer reputation among inner city adolescents: Structure and correlates. *Journal of Research on Adolescence, 6,* 581–603.

Mesquita, B., & Markus, H. (2004). Culture and emotion: Models of agency as sources of cultural variation in emotion. In A. S. Manstead, N. Frijda, & A. Fischer (Eds.), *Feelings and emotions: The Amsterdam symposium* (pp. 341–358). New York: Cambridge University Press.

Muris, P., Merckelbach, H., Meetsers, C., & van den Brand, K. (2002). Cognitive development and worry in normal children. *Cognitive Therapy and Research, 26,* 775–787.

Obradović, J., Stamperdahl, J., Bush, N. R., Adler, N. E., & Boyce, W. T. (2010). Biological sensitivity to context: The interactive effects of stress reactivity and family adversity on socioemotional behavior and school readiness. *Child Development, 81,* 270–289.

Piaget, J. (1972). Intellectual evolution from adolescence to adulthood. *Human Development, 15,* 1–12.

Rutter, M. (1989). Age as an ambiguous variable in developmental research: Some epidemiological considerations from developmental psychopathology. *International Journal of Behavior Development, 12,* 1–34.

Rutter, M. (1981). Stress, coping, and development: Some issues and some questions. *Journal of Child Psychology and Psychiatry, 22,* 323–256.

Saarni, C. (1999). *The development of emotional competence.* New York: Guilford.

Santostefano, S. (1978). *A biodevelopmental approach to clinical child psychology: Cognitive controls and cognitive control therapy.* New York: Wiley.

Scarr, S., & McCartney, K. (1983). How people make their own environments: A theory of genotype environmental effects. *Child Development, 54,* 424–434.

Shields, A. M., Cicchetti, D. L., & Ryan, R. M. (1994). The development of emotional and behavioral self-regulation and social competence among maltreated school-age children. *Development and Psychopathology, 6,* 57–75.

Shipman, K. L., & Zeman, J. L. (2001). Socialization of children's emotion regulation in mother–child dyads: A developmental psychopathology perspective. *Development and Psychopathology, 13,* 317–336.

Steinberg, L., & Avenevoli, S. (2000). The role of context in the development of psychopathology: A conceptual framework and some speculative propositions. *Child Development, 71,* 66–74.

Southam-Gerow, M. A., & Kendall, P. C. (2002). Emotion regulation and understanding: Implications for child psychopathology and therapy. *Clinical Psychology Review, 22,* 189–222.

Sroufe, L. A. (1990). Considering normal and abnormal together: The essence of developmental psychopathology. *Development and Psychopathology, 2,* 335–347.

Sroufe, L. A. (1997). Psychopathology as an outcome of development. *Development and Psychopathology, 9,* 251–268.

Sroufe, L. A., & Rutter, M. (1984). The domain of developmental psychopathology. *Child Development, 55,* 17–29.

Suveg, C., Hoffman, B., Zeman, J., & Thomassin, K. (2009). Common and specific emotion-related predictors of anxiety and depression in youth. *Child Psychiatry and Human Development, 40,* 223–229.

Suveg, C., Sood, E., Barmish, A., Tiwari, S., Hudson, J., & Kendall, P. C. (2008). "I'd rather not talk about it:" Emotion parenting in families of children with an anxiety disorder. *Journal of Family Psychology, 22,* 875–884.

Suveg, C., & Zeman, J. (2004). Emotion regulation in children with anxiety disorders. *Journal of Clinical Child and Adolescent Psychology, 33,* 750–759.

Thompson, R. (1994). Emotion regulation: A theme in search of definition. In N. A. Fox (Ed.), *Emotion regulation: Biological and behavioral considerations. Monographs of the Society for Research in Child Development* (pp. 25–52). Chicago: University of Chicago Press.

Vasey, M. W., Crnic, K. A., & Carter, W. G. (1994). Worry in childhood: A developmental perspective. *Cognitive Therapy and Research, 18,* 529–549.

Waddington, J. C. (1957). *The strategy of genes.* London: Allen and Unwin.

Werner, E. E., & Smith, R. S. (Eds.). (1992). *Overcoming the odds: High risk children from birth to adulthood.* Ithaca, NY: Cornell University Press.

Zeman, J., Perry-Parrish, C., & Cassano, M. (2010). Parent–child discussions of anger and sadness: The importance of parent and child gender [Special issue]. *New Directions in Child and Adolescent Development: 128,* 65–83.

17
Externalizing Disorders

EVA R. KIMONIS

University of South Florida
Tampa, Florida

PAUL J. FRICK

University of New Orleans
New Orleans, Louisiana

Symptoms of common mental disorders in children and adolescents have been conceptually organized into two broad dimensions. One dimension, which is the focus of this chapter, has been labeled as undercontrolled or externalizing and includes various acting out, disruptive, delinquent, hyperactive, and aggressive behaviors. The second dimension has been labeled as overcontrolled or internalizing and includes such behaviors as social withdrawal, anxiety, and depression (see Ollendick & Sander, this volume). The distinction between internalizing and externalizing problems is well supported by a number of factor analytic studies (Achenbach, 1995; Lahey et al., 2008).

Within the externalizing dimension, there are two major categories of behavior: (1) problems of inattention, impulsivity, and hyperactivity associated with a diagnosis of attention-deficit/ hyperactivity disorder (ADHD), and (2) conduct problems and aggressive behavior associated with a diagnosis of oppositional defiant disorder (ODD) or conduct disorder (CD). These two domains of externalizing problems are separated in factor analyses and exhibit different correlates (Lahey et al., 2008; Waschbusch, 2002). For example, ADHD is specifically linked with poor academic achievement, problems in executive functioning, and parental inattention and impulsivity, whereas conduct problems are specifically associated with socioeconomic disadvantage, dysfunctional family backgrounds, and parental criminality and antisocial behavior. However, twin research suggests that shared environmental risk factors, such as parent–child conflict, may act as a common vulnerability for the development of both ADHD and conduct problems (Burt, Krueger, McGue, & Iacono, 2003). The importance of these correlates for understanding the two types of externalizing disorders is discussed in later sections of this chapter.

Although research supports distinguishing between these two forms of externalizing disorders, and the following sections provide somewhat separate reviews of them, they do overlap considerably. For example, approximately half of children diagnosed with ADHD have a co-occurring conduct problem diagnosis (Waschbusch, 2002), and between 65 and 90% of children with either ODD or CD have a co-occurring ADHD diagnosis (Abikoff & Klein, 1992). Awareness of the overlap between these disorders is important for understanding and interpreting research in this area because many studies fail to control for their co-occurrence. As a result, it is often unclear whether the correlates documented in research are due to one or the other type of externalizing disorder or both (Lilienfeld & Waldman, 1990). Further, children with both ADHD and conduct disorders show a more persistent course of ADHD (Barkley, Fischer,

Smallish, & Fletcher, 2002; Broidy et al., 2003; Frick & Loney, 1999). Finally, the presence or absence of comorbidity also influences which type or treatment will be most effective (Arnold et al., 2004; Frick, 2001).

Attention-Deficit/Hyperactivity Disorder

Definition and Description

Diagnosis The primary feature of ADHD is extreme and maladaptive levels of motor activity. It is the most common childhood behavioral disorder; the worldwide prevalence of ADHD is estimated at 5.3%, using the American Psychiatric Association's (APA) *Diagnostic and Statistical Manual of Mental Disorders* (*DSM*) or the World Health Organization's (WHO, 1992) *International Classification of Diseases* (*ICD*) diagnostic criteria (Polanczyk, Silva de Lima, Horta, Biederman, & Rohde, 2007). ADHD has been recognized in the psychiatric literature since the mid-19th century, although there has been longstanding debate concerning its primary cause and the best method for diagnosing it in children. This debate is reflected in numerous changes in its clinical designation (e.g., minimal brain dysfunction, hyperactive child syndrome) and in the diagnostic criteria used over the years.

In the most recent revision of the *DSM* (*DSM–IV–TR*; APA, 2000), ADHD is characterized by two core symptom dimensions—an inattention-disorganization cluster (e.g., not listening when spoken to directly, easily distracted by extraneous stimuli) and a hyperactivity-impulsivity cluster (e.g., excessive talking or activity, difficulty awaiting turn). These two dimensions were identified through many factor analytic studies conducted with both clinic-referred and community-based samples (Lahey, Applegate, McBurnett, & Biederman, 1994). As with all childhood disorders, some degree of ADHD symptoms is normal in childhood; ADHD may be best viewed as an extreme variation of an underlying trait dimension (Willcutt, Pennington, & DeFries, 2000). According to the *DSM–IV–TR*, the following criteria are required to make a diagnosis (APA, 2000):

- Severity (six or more behavioral symptoms),
- Duration (problems are evident before age 7 and persist for at least 6 months),
- Pervasiveness (impairment present in two or more settings),
- Impairment (clear evidence of impaired social, academic, or occupational functioning).

Several changes to the diagnostic criteria for ADHD are currently under consideration for DSM–5 (Frick & Moffitt, 2010). First, several modifications are being considered to make the diagnosis more valid for adults (Barkley, Murphy, & Fischer, 2008). These changes include lowering the symptom threshold for adults, providing examples of how symptoms may be manifested in adults, and enhancing the number of impulsivity symptoms included in the criteria.

Second, rather than requiring the presence of maladaptive symptoms before age 7, the DSM–5 is considering raising this to noticeable symptoms present by age 12. This proposed change was based on a review of the literature suggesting that (a) only about 50% of adults with ADHD recalled an onset before age 7 but 95% recalled an onset before age 12; (b) individuals who met criteria for ADHD but not the age of 7 onset resembled those with the full diagnosis in terms of neuropsychological profile, comorbidity, substance use, personality traits, and impairment; and (c) response to treatment with stimulants was similar among children, adolescents, and adults whether or not they met the age of onset criterion (Kieling et al., 2010).

Third, another major change to the definition of ADHD that is being considered for DSM–5 is a method for improving and refining the subtypes of the disorder that are recognized in the manual. That is, research generally suggests that those with ADHD are a highly heterogeneous group and that there are several important subgroups that can be defined within the broad category (Martel, Goth-Owens, Martinez-Torteya, & Nigg, 2010). However, research has suggested that the current method of defining subtypes in the *DSM–IV–TR* has a number of significant limitations.

Subtypes The *DSM–IV–TR* (APA, 1994) created three subtypes of ADHD. The most common subtype, comprising about 55% of all children referred for treatment, is the combined type (ADHD-CT; Lahey, Applegate, Barkley et al., 1994). These children exhibit at least six symptoms of both inattention/disorganization and impulsivity/hyperactivity. Not surprising given the prevalence rate, much of ADHD research focuses on this subtype.

The second subtype is the predominantly inattentive type (ADHD-PI; APA, 2000). Approximately 27% of children in treatment for ADHD exhibit this subtype (Lahey, Applegate, McBurnett et al., 1994). These children show six or more problems with inattention/disorganization but fewer than six symptoms of impulsivity/hyperactivity. Compared to those diagnosed with ADHD-CT, children with ADHD-PI (a) demonstrate fewer conduct problems and less aggression, (b) experience less rejection from peers, (c) experience higher rates of anxiety and depression, and (d) respond better to lower doses of stimulant medication (Carlson & Mann, 2000; Lahey, Carlson, & Frick, 1997). This subtype often exhibits different cognitive and attentional difficulties from other children with ADHD, such as slow retrieval and information processing (as opposed to fast and impulsive processing of information) and low levels of alertness (Hartman, Willcutt, Rhee, & Pennington, 2004; McBurnett, Pfiffner, & Frick, 2001).

The third and least common ADHD subtype is the predominantly hyperactive/impulsive type (ADHD-PHI). Accounting for about 18% of children diagnosed with ADHD, those in this category show six or more symptoms of hyperactivity/impulsivity without problems of inattention/disorganization (Lahey, Applegate, Barkley et al., 1994). Barkley (1997) proposed that this subtype is a developmental precursor to the ADHD-CT subtype for children who have not yet experienced demands for sustained attention. Consistent with this hypothesis, a study of children diagnosed with ADHD found that the average age of the ADHD-PHI subgroup was 5.68 years, compared to 8.52 years for the ADHD-CT and 9.80 years for the ADHD-PI type (Lahey, Applegate, McBurnett, & Biederman, 1994). ADHD-PHI youth whose symptoms persist over development tend to shift to ADHD-CT following entry into school, likely due to the increased demands placed on them (Lahey, Pelham, Loney, Lee, & Wilcutt, 2005). Additionally, when controlling for conduct disorders, a diagnosis of ADHD-PHI earlier in development appears to predict ODD symptoms later in development (Burke, Loeber, Lahey, & Rathouz, 2005).

As seen with the revisions currently under consideration for DSM–5, there are several criticisms of this method of subtyping (Frick & Moffitt, 2010). The most common criticism is the instability of subtype membership across time, with most children showing subtype changes when followed longitudinally (Lahey et al., 2005). A second criticism is that the magnitude of differences among the subtypes, particularly between the predominantly inattentive subtype and the other two, warrant designation as separate disorders (Milich, Balentine, & Lynam, 2001). A third criticism is that the subtypes should be defined by different cognitive styles rather than the degree of alignment with different symptom clusters. For example, some researchers argue that the ADHD-PI subtype should be defined by a sluggish cognitive tempo (e.g., drowsiness, lethargy, hypoactivity; Carlson & Mann, 2003).

In the face of such objections, the DSM–5 task force is considering several changes for subtyping children with ADHD. First, the existing *DSM–IV–TR* subtypes would be clearly described as "Subtypes Based on Current Presentation" (within the past 6 months) to emphasize their lack of longitudinal stability. Second, a new subtype is under consideration—"Inattentive Presentation (Restrictive)"—in which six or more symptoms of inattention/disorganization but no more than two symptoms of hyperactivity/impulsivity have been present within the past 6 months. In an effort to increase the divergence among the subtypes, those children with three to five hyperactive/impulsive symptoms (less than the required six for the combined type) are precluded from a diagnosis of "Inattentive Presentation (Restrictive)" type; instead these children would still be classified as the PI type.

Developmental Course   Research suggests that ADHD symptoms emerge early in development, with symptoms of overactivity emerging as early as 3 to 4 years of age (Loeber, Green, Lahey, Christ, & Frick, 1992). Although many children swiftly learn to control such behavior upon entry into school, about half of the most hyperactive and disruptive preschoolers are diagnosed with ADHD by age 6 (Campbell, Ewing, Breaux, & Szumowski, 1986). ADHD prevalence rates in preschool age children range from approximately 2% in community children to 60% in clinic-referred children (Keenan & Wakschlag, 2000; Lavigne et al, 1996). For years the prevailing scientific view was that these children would "outgrow" the disorder by adolescence or early adulthood (Lambert, 1988). This assumption has recently been challenged by several prospective longitudinal studies that followed children diagnosed with ADHD into adulthood (Barkley et al., 2002; Faraone, Biederman, & Mick, 2006). These studies suggest that ADHD in childhood confers risk for long-term problematic outcomes.

Several general statements can be made about the current understanding of the developmental course of ADHD. First, for children diagnosed with ADHD, between 50 and 70% experience clinically significant symptoms into adolescence and between 30 and 50% into adulthood (Langley et al., 2010; Lara et al., 2009). Childhood predictors of problem persistence include ADHD-CT subtype, symptom severity, comorbid psychopathology, and parental psychopathology, such as conduct disorder/antisocial personality disorder or mood disorders (Langley et al., 2010; Molina et al., 2009). Second, even when core symptomatology has lessened to the point of no longer meeting diagnostic criteria, many adults who were diagnosed with ADHD as children continue to experience significant impairments in their social, occupational, financial, psychological, or neurocognitive functioning (Balint et al., 2009; Faraone et al., 2006). Third, the manifestation of ADHD symptoms varies across development. For example, the presentation of inattention/disorganization symptoms appears more consistent from childhood to adolescence and adulthood than hyperactive/impulsive symptoms (Hart et al., 1995). This may, however, be partly due to developmental variations in the expression of hyperactive/impulsive symptoms, such that they manifest as driving problems in adolescence (Barkley & Cox, 2007) or relationship instability in adulthood (Biederman et al., 2006).

Comorbidity and Co-occurring Problems   As noted earlier, many children with ADHD present with comorbid disorders and co-occurring adjustment problems (not always severe enough to warrant a separate diagnosis). The presence of comorbid disorders strongly predicts later maladjustment (Connor, Steeber, & McBurnett, 2010). For example, major conduct problems among children diagnosed with ADHD are associated with criminal offending and substance abuse in adulthood (Weiss & Hechtman, 1993). Between 30 and 50% of children with ADHD have significant academic problems such as learning disabilities and early school dropout (Jensen, Martin, & Cantwell, 1997). Compounding academic challenges, a high percentage of these children also experience social difficulties such as peer rejection (Miller-Johnson, Coie, Maumary-Gremaud, & Bierman, 2002). Tobacco use and substance abuse in later development are also more common than among non-ADHD children, even after controlling for other disruptive behavior problems (Burke, Loeber, White, Stouthamer-Loeber, & Pardini, 2007). Between 30 and 50% of this population has comorbid emotional disorders, such as clinical anxiety or depression (Jensen et al., 1997; Schatz & Rostain, 2006). Other frequently co-occurring conditions include tics and sleep disorders (Gau et al., 2010). Taken together, the above findings suggest that comorbid diagnoses are the rule rather than the exception for children diagnosed with ADHD.

Several differences exist between families of children with and without ADHD. In a review of studies examining family functioning, Johnston and Mash (2001) found that having a child with ADHD in the home is associated with poorer parenting; marital and parent–child conflicts; and increased parental stress, self-blame, social isolation, and psychopathology. Such difficulties are exacerbated by a child's comorbid oppositional and conduct problems (Deault, 2010). It is unclear whether these familial problems precede the child's development of ADHD or vice versa—or whether the relationship is instead reciprocal. That is, constant household stressors and challenges involved in parenting a child with ADHD may increase the likelihood that parents will engage in dysfunctional and ineffective parenting strategies (Fischer, 1990). Some researchers suggest familial factors are less responsible for the onset of ADHD than its maintenance (Johnston & Mash, 2001). Other researchers hypothesize that negative family dynamics more strongly predict the development and maintenance of co-occurring problems in children with ADHD (e.g., conduct problems; Langley et al., 2010; Pálmason et al., 2010).

Cultural and Gender Issues   Historically, ADHD research has been dominated by researchers from the United States, leading to the impression that it is largely an American disorder. To test this assumption, Faraone, Sergeant, Gillberg, and Biederman (2003) reviewed studies reporting on the prevalence of ADHD across countries and cultures according to *DSM–III* (APA, 1980), *DSM–III–R* (APA, 1987), or *DSM–IV* criteria. They concluded that ADHD prevalence was roughly equivalent in U.S. and non-U.S. study populations. Another study by Polanczyk et al. (2007) found that prevalence rates were similar in Europe and North America, while ADHD was less common in the Middle East and more common in Africa than in North America and Europe. Other studies also find divergent rates in non-U.S. samples (Verhulst, Van der Ende, Ferdinand, & Kasius, 1997), which may reflect differences in (a) diagnostic criteria used to establish disorder, with the highest prevalence rates reported for *DSM–IV* criteria (Faraone et al., 2003); (b) informants used to assess symptoms (e.g., parents vs. teachers); or (c) the population surveyed (e.g., age range, gender), rather than true geographic variations in ADHD. Within the United States, studies do not find consistent differences in prevalence rates across different cultural groups (Barkley, 1996).

Across the globe, boys are more likely than girls to be diagnosed with ADHD. Male-to-female ratios range from 2:1 to 6:1 in community samples and from 4:1 to 9:1 in clinic-referred samples (Barkley, 1996). There is emerging evidence that the ratio differs across ADHD subtypes, with the greatest gender balance seen in the ADHD-PI subtype (Biederman et al., 2002; Lahey, Applegate, Barkley et al., 1994). Among children diagnosed with ADHD, there are no significant gender differences in symptom presentation, co-occurring adjustment problems, or clinical course (Gershon, 2002). The most consistent differences are a stronger family history of ADHD for boys, particularly with the father, and less severe hyperactivity and fewer conduct problems for girls, although they exhibit greater verbal intellectual impairments (Rucklidge & Tannock, 2001). Interestingly, comorbid psychopathology persists into adolescence more often for girls than boys (Monuteaux, Mick, Faraone, & Biederman, 2010).

Etiology

The core symptoms of ADHD have been associated with a neurological deficit, although documentation of such a deficit is neither sufficient nor necessary for a diagnosis since the diagnostic criteria for ADHD are purely behavioral. The child's psychosocial context (e.g., family environment, quality of educational services)—while not critical to many etiological theories—largely influences the severity and level of impairment of the child's symptoms and the development of co-occurring problems. Intervening in the child's psychosocial context (e.g., improving parenting skills, improving the child's educational environment) to limit the impairment associated with ADHD and prevent the development of secondary problems is critical for effectively treating children with ADHD, a point that is discussed later in this chapter.

Core Deficit   There are many theories on the core cognitive deficit leading to ADHD symptoms. However, the most extensive and best articulated are Barkley's (1997) and Nigg's (2006) theories. These authors posit that ADHD results from a core deficit in behavioral inhibition—defined as the ability to inhibit a prepotent response long enough to consider the consequences of the response; to stop an ongoing response in reaction to environmental feedback; and to suppress stimuli that might interfere with a primary response (i.e., interference control). According to Barkley (1997), this deficit in behavioral inhibition leads to secondary impairments in several executive functions. Executive functions are cognitive actions that are self-directed and allow for self-regulation. Executive functions depend on behavioral inhibition for their adequate performance and include; (a) working memory (e.g., maintaining events in the mind, hindsight, forethought), (b) self-regulation of affect, motivation, and arousal (e.g., self-control of emotions, social perspective taking); (c) internalization of speech (e.g., problem solving, moral reasoning); and (d) reconstitution (e.g., verbal and behavioral fluency).

These impairments explain a number of the self-regulation problems that are exhibited by children with ADHD. That is, the deficit in behavioral inhibition and the resulting impairments in executive functions cause the behavior of individuals with ADHD to be controlled by the immediate context rather than internal representations of information (Nigg, 2006). Characteristics of the child's immediate context, such as the novelty of the task, the intrinsic interest of the child in the activity, the child's level of fatigue, and the degree of immediate reinforcement present, can have a strong influence on the child's behavior (Barkley, 1996, 1997). These deficits also explain both the core symptoms of inattention/disorganization and hyperactivity/impulsivity as well as several secondary features, such as impaired sense of time and greater emotional reactivity. Neurological deficits are theorized to be a mediating process rather than the cause behind the child's behavioral symptom profile (Nigg, 2006).

Neurological Substrates   Neuroimaging studies suggest several important differences in the brains of children with ADHD. Structurally, those with ADHD show on average a 5% reduction in total brain volume, with greater reductions in the prefrontal cortices, corpus callosum, basal ganglia, and cerebellum (Giedd, Blumenthal, Molloy, & Castellanos, 2001; Swanson & Castellanos, 2002). Although the prefrontal cortex is generally one of the last areas of the brain to fully mature, it appears to mature at an even slower rate for children with ADHD (Shaw et al., 2007). This same study found that the motor cortex reaches its peak thickness slightly faster in children with ADHD than controls. Neuroimaging studies in those with ADHD report underactivation of frontostriatal networks, primarily right inferior prefrontal regions of the brain and associated regions and pathways connecting to this region from the caudate and striatal regions (Nigg, 2006). These findings seem to be strongest for those children with ADHD-CT (Loo & Barkley, 2005). Importantly, the implicated brain areas have been linked with deficits in emotion regulation, inhibition, and executive functions and, thus, could explain the core deficits described previously (Barkley, 1997; Nigg, 2006). Stimulant medication, which is effective at reducing symptoms of ADHD, also increases activity in the prefrontal regions of the brain, thus providing a rationale for the method of action of this medication in reducing core symptoms (Lou, Henrikson, Bruhn, Borner, & Nielson, 1989).

Despite these promising findings, research on the neurological underpinnings of ADHD is limited in several ways. First, as in earlier research, it is still evident that many of those with

ADHD do not show clear deficits in brain structure or function. Second, findings are not always consistent across studies. For example, some studies find more defuse abnormalities in cerebral blood flow that are not limited to prefrontal regions of the brain in adults with ADHD (Zametkin et al., 1990); other studies find that diminished blood flow is limited to adolescent girls, and not boys, with ADHD (Ernst et al., 1994; Zametkin et al., 1993). However, some of these inconsistencies may reflect differences in the sample studied (e.g., variations in which subtypes and comorbid conditions are included). Third, these studies do not indicate what causes the neurological deficits.

Causes of the Neurological Abnormalities   There are several different pathways through which a neurological deficit can develop in the brain systems involved in inhibition. One of these pathways may be via an inherited deficit. Family and adoption studies find evidence for the familial transmission of ADHD symptoms (e.g., Faraone & Biederman, 2000; Sprich, Biederman, Crawford, Mundy, & Faraone, 2000). A review of twin studies estimated that approximately 76% of the variance in measures of ADHD can be attributed to genetic influences, making it one of the most heritable forms of childhood psychopathology (Faraone et al., 2005). Familial transmission of ADHD may be subtype specific. A meta-analysis found that relatives of children with ADHD-PI tend to have only this subtype, whereas relatives of children with ADHD-CT have both ADHD-CT and ADHD-PI (Stawicki, Nigg, & von Eye, 2006).

Molecular genetics studies implicate several viable candidate genes, such as *DAT1*, *DRD4*, *DRD5*, *SLC6A4* (*5HTTLPR* long), *HTR1B*, and *SNAP25* (Forero, Arboleda, Vasquez, & Arboleda, 2009; Gizer, Ficks, & Waldman, 2009), each of which may have a small effect in increasing the risk for developing ADHD (Faraone et al., 2005). This research suggests a polygenetic contribution to susceptibility to ADHD. The influence of various genes may be moderated by such factors as ADHD subtype, gender, and comorbidity, explaining some of the inconsistencies in molecular genetic findings. For example, *DAT1* may be specifically associated with ADHD without comorbid conduct problems (Sharp, McQuillin, & Gurling, 2009). Other research suggests that common genes may confer risk for ADHD as well as other psychiatric disorders. One study found significant overlap between genetic factors for ADHD and major depressive disorder, interpreted as reflecting a common genetic pathway to both disorders (Cole, Ball, Martin, Scourfield, & McGuffin, 2009).

Environmental factors may also play a role in the development of ADHD (Benerjee, Middleton, & Faraone, 2007). There is evidence that biological trauma may influence the development of ADHD in some children. For example, children with ADHD are more likely to have been born premature than other children and have higher rates of obstetric complications (Johnson et al., 2010). Additionally, prenatal exposure to environmental toxins, such as alcohol and tobacco, lead, manganese, mercury, and polychlorinated biphenyls, are linked to ADHD symptoms (Benerjee et al., 2007; Stein, Schettler, Wallinga, & Valenti, 2002). Genetic vulnerabilities may also interact with environmental factors to predict ADHD symptomatology (Neuman et al., 2007). Like other forms of psychopathology, there probably are multiple developmental pathways to ADHD and related neurological deficits (Nigg, 2006).

Empirically Validated Treatments

Many treatment approaches have been attempted with ADHD, most of which have gained only limited support for their efficacy (Barkley, 2006). Only two treatments consistently demonstrate efficacy in controlled treatment outcomes studies. These evidence-based treatments (EBT) include pharmacologic intervention and behavioral therapy focusing on developing structured contingency management systems within the child's home and school environments (Pelham & Fabiano, 2008).

The use of stimulant medication as a pharmacologic intervention has robust support in the literature, with over 30 years of research indicating that it leads to significant improvements in ADHD symptoms in 70 to 80% of children (see Swanson, McBurnett, Christian, & Wigal, 1995, for a review). Stimulant medication not only reduces the core symptoms of ADHD but also alleviates many secondary problems, such as conduct problems, aggression, and social and academic problems (Richters et al., 1995; Swanson et al., 1995). With appropriate and carefully monitored trials, the side effects of stimulant medication are fairly mild. The most common side effects are appetite suppression and increased irritability (Barkley, McMurray, Edelbrock, & Robbins, 1990). Although much of the treatment research has been conducted with preadolescent children with ADHD, there is growing support for the efficacy of stimulant medication for reducing symptoms of ADHD in preschool children (Greenhill et al., 2006) and adults (Dowson, 2006). Only a small proportion of affected adults are actually treated, however (Biederman, Spencer, & Wilens, 2004).

The majority of research on pharmacologic intervention focuses on one particular stimulant medication, methylphenidate (Ritalin). However, controlled treatment outcome studies find similar response profiles for other stimulant medications. Also, while stimulants are the pharmacologic EBT for ADHD, a number of nonstimulant medications have also been used, including noradrenergic reuptake inhibitors, tricyclic antidepressants, and antihypertensive agents (Biederman et al., 2004). The limited research on these nonstimulant medications suggests that they are superior to placebo in reducing symptoms of ADHD, although it is unclear whether they are superior in efficacy to the more extensively researched stimulant medications (Biederman et al., 2004).

Despite robust findings for the efficacy of medication (Swanson et al., 1995), pharmacologic interventions for children with ADHD are limited in several important ways. First, many parents report negative feelings about the use of medications, reflected in poor and inconsistent adherence to treatment regimens or even refusal of this form of treatment (Pappadopulos et al., 2009; Richters et al., 1995). Second, a considerable proportion (10 to 20%) of children with ADHD are left with no significant improvement in symptoms with pharmacologic intervention and, even for those who do show improvement, their behavior is often not brought within what would be considered a normal range (Pelham, 1993; Wells et al., 2000). Third, and most importantly, stimulants are most beneficial in the short term, and there is little evidence that they have a long-term benefit for improving outcomes in adolescence or adulthood or once they are discontinued (Pelham et al., 2000; Swanson et al., 1995). Considering that the largest controlled treatment study to date found that only a minority of youth (38%) continued taking medication posttreatment and into adolescence (Molina et al., 2009), symptoms will persist unless other intervention approaches are considered.

Several studies have reported superior performance for pharmacologic intervention over behavioral interventions (Abikoff et al., 2004; Hinshaw, Klein, & Abikoff, 2007). These findings have had a significant influence on some guidelines for the treatment of ADHD and the preference for pharmacologic treatment over behavioral interventions (Leslie & Wolraich, 2007). For example, the American Academy of Child and Adolescent Psychiatry (2007) promotes pharmacologic treatment as the initial and only intervention for ADHD, except when symptoms are mild and minimally impairing or when parents reject medication. Preliminary research, however, suggests that when behavioral interventions are used first they may be effective at treating a majority of children with ADHD, and that most children first treated with stimulant medication will require an additional behavioral intervention (Dopfner et al., 2004).

Of the psychosocial interventions available for the treatment of ADHD, behavioral parent training (BPT) and behavioral classroom management (BCM) have garnered the most empirical support (Pelham & Fabiano, 2008). BPT involves teaching parents intensive behavior management skills and related concepts (e.g., effective commands, token economies in the home, effective discipline) and may also include teaching parents strategies for working effectively with teachers and advocating for their child with school personnel, as well as methods for managing stress, anger, and negative moods to enhance parenting abilities. BCM involves training teachers on how to establish behavioral classroom management techniques (e.g., daily report cards, classroom token economies). More recently, intensive peer-focused behavioral interventions that are typically implemented in recreational settings, such as in summer camp programs (e.g., MTA Cooperative Group, 1999a; 1999b), have also been identified as a well-established treatment (Pelham & Fabiano, 2008). It is also common for studies to combine these behavioral interventions to create more comprehensive and individualized behavioral management programs since interventions will only be effective in those settings to which they are applied.

The most prominent and widely cited treatment study is the Collaborative Multimodal Treatment Study of Children with ADHD, which is a longitudinal multisite treatment study of 579 children ages 7 to 9.9 years diagnosed with ADHD-CT (excluding ADHD-PI and ADHD-HI) funded by the National Institute of Mental Health (NIMH). The controlled treatment trial compared the efficacy of pharmacologic and behavioral interventions across four randomly assigned treatment groups: (1) psychosocial treatment only, (2) stimulant medication only, (3) combined psychosocial and stimulant medication treatment, and (4) standard community treatment (being whatever treatment was typically delivered in that specific community). At the end of the 14-month intervention period, all groups showed improvement relative to the baseline assessment that was maintained 8 years posttreatment, although youth with ADHD continued to function more poorly than their non-ADHD counterparts across development, despite intensive treatment (Molina et al., 2009). Medication and combined treatment groups initially showed greater reduction in ADHD and ODD symptoms and greater improvement in overall adjustment (Conners et al., 2001; Swanson et al., 2001). Combined treatment was also found to be more effective for children with coexisting anxiety problems (Jensen et al., 2001; March et al., 2000) and children of ethnic minority backgrounds (Arnold et al., 2003). However, any differences in treatment efficacy dissipated by 22 months posttreatment (Jensen et al, 2007). Instead, the severity of the child's clinical presentation of ADHD symptoms in the first 3 years of the study, and not treatment group assignment, best predicted outcomes 8 years posttreatment (Molina et al., 2009).

Summary of Treatment for ADHD

The intervention approach used in the MTA study provides an excellent example of applying evidence-based practices for treating children with ADHD (although see Barkley, 2000; Greene & Ablon, 2001; Pelham, 1999, for critiques of the intervention). Despite limited findings for the long-term efficacy of ESTs, the initial findings of this large-scale treatment trial, combined with findings from other treatment studies, support the efficacy of both stimulant medication and behavioral interventions. That is, pharmacologic and behavioral interventions are currently the state-of-the-art treatment for children with ADHD, with some support for combining them to optimize the effects for some children (Pelham et al., 2000). Pharmacologic intervention may be superior to behavioral intervention for treating DSM-based behavioral symptoms, while behavioral treatments may be more effective at treating general functioning and adaptive skills (Pelham et al., 2008; Wells et al., 2006). There is mixed support for the greater cost-effectiveness of one form of intervention over the other (Jensen et al., 2005; Pelham, Foster, & Robb, 2007). At the least, early intervention is critical for preventing the later development of defiant, aggressive, and rule-breaking behaviors (e.g., McCain & Kelley, 1993; McGoey & DuPaul, 2000).

Unfortunately, despite the well-documented efficacy for these two treatment modalities, there continues to be a proliferation of unproven therapies with limited evidence for their effectiveness.

These have ranged from biofeedback programs to specialized diets (Lilienfeld, 2005; Loo & Barkley, 2005; Waschbusch & Hill, 2003). The popularity of these unproven approaches to intervention is likely due to strong biases against the two EBTs. Many parents, and even many professionals, have strong negative feelings about the use of medication for controlling children's behavioral problems. Furthermore, most parents report having tried a system of rewards and punishments in an effort to control their children's behavior, albeit not at the level of consistency and intensity needed to bring about meaningful changes in the child's behavior. As a result, they are often reluctant to agree to interventions focusing on behavior management strategies. These biases often lead to the unfortunate outcome that many children with ADHD do not receive the optimal treatment: a combination of a carefully controlled trial of stimulant medication and an intensive behavior management program.

Oppositional Defiant Disorder and Conduct Disorder

Definition and Description

Diagnosis Conduct disorder is defined as a repetitive and persistent pattern of behavior that violates the rights of others and age-appropriate societal norms or rules. Between 2 and 16% of youth in community settings present with conduct problems, with higher estimates within clinic settings (Boylan, Vaillancourt, Boyle, & Szatmari, 2007; Loeber, Burke, Lahey, Winters, & Zera, 2000). Conduct problems are the most common reason for referral of children and adolescents to outpatient mental health clinics and residential treatment centers (Frick & Silverthorn, 2001). Much research has focused on understanding and treating this externalizing psychopathology, particularly as severe conduct problems often lead to delinquency and violence (Broidy et al., 2003; Moffitt, 2003).

The *DSM–IV–TR* specifies two disorders involving conduct problem behavior. Oppositional defiant disorder is defined as:

- A recurrent pattern of negativistic, defiant, disobedient, and hostile behavior toward authority figures
- A pattern that persists for at least 6 months
- A pattern characterized by the frequent occurrence of at least four of the following behaviors: losing temper, arguing with adults, actively defying or refusing to comply with requests or rules of adults, deliberately doing things that will annoy other people, blaming others for his or her own mistakes or misbehavior, being touchy or easily annoyed by others, being angry and resentful, or being spiteful or vindictive (APA, 2000, p. 100)

Conduct disorder is defined as:

- A repetitive and persistent pattern of behavior that violates the rights of others or major age appropriate societal norms or rules are violated
- These behaviors fall into four main groupings: aggressive conduct that threatens physical harm to other people or animals, nonaggressive conduct that causes property loss or damage, deceitfulness and theft, and serious violations of rules
- Three or more characteristic behaviors must have been present during the past 12 months (APA, 2000, pp. 934–994)

Researchers have debated about the best way to conceptualize the relationship between these two disorders. Initial ODD symptoms appear to be a strong predictor of CD symptoms later in development (APA, 2000). Oppositional defiant disorder youth typically begin demonstrating mild oppositional and argumentative behaviors between the ages of 3 and 8. Over the course of childhood, the behaviors gradually escalate into increasingly frequent and severe patterns of conduct problems (Shaw, Gilliom, Ingoldsby, & Nagin, 2003). Some research suggests that risk factors for future conduct problems can be identified in the mother during pregnancy or shortly after birth, and that symptoms manifest in the first 2 years of life (Petitclerc, Boivin, Dionne, Zoccolillo, & Tremblay, 2009). It must be noted, however, that approximately 40% of children with ODD do not later exhibit more severe conduct problems (Shaw et al., 2003). Those who do progress from ODD to CD do not *change* the types of behaviors they display but instead *add* the more severe conduct problem behaviors to their existing behavioral repertoire (Kim-Cohen et al., 2009) and, typically, ODD symptoms are retained (Loeber, Lahey, & Thomas, 1991).

Developmental Course   Conduct problems are relatively stable across development (Broidy et al., 2003; Shaw et al., 2003). In one study approximately half of the children diagnosed with CD at an initial assessment were rediagnosed with the disorder at a follow-up assessment up to 5 years later (Frick & Loney, 1999). Severe conduct problems that persist into adulthood are often diagnosed as antisocial personality disorder (APD), which is diagnosed when an individual age 18 or older displays a chronic pattern of recklessness, impulsivity and irresponsibility, deceitfulness, criminal behavior, and lack of remorse. Robins (1966) found that 31% of boys and 17% of girls referred to a mental health clinic for CD symptoms were diagnosed with an antisocial disorder as adults. In addition, 43% of the boys with CD and 12% of girls were later imprisoned at least once as an adult. Further, APD in adulthood is more common among children with co-occurring CD and ADHD (Hofvander, Ossowski, Lundstrom, & Anckarsater, 2009).

Many youth with early-starting conduct problems remit from these behaviors over the course of development (Raine et al., 2005; Robins, 1966), particularly those diagnosed when they were preschoolers (Kim-Cohen et al., 2009). However, even when CD symptoms remit these children continue to show adjustment problems later in development (Kim-Cohen et al., 2009). Although they have received less empirical attention, factors related to desistance from antisocial behavior include decreased exposure to risk factors known to contribute to conduct problems and increased exposure to positive factors that protect against them (Loeber, Pardini, Stouthamer-Loeber, & Raine, 2007). Positive factors most often identified as contributing to desistance are normative developmental processes, such as increased physical and mental maturity (Glueck & Glueck, 1940); identity formation (Neugarten & Neugarten, 1996); formation of social controls, such as getting a job or developing bonds with others (e.g., through romantic relationships; Laub & Sampson, 2001; Moffitt, 1993); and development of internal controls that deter criminal involvement, such as greater perceived likelihood of detection and sanctions (Loeber et al., 2007; Mulvey et al., 2004; Stouthamer-Loeber, Wei, Loeber, & Masten, 2004).

Co-occurring Problems   Conduct problems can co-occur with several psychiatric disorders other than ADHD. Anxiety and depression are common among youth with ODD and CD (Boylan et al., 2007). Approximately one third of community children and three quarters of clinic-referred children with CD have a comorbid depressive or anxiety disorder (Russo & Beidel, 1994; Zoccolillo, 1993). The development of internalizing problems, particularly depression, is likely attributable to regular interpersonal conflicts (e.g., with parents, peers, teachers, and police) and other stressors (e.g., family dysfunction, school failure), some of which result from the child's problematic behavior (Frick, Lilienfeld, Ellis, Loney, & Silverthorn, 1999). Recent research suggests that much of the overlap between CD, social skills problems, peer rejection, academic problems, and depression or anxiety is attributable to co-occurring ODD (Burke et al., 2005; Maughan, Rowe, Messer, Goodman, & Meltzer, 2004) or ADHD (Fergusson & Horwood, 1995; Miller-Johnson et al., 2002).

For ODD, factor analyses suggest that symptoms can be separated into three distinct dimensions: angry/irritable mood, defiant/headstrong behavior, and vindictiveness/spitefulness (Stingaris & Goodman, 2009). A study of a nationally representative sample of British youth found that these dimensions predicted distinct outcomes. Both vindictive and headstrong behavior among ODD children predicted the development of CD, with vindictive behavior in particular linked to marked aggression (Stingaris & Goodman, 2009). This study and others also found that irritability in ODD children predicted later anxiety or depressive disorders (e.g., Burke, Hipwell, & Loeber, 2010; Loeber, Burke, & Pardini, 2009).

Subtypes of Conduct Disorders   Much of the stability in CD found in large samples is accounted for by a small group of children who show particularly severe and stable conduct problems (Broidy et al., 2003; Moffitt, 2003). There have been many attempts to uncover characteristics that distinguish between more severe and chronic forms of conduct problems and more benign and transient forms. Similar to ADHD, one of the more consistent predictors of poor outcome is the initial severity of the disorder. The frequency and intensity of the behavior exhibited, the variety of different types of symptoms displayed, and the presence of symptoms in more than one setting are all linked with a more severe and persistent form of CD (Loeber, 1991). Children with comorbid ADHD and intellectual deficits also have worse outcomes than children with either disorder alone (Farrington, 1991; Waschbusch, 2002). Family dysfunction and socioeconomic adversity have also been linked with poorer outcomes for children with conduct problems (Frick & Loney, 1999; Moffitt, 1990).

Perhaps one of the most consistent predictors of poor outcome is the age at which the child begins to show serious conduct problems (Frick & Loney, 1999; Moffitt, 1990, for reviews). For example, in a prospective study of the adult outcomes of a birth cohort in New Zealand, Moffitt, Caspi, Harrington, and Milne (2002) compared two groups of adults who had severe conduct problems as youth. One group who began showing serious problems prior to puberty made up only 10% of the birth cohort but accounted for 43% of violent convictions, 40% of the drug convictions, and 62% of the convictions for violence against women in the sample. The second group, whose conduct problems emerged in adolescence (26% of the sample), showed less temperamental and psychosocial adversity than the childhood-onset group (Moffitt, Caspi, Dickson, Silva, & Stanton, 1996; Moffitt et al., 2002). The adolescent-onset youth were also 50 to 60% less likely to be convicted of an offense than the childhood-onset group, and their offenses tended to be less serious (e.g., minor theft, public drunkenness) and less violent (e.g., accounting for 50% of the convictions for property offenses). Although these data did not use a diagnosis of CD to form their groups and instead used operational definitions of "significant conduct problems," these data influenced the *DSM–IV–TR* criteria to parse CD into childhood-onset and adolescent-onset subtypes depending on whether severe behavior problems begin before or after the age of 10.

More recent research considers the presence of callous and unemotional traits (e.g., lacking empathy and guilt; constricted emotions) to designate a distinct group of children with severe and chronic conduct problems and aggressive behaviors (Frick, Cornell, Barry, Bodin, & Dane, 2003). In fact, for the next revision of the *DSM*, there is consideration of adding a specifier to the diagnosis of CD defined as "with Significant Callous-Unemotional Traits" that can be used in combination with existing age at onset and severity specifiers (Frick & Moffitt, 2010; Moffitt et al., 2008). If a child meets full diagnostic criteria for CD, this specifier would be applied if two or more of the following four characteristics are present over at least 12 months and in more than one relationship or setting: lack of remorse or guilt; lack of concern for others' feelings; lack of concern over poor performance at school, work, or in other important activities; and shallow or deficient emotions.

Callous-unemotional (CU) traits are more common in the childhood-onset group (Moffitt et al., 2002) and are present in about one third of these children (Christian, Frick, Hill, Tyler, & Frazer, 1997). This minority of children consistently show a more severe, aggressive, and stable pattern of behavioral problems among youth with conduct problems (Frick & Dickens, 2006). For example, clinic-referred children with conduct problems and CU traits show a greater number and variety of conduct problems, more police contacts, and stronger family histories of APD than their non-CU counterparts (Christian et al., 1997). The utility of CU traits for predicting a more severe pattern of conduct problems has been found in samples of preschool children (Kimonis, Frick, Boris et al., 2006), elementary school-aged children (Frick, Stickle, Dandreaux, Farrell, & Kimonis, 2005), and adolescents (Kruh, Frick, & Clements, 2005). This has also been found to be true for both boys and girls (Marsee, Silverthorn, & Frick, 2005). Callous-unemotional traits have been associated with severity of antisocial behavior in several different countries such as Australia (Dadds, Fraser, Frost, & Hawes, 2005), the United Kingdom (Moran, Ford, Butler, & Goodman, 2008; Viding, Simmonds, Petrides, & Frederickson, 2009), Belgium (Roose, Bijttebier, Decoene, Claes, & Frick, 2010), Germany (Essau, Sasagawa, & Frick, 2006), Greek Cyprus (Fanti, Frick, & Georgiou, 2009), and Israel (Somech & Elizur, 2009). Importantly, research has also shown that youth with CU traits have a differential treatment response compared to other antisocial youth (Hawes & Dadds, 2005; Waschbusch, Carrey, Willoughby, King, & Andrade, 2007). Finally, CU traits are also relatively stable across development (Frick, Kimonis, Dandreaux, & Farell, 2003; Obradovic, Pardini, Long, & Loeber, 2007).

Cultural and Gender Issues

There is evidence that aggressive and violent behavior varies in rate across cultures. For example, the United States has 4 to 73 times the rates of violence found in other industrialized nations (Fingerhut & Kleinman, 1990). This high rate of violence in the United States has been linked to various factors, such as greater exposure in childhood to violence within the home, neighborhood, and through media portrayals (Anderson et al., 2010; Huesmann, Moise-Titus, Podolski, & Eron, 2003), cultural glorification of violence, and the availability of handguns (O'Donnell, 1995).

However, the differences in the rates of ODD and CD across cultures is less clear. Canino, Polanczyk, Bauermeister, Rohde, and Frick (2010) conducted a meta-analysis of the worldwide prevalence of both ODD and CD, including only studies that used (a) probability school or community household samples, and (b) either *DSM–III–R* or *DSM–IV* criteria. The overall pooled prevalence for children and adolescents ages 6 to 18 was 3.2% for CD and 3.3% for ODD. Importantly, geographic location of the country, as a marker for culture, did not moderate the prevalence estimates for either diagnosis. For CD, prevalence rates were lower when using the *DSM–III–R* (vs. *DSM–IV*) definition, which requires impairment to make the diagnosis. For ODD, children younger than age 12 showed a higher prevalence of the disorder.

Although there do not appear to be clear differences in conduct problems across countries, there are clear gender differences, with most studies showing that boys are more likely to show conduct problems than girls (see Silverthorn & Frick, 1999, for a review). However, gender differences vary somewhat across development. For example, for preschool children gender differences are small and sometimes nonexistent (Keenan & Shaw, 1997), whereas throughout childhood there is a male to female ratio of about 4:1 (Silverthorn & Frick, 1999). This ratio closes to about 2:1 in adolescence, when both boys and girls show a dramatic increase in rates of ODD and CD (Loeber et al., 2000). It is unclear whether developmental changes in prevalence rates are real differences or an artifact of diagnostic criteria that are not sensitive to gender differences in the expression of conduct problems. For example, some argue that girls are less often diagnosed with severe conduct problems than boys because they manifest more indirect or relational aggression (i.e., spreading rumors, hurting others in the context of a relationship) than physical aggression (Crick & Grotpeter, 1995; Underwood, 2003). Others argue that girls manifest similar types of behaviors as boys, but that they should be diagnosed using more lenient criteria that compares girls to other girls rather than to mixed samples of girls and boys (Zoccolillo, 1993). Still others argue that girls manifest similar antisocial behaviors to boys but are less likely to experience the necessary pathogenic processes (e.g., impulsivity, deficits in conscience) that can lead to the development of antisocial behavior (Moffitt & Caspi, 2001; Silverthorn & Frick, 1999).

Boys and girls with conduct problems generally show similar risk factors (Fergusson & Horwood, 2002; Lahey et al., 2000), although there has been significantly less research on the applicability of CD subtypes to girls. Consistently, childhood-onset conduct problems are less common in girls than boys. For example, in an entire birth cohort of New Zealand children, only six girls with childhood-onset CD were identified compared to larger groups of adolescent-onset girls ($N = 78$), childhood-onset boys ($N = 47$), and adolescent-onset boys ($N = 122$; Moffitt & Caspi, 2001). Similarly, in an adjudicated sample of adolescent boys and girls, an almost equal number of boys had a childhood-onset (46%) or adolescent-onset (54%) of severe antisocial behavior, whereas 94% of girls had an adolescent-onset to their antisocial behavior (Silverthorn, Frick, & Reynolds, 2001).

Despite the predominance of the adolescent-onset subtype in antisocial girls, girls with severe conduct problems show a large number of dispositional and contextual risk factors, similar to childhood-onset boys. They also show poor outcomes in adulthood, such as high rates of criminality, violence, antisocial personality, and other psychiatric disorders (Zoccolillo, 1993). To explain these findings, Silverthorn and Frick (1999) proposed a delayed-onset pathway to serious conduct problems in girls. That is, girls who develop serious conduct problems in adolescence often show many risk factors that may have been present in childhood and predate their behavioral problems. However, the onset of conduct problems may be delayed until adolescence, coinciding with biological (e.g., hormonal changes associated with puberty) and psychosocial (e.g., less parental monitoring and supervision; greater contact with deviant peers) changes that encourage antisocial behavior in girls with predisposing vulnerabilities (e.g., CU traits, problems in emotional regulation).

In an initial test of this theory, adjudicated adolescent girls with an adolescent onset to their antisocial behavior also showed high levels of CU traits and problems with impulse control, which was more similar to childhood-onset boys than to adolescent-onset boys (Silverthorn et al., 2001). Despite this initial positive finding, additional tests of this model have been more mixed (Lahey et al., 2006; White & Piquero, 2004).

Etiology: Developmental Pathways to Severe Conduct Problems

A large number of factors have been identified that increase a child's risk for developing conduct problems. These range from individual risk factors (e.g., poor impulse control, poor emotional regulation, low intelligence, lack of social skills), to problems in the child's immediate psychosocial context (e.g., exposure to toxins, poverty, parental psychopathology, inadequate parental discipline, association with a deviant peer group, parental prenatal smoking), to problems in the child's broader psychosocial context (e.g., living in a high crime neighborhood, exposure to violence, lack of educational and vocational opportunities; see Dodge & Pettit, 2003; Frick, 2006, for reviews). It has been difficult to weave this broad array of risk factors into a coherent, yet comprehensive, causal model for conduct problems both because of the sheer number of factors and because they involve so many different types of causal processes. Risk factors are also typically not independent of one another and likely operate in a transactional (e.g., one risk factor having an influence on another risk factor) or multiplicative fashion (Dodge & Pettit, 2003). For example, Jaffee et al. (2005) found that childhood-onset conduct problems were more common in children with a genetic vulnerability to problem behavior who were also exposed to maltreatment. Altogether, this body of research suggests that youth with conduct problems are a highly heterogeneous group, for whom there are multiple developmental pathways (Frick, 2006; Moffitt, 2003).

As a result, the development of conduct problems for any given child is likely the result of a number of different risk factors that interact to increase that child's risk level. Another complicating factor is the possibility that the causal mechanisms leading to conduct problems differ across subgroups of youth exhibiting antisocial behavior. For example, the distinction between childhood- and adolescent-onset CD not only has important predictive utility, as mentioned previously, but the two groups also show different correlates that could suggest divergent etiologies. Childhood-onset CD is linked with a host of co-occurring problems, including aggression, cognitive and neuropsychological disturbances (e.g., executive functioning deficits, autonomic nervous system irregularities), impulsivity, social alienation, and more dysfunctional family backgrounds compared with adolescent-onset CD (Dandreaux & Frick, 2009; Moffitt, 2006), although, as noted previously, these findings may not be as consistent for girls. There also appears to be a strong genetic contribution to the childhood-onset subtype of CD (Moffitt, 2003, 2006).

A greater emphasis is placed on social causes for the development of the adolescent-onset subtype (Moffitt, 2003, 2006). The onset and course of this type of CD seem to be highly influenced by associations with delinquent peers, who encourage these youth to engage in delinquent activities to achieve social status and to reject traditional status hierarchies and religious rules (Moffitt, 2003; Moffitt & Caspi, 2001). This process appears to be an exaggeration of the normal developmental process involving separation and individuation that is crucial to identity formation in adolescence. For these youth, engaging in forbidden behaviors with peers can engender feelings of independence, maturity, and adult status, albeit in a misguided manner (Moffitt, 2003). Also, there are typically fewer adjustment problems in adulthood due to enduring psychosocial vulnerabilities (e.g., neuropsychological impairments, deficits in social skills), and they are usually a direct consequence of their antisocial behaviors (e.g., poor educational attainment, criminal record, early marriage; Moffitt et al., 2002).

As mentioned previously, the presence of CU traits designates a more severe group of children within the childhood-onset group. These traits may also distinguish a group of children with different causal processes leading to their behavioral problems (see Frick, 2006; Frick & Morris, 2004, for reviews). For example, some research suggests that the genetic influence to childhood-onset CD is largely accounted for by youth with significant levels of CU traits (Larsson, Andershed, & Lichtenstein, 2006; Taylor, Loney, Bobadilla, Iacono, & McGue, 2003). A large twin study found that the genetic influences on conduct problems were over twice as great for children high on CU traits as for children low on CU traits (Viding, Blair, Moffitt, & Plomin, 2005). Differences in heritability could not be attributed to differences in the severity of conduct problems or levels of impulsivity/hyperactivity (Viding, Jones, Frick, Moffitt, & Plomin, 2008). Viding et al. (2005) further reported that the influence of shared environment was substantial for the group low on CU traits but negligible for youth high on CU traits. Differences in heritability are theorized to be a function of deficits in amygdala functioning in youth with CU CD (Blair, Mitchell, & Blair, 2005), which has been supported by recent brain imaging studies (Jones, Laurens, Herba, Barker, & Viding, 2009; Marsh et al., 2008).

Children with conduct problems who display CU traits tend to be more fearless (Pardini, 2006), thrill and adventure seeking (Frick, Cornell, Bodin et al., 2003; Frick et al., 1999), and show less trait anxiety than other youth with the same level of conduct problems (Essau et al., 2006; Frick, Cornell, Bodin et al., 2003). They also show a decreased sensitivity to punishment cues in laboratory and social settings (Blair, Peschardt, Budhani, Mitchell, & Pine, 2006; Dadds & Hawes, 2006), lower resting and stress-induced cortisol levels (Loney, Butler, Lima, Counts, & Eckel, 2006; O'Leary, Loney, & Eckel, 2007), and are less reactive to threatening and emotionally distressing stimuli than other children with conduct problems (Blair, 1999; Kimonis, Frick, Fazekas, & Loney, 2006; Loney, Frick, Clements, Ellis, & Kerlin, 2003).

This temperamental style, characterized by low fear and low emotional reactivity to aversive stimuli, can place a child at risk for missing some of the early precursors to empathic concern, which require emotional arousal evoked by the misfortune and distress of others (Blair, 1995). It could also lead a child to be relatively insensitive to the prohibitions and sanctions of parents and other socializing agents (Frick & Morris, 2004; Kochanska, 1993). Finally, it could create an interpersonal style in which the child becomes so focused on the potential rewards and gains of aggression or other antisocial means to solve interpersonal conflicts that he or she ignores the potentially harmful effects of this behavior on him- or herself and others. Thus, low fearfulness and low emotional reactivity to aversive stimuli may be fundamental characteristics that lead to the development of CU traits (Frick & White, 2008). In support of these hypotheses, antisocial and delinquent youth with CU traits are less distressed by the negative effects of their behavior on others (Blair, Jones, Clark, & Smith, 1997; Pardini, Lochman, & Frick, 2003), are more impaired in their moral reasoning and empathic concern towards others (Blair, 1999; Pardini et al., 2003), expect more instrumental gain (e.g., obtaining goods or social goals) from their aggressive actions (Pardini et al., 2003), and are more predatory in their violence than antisocial youth without these traits (Caputo, Frick, & Brodsky, 1999; Kruh et al., 2005).

In contrast, children with childhood-onset conduct problems without CU traits are more highly reactive to emotional and threatening stimuli (Kimonis, Frick, Fazekas et al., 2006; Loney et al., 2003), more distressed by the negative effects of their behavior on themselves and others (Frick, Cornell, Bodin, et al., 2003; Pardini et al., 2003), and are more likely to attribute hostile intent to the actions of peers compared with those high on CU traits. These findings suggest that children with conduct problems without CU traits may have greater difficulties with behavioral and emotional regulation that are related to high levels of emotional reactivity. Studies find that the aggressive and antisocial behavior of children with conduct problems without CU traits is more strongly associated with dysfunctional parenting practices (Hipwell et al., 2007; Oxford, Cavell, & Hughes, 2003; Wootton, Frick, Shelton, & Silverthorn, 1997) and deficits in intelligence (Loney, Frick, Ellis, & McCoy, 1998) than for children high on CU traits. Emotional regulation problems can lead to impulsive and unplanned aggressive acts for which the child may be remorseful afterward but over which he or she still has little control. They can also lead to a higher susceptibility to anger due to perceived provocations from peers, leading to violent and aggressive acts within the context of high emotional arousal (Kruh et al., 2005).

Empirically Validated Treatments

Given the link between conduct problems and later violence and delinquency, it is not surprising that the treatment of antisocial and aggressive behavior in youth has been the focus of a large number of controlled treatment outcome studies. Several reviews of this literature have identified four treatments that have proven effective in controlled outcome studies (see Eyberg, Nelson, & Boggs, 2008, and Frick, 2006, for more extended discussions).

The first intervention involves the use of contingency management programs. The basic components of contingency management programs are: (a) establishing clear behavioral goals that gradually shape a child's behavior in those areas of specific concern for the child, (b) monitoring the child's progress toward these goals, (c) reinforcing appropriate steps toward reaching these goals, and (d) providing consequences for inappropriate behavior. These programs can bring about behavioral changes for children with conduct problems in a number of different settings, such as at home (Ross, 1981), school (Abramowitz & O'Leary, 1991), and in residential treatment centers (Lyman & Campbell, 1996).

The second effective treatment is parent management training (PMT), which is sometimes called "behavioral parent training," as described above as an effective psychosocial intervention for ADHD. A critical goal of PMT programs is to teach parents how to develop and implement structured contingency management programs to alter their child's behavior in the home (Kazdin, 2005; Kazdin & Whitley, 2003). However, PMT programs also focus on (a) improving the quality of parent–child interactions (e.g., having parents more involved in their children's activities, improving parent–child communication, increasing parental warmth and responsiveness); (b) changing antecedents to behavior that enhance the likelihood that positive prosocial behaviors will be displayed by children (e.g., how to time and present requests, providing clear and explicit rules and expectations); (c) improving parents' ability to monitor and supervise their children; and (d) using more effective discipline strategies (e.g., being more consistent in discipline, using a variety of approaches to discipline). The effectiveness of this type of intervention has been the most consistently documented of any technique used to treat children with severe conduct problems (Kazdin, 1995; Kazdin & Whitley, 2003).

The third type of intervention that has proven effective in treating children with conduct problems is a cognitive-behavioral approach, which is designed to overcome deficits in social cognition and social problem-solving experienced by many children and adolescents with conduct problems. For example, as mentioned previously, some children with conduct problems tend to attribute hostile intent to ambiguous interactions with peers that make them more likely to act aggressively toward peers. Other aggressive children overestimate the likelihood that their aggressive behavior will lead to positive results (e.g., enhanced status, obtaining a desired toy), and this cognitive bias makes them more likely to select aggressive alternatives when solving peer conflict (Dodge, Lochman, Harnish, Bates, & Pettit, 1997). Most cognitive-behavioral skills-building programs teach the child to inhibit impulsive or angry responding. This allows the child to go through a series of problem-solving steps (e.g., how to recognize problems, consider alternative responses and select the most adaptive one) and overcome deficits in the way they process social information (Larson & Lochman, 2003).

For the large proportion of children who have conduct problems and comorbid ADHD, the final intervention that has proven to have some effectiveness in reducing conduct problems is the use of stimulant medication. The impulsivity associated with ADHD may directly lead to some of the aggressive and other poorly regulated behaviors of children with severe conduct problems. The presence of ADHD may also indirectly contribute to the development of conduct problems through its effect on (a) children's interactions with peers and significant others (e.g., parents and teachers), (b) parents' ability to use effective socialization strategies, or (c) a child's ability to perform academically. Therefore, for many children and adolescents with conduct problems, reducing ADHD symptoms is an important treatment goal. The effectiveness of stimulants for reducing conduct problems in children with ADHD has been demonstrated in several controlled medication trials (Hinshaw, Heller, & McHale, 1992; Pelham et al., 1993).

Limitations   Each of these interventions have substantial limitations (Brestan & Eyberg, 1998; Kazdin, 1995). First, a significant proportion of children with severe conduct problems do not show a positive response to these interventions and, for those who do respond positively, their behavior problems are often not reduced to a normal level. Second, treatment is most effective with younger children (prior to age 8) with less severe behavioral disturbances. Third, the generalizability of treatment effects across settings tends to be poor. That is, treatments that are effective in changing a child's behavior in one setting (e.g., mental health clinics) often do not bring about changes in the child's behavior in other settings (e.g., schools). Fourth, improvements in behavior are often difficult to maintain over time.

Given these limitations, there has been an increasing focus on trying to improve treatments by integrating our knowledge about the causes of conduct problems with the development of innovative approaches to treatment (Frick, 2001; 2006). Each of the four treatments described previously targets basic processes that research has shown to be important in the development of conduct problems (e.g., family dysfunction, problems in impulse control). However, these treatments have ignored the fact that severe conduct problems are generally caused by many different and interacting processes. As a result, any single intervention is not likely to be effective for all children with ODD or CD.

Empirically Supported Principles   Based on this research, there is not likely to be any single "best" treatment for severe conduct problems. Instead, interventions must be tailored to the individual needs of children with ODD or CD, and these needs will likely differ depending on the specific mechanisms underlying the child's behavioral disturbance. For example, interventions for children in the adolescent-onset pathway will likely be somewhat different from interventions for children in the childhood-onset pathway. Even within the childhood-onset pathway, the focus of intervention may be different depending on the presence or absence of CU traits (see Frick, 2001; 2006, for examples).

Youth with CU CD may be in greatest need of intensive interventions because of their chronic and severe pattern of antisocial behavior across development. Preliminary research suggests some promising interventions for these youth. For example, exposure of antisocial school-aged children to a treatment program enhancing warm and involved parenting resulted in a reduction in CU traits and antisocial behaviors 1 year later (Pardini, Lochman, & Powell, 2007). Also, a parenting intervention with clinic-referred boys with a primary diagnosis of ODD that taught methods for using positive reinforcement, rather than punishment-oriented behavior modification, to encourage prosocial behaviors found a significant reduction in disruptive behaviors for children high on CU traits (Hawes & Dadds, 2005). Similarly, an intensive treatment program administered to incarcerated adolescents high on CU traits that utilized reward-oriented approaches, taught empathy skills, and targeted the youth's interests led to reductions in recidivism over a 2-year follow-up period (Caldwell, Skeem, Salekin, & Van Rybroek, 2006).

One approach to treatment that incorporates research on developmental models of conduct problems is multisystemic therapy (MST), which was originally developed as a general approach to intervention for psychopathological conditions (Henggeler & Borduin, 1990) but has been applied extensively to the treatment of severe antisocial behavior in children and adolescents (Henggeler, Schoenwald, Borduin, Rowland, & Cunningham, 2009) and more recently for the treatment of juveniles who sexually offend (Henggeler, Letourneau et al., 2009). The orientation of MST is an expansion of a systems orientation to family therapy. In systemic family therapy, problems in children's adjustment are viewed as being embedded within the larger family context. Multisystemic therapy expands this notion to include other contexts, such as the child's peer, school, and neighborhood contexts. Most importantly, MST is an intervention framework that emphasizes a comprehensive and individualized approach to intervention that is consistent with the treatment principles outlined above and is delivered in the youth's natural environment.

Multisystemic theory involves an initial comprehensive assessment that seeks to understand the level and severity of the child or adolescent's presenting problems and to understand how these problems may be related to factors in the child's familial, peer, and cultural environments. The information from this assessment is used to outline an individualized treatment plan based on the specific needs of the child and his or her family. Unlike the individual interventions described previously, MST does not emphasize the use of specific techniques. Instead, it emphasizes several principles that follow from its orientation to intervention. These principles include:

- The identified problems in the child are understood within the child's familial, peer, and cultural contexts.
- Therapeutic contacts emphasize positive (strength-oriented) levers for change.
- Interventions promote responsible behavior among family members.
- Interventions are present focused and action oriented, targeting specific and well-defined problems.
- Interventions target sequences of behavior within and between multiple systems.
- Interventions must be developmentally appropriate.
- Interventions are designed to require daily or weekly effort by family members.
- Intervention effectiveness must be evaluated continuously from multiple perspectives.
- Interventions are designed to promote maintenance of therapeutic change by empowering caregivers.

A critical component of MST is a system of intensive supervision for the therapists implementing the treatment to determine how these principles should be implemented to meet the needs of each individual case and to ensure that the principles are followed throughout the intervention (Henggeler, Schoenwald et al., 2009).

One of the important contributions of MST to the treatment outcome literature is its demonstration that individualized interventions can be rigorously evaluated through controlled treatment outcome studies. To illustrate the individualized nature of the treatment, the length of treatment with MST ranged from 5 to 54 hr (mean, 23 hr). In addition to this variation in intensity, the way in which these hours were utilized varied depending on the needs of the clients. Eighty-three percent of the MST group participated in family therapy and 60% participated in some form of school intervention, which included facilitation of parent–teacher communication, academic remediation, or help in classroom behavior management. In 57% of the cases, there was some form of peer intervention, which included coaching and emotional support for integration into prosocial peer groups (e.g., scouts, athletic teams) or direct intervention with peers. In 28% of the cases, there was individual therapy with the adolescent, which typically involved some form of cognitive-behavioral, skills-building intervention. Finally, in 26% of the cases the adolescent's parents became involved in marital therapy.

Findings from controlled treatment outcome studies on the effectiveness of MST in reducing antisocial and aggressive behavior among even severely disturbed youth have been quite promising. For example, one study found that adolescent repeat offenders who underwent MST had lower rearrest rates 4 years later when compared with a control group of offenders who received traditional outpatient services, typically focusing on individual psychotherapy (26 vs. 71%; Borduin et al., 1995). This efficacy was maintained in a long-term follow-up 10 to 16 years after treatment. The MST participants had significantly lower rates of criminal recidivism (50 vs. 81%, respectively), fewer arrests, and less time in secure confinement over this extended follow-up period (Schaeffer & Borduin, 2005). Another controlled treatment outcome study found that adolescent offenders with multiple arrests who were randomly assigned to receive MST had half as many arrests and spent an average of 73 fewer days incarcerated than adolescents who received standard services provided by the juvenile justice system (Henggeler, Melton, & Smith, 1992). These studies and others (e.g., Curtis, Ronan, & Borduin, 2004; Henggeler, Schoenwald et al., 2009) illustrate the promise of MST for treating youth with serious conduct problems.

Conclusions

Externalizing disorders are one of the most common reasons children are referred to mental health clinics for treatment. Children with disorders such as ADHD, ODD, and CD often cause significant disruption to those around them, particularly parents and teachers, who are most likely to refer them for treatment. Further, children with these problems are at increased risk for a number of longer-term problems in adjustment, such as delinquency, substance abuse, and depression. Fortunately, there is a large body of research on externalizing disorders, which has led to great advances in our understanding of their causes and the development of effective interventions to treat them in youth. Unfortunately, this research is often not translated well into practice and, as a result, many children with these disorders do not receive state-of-the-art treatment. There are several reasons for this research-to-practice gap, such as practitioners not remaining current on this research or not being trained in the most current theories and approaches to treatment, or alternatively, from research not being conducted or presented in a way that is useful to practicing psychologists, or a combination of the two. In either case, the quality of services provided to children with disruptive behaviors depends heavily on advances in research and our ability to translate these findings into widely used applications. The focus of this chapter was to summarize research on children with externalizing disorders in a way that promotes such a translation.

References

Abikoff, H., Hechtman, L., Klein, R. G., Weiss, G., Fleiss, K., Cousins, L., … Pollack, S. (2004). Symptomatic improvement in children with ADHD treated with long-term methylphenidate and multimodal psychosocial treatment. *Journal of the American Academy of Child and Adolescent Psychiatry, 43*(7), 802–811.

Abikoff, H., & Klein, R. G. (1992). Attention-deficit hyperactivity and conduct disorder: Comorbidity and implications for treatment. *Journal of Consulting and Clinical Psychology, 60*, 881–892.

Abramowitz, A. J., & O'Leary, S. G. (1991). Behavioral interventions for the classroom: Implications for students with ADHD. *School Psychology Review, 20*, 220–234.

Achenbach, T. M. (1995). Diagnosis, assessment, and comorbidity in psychosocial treatment research. *Journal of Abnormal Psychology, 23*, 45–65.

American Academy of Child and Adolescent Psychiatry. (2007). Practice parameters for the assessment and treatment of children and adolescents with attention-deficit/hyperactivity disorder. *Journal of the American Academy of Child and Adolescent Psychiatry, 46*, 894–921.

American Psychiatric Association. (1980). *Diagnostic and statistical manual of mental disorders* (3rd. ed.). Washington, DC: Author.

American Psychiatric Association. (1987). *Diagnostic and statistical manual of mental disorders* (3rd rev. ed.). Washington, DC: Author.

American Psychiatric Association. (1994). *Diagnostic and statistical manual of mental disorders* (4th ed.). Washington, DC: Author.

American Psychiatric Association. (2000). *Diagnostic and statistical manual of mental disorders* (4th ed., text rev.). Washington, DC: Author.

Anderson, C. A., Shibuya, A., Ihori, N., Swing, E. L., Bushman, B. J., Sakamoto, A., Rothstein, H. R., & Saleem, M. (2010). Violent video game effects on aggression, empathy, and prosocial behavior in Eastern and Western countries. *Psychological Bulletin, 136*, 151–173.

Arnold, L. E., Chuang, S., Davies, M., Abikoff, H. B., Conner, C. K., Elliott, G. R., … Wigal, T. (2004). Nine months of multicomponent behavioral treatment for ADHD and effectiveness of MTA fading procedures. *Journal of Abnormal Child Psychology, 32*(1), 39–51.

Arnold, L. E., Elliott, M., Sachs, L., Bird, H., Kraemer, H. C., Wells, K. C., … Wigal, T. (2003). Effects of ethnicity on treatment attendance, stimulant response/dose, and 14-month outcome in ADHD. *Journal of Consulting and Clinical Psychology, 71*(4), 713–727.

Balint, S., Czobor, P., Komlosi, S., Meszaros, A., Simon, V., & Bitter, I. (2009). Attention deficit hyperactivity disorder (ADHD): gender- and age-related differences in neurocognition. *Psychological Medicine, 39*(8), 1337–1345.

Barkley, R. A. (1996). Attention-deficit/hyperactivity disorder. In E. J. Mash & R. A. Barkley (Eds.), *Child psychopathology* (pp. 63–112). New York: Guilford.

Barkley, R. A. (1997). Behavioral inhibition, sustained attention, and executive functions: Constructing a unifying theory of ADHD. *Psychological Bulletin, 121,* 65–94.

Barkley, R. A. (2000). Commentary on the Multimodal Treatment Study of children with ADHD. *Journal of Abnormal Child Psychology, 28,* 595–599.

Barkley, R. A. (2006). *Attention-deficit hyperactivity disorder: A handbook for diagnosis and treatment* (3rd vol.). New York: Guilford.

Barkley, R. A., & Cox, D. (2007). A review of driving risks and impairments associated with attention-deficit/hyperactivity disorder and the effects of stimulant medication on driving performance. *Journal of Safety Research, 38*(1), 113–128.

Barkley, R. A., Fischer, M., Smallish, L., & Fletcher, K. (2002). The persistence of attention-deficit/hyperactivity disorder into young adulthood as a function of reporting source and definition of disorder. *Journal of Abnormal Psychology, 111,* 279–289.

Barkley, R. A., McMurray, M. B., Edelbrock, C. S., & Robbins, K. (1990). Side effects of methylphenidate in children with attention deficit hyperactivity disorder: A systematic, placebo-controlled evaluation. *Pediatrics, 86,* 184–192.

Barkley, R. A., Murphy, K. R., & Fischer, M. (2008). *ADHD in adults: What the science says.* New York: Guilford.

Benerjee, T. D., Middleton, F., & Faraone, S. V. (2007). Environmental risk factors for attention-deficit hyperactivity disorder. *Acta Paediatrica, 96*(9), 1269–1274.

Biederman, J., Faraone, S. V., Spencer, T. J., Mick, E., Monuteaux, M. C., & Aleardi, M. (2006). Functional impairments in adults with self-reports of diagnosed ADHD: A controlled study of 1001 adults in the community. *Journal of Clinical Psychiatry, 67*(4), 524–540.

Biederman, J., Mick, E., Faraone, S. V., Braaten, E., Doyle, A., Spencer, T., … Johnson, M. A. (2002). Influence of gender on attention deficit hyperactivity disorder in children referred to a psychiatric clinic. *American Journal of Psychiatry, 159,* 36–42.

Biederman, J., Spencer, T., & Wilens, T. (2004). Evidence-based pharmacotherapy for attention-deficit hyperactivity disorder. *International Journal of Neuropsychopharmacology, 7,* 77–97.

Blair, R. J. R. (1995). A cognitive developmental approach to morality: Investigating the psychopath. *Cognition, 57,* 1–29.

Blair, R. J. R. (1999). Responsiveness to distress cues in the child with psychopathic tendencies. *Personality and Individual Differences, 27,* 135–145.

Blair, R. J. R., Jones, L., Clark, F., & Smith, M. (1997). The psychopathic individual: A lack of responsiveness to distress cues? *Psychophysiology, 34,* 192–198.

Blair, R. J. R., Mitchell, D. G. V., & Blair, K. (2005). *The psychopath: Emotion and the brain.* Malden, MA: Blackwell.

Blair, R. J. R., Peschardt, K. S., Budhani, S., Mitchell, D. G. V., & Pine, D. S. (2006). The development of psychopathy. *Journal of Child Psychology and Psychiatry and Allied Disciplines, 47*(3), 262–275.

Borduin, C. M., Mann, B. J., Cone, L. T., Henggeler, S. W., Fucci, B. R., & Blaske, D. M. (1995). Multisystemic treatment of serious juvenile offenders: Long term prevention of criminality and violence. *Journal of Consulting and Clinical Psychology, 63,* 569–578.

Boylan, K., Vaillancourt, T., Boyle, M., & Szatmari, P. (2007). Comorbidity of internalizing disorders in children with oppositional defiant disorder. *European Journal of Child Adolescent Psychiatry, 16,* 484–494.

Brestan, E. V., & Eyberg, S. M. (1998). Effective psychosocial treatments for conduct disordered children and adolescents. *Journal of Clinical Child Psychology, 27,* 180–189.

Broidy, L. M., Nagin, D. S., Tremblay, R. E., Bates, J. E., Brame, B., & Dodge, K. A. (2003). Developmental trajectories of childhood disruptive behaviors and adolescent delinquency: A six-site, cross-national study. *Developmental Psychology, 39*(2), 222–245.

Burke, J. D., Hipwell, A. E., & Loeber, R. (2010). Dimensions of oppositional defiant disorder as predictors of depression and conduct disorder in preadolescent girls. *Journal of the American Academy of Child and Adolescent Psychiatry, 49*(5), 484–492.

Burke, J. D., Loeber, R., Lahey, B. B., & Rathouz, P. J. (2005). Developmental transitions among affective and behavioral disorders in adolescent boys. *Journal of Child Psychology and Psychiatry, 46*(11), 1200–1210.

Burke, J. D., Loeber, R., White, H. R., Stouthamer-Loeber, M., & Pardini, D. (2007). Inattention as a key predictor of tobacco use in adolescence. *Journal of Abnormal Psychology, 116*(2), 249–259.

Burt, S. A., Krueger, R. F., McGue, M., & Iacono, W. (2003). Parent-child conflict and the comorbidity among childhood externalizing disorders. *Archives of General Psychiatry, 60*(5), 505–513.

Caldwell, M., Skeem, J., Salekin, R., & Van Rybroek, G. (2006). Treatment response of adolescent offenders with psychopathy features: A 2-year follow-up. *Criminal Justice and Behavior, 33*, 571–596.

Campbell, S. B., Ewing, L. J., Breaux, A. M., & Szumowski, E. K. (1986). Parent-referred problem three-year-olds: Follow-up at school entry. *Journal of Child Psychology and Psychiatry, 27*(473–488).

Canino, G., Polanczyk, G., Bauermeister, J. J., Rohde, L. A., & Frick, P. J. (2010). Does the prevalence of CD and ODD vary across cultures? *Social Psychiatry and Psychiatric Epidemiology, 45*, 695–704.

Caputo, A. A., Frick, P. J., & Brodsky, S. L. (1999). Family violence and juvenile sex offending: Potential mediating roles of psychopathic traits and negative attitudes toward women. *Criminal Justice and Behavior, 26*, 338–356.

Carlson, C. L., & Mann, M. (2000). Attention-deficit/hyperactivity disorder, predominantly inattentive subtype. *Child and Adolescent Psychiatric Clinics of North American, 9*, 499–510.

Carlson, C. L., & Mann, M. (2003). Sluggish cognitive tempo predicts a different pattern of impairment in the attention deficit hyperactivity disorder type. *Journal of Clinical Child and Adolescent Psychology, 31*, 123–129.

Christian, R. E., Frick, P. J., Hill, N. L., Tyler, L., & Frazer, D. R. (1997). Psychopathy and conduct problems in children: II. Implications for subtyping children with conduct problems. *Journal of the American Academy of Child and Adolescent Psychiatry, 36*, 233–241.

Cole, J., Ball, H. A., Martin, N. C., Scourfield, J., & McGuffin, P. (2009). Genetic overlap between measures of hyperactivity/inattention and mood in children and adolescents. *Journal of the American Academy of Child and Adolescent Psychiatry, 48*(11), 1094–1101.

Conners, C. K., Epstein, J. N., March, J., Angold, A., Wells, K. C., Klaric, J., ... Wigal, T. (2001). Multimodal treatment of ADHD in the MTA: An alternative outcome analysis. *Journal of the American Academy of Child and Adolescent Psychiatry, 40*, 159–167.

Connor, D. F., Steeber, J., & McBurnett, K. (2010). A review of attention-deficit/hyperactivity disorder complicated by symptoms of oppositional defiant disorder or conduct disorder. *Journal of Developmental and Behavioral Pediatrics, 31*(5), 427–440.

Crick, N. R., & Grotpeter, J. K. (1995). Relational aggression, gender, and social-psychological adjustment. *Child Development, 66*, 710–722.

Curtis, N. M., Ronan, K. R., & Borduin, C. M. (2004). Multisystemic treatment: A meta-analysis of outcome studies. *Journal of Family Psychology, 18*(3), 411–419.

Dadds, M. R., Fraser, J., Frost, A., & Hawes, D. (2005). Disentangling the underlying dimensions of psychopathy and conduct problems in childhood: A community study. *Journal of Consulting and Clinical Psychology, 73*, 400–410.

Dadds, M. R., & Hawes, D. J. (2006). *Integrated family intervention for child conduct problems: A behaviour-attachment-systems intervention for parents.* Bowen Hills, QLD Australia: Australian Academic Press.

Dandreaux, D. M., & Frick, P. J. (2009). Developmental pathways to conduct problems: A further test of the childhood and adolescent-onset distinction. *Journal of Abnormal Child Psychology, 37*, 375–385.

Deault, L. C. (2010). A systematic review of parenting in relation to the development of comorbidities and functional impairments in children with attention-deficit/hyperactivity disorder (ADHD). *Child Psychiatry and Human Development, 41*(2), 168–192.

Dodge, K. A., Lochman, J. E., Harnish, J. D., Bates, J. E., & Pettit, G. S. (1997). Reactive and proactive aggression in school children and psychiatrically impaired chronically assaultive youth. *Journal of Abnormal Psychology, 106*(1), 37–51.

Dodge, K. A., & Pettit, G. S. (2003). A biopsychosocial model of the development of chronic conduct problems in adolescence. *Developmental Psychology, 39*, 349–371.

Dopfner, M., Breuer, D., Schurmann, S., Metternich, T. W., Rademacher, C., & Lehmkuhl, G. (2004). Effectiveness of an adaptive multimodal treatment in children with attention-deficit hyperactivity disorder-global outcome. *European Child and Adolescent Psychiatry, 13*(Suppl. 1), I117–I129.

Dowson, J. H. (2006). Pharmacological treatment for attention-deficit hyperactivity disorder (ADHD) in adults. *Current Psychiatry Reviews, 2*, 317–331.

Ernst, M., Liebenauer, L. L., King, A. C., Fitzgerald, G. A., Cohen, R. M., & Zametkin, A. J. (1994). Reduced brain metabolism in hyperactive girls. *Journal of the American Academy of Child and Adolescent Psychiatry, 33*, 858–868.

Essau, C. A., Sasagawa, S., & Frick, P. J. (2006). Callous-unemotional traits in community sample of adolescents. *Assessment, 13*, 454–469.

Eyberg, S. M., Nelson, M. M., & Boggs, S. R. (2008). Evidence-based psychosocial treatments for child and adolescent with disruptive behavior. *Journal of Clinical Child and Adolescent Psychology, 37*, 215–237.

Fanti, K. A., Frick, P. J., & Georgiou, S. (2009). Linking callous-unemotional traits to instrumental and non-instrumental forms of aggression. *Journal of Psychopathology and Behavioral Assessment, 31*(4), 285–298.

Faraone, S. V., & Biederman, J. (2000). Nature, nurture, and attention deficit hyperactivity disorder. *Developmental Research, 20,* 568–581.

Faraone, S. V., Biederman, J., & Mick, E. (2006). The age-dependent decline of attention deficit hyperactivity disorder: a meta-analysis of follow-up studies. *Psychological Medicine, 36*(2), 159–165.

Faraone, S. V., Perlis, R. H., Doyle, A. E., Smoller, J. W., Goralnick, J. J., Holmgren, M. A., & Sklar, P. (2005). Molecular genetics of attention-deficit/hyperactivity disorder. *Biological Psychiatry, 57,* 1313–1323.

Faraone, S. V., Sergeant, J., Gillberg, C., & Biederman, J. (2003). The worldwide prevalence of ADHD: Is it an American condition? *World Psychiatry, 2,* 104–113.

Farrington, D. P. (1991). Childhood aggression and adult violence: Early precursors and later-life outcomes. In D. J. Pepler & K. H. Rubin (Eds.), *The development and treatment of childhood aggression* (pp. 5–29). Hillsdale, NJ: Erlbaum.

Fergusson, D. M., & Horwood, L. J. (1995). Early disruptive behavior, IQ, and later school achievement and delinquent behavior. *Journal of Abnormal Child Psychology, 23*(2), 183–199.

Fergusson, D. M., & Horwood, L. J. (2002). Male and female offending trajectories. *Development and Psychopathology, 14,* 159–177.

Fingerhut, L. A., & Kleinman, J. C. (1990). International and interstate comparisons of homicide among young males. *Journal of the American Medical Association, 263,* 3292–3295.

Fischer, M. (1990). Parenting stress and the child with attention deficit hyperactivity disorder. *Journal of Clinical Child Psychology, 19,* 337–346.

Forero, D. A., Arboleda, G. H., Vasquez, R., & Arboleda, H. (2009). Candidate genes involved in neural plasticity and the risk for attention-deficit hyperactivity disorder: a meta-analysis of 8 common variants. *Journal of Psychiatry Neuroscience, 34*(5), 361–366.

Frick, P. J. (2001). Effective interventions for children and adolescents with conduct disorder. *Canadian Journal of Psychiatry, 46,* 26–37.

Frick, P. J. (2006). Developmental pathways to conduct disorder. *Child Psychiatric Clinics of North America, 15,* 311–332.

Frick, P. J., Cornell, A. H., Barry, C. T., Bodin, S. D., & Dane, H. A. (2003). Callous-unemotional traits and conduct problems in the prediction of conduct problem severity, aggression, and self-report of delinquency. *Journal of Abnormal Child Psychology, 31,* 457–470.

Frick, P. J., Cornell, A. H., Bodin, S. D., Dane, H. A., Barry, C. T., & Loney, B. R. (2003). Callous-unemotional traits and developmental pathways to severe conduct problems. *Developmental Psychology, 39,* 246–260.

Frick, P. J., & Dickens, C. (2006). Current perspectives on conduct disorder. *Current Psychiatry Reports, 8*(1), 59–72.

Frick, P. J., Kimonis, E. R., Dandreaux, D. M., & Farell, J. M. (2003). The 4 year stability of psychopathic traits in non-referred youth. *Behavioral Sciences and the Law, 21*(6), 713–736.

Frick, P. J., Lilienfeld, S. O., Ellis, M. L., Loney, B. R., & Silverthorn, P. (1999). The association between anxiety and psychopathy dimensions in children. *Journal of Abnormal Child Psychology, 27*(5), 383–392.

Frick, P. J., & Loney, B. R. (1999). Outcomes of children and adolescents with conduct disorder and oppositional defiant disorder. In H. C. Quay & A. Hogan (Eds.), *Handbook of disruptive behavior disorders* (pp. 507–524). New York: Plenum.

Frick, P. J., & Moffitt, T. E. (2010). *A proposal to the DSM-V Childhood Disorders and the ADHD and Disruptive Behavior Disorders Work Groups to include a specifier to the diagnosis of conduct disorder based on the presence of callous-unemotional traits.* Washington, DC: APA.

Frick, P. J., & Morris, A. S. (2004). Temperament and developmental pathways to conduct problems. *Journal of Clinical Child and Adolescent Psychology, 33,* 54–68.

Frick, P. J., & Silverthorn, P. (2001). Psychopathology in children. In P. B. Sutker & H. E. Adams (Eds.), *Comprehensive handbook of psychopathology* (3rd ed., pp. 881–920). New York: Kluwer.

Frick, P. J., Stickle, T. R., Dandreaux, D. M., Farrell, J. M., & Kimonis, E. R. (2005). Callous-unemotional traits in predicting the severity and stability of conduct problems and delinquency. *Journal of Abnormal Child Psychology, 33*(4), 471–487.

Frick, P. J., & White, S. F. (2008). Research review: The importance of callous-unemotional traits for developmental models of aggressive and antisocial behavior. *Journal of Child Psychology and Psychiatry, 49*(4), 359–375.

Gau, S. S., Ni, H. C., Shang, C. Y., Soong, W. T., Wu, Y. Y., Lin, L. Y., & Chiu, Y. N. (2010). Psychiatric comorbidity among children and adolescents with and without persistent attention-deficit hyperactivity disorder. *Aust N Z J Psychiatry, 44*(2), 135–143.

Gershon, J. (2002). A meta-analytic review of gender differences in ADHD. *Journal of Attentional Disorders, 5*, 143–154.

Giedd, J. N., Blumenthal, J., Molloy, E., & Castellanos, F. X. (2001). Brain imaging of attention deficit/hyperactivity disorder. *Annals of the New York Academy of Sciences, 931*, 33–49.

Gizer, I. R., Ficks, C., & Waldman, I. D. (2009). Candidate gene studies of ADHD: A meta-analytic review. *Human Genetics, 126*(1), 51–90.

Glueck, S., & Glueck, E. (1940). *Juvenile delinquents grown up*. Oxford, England: Commonwealth Fund.

Greene, R. W., & Ablon, J. S. (2001). What does the MTA study tell us about effective psychosocial treatment for ADHD? *Journal of Clinical Child Psychology, 30*, 114–121.

Greenhill, L. L., Kollins, S., McCracken, J., Riddle, M., Swanson, J., Wigal, S., … Cooper, T. (2006). Efficacy and safety of immediate-release methylphenidate treatment for preschoolers with ADHD. *Journal of the American Academy of Child and Adolescent Psychiatry, 45*, 1284–1293.

Hart, E. L., Lahey, B. B., Loeber, R., Applegate, B., Green, S. M., & Frick, P. J. (1995). Developmental change in attention-deficit hyperactivity disorder in boys: A four-year longitudinal study. *Journal of Abnormal Child Psychology, 23*, 729–749.

Hartman, C. A., Willcutt, E. G., Rhee, S. H., & Pennington, B. F. (2004). The relation between sluggish cognitive tempo and DSM-IV ADHD. *Journal of Abnormal Child Psychology, 32*, 491–503.

Hawes, D. J., & Dadds, M. R. (2005). The treatment of conduct problems in children with callous-unemotional traits. *Journal of Consulting and Clinical Psychology, 73*(4), 737–741.

Henggeler, S. W., & Borduin, C. M. (1990). *Family therapy and beyond: A multisystemic approach to treating the behavior problems of children and adolescents*. Pacific Grove, CA: Brooks/Cole.

Henggeler, S. W., Letourneau, E. J., Chapman, J. E., Borduin, C. M., Schewe, P. A., & McCart, M. R. (2009). Mediators of change for multisystemic therapy with juvenile sexual offenders. *Journal of Consulting and Clinical Psychology, 77*(3), 451–462.

Henggeler, S. W., Melton, G. B., & Smith, L. A. (1992). Family preservation using multisystemic therapy: An effective alternative to incarcerating juvenile offenders. *Journal of Consulting and Clinical Psychology, 60*, 953–961.

Henggeler, S. W., Schoenwald, S. K., Borduin, C. M., Rowland, M. D., & Cunningham, P. B. (2009). *Multisystemic therapy for antisocial behavior in children and adolescents* (Vol. 2nd). New York: Guilford.

Hinshaw, S. P., Heller, T., & McHale, J. P. (1992). Covert antisocial behavior in boys with attention-deficit hyperactivity disorder: External validation and effects of methylphenidate. *Journal of Consulting and Clinical Psychology, 60*, 274–281.

Hinshaw, S. P., Klein, R. G., & Abikoff, H. (2007). Childhood attention deficit hyperactivity disorder: Nonpharmacological treatments and their combination with medication. In P. E. Nathan & J. M. Gorman (Eds.), *A guide to treatments that work* (Vol. 3rd, pp. 3–27). New York: Oxford University Press.

Hipwell, A. E., Pardini, D. A., Loeber, R., Sembower, M., Keenan, K., & Stouthamer-Loeber, M. (2007). Callous-unemotional behaviors in young girls: Shared and unique effects relative to conduct problems. *Journal of Clinical Child and Adolescent Psychology, 36*(3), 293–304.

Hofvander, B., Ossowski, D., Lundstrom, S., & Anckarsater, H. (2009). Continuity of aggressive antisocial behavior from childhood to adulthood: The question of phenotype definition. *International Journal of Law Psychiatry, 32*(4), 224–234.

Huesmann, L. R., Moise-Titus, J., Podolski, C. L., & Eron, L. D. (2003). Longitudinal relations between children's exposure to TV violence and their aggressive and violent behavior in young adulthood: 1977–1992. *Developmental Psychology, 39*, 201–221.

Jaffee, S., Caspi, A., Moffitt, T. E., Dodge, K. A., Rutter, M., & Taylor, A. (2005). Nature × nurture: Genetic vulnerabilities interact with physical maltreatment to promote conduct problems. *Development and Psychopathology, 17*, 67–84.

Jensen, P. S., Arnold, L. E., Swanson, J. M., Vitello, B., Abikoff, H. B., … Hur, K. (2007). 3-year follow-up of the NIMH MTA study. *Journal of the American Academy of Child & Adolescent Psychiatry, 46*, 989–1002.

Jensen, P. S., Garcia, J. A., Glied, S., Foster, M., Schlander, M., Hinshaw, S., … Wells, K. (2005). Cost-effectiveness of ADHD treatments: Findings from the multimodal treatment study of children with ADHD. *American Journal of Psychiatry, 162*(9), 1628–1636.

Jensen, P. S., Hinshaw, S. P., Swanson, J. M., Greenhill, L. L., Conners, C. K., Arnold, L. E., … Wigal, T. (2001). Findings from the NIMH Multimodal Treatment Study of ADHD (MTA): Implications and applications for primary care providers. *Journal of Developmental and Behavioral Pediatrics, 22*(1), 60–73.

Jensen, P. S., Martin, D., & Cantwell, D. P. (1997). Comorbidity in ADHD: Implications for research, practice, and DSM-IV. *Journal of the American Academy of Child and Adolescent Psychiatry, 36*, 1065–1079.

Johnson, S., Hollis, C., Kochhar, P., Hennessy, E., Wolke, D., & Marlow, N. (2010). Psychiatric disorders in extremely preterm children: longitudinal finding at age 11 years in the EPICure Study. *Journal of the American Academy of Child and Adolescent Psychiatry, 49*(5), 453–463.

Johnston, C., & Mash, E. J. (2001). Families of children with attention-deficit/hyperactivity disorder: Review and recommendations for future research. *Clinical Child and Family Psychology Review, 4*, 183–207.

Jones, A. P., Laurens, K. L., Herba, C., Barker, G., & Viding, E. (2009). Amygdala hypoactivity to fearful faces in boys with conduct problems and callous-unemotional traits. *American Journal of Psychiatry, 166*, 95–102.

Kazdin, A. E. (1995). *Conduct disorders in childhood and adolescence* (2nd ed.). Thousand Oaks, CA: Sage.

Kazdin, A. E. (2005). *Parent management training: Treatment for oppositional, aggressive, and antisocial behavior in children and adolescents.* New York: Oxford University Press.

Kazdin, A. E., & Whitley, M. K. (2003). Treatment of parental stress to enhance therapeutic change among children referred for aggressive and antisocial behavior. *Journal of Consulting and Clinical Psychology, 71*, 504–515.

Keenan, K., & Shaw, D. S. (1997). Developmental and social influences on young girls' behavioral and emotional problems. *Psychological Bulletin, 121*, 95–113.

Keenan, K., & Wakschlag, L. S. (2000). More than the terrible twos: The nature and severity of behavior problems in clinic-referred preschool children. *Journal of Abnormal Child Psychology, 28*, 33–46.

Kieling, C., Kieling, R. R., Rohde, L. A., Frick, P. J., Moffitt, T., Nigg, J. T., ... Castellanos, F. X. (2010). The age at onset of attention deficit hyperactivity disorder. *American Journal of Psychiatry, 167*(1), 14–16.

Kim-Cohen, J., Arseneault, L., Newcombe, R., Adams, F., Bolton, H., Cant, L., & Moffitt, T. E. (2009). Five-year predictive validity of DSM-IV conduct disorder research diagnosis in 4(1/2)–5-year-old children. *European Child and Adolescent Psychiatry, 18*(5), 284–291.

Kimonis, E. R., Frick, P. J., Boris, N. W., Smyke, A. T., Cornell, A. H., Farrell, J. M., & Zeanah, C. H. (2006). Callous-unemotional features, behavioral inhibition, and parenting: Independent predictors of aggression in a high-risk preschool sample. *Journal of Child and Family Studies, 15*(6), 745–756.

Kimonis, E. R., Frick, P. J., Fazekas, H., & Loney, B. R. (2006). Psychopathy, aggression, and the processing of emotional stimuli in non-referred girls and boys. *Gender and Psychopathy, 24*(1), 21–37.

Kochanska, G. (1993). Toward a synthesis of parental socialization and child temperament in early development of conscience. *Child Development, 64*, 325–347.

Kruh, I. P., Frick, P. J., & Clements, C. B. (2005). Historical and personality correlates to the violence patterns of juveniles tried as adults. *Criminal Justice and Behavior, 32*, 69–96.

Lahey, B. B., Applegate, B., Barkley, R. A., Garfinkel, B., McBurnett, K., Kerdyck, L., ... Newcorn, J. (1994). DSM-IV field trials for oppositional defiant disorder and conduct disorder in children and adolescents. *American Journal of Psychiatry, 151*, 1163–1171.

Lahey, B. B., Applegate, B., McBurnett, K., & Biederman, J. (1994). DSM-IV field trials for attention deficit hyperactivity disorder in children and adolescents. *American Journal of Psychiatry, 151*(11), 1673–1685.

Lahey, B. B., Carlson, C. L., & Frick, P. J. (1997). Attention deficit disorder without hyperactivity. In T. A. Widiger, A. J. Frances, H. A. Pincus, R. Ross, M. B. First, & W. Davis (Eds.), *DSM-IV sourcebook* (Vol. 3, pp. 163–188). Washington, DC: American Psychiatric Association.

Lahey, B. B., Pelham, W. E., Loney, J., Lee, S. S., & Wilcutt, E. (2005). Instability of the DSM-IV subtypes of ADHD from preschool through elementary school. *Archives of General Psychiatry, 62*, 896–902.

Lahey, B. B., Rathouz, P. J., Van Hulle, C. A., Urbano, R. C., Krueger, R. F., Applegate, B., ... Waldman, D. (2008). Testing structural models of DSM-IV symptoms of common forms of child and adolescent psychopathology. *Journal of Abnormal Child Psychology, 36*, 187206.

Lahey, B. B., Schwab-Stone, M., Goodman, S. H., Waldman, I. D., Canino, G., Rathouz, P. J., ... Jensen, P. S. (2000). Age and gender differences in oppositional behavior and conduct problems: A cross-sectional household study of middle childhood and adolescence. *Journal of Abnormal Psychology, 109*, 488–503.

Lahey, B. B., Van Hulle, C. A., Waldman, I. D., Rodgers, J. L., D'Onofrio, B. M., Pedlow, S., ... Keenan, K. (2006). Testing descriptive hypotheses regarding sex differences in the development of conduct problems and delinquency. *Journal of Abnormal Child Psychology, 34*(5), 737–755.

Lambert, N. M. (1988). Adolescent outcomes for hyperactive children. *American Psychologist, 13*, 786–799.

Langley, K., Fowler, T., Ford, T., Thapar, A. K., van den Bree, M., Harold, G., ... Thapar, A. (2010). Adolescent clinical outcomes for young people with attention-deficit hyperactivity disorder. *British Journal of Psychiatry, 196*, 235–240.

Lara, C., Fayyad, J., de Graaf, R., Kessler, R. C., Aguilar-Gaxiola, S., Angermeyer, M., ... Sampson, N. (2009). Childhood predictors of adult attention-deficit/hyperactivity disorder: Results from the World Health Organization World Mental Health Survey initiative. *Biological psychiatry, 65*(1), 46–54.

Larson, J., & Lochman, J. E. (2003). *Helping schoolchildren cope with anger*. New York: Guilford.

Larsson, H., Andershed, H. A., & Lichtenstein, P. (2006). A genetic factor explains most of the variation in the psychopathic personality. *Journal of Abnormal Psychology, 115*(2), 221–230.

Laub, J. H., & Sampson, R. J. (2001). Understanding desistance from crime. *Crime and Justice, 28*(1), 1–69.

Lavigne, J. V., Gibbons, R. D., Christoffel, K. K., Aremd, R., Rosenbaum, D, Binns, H., ... Isaacs, C. (1996). Prevalence rates and correlates of psychiatric disorders among preschool children. *Journal of the American Academy of Child and Adolescent Psychiatry, 35*, 204–214.

Leslie, L. K., & Wolraich, M. L. (2007). ADHD service use patterns in youth. *Ambulatory Pediatrics, 7*(Suppl. 1), 107–120.

Lilienfeld, S., & Waldman, I. D. (1990). The relation between childhood attention-deficit hyperactivity disorder and adult antisocial behavior reexamined: The problem of heterogeneity. *Clinical Psychology Review, 10*, 699–725.

Lilienfeld, S. O. (2005). Scientifically unsupported and supported interventions for childhood psychopathology: A summary. *Pediatrics, 115*, 761–764.

Loeber, R. (1991). Antisocial behavior: More enduring than changeable? *Journal of the American Academy of Child and Adolescent Psychiatry, 30*, 393–397.

Loeber, R., Burke, J. D., Lahey, B. B., Winters, A., & Zera, M. (2000). Oppositional defiant and conduct disorder: A review of the past 10 years, part I. *Journal of the American Academy of Child and Adolescent Psychiatry, 39*(12), 1468–1482.

Loeber, R., Burke, J. D., & Pardini, D. A. (2009). Development and etiology of disruptive and delinquent behavior. *Annual Review of Clinical Psychology, 5*, 291–310.

Loeber, R., Green, S. M., Lahey, B. B., Christ, M. A. G., & Frick, P. J. (1992). Developmental sequences in the age of onset of disruptive child behavior. *Journal of Child and Family Studies, 1*, 21–41.

Loeber, R., Lahey, B. B., & Thomas, C. (1991). Diagnostic conundrum of oppositional defiant disorder and conduct disorder. *Journal of Abnormal Psychology, 100*, 379–390.

Loeber, R., Pardini, D. A., Stouthamer-Loeber, M., & Raine, A. (2007). Do cognitive, physiological, and psychosocial risk and promotive factors predict desistance from delinquency in males? *Development and Psychopathology, 19*(3), 867–887.

Loney, B. R., Butler, M. A., Lima, E. N., Counts, C. A., & Eckel, L. A. (2006). The relation between salivary cortisol, callous-unemotional traits, and conduct problems in an adolescent non-referred sample. *Journal of Child Psychology and Psychiatry, 47*(1), 30–36.

Loney, B. R., Frick, P. J., Clements, C. B., Ellis, M. L., & Kerlin, K. (2003). Callous-unemotional traits, impulsivity, and emotional processing in antisocial adolescents. *Journal of Clinical Child and Adolescent Psychology, 32*, 139–152.

Loney, B. R., Frick, P. J., Ellis, M., & McCoy, M. G. (1998). Intelligence, psychopathy, and antisocial behavior. *Journal of Psychopathology and Behavioral Assessment, 20*, 231–247.

Loo, S. K., & Barkley, R. A. (2005). Clinical utility of EEG in attention deficit hyperactivity disorder. *Applied Neuropsychology, 12*(2), 64–76.

Lou, H. C., Henrikson, L., Bruhn, P., Borner, H., & Nielson, J. B. (1989). Striatal dysfunction in attention deficit and hyperkinetic disorder. *Archives of Neurology, 46*, 48–52.

Lyman, R. D., & Campbell, N. R. (1996). *Treating children and adolescents in residential and inpatient settings.* Thousand Oaks, CA: Sage.

March, J. S., Swanson, J. M., Arnold, E., Hoza, B., Conners, K., Hinshaw, S. P., ... Pelham, W. E. (2000). Anxiety as a predictor and outcome variable in the multimodal treatment study of children with ADHD (MTA). *Journal of Abnormal Child Psychology, 28*, 527–541.

Marsee, M. A., Silverthorn, P., & Frick, P. J. (2005). The association of psychopathic traits with aggression and delinquency in non-referred boys and girls. *Behavioral Sciences and the Law, 23*(6), 803–817.

Marsh, A. A., Finger, E. C., Mitchell, D. G., Reid, M. E., Sims, C., Kosson, D. S., ... Blair, R J. (2008). Reduced amygdala response to fearful expressions in children and adolescents with callous-unemotional traits and disruptive behavior disorders. *American Journal of Psychiatry, 165*, 712–720.

Martel, M. M., Goth-Owens, T., Martinez-Torteya, C., & Nigg, J. T. (2010). A person-centered personality approach to heterogeneity in attention-deficit/hyperactivity disorder (ADHD). *Journal of Abnormal Psychology, 119*(1), 186–196.

Maughan, B., Rowe, R., Messer, J., Goodman, R., & Meltzer, H. (2004). Conduct disorder and oppositional defiant disorder in a national sample: Developmental epidemiology. *Journal of Child Psychology and Psychiatry, 45*(3), 609–621.

McBurnett, K., Pfiffner, L. T., & Frick, P. J. (2001). Symptom properties as a function of ADHD type: An argument for continued study of sluggish cognitive tempo. *Journal of Abnormal Child Psychology, 29*(3), 207–213.

McCain, A. P., & Kelley, M. L. (1993). Managing the classroom behavior of an ADHD preschooler: The efficacy of a school-home note intervention. *Child and Family Behavior Therapy, 15*, 33–44.

McGoey, K. E., & DuPaul, G. J. (2000). Token reinforcement and response cost procedures: Reducing the disruptive behavior of preschool children with ADHD. *School Psychology Quarterly, 15*, 330–343.

Milich, R., Balentine, A. C., & Lynam, D. R. (2001). ADHD combined type and ADHD predominantly inattentive type are distinct and unrelated disorders. *Clinical Psychology: Science and Practice, 8*(4), 463–488.

Miller-Johnson, S., Coie, J. D., Maumary-Gremaud, A., & Bierman, K. L. (2002). Peer rejection and aggression and early starter models of conduct disorder. *Journal of Abnormal Child Psychology, 30*(3), 217–230.

Moffitt, T. E. (1990). Juvenile delinquency and attention deficit disorder: Boys' developmental trajectories from age 3 to age 15. *Child Development, 61*, 893–910.

Moffitt, T. E. (1993). Adolescence-limited and life-course persistent antisocial behavior: A developmental taxonomy. *Psychological Review, 100*, 674–701.

Moffitt, T. E. (2003). Life-course persistent and adolescence-limited antisocial behavior: A 10-year research review and research agenda. In B. B. Lahey, T. E. Moffitt & A. Caspi (Eds.), *Causes of conduct disorder and juvenile delinquency* (pp. 49–75). New York: Guilford.

Moffitt, T. E. (2006). Life-course-persistent versus adolescence-limited antisocial behavior. In D. Cicchetti & D. J. Cohen (Eds.), *Developmental psychopathology*, Vol 3: *Risk, disorder, and adaptation* (2nd ed., pp. 570–598). Hoboken, NJ: Wiley.

Moffitt, T. E., Arseneault, L., Jaffee, S. R., Kim-Cohen, J., Koenen, K. C., Odgers, C. L., … Viding, E. (2008). Research review: DSM-V conduct disorder: Research needs for an evidence base. *Journal of Child Psychology and Psychiatry, 49*(1), 3–33.

Moffitt, T. E., & Caspi, A. (2001). Childhood predictors differentiate life-course persistent and adolescence-limited antisocial pathways among males and females. *Development and Psychopathology, 13*(2), 355–375.

Moffitt, T. E., Caspi, A., Dickson, N., Silva, P., & Stanton, W. (1996). Childhood-onset versus adolescent-onset antisocial conduct problems in males: Natural history from ages 3 to 18 years. *Development and Psychopathology, 8*, 399–424.

Moffitt, T. E., Caspi, A., Harrington, H., & Milne, B. J. (2002). Males on the life-course persistent and adolescent-limited antisocial pathways: Follow-up at age 26 years. *Development and Psychopathology, 14*, 179–207.

Molina, B. S. G., Hinshaw, S. P., Swanson, J. M., Arnold, L. E., Vitiello, B., Jensen, P. S., … MTA Cooperative Group. (2009). The MTA at 8 years: Prospective follow-up of children treated for combined-type ADHD in a multisite study. *Journal of the American Academy of Child & Adolescent Psychiatry, 48*(5), 484–500.

Monuteaux, M. C., Mick, E., Faraone, S. V., & Biederman, J. (2010). The influence of sex on the course and psychiatric correlates of ADHD from childhood to adolescence: A longitudinal study. *Journal of Child Psychology and Psychiatry, 51*(3), 233–241.

Moran, P., Ford, T., Butler, G., & Goodman, R. (2008). Callous and unemotional traits in children and adolescents living in Great Britain. *British Journal of Psychiatry, 192*(1), 65–66.

MTA Cooperative Group. (1999a). 14-month randomized clinical trial of treatment strategies for attention deficit hyperactivity disorder. *Archives of General Psychiatry, 56*, 1073–1086.

MTA Cooperative Group. (1999b). Moderators and mediators of treatment response for children with attention-deficit/hyperactivity disorder: The multimodal treatment study of children with ADHD. *Archives of General Psychiatry, 56*, 1088–1096.

Mulvey, E., Steinberg, L., Fagan, J., Cauffman, E., Piquero, A., Chassin, L., … Losoya, S. H. (2004). Theory and research on desistance from antisocial activity among adolescent serious offenders. *Journal of Youth Violence and Juvenile Justice, 2*, 213–236.

Neugarten, B. L., & Neugarten, D. A. (1996). *The meanings of age: Selected papers of Bernice L. Neugarten.* Chicago: University of Chicago Press.

Neuman, R. J., Lobos, E., Reich, W., Henderson, C. A., Sun, L. W., & Todd, R. D. (2007). Prenatal smoking exposure and dopaminergic genotypes interact to cause a severe ADHD subtype. *Biological Psychiatry, 61*(2), 1320–1328.

Nigg, J. T. (2006). *What causes ADHD? Understanding what goes wrong and why.* New York: Guildford.

Obradovic, J., Pardini, D., Long, J., & Loeber, R. (2007). Measuring interpersonal callousness in boys from childhood to adolescence. An examination of longitudinal invariance and temporal stability. *Journal of Clinical Child and Adolescent Psychiatry, 36,* 276–292.

O'Donnell, C. R. (1995). Firearms deaths among children and youth. *American Psychologist, 50,* 771–776.

O'Leary, M. M., Loney, B. R., & Eckel, L. A. (2007). Gender differences in the association between psychopathic personality traits and cortisol response to induced stress. *Psychoneuroendocrinology, 32*(2), 183–191.

Oxford, M., Cavell, T. A., & Hughes, J. N. (2003). Callous-unemotional traits moderate the relation between ineffective parenting and child externalizing problems: A partial replication and extension. *Journal of Clinical Child and Adolescent Psychology, 32,* 577–585.

Pálmason, H., Moser, D., Sigmund, J., Vogler, C., Hanig, S., Schneider, A., ... Freitag, C. M. (2010). Attention-deficit/hyperactivity disorder phenotype is influenced by a functional catechol-O-methyltransferase variant. *Journal of Neural Transmission, 117*(2), 259–267.

Pappadopulos, E., Jensen, P. S., Chait, A. R., Arnold, L. E., Swanson, J. M., Greenhill, L. L., ... Newcorn, J. H. (2009). Medication adherence in the MTA: Saliva methylphenidate samples versus parent report and mediating effect of concomitant behavioral treatment. *Journal of the American Academy of Child Adolescent Psychiatry, 48*(5), 501–510.

Pardini, D. A. (2006). The callousness pathway to severe and violent delinquency. *Aggressive Behavior, 32,* 1–9.

Pardini, D. A., Lochman, J. E., & Frick, P. J. (2003). Callous/unemotional traits and social-cognitive processes in adjudicated youths. *Journal of the American Academy of Child and Adolescent Psychiatry, 42*(3), 364–371.

Pardini, D. A., Lochman, J. E., & Powell, N. (2007). The development of callous-unemotional traits and antisocial behavior in children: Are there shared and/or unique predictors? *Journal of Clinical Child and Adolescent Psychology, 36,* 319–333.

Pelham, W. E. (1993). Pharmacotherapy for children with attention-deficit hyperactivity disorder. *School Psychology Review, 22,* 199–227.

Pelham, W. E. (1999). The NIMH multimodal treatment study for attention-deficit hyperactivity disorder: Just say yes to drugs alone? *Canadian Journal of Psychiatry, 44,* 765–775.

Pelham, W. E., Carlson, C., Sams, S. E., Vallan, G., Dixon, M. J., & Hoza, B. (1993). Separate and combined effects of methylphenidate and behavior modification on boys with attention deficit-hyperactivity disorder in the classroom. *Journal of Consulting and Clinical Psychology, 61,* 506–515.

Pelham, W. E., & Fabiano, G. A. (2008). Evidence-based psychosocial treatments for attention-deficit/hyperactivity disorder. *Journal of Clinical Child and Adolescent Psychology, 37,* 184–214.

Pelham, W. E., Foster, E. M., & Robb, J. A. (2007). The economic impact of attention-deficit/hyperactivity disorder in children and adolescents. *Ambulatory Pediatrics, 7,* 121–131.

Pelham, W. E., Gnagy, E. M., Greiner, A. R., Hoza, B., Hinshaw, S. P., Swanson, J. M., ... McBurnett, K. (2000). Behavioral versus behavioral and pharmacological treatment in ADHD children attending a summer treatment program. *Journal of Abnormal Child Psychology, 28,* 507–526.

Petitclerc, A., Boivin, M., Dionne, G., Zoccolillo, M., & Tremblay, R. E. (2009). Disregard for rules: The early development and predictors of a specific dimension of disruptive behavior disorders. *Journal of Child Psychology and Psychiatry, 50*(12), 1477–1484.

Polanczyk, G., Silva de Lima, M., Horta, B. L., Biederman, J., & Rohde, L. A. (2007). The worldwide prevalence of ADHD: A systematic review and metaregression analysis. *American Journal of Psychiatry, 164,* 942–948.

Raine, A., Moffitt, T. E., Caspi, A., Loeber, R., Stouthamer-Loeber, M., & Lynam, D. (2005). Neurocognitive impairments in boys on the life-course persistent antisocial path. *Journal of Abnormal Psychology, 114*(1), 38–49.

Richters, J. E., Arnold, L. E., Jensen, P. S., Abikoff, H., Conners, C. K., Greenhill, L. L., ... Swanson, J. M. (1995). The National Institute of Mental Health collaborative multisite multimodal treatment study of children with attention deficit hyperactivity disorder (MTA): I. Background and rationale. *Journal of the American Academy of Child and Adolescent Psychiatry, 34,* 987–1000.

Robins, L. N. (1966). *Deviant children grown up.* Baltimore, MD: Williams and Wilkins.

Roose, A., Bijttebier, P., Decoene, S., Claes, L., & Frick, P. J. (2010). Assessing the affective features of psychopathy in adolescence: A further validation of the inventory of callous and unemotional traits. *Assessment, 17*(1), 44–57.

Ross, A. O. (1981). *Child behavior therapy: Principles, procedures, and empirical basis.* New York: Wiley.

Rucklidge, J. J., & Tannock, R. (2001). Psychiatric, psychosocial, and cognitive functioning of female adolescents with ADHD. *Journal of the American Academy of Child and Adolescent Psychiatry, 40*, 530–540.

Russo, M. F., & Beidel, D. C. (1994). Comorbidity of childhood anxiety and externalizing disorders: Prevalence, associated characteristics, and validation issues. *Clinical Psychology Review, 14*, 199–221.

Schaeffer, C. M., & Borduin, C. M. (2005). Long-term follow-up to a randomized clinical trial of multisystemic therapy with serious and violent juvenile offenders. *Journal of Consulting and Clinical Psychology, 73*, 445–453.

Schatz, D. B., & Rostain, A. L. (2006). ADHD with comorbid anxiety: A review of the current literature. *Journal of Attention Disorders, 10*, 141–149.

Sharp, S. I., McQuillin, A., & Gurling, H. M. (2009). Genetics of attention-deficit hyperactivity disorder (ADHD). *Neuropharmacology, 57*(7–8), 590–600.

Shaw, D. S., Gilliom, M., Ingoldsby, E. M., & Nagin, D. S. (2003). Trajectories leading to school-age conduct problems. *Developmental Psychology, 39*, 201–221.

Shaw, P., Eckstrand, K., Sharp, W., Blumenthal, J., Lerch, J. P., Greenstein, D., … Rapoport, J. L. (2007). Attention-deficit/hyperactivity disorder is characterized by a delay in cortical maturation. *Proceedings of the National Academy of Sciences, 104*, 19649–19654.

Silverthorn, P., & Frick, P. J. (1999). Developmental pathways to antisocial behavior: The delayed-onset pathway in girls. *Development and Psychopathology, 11*, 101–126.

Silverthorn, P., Frick, P. J., & Reynolds, R. (2001). Timing of onset and correlates of severe conduct problems in adjudicated girls and boys. *Journal of Psychopathology and Behavioral Assessment, 23*, 171–181.

Somech, L. Y., & Elizur, Y. (2009). Adherence to honor code mediates the prediction of adolescent boys' conduct problems by callousness and socioeconomic status. *Journal of Clinical Child and Adolescent Psychology, 38*(5), 606–618.

Sprich, S., Biederman, J., Crawford, M. H., Mundy, E., & Faraone, S. V. (2000). Adoptive and biological families of children and adolescents with ADHD. *Journal of the American Academy of Child and Adolescent Psychiatry, 39*, 1432–1437.

Stawicki, J. A., Nigg, J. T., & von Eye, A. (2006). Family psychiatric history evidence on the nosological relations of DSM-IV ADHD combined and inattentive subtypes: New data and meta-analysis. *Journal of Child Psychology and Psychiatry, 47*(9), 935–945.

Stein, J., Schettler, T., Wallinga, D., & Valenti, M. (2002). In harm's way: Toxic threats to child development. *Journal of Developmental and Behavioral Pediatrics, 23*, 13–22.

Stingaris, A., & Goodman, R. (2009). Longitudinal outcome of youth oppositionality: Irritable, headstrong, and hurtful behaviors have distinctive predictions. *Journal of the American Academy of Child & Adolescent Psychiatry, 48*(4), 404–412.

Stouthamer-Loeber, M., Wei, E., Loeber, R., & Masten, A. (2004). Desistance from persistent serious delinquency in the transition to adulthood. *Development and Psychopathology, 16*, 897–918.

Swanson, J. M., & Castellanos, F. X. (2002). Biological bases of ADHD: Neuroanatomy, genetics, and pathophysiology. In P. S. Jensen & J. R. Cooper (Eds.), *Attention-deficit hyperactivity disorder: State of the science, best practices* (pp. 7-1–7-20). Kingston, NJ: Civic Research Institute.

Swanson, J. M., Kraemer, H. C., Hinshaw, S. P., Arnold, L. E., Conners, C. K., Abikoff, H. B., … Wu, M. (2001). Clinical relevance of the primary findings of the MTA: Success rates based on severity of ADHD and ODD symptoms at the end of treatment. *Journal of the American Academy of Child and Adolescent Psychiatry, 40*(2), 168–179.

Swanson, J. M., McBurnett, K., Christian, D. L., & Wigal, T. (1995). Stimulant medication and treatment of children with ADHD. In T. H. Ollendick & R. J. Prinz (Eds.), *Advances in clinical child psychology* (pp. 265–322). New York: Plenum.

Taylor, J., Loney, B. R., Bobadilla, L., Iacono, W. G., & McGue, M. (2003). Genetic and environmental influences on psychopathy trait dimensions in a community sample of male twins. *Journal of Abnormal Child Psychology, 31*(6), 633–645.

Underwood, M. K. (2003). *Social aggression among girls.* New York: Guilford.

Verhulst, F. C., Van der Ende, J., Ferdinand, R. F., & Kasius, M. C. (1997). The prevalence of DSM-III-R diagnoses in a national sample of Dutch adolescents. *Archives of General Psychiatry, 54*, 329–336.

Viding, E., Blair, R. J. R., Moffitt, T. E., & Plomin, R. (2005). Evidence for a substantial genetic risk for psychopathic traits in 7-year-olds. *Journal of Child Psychology and Psychiatry, 46*(6), 592–597.

Viding, E., Jones, A. P., Frick, P. J., Moffitt, T. E., & Plomin, R. (2008). Heritability of antisocial behaviour at 9: Do callous-unemotional traits matter? *Developmental Science, 11*(1), 17–22.

Viding, E., Simmonds, E., Petrides, K. V., & Frederickson, N. (2009). The contribution of callous-unemotional traits and conduct problems to bullying in early adolescence. *Journal of Child Psychology and Psychiatry, 50*(4), 471–481.

Waschbusch, D. A. (2002). A meta-analytic examination of comorbid hyperactive-impulsive-attention problems and conduct problems. *Psychological Bulletin, 128*, 118–150.

Waschbusch, D. A., Carrey, N. J., Willoughby, M. T., King, S., & Andrade, B. F. (2007). Effects of methylphenidate and behavior modification on the social and academic behavior of children with disruptive behavior disorders: The moderating role of callous/unemotional traits. *Journal of Clinical Child and Adolescent Psychology, 36*, 629–644.

Waschbusch, D. A., & Hill, G. P. (2003). Empirically supported, promising, and unsupported treatments for children with attention-deficit/hyperactivity disorder. In S. O. Lilienfeld, S. J. Lynn & J. M. Lohr (Eds.), *Science and Pseudoscience in Clinical Psychology* (pp. 333–362). New York: Guilford.

Weiss, G., & Hechtman, L. T. (1993). *Hyperactive children grown up: ADHD in children, adolescents, and adults.* New York: Guilford.

Wells, K. C., Chi, T. C., Hinshaw, S. P., Epstein, J. N., Pfiffner, L. J., Nebel-Schwain, M., … Wigal, T. (2006). Treatment-related changes in objectively measured parenting behaviors in the Multimodal Treatment Study of Children with ADHD. *Journal of Consulting and Clinical Psychology Review, 74*, 649–657.

Wells, K. C., Pelham, W. E., Kotkin, R. A., Hoza, B., Abikoff, H. B., Abramowitz, A., … Schiller, E. (2000). Psychosocial treatment strategies in the MTA study: Rationale, methods, and critical issues in design and implementation. *Journal of Abnormal Child Psychology, 28*, 483–505.

White, N. A., & Piquero, A. R. (2004). A preliminary empirical test of Silverthorn and Prick's delayed-onset pathway in girls using an urban, African-American, US-based sample: Comment. *Criminal Behaviour and Mental Health, 14*(4), 291–309.

Willcutt, E. G., Pennington, B. F., & DeFries, J. C. (2000). Etiology of inattention and hyperactivity/impulsivity in a community sample of twins with learning difficulties. *Journal of Abnormal Child Psychology, 28*, 149–159.

Wootton, J. M., Frick, P. J., Shelton, K. K., & Silverthorn, P. (1997). Ineffective parenting and childhood conduct problems: The moderating role of callous-unemotional traits. *Journal of Consulting and Clinical Psychology, 65*, 301–308.

World Health Organization. (1992). *The ICD-10 classification of mental and behavioural disorders: Clinical description and diagnostic guidelines.* Geneva: Author.

Zametkin, A. J., Liebenauer, L. L., Fitzgerald, G. A., King, A. C., Minkunas, D. V., Herscovitch, P., … Cohen, R. M. (1993). Brain metabolism in teenagers with attention deficit hyperactivity disorder. *Archives of General Psychiatry, 50*, 333–340.

Zametkin, A. J., Nordahl, T. E., Gross, M., King, A. C., Semple, W. E., Rumsey, J., … Cohn, R. M. (1990). Cerebral glucose metabolism in adults with hyperactivity of childhood onset. *New England Journal of Medicine, 323*, 1361–1366.

Zoccolillo, M. (1993). Gender and the development of conduct disorder. *Development and Psychopathology, 5*, 65–78.

18
Internalizing Disorders

THOMAS H. OLLENDICK

Virginia Polytechnic Institute and State University
Blacksburg, Virginia

JANAY B. SANDER

The University of Texas at Austin
Austin, Texas

Internalizing disorders in childhood and adolescence include the anxiety and affective disorders. As such, they consist of problems related to worry, fear, shyness, low self-esteem, sadness, and depression. These "emotional" problems have frequently been found to be interrelated in clinical settings and to be associated statistically with one another in factor analytic studies. Internalizing problems can be contrasted with externalizing problems—problems frequently associated with inattention, bad conduct, and opposition and defiance (see Kimonis & Frick, this volume). It is of historic interest to note that these two broad dimensions of childhood and adolescent problems have been recognized for many years. Karen Horney (1945), for example, spoke of children who "move against the world" (i.e., externalizing disorder children) and those who "move away from the world" (i.e., internalizing disorder children) (p. 27).

Although there is little question about the existence of internalizing problems in childhood and adolescence and their detrimental effects on the growing child and adolescent (Ollendick & King, 1994), there is considerable controversy about whether they constitute a single broadband internalizing set of problems or whether they constitute multiple, narrow-band psychiatric disorders. At the heart of this issue is the frequent observation that anxiety disorders and affective disorders frequently co-occur with one another (i.e., are comorbid disorders) and that they are rarely observed in their "pure" forms, at least in childhood and adolescence (Seligman & Ollendick, 1998). For example, in an early study, Last, Strauss, and Francis (1987) found that 73% of separation anxious children and adolescents and 79% of overanxious children and adolescents presented at their outpatient clinic for *anxious* children with one or more additional psychiatric disorders, including major depressive disorders. Similarly, Kovacs, Feinberg, Crouse-Novak, Paulauskas, and Finkelstein (1984) demonstrated early on that a majority of children and adolescents who presented at their outpatient clinic for *depressed* children were diagnosed with concurrent disorders. In fact, 79% of youths with a major depressive disorder and 93% of the youths who presented with dysthymic disorder had a concurrent psychiatric disorder, of which one of the most common was an anxiety disorder. Of importance for the developmental sequence of these disorders, Kovacs et al. reported that anxiety disorders tended to precede the depressive disorders when these two conditions were present in the same child or adolescent. Last, Perrin, Hersen, and Kazdin (1992) have reaffirmed these rates of comorbidity and developmental sequelae, as have Seligman and Ollendick (1998).

Although the major anxiety and affective disorders in childhood and adolescence overlap, we will present them as separate diagnostic entities in this chapter, consistent with nosological approaches, such as the *Diagnostic and Statistical Manual of Mental Disorders* (fourth edition text revision, *DSM–IV-TR*; American Psychiatric Association [APA], 2000) and the *International Classification of Diseases* 10th edition (*ICD–10*; World Health Organization, 1992). In doing so, this chapter will point out areas of overlap and draw distinctions between them. We recognize this decision is not without controversy, but it is consistent with much of clinical practice and research, and it allows us to present information about the disorders in a coherent and organized manner.

Anxiety Disorders in Children and Adolescents

Phenomenology

For children and adults alike, anxiety is a normal and common emotional response to a perceived threat to one's physical or emotional well-being. Feeling fearful and fleeing from a genuinely dangerous situation is adaptive. However, if the anxiety response is elicited by a situation or object that is not truly dangerous, then the anxiety and the avoidance associated with it are not adaptive. A diagnosis of an anxiety disorder may be warranted if the anxiety response is excessive in frequency, intensity, or duration and if it results in significant impairment in functioning. Excessive anxiety is distressing to children and adolescents, and the associated avoidance interferes with their ability to engage in developmentally appropriate tasks and activities. Alarmingly, anxiety disorders are one of the most common psychological difficulties experienced by children and adolescents, and these disorders tend to persist into late adolescence and adulthood unless effective treatment is received (Ollendick & March, 2004).

Consistent with Lang's (1979) tripartite model, anxiety is best viewed as a multidimensional construct involving *physiological* features such as increased heart rate and respiration, *cognitive* ideation including catastrophic and unhelpful thoughts (e.g., "I can't do this," "What if something terrible happens?"), and *behavioral* responses such as avoidance of the anxiety-provoking object or situation. Furthermore, there are developmental differences in the expression of anxiety. For example, young children may avoid objects or situations that scare them; however, they may have difficulty identifying the exact cognitions associated with the feared situation. Young children may also have trouble relating or connecting their physiological symptoms to their anxiety. For example, a child with separation anxiety might insist that the reason she is sick with a headache and stomach ache when she has to go to school is that she has come down with a physical illness such as the flu, not because she is fearful about separation from her caretaker.

Developmental Considerations   As noted, for most children and adolescents, fears and worries are a normal part of development. Accordingly, clinicians assessing anxiety in children need to be aware of what constitutes "normal" fears at each level of development. For example, young infants and toddlers tend to fear aspects of their immediate environment such as loud noises, unfamiliar people, separation from caregivers, or heights. Fears of animals, being alone, and of the dark begin to emerge during the preschool years. As cognitive abilities continue to develop during the early school years, children's fears begin to include abstract, imaginary, or anticipatory fears such as fear of failure or evaluation, death, bodily injury, and supernatural phenomena. Finally, concerns about death, danger, social comparison, personal conduct, and physical appearance extend from adolescence to adulthood (Gullone, 2000; Ollendick, King, & Muris, 2002).

Developmentally normal fears are, by definition, age appropriate and transitory in nature. In contrast, a diagnosis of an anxiety disorder is warranted when a child experiences anxiety that is not typical of a child his or her age and when a child experiences anxiety that is severe and causes considerable distress or impairs a child's functioning at home, school, or in peer and family relationships.

Gender Differences   Research examining the prevalence of anxiety disorders in boys and girls has produced mixed results. Studies using community samples have found that girls are more likely to report anxiety than boys (Essau, Conradt, & Petermann, 2000; McGee et al., 1990). In contrast, gender differences are usually not found in clinical samples (Strauss & Last, 1993). There are at least two explanations for this discrepancy. First, societal expectations of gender-appropriate behavior for boys and girls may mean that girls are more likely to report anxiety symptoms than boys. Alternatively, anxiety symptoms may be more common in girls, and the equal ratio of males to females in clinic samples may indicate that boys experiencing anxiety are more likely to be referred for treatment than girls with similar symptoms.

The direction and size of the gender difference is also dependent on the diagnostic category being considered. Generalized anxiety disorder (GAD) appears to be similarly prevalent in boys and girls during childhood, although in adolescence it is more common among females than males (Cohen et al., 1993; Werry, 1991). Research concerning gender differences for separation anxiety disorder (SAD) has been mixed. Although some studies find no gender differences for SAD (Cohen et al., 1993; Last et al., 1992), most studies find that girls outnumber boys for SAD symptoms (e.g., Anderson, Williams, McGee, & Silva, 1987; Kashani, Orvaschel, Rosenberg, & Reid, 1989). The research on social phobia is less clear, although few gender differences have been noted (Beidel & Morris, 1995; Ollendick & Ingman, 2001)

Prevalence

Estimated prevalence rates for the childhood anxiety disorders using *DSM* criteria have been found to vary considerably but typically range between 7 and 12% (Anderson et al., 1987; Kashani et al., 1987, 1989; Moreau & Weissman, 1992). For example, Anderson et al. (1987) showed that 7.4% of 792 children in the Dunedin, New Zealand, longitudinal study met criteria for an anxiety disorder when they were 11 years of age. At 15 years of age, McGee et al. (1990) reported that 10.7% of the adolescents in this same sample met criteria for an anxiety disorder. A 3.3% increase in the anxiety disorders was evident over the 4-year period of time. Similar prevalence rates for the anxiety disorders have been found by a host of other researchers, with many indicating that the prevalence of some anxiety disorders increases with age (e.g., GAD, social phobia, panic disorder), whereas others tend to decrease with age (e.g., SAD, specific phobia). Thus, overall prevalence rates vary by gender and age. They also vary by the diagnostic category being considered, as we shall see next.

Diagnostic Categories

Separation Anxiety Disorder   The *DSM–IV-TR* describes SAD as developmentally inappropriate and excessive anxiety associated with separation from home or from those to whom the individual is attached (APA, 2000). Often children with SAD worry about danger or harm coming to themselves (e.g., being kidnapped) or their loved one (e.g., becoming ill) when they are separated. Children with SAD exhibit distress when they are separated from their attachment figures and will undertake steps to avoid being apart from them. This may result in children refusing to attend school, go to church day camps, or sleep away from home. The evidence indicates that as children become older, the prevalence of SAD declines. For example, in the Dunedin study, it was shown that the 12-month prevalence rate for SAD was 3.5% for the 11-year-old children but 2.0% for the 15-year-old adolescents. In adolescence, this disorder seems to become less common compared to other disorders such as GAD, social phobia, and panic disorder (Mattis & Ollendick, 2002).

Generalized Anxiety Disorder   GAD is characterized as excessive anxiety and worry, which occurs more days than not for at least 6 months. These children find it difficult to control their worries about a number of events or activities. To meet criteria for GAD, children need to experience at least one associated physiological symptom, although typically these children report multiple physical symptoms. Physical symptoms include stomach aches or nausea, headaches, muscle tension, restlessness, irritability, fatigue, and sleep disturbance. The *DSM–IV–TR* category of GAD in children replaced overanxious disorder (OAD; in *DSM–III–R*; American Psychiatric Association, 1980). As noted above, there is some evidence to suggest that the prevalence of OAD/GAD increases with age (Kashani et al., 1989; Strauss, 1994).

Specific Phobia   Specific phobia (SP) is defined as persistent fear of a specific object or situation that is excessive or unreasonable. Phobias of certain animals or insects, the dark, heights, storms, and medical procedures are among the most common in children. There are four major types of specific phobia: animal, environmental, situational, and blood-injury-injection. A recent study conducted in Germany reported a prevalence rate of 2.5% in 12- to 17-year-olds (Essau et al., 2000). Studies in the United States have reported prevalence rates ranging from 3.6 to 9% (Costello et al., 1988; Kashani et al., 1987; Kessler et al., 1994). Taken together, studies suggest a prevalence rate of about 5% for specific phobia in children and adolescents (Ollendick, Hagopian, & King, 1997; Ollendick, Raishevich, Davis, Sirbu, & Ost, 2010).

Social Phobia   Social phobia in children, like in adults, is characterized by a marked or persistent fear of social situations or performance situations. Typically, in these situations, the child is exposed to unfamiliar people or is scrutinized by others. Social phobia is a disorder with a later age of onset (usually around 11 years of age), being rarely diagnosed in children younger than 10 years old (Davidson, Hughes, George, & Blazer, 1993). Of the changes in diagnostic criteria from the *DSM–III–R* to *DSM–IV*, the difference between the previous category of avoidant disorder and the new category of social phobia has been found to be the most significant (Kendall & Warman, 1996). This disparity has made comparison of prevalence rates across studies using these two systems more difficult. Using the *DSM–III–R*, Anderson et al. (1987) found that less than 1% of children aged 11 years and none of the 15-year-olds in the Dunedin study were diagnosed with avoidant disorder. A later study using *DSM–IV* criteria reported that 6.3% of adolescents were diagnosed with social phobia. Although these results may suggest an increase in prevalence with age, it is more likely that these results reflect changes in diagnostic criteria from *DSM–III–R* to *DSM–IV* (Schniering, Hudson, & Rapee, 2000).

Obsessive-Compulsive Disorder   Obsessive-compulsive disorder (OCD) is characterized by obsessions, which are recurrent thoughts, images, or impulses that are intrusive and result in an increase in anxiety. These obsessions are most often, though not always, accompanied by compulsions, which are repetitive behaviors that reduce anxiety (e.g., washing hands or checking). Epidemiological data on the prevalence of OCD in prepubertal children have been reported to be less than 1% (Heyman et al., 2001). The prevalence rates for adolescents, however, range from 1.9 to 3.6% (Cook et al., 2001). The results of the Heyman et al. (2001) study suggest that prevalence may increase with age.

Differential Diagnosis and Comorbidity

Although recent research using the *DSM* classification system has facilitated the communication of knowledge between researchers and clinicians, the overlap in diagnostic criteria between some of these nosological categories has generated controversy. Briefly, the major problem, as we noted earlier, is the co-occurrence of multiple disorders (i.e., comorbidity) in the same child or adolescent. Some authors (e.g., Caron & Rutter, 1991) have argued that the categorical system of diagnosis does not accurately reflect the true nature of childhood anxiety and suggest that a dimensional approach may be preferred in dealing with the overarching issue of comorbidity. Others, however, maintain that the current diagnostic system is sufficiently precise and that we need more refined research to clarify the boundaries among the various anxiety disorders (cf. Ollendick & March, 2004). Although all decisions regarding the upcoming DSM–5 have not yet been determined, it is probable that it will take an intermediate position and welcome both the categorical and dimensional aspects of disorders, both in childhood and adulthood (see Widiger, this volume). Nonetheless, the shifts in nosology do not appear to be substantial ones, and the categorical system will likely prevail. Undoubtedly, there are positive aspects to both dimensional and categorical systems, depending on the intended use of the information obtained from these somewhat disparate approaches. Thus, we believe such developments, even in their limited form, are welcome ones.

In clinical populations, the most common comorbidity with any specific anxiety disorder is another type of anxiety disorder (Kendall, Brady, & Verduin, 2001). Across epidemiological and clinical studies using varied methodologies, disorders have been found to co-occur with one another at rates higher than chance (Caron & Rutter, 1991). Evidence of significant comorbidity is troubling because children with comorbid disorders tend to have a greater severity and persistence of symptoms, have more interpersonal problems, and may be more refractory to change and clinically challenging for therapists (Manassis & Monga, 2001).

In addition to comorbidity with other anxiety disorders, anxious children may also exhibit high rates of depression (Brady & Kendall, 1992; Seligman & Ollendick, 1998), as noted previously. Using a large cohort of 1,710 adolescents, the Oregon Adolescent Depression project found that 49% of the adolescents with an anxiety disorder also had comorbid depressive disorders using *DSM* criteria (Lewinsohn, Hops, Roberts, Seeley, & Andrews, 1993). Similarly, high rates of comorbidity were found in the Dunedin, New Zealand, sample of youths (Anderson et al., 1987; McGee, Feehan, Williams, & Anderson, 1992; McGee et al., 1990). This series of studies also found that the rates of comorbid mood disorders increased as the children became older. Rates of comorbidity of anxiety and depressive disorders were higher among adolescents than among younger children.

Rates of comorbidity between anxiety and externalizing problems such as attention-deficit/ hyperactivity disorder (ADHD) are also high (Caron & Rutter, 1991). Studies examining this relationship have found that between 13 and 24% of children with an anxiety disorder also have ADHD, oppositional defiant disorder, or conduct disorder (Keller et al., 1992; Last et al., 1987). Consistent with these findings, Kendall et al. (2001) reported that 25% of their clinical sample of anxious children also met *DSM* criteria for one of these three disruptive behavior disorders.

Developmental Course and Prognosis

A common misconception is that children and adolescents will outgrow their worries and fears. Although this may be true of developmentally normal fears and everyday concerns, research suggests that anxiety disorders tend to persist unless treated. For example, Pfeffer, Lipkins, Plutchik, and Mizruchi (1988) found that for children aged 6 to 12 years who were diagnosed with OAD, 70.6% still met this diagnosis 2 years later. Similarly, in the Dunedin study, longitudinal results showed that girls diagnosed with an anxiety or depressive disorder at one age were more likely to continue to meet diagnostic criteria in subsequent years (McGee et al., 1990, 1992).

Anxiety disorders have been shown to persist not only over time but also to be associated with the development of more severe symptomatology (Albano, Chorpita, & Barlow, 1996). Older children tend to report more severe anxiety and comorbid symptomatology than do younger children with the same diagnosis (Strauss, Lease, Last, & Francis, 1988). Similarly, many adults with anxiety disorders report a lifelong history of anxiety symptoms beginning in childhood

(Markowitz, Weissman, Ouellette, Lish, & Klerman, 1989; Ollendick, Lease, & Cooper, 1993). For example, a longitudinal study conducted in the United States found that children with an anxiety disorder were at greater risk for future anxiety disorders, and they were at increased risk of developing dysthymic disorders as well (Lewinsohn et al., 1993; Orvaschel, Lewinsohn, & Seeley, 1995).

Etiological Theories of Childhood Anxiety

Understanding the development of anxiety and its disorders requires us to consider the potential for complex, reciprocal interactions and transactions between many etiological factors over the course of a child's development, consistent with a developmental psychopathology approach (see Zeman & Suveg, this volume). Empirical efforts to explain the development and maintenance of anxiety have focused on the interaction between personal characteristics of the child (e.g., genetic vulnerability, behavioral inhibition, cognitive processes) and interpersonal factors such as attachment to caregivers and learning processes that occur within the family. Some of these etiological factors will now be addressed briefly.

Biological and Familial Factors   Family studies using both referred and nonreferred samples show that the parents of anxious children, and the children of anxious parents, are more likely to experience anxiety problems than nonclinical controls (McClure, Brennan, Hammen, & Le Brocque, 2001). Although family studies have demonstrated that anxiety disorders tend to run in families, the mechanism of transmission remains unanswered. Twin studies help to distinguish whether this mechanism is genetic, environmental, or a combination of the two. Although specific heritability estimates vary across studies, almost all twin studies support the conclusion that there is a heritable genetic risk for anxiety disorders (see Thapar & McGuffin, 1995, for a review). However, rather than a risk toward developing a specific anxiety disorder, the research is strongest for a genetic vulnerability toward either an anxiety or a depressive disorder (Eley & Stevenson, 1999; Kendler et al., 1995).

One of the proposed mechanisms by which a predisposition for anxiety is transmitted genetically is via inherited temperamental characteristics such as behavioral inhibition (BI). Kagan, Reznick, and Snidman (1987) found BI to occur in about 15 to 20% of children, and that children with BI tended to react with withdrawal, avoidance, or distress when confronted with unfamiliar people, situations, or objects. Behavioral inhabition has also been shown to be a risk factor for later childhood anxiety problems (Biederman et al., 2001). However, it is important to remember that not all behaviorally inhibited children develop anxiety disorders, and it is best conceptualized as one possible predisposing factor that may lead to anxiety given the "right" set of other contextual conditions (Ollendick & Hirshfeld-Becker, 2002).

Learning Influences   The theory of classical conditioning can be invoked to help explain the development of certain fears and phobias, as well as anxiety disorders in general. For example, a child might develop a dog phobia after the previously neutral stimulus (a dog) was associated with the pain of being bitten (unconditioned stimuli), resulting in a conditioned fear response. However, classical conditioning theory alone cannot explain why some individuals who experience a pairing of trauma or pain with a particular object or situation do not develop a phobia (Ollendick & Cerny, 1981). In more recent years, theorists have integrated information-processing theories with classical conditioning theory suggesting that an individual's internal representation and subsequent evaluation of the unconditioned stimuli mediate the strength of the conditioned response (Davey, 1992). For example, Reiss (1980) suggested that a person's anticipation of social or physical danger, or the expectation of anxiety, might make a person more susceptibility to traumatic conditioning.

Operant conditioning theory suggests that behaviors that are reinforced are more likely to occur again and behaviors that are followed by punishment are less likely to occur again (Skinner, 1938). Furthermore, the concept of negative reinforcement is frequently used to explain how avoidant behavior maintains anxiety symptoms over time. Specifically, when an anxious child avoids a feared situation, the child is reinforced by the resultant reduction in anxiety symptoms. The child therefore learns that to prevent experiencing the unpleasantness of anxiety, he or she needs to avoid the feared situation or object.

Operant conditioning principles can also be used to explain the process by which a child's nonanxious behavior gradually decreases in frequency, while the anxious behavior increases (Ollendick, Vasey, & King, 2000). For example, Barrett, Rapee, Dadds, and Ryan (1996) found that parents of clinically anxious children attended more to the anxious and avoidant behaviors of their children than to their brave, coping behaviors. Although this study was unable to clarify whether this pattern of parenting behavior existed prior to or after the development of their child's anxiety, it does indicate that positive reinforcement from parents may serve to maintain the problem.

Childhood anxiety has also been shown to develop as a result of vicarious learning and modeling. Bandura (1999) suggested that behaviors might be acquired, facilitated, reduced, or eliminated by observing the behavior of others. Accordingly, fears may appear after the child has observed their parents or peers reacting fearfully to certain objects or situations. Silverman, Cerny, Nelles, and Burke (1988) studied a group of anxious parents and their children and found that children's anxious behaviors were associated with heightened levels of avoidance evidenced by their parents. Interestingly, these researchers noted that anxiety disorders showing the most pronounced avoidance behaviors (social and simple phobia and agoraphobia) seem to have the highest rates of familial risk.

Cognitive and Information-Processing Biases   Cognitive theorists suggest that when processing information, anxious people tend to overestimate the threat of danger and underestimate their abilities to cope with that threat (Beck, 1976, 1991). Using a variety of methodologies, attentional biases toward threat-related stimuli have been demonstrated for clinically and non-clinically anxious adults (Pury & Mineka, 2001; Wood, Mathews, & Dalgleish, 2001). Similar research has found evidence of attentional bias toward threat related cues in both clinically anxious (Taghavi, Neshat-Doost, Moradi, Yule & Dalgleish, 1999) and nonclinically anxious children (Kindt, Brosschot, & Everaerd, 1997).

Findings of biased attention in anxious children have been complemented by research examining the process of threat interpretation (Cowart & Ollendick, 2010). For example, a series of studies by Barrett and colleagues (Barrett, Rapee, Dadds, & Rapee, 1996; Dadds & Barrett, 1996; Dadds, Barrett, Rapee, & Ryan, 1996) demonstrated that clinically anxious children tended to interpret ambiguous vignettes of social and physical situations as threatening compared to non-clinical controls.

The Parent–Child Relationship   An increasing number of studies have examined the relations between parenting behavior and anxiety in children. Parents of clinic-referred anxious children have been found to be more controlling (Dumas, LaFreniere, & Sereketich, 1995), more restrictive (Krohne & Hock, 1991), more overinvolved emotionally (Hirshfeld, Biederman, Brody, Faraone, & Rosenbaum, 1997), less accepting (Ollendick & Horsch, 2007), and less granting of psychological autonomy (Siqueland, Kendall, & Steinberg., 1996) than are parents of nonreferred children. Because these studies are cross-sectional, however, it is impossible to draw firm conclusions about whether relations between parent behavior and anxiety represent cause or effect, or, for that matter, whether it is more reciprocal in nature. This latter possibility is more consistent with a developmental psychopathology perspective (for extended discussion of these issues, see Rapee, 1997, and Dadds and Roth, 2001, and Zeman & Suveg, this volume).

Assessment

Only a brief overview of assessment practices is provided here (for a more complete review of assessment practices with anxious youths, see Silverman & Ollendick, 2008, and Silverman & Treffers, 2001). Anxiety, of course, is recognized as a multidimensional construct and as such a multi-informant and multimethod approach to the assessment of childhood anxiety is recommended. Diagnostic interviews with the child and the child's parent(s) are one of the best methods for distinguishing normal, developmentally appropriate fears and anxieties from problematic anxiety disorders. The most commonly used diagnostic interview to assess youth with anxiety disorders is the Anxiety Disorders Interview Schedule for Children (ADIS-C/P) (Silverman & Albano, 1996). This interview can be used to solicit detailed information about a range of individual anxiety symptoms, interference in daily functioning, school refusal behavior, interpersonal functioning, and avoided situations. In addition to the interviews, the child and her or his parents are usually asked to complete self-report questionnaires, and responses on these questionnaires can be compared to available normative data.

The Multidimensional Anxiety Scale for Children (MASC; March, Parker, Sullivan, Stallings, & Connor, 1997), the Revised Children's Manifest Anxiety Scale (Reynolds & Richmond, 1985), and the Fear Survey Schedule for Children–Revised (Ollendick, 1983) are examples of questionnaires that are frequently used in this regard. Parents and teachers can complete ratings scales such as the Child Behavior Checklist (CBCL) and Teacher Report Form (TRF; Achenbach, 1991). These scales have the advantage of measuring anxiety or depression symptoms as well as externalizing and other related problems. In addition to these measures, it is recommended that behavioral observation, cognitive assessment, and physiological assessment be considered.

Interventions

Pharmacologic Interventions   There have been a limited number of controlled pharmacologic treatment trials for anxiety in children and adolescents. Labellarte, Ginsburg, Walkup, and Riddle (1999), as well as Ollendick and March (2004), conducted extensive reviews of psychopharmacologic treatments for anxiety disorders in children and concluded that selective serotonin reuptake inhibitors (SSRIs) represent the first-line medical treatment for childhood anxiety disorders (as well as affective disorders). Serotonergic and tricyclic antidepressants are second-line anxiety agents, and buspirone may be used as a second- or third-line anxiety treatment. Medication alone is rarely the treatment of choice for children with anxiety disorders, and typically medication is used in combination with psychological treatment (Ollendick & March, 2004).

Psychosocial Interventions   Cognitive-behavioral therapy (CBT) for childhood anxiety has the strongest empirical support (Ollendick & King, 1998). CBT consists of four main strategies. First, *exposure* requires the child to approach the object or situation she or he fears or worries about, either directly (in vivo) or imaginally. Exposure is typically conducted in a graduated and progressive manner. Exposure may also take the form of systematic desensitization in which the child receives relaxation training and then practices relaxation while facing his or her feared situations in vivo or imaginally. In vivo and imaginal desensitization are both effective treatments for childhood anxiety disorders, although in vivo procedures are generally viewed as more effective than imaginal ones (Seligman & Ollendick, 2011).

The second strategy implemented to treat childhood anxiety is *modeling*. Modeling involves a person demonstrating approach behavior in situations that the child finds anxiety provoking. Variants of modeling include filmed modeling where the child watches a videotape, live modeling where the person modeling is in the presence of the anxious child, and participant modeling where a model interacts with the child and guides him or her to approach the feared situation. In their review of nine controlled studies that examined the efficacy of modeling as a treatment for childhood fears and phobias, Ollendick and King (1998) concluded that filmed modeling and live modeling are moderately effective procedures and that participant modeling is a highly effective treatment for childhood fears and phobias.

Progressive exposure and modeling assume that fear must be reduced before approach behavior will occur. In contrast, the third CBT strategy—*contingency management*—based on the principles of operant conditioning, encourages increases in approach behavior by altering the consequences of a child's behavior in the anxiety provoking situations. Contingency management involves modifying the antecedents of anxiety or the consequences of anxious behavior through positive reinforcement, punishment, extinction, and shaping. For example, positive reinforcement for "courageous" or approach behaviors to the feared or dreaded stimulus are frequently used in such programs. These procedures are implemented by the therapist during the therapy session and are often taught to parents and teachers for use in the home, school, and other community settings. Treatments involving reinforced practice have been shown to be superior to no treatment or wait-list control conditions and other treatments (verbal coping skills, modeling) in reducing phobic symptoms. As such, reinforced practice is considered to be a well-established treatment for childhood fears and phobias (Ollendick & King, 1998).

The fourth strategy used in CBT is primarily a *cognitive* or information-processing strategy. Cognitive interventions include techniques such as identifying self-talk, cognitive restructuring, and problem solving, and they are usually taught in combination with one or more of the behavioral strategies reviewed above. Consequently, most published studies have examined treatments combining cognitive and behavioral interventions and very few have examined the effectiveness of cognitive strategies in isolation. These integrated CBT programs are the most widely used treatments for children suffering from the most common anxiety disorders.

Kendall, Kane, Howard, and Siqueland (1989), for example, pioneered an integrated cognitive-behavioral treatment program for anxiety in children called "Coping Cat." The four coping strategies taught to anxious children were summarized in the acronym FEAR, which helped children remember the steps to take when they felt anxious: *F*eeling frightened, *E*xpect good things to happen, *A*ctions and attitudes to take, and *R*eward yourself. A host of randomized control clinical trials provide strong evidence that individual CBT programs such as Coping Cat and its variants are more effective than a wait-list and credible placebo conditions for reducing anxiety related to social phobia, SAD, GAD, and school refusal (see recent review by Ollendick, Jarrett, Grills-Taquechel, Seligman, & Wolff, 2008). In general, these studies suggest that approximately two-thirds of youth recover from their anxiety diagnosis at the end of treatment. Moreover, long-term outcome studies suggest that these gains are maintained over time and, in at least some instances, continued improvement is seen.

Studies have also examined the impact of incorporating parents in the therapeutic process. For example, teaching parents better strategies to manage their own anxiety and informing parents about strategies their children are learning to manage their anxiety may lead to better treatment outcomes than interventions that focus solely on the child (Barrett et al., 1996; Cobham, Dadds, & Spence, 1998). Also, preliminary findings by Cobham et al. (1998) suggest that anxious children who also have an anxious parent benefit the most from combined parent–child interventions. A recent study by Suveg et al. (2009) confirmed this finding with a family-based supportive approach. Although both individual- and family-based approaches were equally effective in reducing symptoms of anxiety, the latter approach also resulted in changes in family functioning that might maintain the anxiety problems.

Although group interventions for anxiety in children have been used for some time (Ollendick & King, 1998), it is only recently that group CBT has been investigated in controlled clinical trials. A series of studies by different research teams suggests that group format CBT is more effective in reducing anxiety than wait-list and placebo conditions (Barrett, 1998; Flannery-Schroeder & Kendall, 2000; Mendlowitz et al., 1999; Shortt, Barrett, & Fox, 2001; Silverman et al., 1999). The question as to whether group CBT is more, less, or equally as effective as individual CBT awaits large-scale studies.

Summary

Anxiety is a common problem in childhood and adolescence. Anxiety problems are frequently comorbid with other anxiety disorders, depression, or externalizing behaviors and have a poor prognosis if not treated. Several etiological theories have been proposed to explain the development and maintenance of anxiety. Although research indicates a familial risk of anxiety, most anxiety problems can be conceptualized as an interaction between temperament and environmental and contextual factors. Anxiety in children and adolescents can be reliably assessed, and promising cognitive-behavioral and pharmacologic treatments are available.

Depressive Disorders

Phenomenology

Depressive disorders also affect a significant number of children and adolescents, and there are important developmental factors to consider when making a diagnosis and planning for treatment with youths who have these disorders (Duggal, Carlson, Sroufe, & Egeland, 2001). A thorough understanding of risk factors, development, family factors, and individual cognitive variables, as well as comorbid disorders, assists in both assessment and treatment of depression in youth (Stark, Sander, Yancy, Bronik, & Hoke, 2000). The literature base spans approximately 30 years, describing symptoms of depression in children and adolescents and empirical evaluations of its treatment (Costello, Erkanli, & Angold, 2006; Weisz, McCarty, & Valeri, 2006).

Developmental Considerations   In general, many children and some adolescents who are depressed do not report feeling sad or "depressed," and developmentally appropriate language is needed to understand and communicate with them about their experiences. Children may not always look "depressed" either, so with mild or moderate levels of clinical symptoms an untrained observer, including parents or teachers, may fail to recognize signs of depression. In particular, children tend to express their negative emotions as irritability or anhedonia (i.e., things that once were fun or reinforcing no longer are), rather than as depressed or sad mood, as with older adolescents and adults (Hammen & Rudolph, 1996). Children may also lack the emotional vocabulary to describe their irritable or flat affect and other depressive symptoms in terms of feelings, and even if they know how to voice their experiences, dysthymia poses unique problems for children. A child who has dysthymia, a milder but more chronic set of symptoms over a period of at least 12 months (APA, 1994), may not have the cognitive-developmental awareness that their depressive symptoms are different from the emotions of other children, or even their own predepression life. Although some researchers and clinicians suggest that the observed developmental differences in symptoms warrant different diagnostic categories (not unlike developmental differences between oppositional defiant disorder and conduct disorder), the field appears to have accepted these differences in symptom patterns across development and to embrace them.

Children and adolescents also differ in their perceptions of personal control and resultant depression. A model put forth by Weisz, Southam-Gerow, and McCarty (2001) articulated developmental differences in perceived contingency, control, and competence (CCC) related to depression in children and adolescents. Data were collected in several mental health outpatient centers with 360 child and adolescent participants. The CCC model defined perceived control as one's power to influence or engineer a desired outcome. Contingency was determined by how much one's efforts caused the outcome, considering other possible contributing factors. Competence was defined as the degree to which one actually carried out the necessary behaviors to produce the desired outcomes. Both children and adolescents appeared negatively affected by low perceived control and low perceived competence, but adolescents were also sensitive to the contingency or "fairness" of the circumstances in a more global sense. Such findings may have important implications for current treatments for depression in children versus adolescents.

As in many types of clinical distress and disease, certain factors increase the likelihood that a youth will develop the disorder. In a prospective, longitudinal study by Duggal et al. (2001), significant differences emerged for factors associated with childhood-onset and adolescent-onset depression. Abuse at an early age, higher maternal stress, and less supportive early care differentiated childhood-onset from adolescent-onset depression. In general, adverse family relationships were associated with childhood-onset depression but not adolescent-onset depression. As reported in more recent studies, family functioning is a concern, but it could be family conflict, specifically, that relates to prognosis (Fccny et al., 2009).

Gender Differences   Prevalence rates of depressive disorders are different for boys and girls. The differences change systematically with development, adding an additional factor to consider. Prior to adolescence, there are approximately equal proportions of depressive disorders among boys and girls, hovering near 4 to 6% of boys and girls at any given time (Costello et al., 2006). However, beginning in adolescence and continuing into adulthood, depressive disorders occur more frequently among females than males (Kessler, Avenevoli, & Merikangas, 2001), with ratios upward of two to one (Axelson & Birmaher, 2001). The exact reasons for these gender differences remain unclear. Biological, cultural, and interpersonal factors have been proposed, with no clear causes emerging (Nolen-Hoeksema, 1995). Still, these gender differences have been found to be robust across cultures. For example, in a large study of Mexican youth, Benjet and Hernandez-Guzman (2001) reported that prevalence of depression was similar for boys and girls prepuberty and increased for females postmenarche but not for males postpuberty.

One theory espoused by Shaw, Kennedy, and Joffe (1995) is that girls are more sensitive to interpersonal rejection and more focused on dissatisfying interpersonal relationship qualities than boys. A modeling theory also proposes that the incidence of depression is greater among women of child-rearing age, and that their daughters may learn about depressive symptoms, cognitions, and behaviors from their mothers, thus placing them at higher risk for depressive symptoms (Goodman & Gotlib, 1999). Benjet and Hernandez-Guzman (2001) also explored family factors, self-esteem, parental education, and attitudes about menstruation as potential modifiers in the puberty–depression relationship among young Mexican females but did not find support for modifying effects.

In a thorough review, Beardslee and Gladstone (2001) provided an overview of risk factors for the development of depression in boys and girls. These factors included having a biological relative with a mood disorder, presence of severe stressor, low self-esteem or hopelessness, being female, and low socioeconomic status (poverty). Males and females were characterized, at least partially, by a unique set of risk factors. For boys, but not girls, neonatal and subsequent health problems posed risk for depression; in girls, but not boys, death of a parent by age 9 years, poor academic performance, and family dysfunction were related to risk for depression. In another review, Duggal et al. (2001) indicated that early caregiving patterns, such as household stress and quality of early childhood care, predicted depression for adolescent males but not adolescent females, whereas presence of maternal depression predicted depression in adolescent females but not adolescent males. The patterns of gender differences in prevalence and risk are reasonably well established. Yet, the mechanisms contributing to gender differences remain elusive, and the field is ripe for new ideas and investigations.

Prevalence

Prevalence and incidence rates of depressive disorders vary across studies, and large-scale research is currently available via a meta-analysis. Gathering data from a period of 30 years from 1965 to 1996, Costello et al. (2006) synthesized data from more than 60,000 children that used clinician interviews as the measure of depressive symptoms. Rates were generally consistent, with 5% of children meeting criteria for clinical depression. The lifetime prevalence rates for the spectrum of depressive disorders in adolescents are between 5 and 21% in community samples (Hankin et al., 1998; Kessler & Walters, 1998; Reinherz, Giaconia, Hauf, Wasserman & Silverman, 1999). Of course, rates increase for subclinical levels of depressive symptoms; depressive symptoms are reported by half of children and adolescents at one time or another in their lives (Costello et al., 2006).

Depression is a cyclic, often recurrent, disorder. Emslie and Mayes (2001) reported that 90% of youngsters recovered from a depressive episode within 2 years. Yet, within 6 to 7 years, 25 to 50% of them reexperienced significant symptoms and distress. In addition, within 8 years, 54 to 72% had a recurrent episode of depression. These relapse rates hold true for the treatment studies on depression in youth as well, which we describe in a later section.

Differential Diagnosis and Comorbidity

Another important (if not vexing) factor in the diagnosis and treatment of depression is the existence of comorbid disorders. Comorbid disorders most often include an anxiety disorder, conduct disorder, and substance abuse. Lewinsohn, Zinbarg, Seeley, Lewinsohn, and Sack (1997) reported that depression often co-occurs with the anxiety diagnoses of panic, generalized anxiety, separation anxiety, social phobia, and specific phobia. Although depression may be the first onset with some comorbid disorders (especially with substance abuse disorders), general anxiety disorders such as panic disorder and GAD frequently precede depression (Kessler et al., 2001). In externalizing disorders, such as conduct disorder, a model of comorbidity was presented by Capaldi and colleagues (Capaldi, 1992; Capaldi & Stoolmiller, 1999; DeBaryshe, Patterson, & Capaldi, 1993; Wiesner, Kim, & Capaldi, 2005; see also Wolff & Ollendick, 2006). The model elaborates on how early childhood behavioral challenges, school and social failure, and more serious conduct problems in adolescence eventually lead to depression after many repeated failures over time.

Although anxiety disorders are common comorbid disorders with depression, the two classes of disorders appear to be distinct in children but related through a common construct of negative affectivity (Axelson & Birmaher, 2001; Seligman & Ollendick, 1998). In depressed youth, up to 75% may have a lifetime prevalence of a comorbid anxiety disorder, and between 45 to 50% may have a disruptive behavior disorder or substance use disorder (Avenevoli, Stolar, Dierker, & Merikangas, 2001). Point prevalence rates for children and adolescents with depression and a comorbid anxiety disorder range from 25 to 50%; in contrast, point prevalence rates for anxious youths with depression range between 15 and 20%. In other words, it is more common for depressed children and adolescents to have a comorbid anxiety disorder than for anxious children and adolescents to have a comorbid depressive disorder. Presence of a comorbid disorder appears to relate to severity of symptoms, such that youngsters with major depression and comorbid anxiety possess more severe depressive symptoms (Axelson & Birmaher, 2001).

Comorbidity is particularly relevant in assessment of suicide risk. Youths with substance abuse as either a primary or secondary diagnosis are at increased risk for suicidal behavior. In addition, antisocial behavior, particularly in females, may increase the risk for lethal suicidal behaviors (Wannan & Fombonne, 1998).

Etiological Considerations

Biological Factors   Specific neurotransmitters have been implicated in the onset and course of depression in children and adolescents. One prominent theory suggests that select neurotransmitters, such as the monoamines, norepinephrine, serotonin, and dopamine, are not available at receptor sites in sufficient supply (Wagner & Ambrosini, 2001). Other theories, which have not yet been demonstrated with children, implicate poor growth hormone stimulation, as well as hypothalamic–pituitary–adrenal axis regulation difficulties (Axelson & Birmaher, 2001).

Family and Interpersonal Factors   Family risk factors have historically focused on maternal factors, such as maternal depression or low maternal warmth and availability. More recent models include a more complex conceptualization of family risks for youth depression, including the contribution of fathers and mothers, genetic risk, and other environmental considerations, such as poverty and stressful life events. Goodman and Gotlib's (1999) integrative model of risk for transmission of depression from mother to child considers heritability, depressive maternal affect and symptoms, stress within a household with a depressed parent, and neuroregulatory consequences from that environmental circumstance. In addition, they proposed that the timing, severity, and duration of depressive symptoms interact with the developmental tasks and challenges for children. The Oregon Adolescent Depression Project (Allen, Lewinsohn, & Seeley, 1998) examined prenatal, neonatal, developmental, and family relationship factors in psychopathology. They reported several factors that were correlated with increased risk of adolescent depression, including maternal depression and absence of breastfeeding.

Yet relationship quality with parents may not be the most important consideration across developmental stages. In a study by Williams, Connolly, and Segal (2001), the level of intimacy in romantic relationships predicted risk for depression in adolescents beyond other parental and friendship relationship factors. Sander and McCarty (2005) conducted a comprehensive review of family factors and interventions addressing family factors in depressed youth. Their conclusions were that many factors, including cognitive style of parents, parental psychopathology, emotional availability of parents, coping styles, and family conflict, contribute in important ways to risk for youth depression. Importantly, both mothers and fathers, along with other contextual factors, are important in conceptualizing risk (Sander & McCarty, 2005).

The causal effect of early relationship quality on later depression in children and adolescents is unclear, as is the contribution made by youngsters with a predisposition for depression to the negative quality of their interpersonal interactions. However, depressed youths do appear to have poorer social competence and perceive less support from peers, and they spend less time with peers than do nondepressed youths (Hammen & Rudolph, 1996). Professionals need to acknowledge and integrate interpersonal deficits or struggles, including peer and parental relationships, when conceptualizing and implementing treatment programs for depressed youngsters (Mufson, Weissman, Moreau, & Garfinkel, 1999; Stark et al., 2000). In addition, depression and its associated cognitive distortions appear to be related to interpersonal factors and, therefore, can or should be treated within an interpersonal context (Joiner, Coyne, & Blalock, 1999).

Consistent with research on the role of interpersonal and cognitive variables in depression in youth, a cognitive-interpersonal theory of depression proposes that cognitive style and interpersonal relationship patterns combine to result in depression (Stark et al., 2000). From this perspective, Bowlby's (1980) attachment theory plays an important role. In brief, the early or primary interpersonal relationships are proposed to either buffer or increase risk for cognitive style associated with depression (Stark et al., 2000). According to this theory, early relationship patterns and the caregiver's responsiveness to the child shape the child's expectations of how he or she will be treated by others and how responsive others will be to his or her needs. An unresponsive caregiver, such as a depressed parent, could inadvertently communicate the message that the child's needs are unimportant, thus predisposing the child to adopt a negative self-schema (Duggal et al., 2001; Stark et al., 2000). Others suggest similar cognitive-interpersonal pathways and theoretical integration (Gotlib & Hammen, 1992).

Individual and Cognitive Variables   Among individual variables, cognitive style, including attributional style, has received the most consistent empirical support. In brief, cognitive vulnerability to depression includes several components. It includes the concepts of negative thought patterns, depressive self-schema, and pessimistic attributional style about events (Clark, Beck, & Alford, 1999; Stark, Schmidt, & Joiner, 1996). According to cognitive theory of depression, the self-schema guides information processing and may produce errors in perception that are consistent with a depressive self-schema—typically that the self is unlovable or incompetent (Clark et al., 1999). Attributional style refers to the patterns of causality assigned to events, such as how stable, global, and internal those events are perceived to be (Nolen-Hoeksema, Girgus, & Seligman, 1992). Depressed children and adolescents, in contrast to non-depressed children and adolescents, distort events and make information-processing errors that confirm negatively biased assumptions about the self (Jacobs, Reinecke, Gollan, & Kane, 2008; Stark et al., 1996) and the internal, stable, and global nature of negative events (Nolen-Hoeksema et al., 1992). Developmentally, children as young as 8 to 9 years of age make attributions about causality of events; prior to that age, attributional style in terms of cognitive vulnerability for depression may be unclear (Jacobs et al., 2008) and could be related to developmentally limited understanding of causality as well as the means to articulate the abstract ideas and emotional experiences.

Information-processing errors, such as a bias for depressive information, are evident in children as young as 5 years of age. At the same time, though, there are differences in how children present with cognitive and information-processing errors relative to adolescents. Children may display an inability to recall positive events, rehearse negative information about events, and have lower rates of positive self-descriptions, but in some cases the measures available are less sensitive to these aspects of children's information-processing errors (Jacobs et al., 2008). Adolescents are typically able to articulate and report their cognitive errors, information-processing patterns, and indicate their cognitive vulnerabilities to depression on established measures (Jacobs et al., 2008), which are described below.

Assessment

The scope of this chapter does not allow for thorough review of the assessment process. However, brief recommendations are put forth (see Kendall, Cantwell, & Kazdin, 1989, for a thorough discussion of this topic). Within the field of depression, a common diagnostic interview used for assessing clinical depression is the Kiddie Schedule for Affective Disorders and Schizophrenia (K-SADS; Orvaschel & Puig-Antich, 1987). Different researchers have adopted modified versions of the K-SADS, including present episode, epidemiologic version, and combined versions with updates for the *DSM–IV* (Ambrosini, 2000). The K-SADS is a semistructured diagnostic interview designed to be used by clinically trained interviewers and can be administered to the youth and parent separately. The complete interview is cumbersome and was designed for research. However, the specific prompts and questions can be incorporated into an interview for clinical practice (Stark et al., 2000). Other questionnaires and self-report measures can be administered efficiently and used in community or clinic populations, such as the depression scale of the Behavior Assessment Scale for Children, second edition (BASC-2; Reynolds & Kamphaus, 2004), the Beck Youth Inventory–Depression Scales (BDI-Y; Beck, Beck, & Jolly, 2001), or the Children's Depression Inventory (CDI; Kovacs, 1992), but these are recommended only when used in conjunction with a clinician's interview and other sources of information to determine accurate diagnosis.

Assessment of suicide risk and behavior is important. In adolescents, there may be a precipitating stressor that has compromised developmental tasks such as establishing autonomy, acceptance by their desired peer group, or conflict with important peers or with family members. The clinician must remain attuned to those potential events in relation to increased risk for suicide in youths (Rudd & Joiner, 1998), as well as assess for substance use and antisocial behavior, as discussed previously (Wannan & Fombonne, 1998). Several self-report measures listed above include items and clusters of items that address suicidal risk and should be reviewed immediately following administration.

Interventions

Treatment of depression in youth is a somewhat daunting undertaking, and relapse rates are typically high (40 to 50%) for clinically depressed youths (Asarnow, Jaycox, & Tompson, 2001). There have been several large-scale studies within the past 10 years, as well as a few thorough research synthesis studies on the topic, that are instrumental in advancing treatment for child and adolescent depression (Ollendick & Jarrett, 2009). Even so, the results and conclusions are not decisively clear, and practice guidelines and widespread use of empirically supported interventions remain sparse. There are three main approaches in the treatment of child and adolescent depression: pharmacologic interventions, family or interpersonal psychosocial treatment, and cognitive-behavioral interventions.

Pharmacologic Interventions   As with the anxiety disorders, there have been a limited number of controlled, randomized clinical trials of treatment of depression in children and adolescents, either pharmacologic or psychosocial. Pharmacologically, the most promising results have been obtained with use of SSRIs (e.g., fluoxetine, marketed as Prozac) to reduce depressive symptoms. However, rates of improvement have been from 40% (Wagner & Ambrosini, 2001) to 60% at posttreatment (Reinecke, Curry, & March, 2009). As a class of medications, the SSRIs are most likely to quickly reduce depressive symptoms and have fewer and less detrimental side effects than other antidepressants (Emslie & Mayes, 2001).

In the most extensive multisite medication and psychosocial intervention study with adolescents to date, which included 439 adolescents from 2000 to 2003, the Treatment of Adolescent Depression Study (TADS) team (2004) reported that fluoxetine medication plus cognitive-behavioral treatment was the most effective intervention to alleviate depression in adolescents, with improvement rates at 81% at 3 months posttreatment. Fluoxetine was superior to cognitive-behavioral treatment alone in terms of providing earlier response to treatment and reduction of symptoms (TADS, 2004). Although the cognitive-behavioral interventions incorporated for the TADS study were criticized for being less rigorous than those used in cognitive-behavioral treatment studies (Hollon, Garber, & Shelton, 2005; Stark, Streusand, Arora, & Patel, 2010), the conclusions from the large study do offer cautiously positive indications that medication, for some children and adolescents with depression, may be useful as a treatment component (Reinecke et al., 2009). It should be noted that even when medication was effective, particularly early on, in follow-up studies the relapse rate for medication alone was higher than that of the cognitive-behavioral approach (McCarty & Weisz, 2007).

Psychosocial Interventions   In a synthesis of psychosocial interventions for depressed children and adolescents, Weisz et al. (2006) included 35 studies from 1980 to 2004 to examine efficacy of psychosocial treatment of childhood and adolescent depression. The research synthesis is a helpful approach to consolidate many smaller-scale studies and help interpret how well interventions work when using a similar measure of effect size. An effect size calculation takes into account the means and standard deviations of the treatment and comparison groups, as well as sample size. The overall finding from the synthesis of all psychosocial interventions for depression that were available is a cautiously positive endorsement. Psychosocial interventions as a group certainly seem helpful in the short term (posttreatment). Long-term outcomes are not as positive, as shown below. Taking a closer look at the effective interventions at posttreatment, defined as a moderate effect size of 0.5 or greater in the meta-analysis, McCarty and Weisz (2007) identified nine studies that stood out. They provided a table of each of the nine studies, along with specific components within each treatment approach, since all of them had multiple components and several components in common across interventions. The approaches to treatment in these successful interventions included cognitive-behavioral therapy, interpersonal therapy, cognitive therapy, and family therapy. One point to note is that these were all clinical trials, and the studies with the best treatment outcomes were those with a wait-list condition, rather than a comparison treatment condition. It would be helpful to have data comparing one intervention to another, but that information is not yet available. Nonetheless, these specific studies reflect the most current and efficacious psychosocial treatments that are available.

Cognitive-Behavioral Therapy   Cognitive-behavioral therapy has received the most empirical support among the psychosocial treatments (Curry, 2001). Components of CBT include affective education, planning positive activities, proactive problem solving, social skills training, coping strategies, and cognitive restructuring. Family and interpersonal components may also be included. Cognitive-behavioral therapy has been implemented with children as young as 8 to 9 years of age. Among 15 CBT studies reviewed by Curry (2001), treatment duration ranged from 5 to 16 weeks. Some therapy protocols involved twice weekly sessions, with an average of 11 sessions total. New treatment investigations include an emphasis on family components, combined with cognitive-behavioral approaches (Asarnow et al., 2001; Curry, 2001; Ollendick & Jarrett, 2009).

There are two controlled clinical trials of high scientific rigor that address depression in youth from a cognitive-behavioral perspective. In addition, these studies included samples that are typical of real-world practice with complex, multiple diagnoses and clinical symptoms: the Coping with Depression for Adolescents group treatment (CWD-A; Clarke, Rohde, Lewinsohn, Hops, & Seeley, 1999, Lewinsohn, Clarke, Hops, & Andrews, 1990) and the ACTION program (Stark et al., 2010). The CWD-A group treatment, which was included in the Weisz et al. (2006) research synthesis, is based on cognitive-behavioral principles and has been effective in reducing depressive symptoms in youths with a primary diagnosis of depression (Clarke et al., 1999; Lewinsohn et al., 1990). The most recent empirical investigation of CWD-A is with a sample of 93 girls and boys (age 13 to 17 years) who had comorbid depression and conduct disorder (Rohde, Clarke, Mace, Jorgensen, & Seeley, 2004). Components of treatment included altering cognitions and behaviors, use of a structured intervention session, teaching mood monitoring, social skills, and pleasant activity scheduling. The CWD-A treatment did not appear to address the comorbid conduct disorder symptoms, but it did reduce depressive symptoms in this highly challenging and distressed group of youths at posttreatment (Rohde et al., 2004). The comparison condition was a life-skills training, which included job-seeking and -related skills, for example, and was provided in equal proportion to the CBT components. Both conditions included 16 2-hr sessions over an 8-week period. Attendance was somewhat low in terms of the length of treatment the participants received but was acceptable for the population in the study. At posttreatment, the CBT group had a 39% recovery rate for depression, compared to 19% in the life-skills condition. The difference between conditions was not maintained over time, but the life-skills and CBT groups all had reduced symptoms of depression over a 1-year follow-up. Given the overall challenges of working with this complex clinical picture, these results are notable at posttreatment in terms of some psychosocial interventions that reduced depression.

Another CBT approach is the ACTION program. The ACTION program (Stark et al., 2010) is a cognitive-behavioral group treatment for young adolescent girls (age 9 to 13 years). It has not been included in a research synthesis, but it is nonetheless a well-designed study with two active treatment groups and one wait-list condition. The ACTION program included 158 girls who had a primary diagnosis of depression to qualify to receive treatment as part of the study, but the majority (60%) had dual diagnoses, most often an anxiety disorder (Sander, 2004). The ACTION program is delivered over 11 weeks, with a total of 20 group meetings and 2 individual meetings with the girls. There is a child's workbook and a therapist manual. An individual case conceptualization is created for each girl in treatment so that the therapist incorporates the girl's individual needs throughout the group intervention. There is also a manualized parent component to treatment in the ACTION program, with focus on parental support for the skills and tools the girls learn during the group treatment (Stark et al., 2010). Based on posttreatment diagnostic interviews, 84% and 81% of girls who received CBT or CBT plus parent training, respectively, no longer met diagnostic criteria for any depressive disorder. This was compared to 46% of girls in a minimal contact control condition. One of the key elements of treatment for girls at this particular age, as emphasized by Stark et al. (2010), is the behavioral activation component of CBT. This component includes active problem solving, coping strategies, and pleasant activity scheduling. Although the outcomes have not yet been included in another research synthesis or in terms of treatment effects that would allow for examination of effect sizes, the overall clinical findings are promising.

Interpersonal Therapy   Interpersonal therapy for adolescents (IPT-A) has also received promising empirical support. In IPT-A, focus is on resolving conflicts in current, important, interpersonal relationships and improving communication and relationship skills (Mufson, Moreau, Weissman, & Klerman, 1993). The goals of IPT-A are to reduce depressive symptoms via improving interpersonal functioning. The main areas to consider for improvement in interpersonal areas are grief, role disputes, role transitions, and interpersonal deficits (Mufson et al., 2004). The empirical support for this intervention from one major clinical trial was included in McCarty and Weisz's (2007) summary. In a more recent study, IPT-A was delivered in school clinics located within urban, low-income neighborhoods to a sample (*n* = 57) of predominantly Hispanic children, 12 to 18 years of age. Results indicated IPT-A was beneficial and feasible within these school-based clinics as well as in more controlled settings from earlier clinical trials (Mufson et al., 2004).

Family Therapy   The most promising family therapy approach for youth depression is currently attachment-based family therapy (ABFT; Diamond, Reis, Diamond, Siqueland, & Isaacs, 2002). This intervention was included in the McCarty and Weisz (2007) synthesis of the nine most effective interventions. The treatment objectives of ABFT are not solely to reduce depressive symptoms, but to improve relationships, repair relationally based wounds such as abandonment, and increase empathy among family members. The reduction of family conflict and discord is also important, as is fostering trust among family members.

Suicidality   Managing suicidal risk is very important to include early in treatment. Integrating appropriate intervention to reduce suicidality is a necessary skill when working with depressed youngsters, particularly as outpatients. Managing this risk involves several straight-forward strategies (Rudd & Joiner, 1998). The first is to have a proactive stance and a plan for potential hospitalization to be revised or revisited frequently during suicide risk periods. In addition, treatment progress and goals should be revisited and updated often, particularly noting the changes that co-occur with decreased suicidal ideation. Sessions may need to occur more frequently, and the family's involvement and a phone contact list, as well as availability of emergency 24-hour support, is necessary. Furthermore, full consideration of medication assessment and monitoring, as well as consultation with medical professionals to manage this aspect of treatment, is recommended. In the large-scale TADS (2004) study, the combination of CBT and medication was found to be the most effective in reducing suicidality. The specific addition of CBT with the medication seemed particularly helpful in attaining a quicker reduction in suicidal thoughts (Reinecke et al., 2009).

In summary, although the available treatments for depressed and suicidal children and adolescents show promise, several important caveats should be kept in mind. Overall, recovery rates across broadly defined interventions are generally at or below 50% (Asarnow et al., 2001; Curry, 2001; Ollendick & Jarrett, 2009). The most successful interventions, mainly clinical trials, achieve recovery rates at 80% or better at posttreatment, but long-term follow-up rates are rarely available. Moreover, relapse rates are high. Also, comorbidity has been rarely addressed in treatment efficacy studies, and it remains an important factor to consider in day-to-day clinical practice as well as in major clinical outcome trials (Curry, 2001). Recent studies are including comorbidity as part of the design, rather than focusing on single-diagnosis participants. Psychosocial interventions, particularly the CBT-based approaches, are moving in new directions to reflect a more integrative treatment, incorporating individual, cognitive, relational, and interpersonal factors.

Summary

The research on child and adolescent depression offers a number of exciting and promising findings. Treatment research is ongoing, including new directions involving biological and interpersonal factors. Although efficacious treatments exist, both pharmacologic and psychosocial (primarily CBT, IPT-A, and ABFT), not all youth are being helped by these interventions. Furthermore, the issue of comorbidity has not been adequately addressed nor has the role of culture and ethnicity. The protective factors and risk factors associated with different cultural and ethnic practices have yet to be examined in standard research and clinical practice. These could be pivotal factors in understanding and treating childhood depression in our increasingly diverse society.

Future Directions

The internalizing disorders of children and adolescents represent a major challenge to practicing clinicians and researchers alike. As we have seen, the anxiety and affective disorders are highly prevalent in childhood and adolescence. Their effects are distressing in the short run and can be long lasting.

Although we have attempted to use a developmental psychopathology perspective (see Zeman & Suveg, this volume) on these disorders, it is evident that the field has not yet fully embraced this way of thinking about these problems. As a result, many studies continue to look at single causal pathways and direct, linear outcomes. As we have suggested, it may be more productive to posit that several very different pathways can lead to any one outcome such as depression or anxiety (i.e., the developmental principle of equifinality) and that any one pathway can lead to diverse outcomes (i.e., the principle of multifinality). Thus, a risk factor such as child sexual abuse can and frequently does lead to multiple outcomes, whether they are an internalizing disorder or one of the externalizing disorders (reviewed in Kimonis & Frick, this volume). Tracking this developmental process is undoubtedly a complex and challenging undertaking, but a necessary one. This effort will benefit greatly from carefully planned, multisite, longitudinal studies (Ollendick & King, 1994).

Moreover, the effects of these risk factors may not be direct, and we need to consider conditions that moderate these relations. Direct effects are oftentimes captured by what are referred to as "main effect" models, which imply that a risk factor is directly related to the outcome in a linear fashion. Yet any one risk factor does not invariably result in any one pathological outcome. For example, it is well known that not all sexually abused children have negative outcomes, such as the development of internalizing or externalizing disorders, or at least not the same negative outcomes. Often a significant minority of abused children do not develop any disorders at all, implying a profound interaction between the experience of abuse and some other internal or external moderating conditions (Kazdin & Kagan, 1994). What does seem most important is the context in which the abuse occurs and the interrelated risk factors that are present. As noted by Kazdin and Kagan, "when one begins with the multiplicity of variables that operate, one might better consider nonlinearity to be the better point of departure in our work" (1994, p. 38).

These same issues have important implications for the treatment and prevention of internalizing disorders. Our treatment and prevention programs must move away from a "one-size-fits-all" mentality. Children and adolescents become depressed or anxious through a variety of pathways, and they express these disorders in a variety of ways. We need to take this complexity into consideration in designing, implementing, and evaluating our interventions. Although current empirically supported or evidence-based interventions work with most (50 to 70%) of the children and adolescents and families who come into our practices and research clinics, we must do better. An approach that is individualized and prescriptive, and one that is based in developmental theory and grounded in established principles of behavior change (e.g., exposure, cognitive change, interpersonal relationships), is likely to be most effective, although this remains to be carefully documented.

References

Achenbach, T. M. (1991). *Manual for the child behavior checklist 4–18 and 1991 profile*. Burlington: University of Vermont, Department of Psychiatry.

Albano, A. M., Chorpita, B., & Barlow, D. H. (1996). Anxiety disorders in children and adolescents. In E. J. Mash & R. A. Barkley (Eds.), *Child psychopathology* (pp. 196–241). New York: Guilford.

Allen, N. B., Lewinsohn, P. M., & Seeley, J. R. (1998). Prenatal and perinatal influences on risk for psychopathology in childhood and adolescence. *Development and Psychopathology, 10*, 513–529.

Ambrosini, P. J. (2000). Historical development and present status of the Schedule for Affective Disorders and Schizophrenia for School-Age Children (K-SADS). *Journal of the American Academy of Child and Adolescent Psychiatry, 39*(1), 49–58.

American Psychiatric Association. (1994). *Diagnostic and statistical manual of mental disorders-TR* (4th ed.). Washington, DC: Author.

American Psychiatric Association. (1980). *Diagnostic and statistical manual of mental disorders* (3rd ed.). Washington, DC: Author.

Anderson, J. C., Williams, S., McGee, R., & Silva, A. (1987). DSM-III disorders in pre-adolescent children: Prevalence in a large sample from the general population. *Archives of General Psychiatry, 44*, 69–76.

Asarnow, R., Jaycox, L. H., & Tompson, M. C. (2001). Depression in youth: Psychosocial interventions. *Journal of Clinical Child Psychology, 30*, 33–47.

Avenevoli, S., Stolar, M., Li, J., Dierker, L., & Merikangas, K. R. (2001). Comorbidity of depression in children and adolescents: Models and evidence from a prospective high-risk family study. *Biological Psychiatry, 49*, 1071–1081.

Axelson, D. A., & Birmaher, B. (2001). Relation between anxiety and depressive disorders in childhood and adolescence. *Depression and Anxiety, 14*, 67–78.

Bandura, A. (1999). Self-efficacy: Toward a unifying theory of behavioral change. In R. F. Baumeister (Ed.), *The self in social psychology* (pp. 285–298). New York: Psychology Press.

Barrett, P. M. (1998). Evaluation of cognitive-behavioral group treatments for childhood anxiety disorders. *Journal of Clinical Child Psychology, 27*, 459–468.

Barrett, P. M., Dadds, M. R., & Rapee, R. M. (1996). Family treatment of childhood anxiety: A controlled trial. *Journal of Consulting and Clinical Psychology, 64*, 333–342.

Barrett, P. M., Rapee. R. M., Dadds, M. M., & Ryan, S. M. (1996): Family enhancement of cognitive style in anxious and aggressive children. *Journal of Abnormal Child Psychology, 24*,187–203.

Beardslee, W. R., & Gladstone, T. R. G. (2001). Prevention of childhood depression: Recent findings and future prospects. *Biological Psychiatry, 49*, 1101–1110.

Beck, A. T. (1976). *Cognitive therapy and the emotional disorders.* New York: International Universities Press.

Beck, A. T. (1991). Cognitive therapy: A 30-year retrospective. *American Psychologist, 46*, 368–375.

Beck, J., Beck, A. T., & Jolly, J. B. (2001). *Beck Youth Inventories.* United States: Psychological Corporation (Harcourt Assessment).

Beidel, D. C., & Morris, T. L. (1995). Social phobia. In E. J. Mash & R. A. Barkley (Eds.), *Child psychopathology* (pp. 181–211). New York: Guilford.

Benjet, C., & Hernandez-Guzman, L. (2001). Gender differences in psychological well-being of Mexican early adolescents. *Adolescence, 36*, 47–65.

Biederman, J., Hirshfeld-Becker, D. R., Rosenbaum, J. F., Herot, C., Friedman, D., Snidman, N., … Faraone, S. V. (2001). Further evidence of association between behavioral inhibition and social anxiety in children. *American Journal of Psychiatry, 158*, 1673–1679.

Bowlby, J. (1980). *Attachment and loss:* Vol. III. *Loss, sadness, and depression.* New York: Basic Books.

Brady, E. U., & Kendall, P. C. (1992). Comorbidity of anxiety and depression in children and adolescents. *Psychological Bulletin, 111*, 244–255.

Capaldi, D. (1992). Co-occurrence of conduct problems and depressive symptoms in early adolescent boys: II. A 2-year follow-up at Grade 8. *Development and Psychopathology, 4*(1), 125–144.

Capaldi, D., & Stoolmiller, M. (1999). Co-occurrence of conduct problems and depressive symptoms in early adolescent boys: III. Prediction to young-adult adjustment. *Development and Psychopathology, 11*(1), 59–84.

Caron, C., & Rutter, M. (1991). Comorbidity in child psychopathology: Concepts, issues and research strategies. *Journal of Child Psychology and Psychiatry, 32*, 1063–1080.

Clark, D. A., Beck, A. T., & Alford, B. A. (1999). *Scientific foundations of cognitive theory and therapy of depression.* New York: Wiley.

Clarke, G. N., Rohde P., Lewinsohn, P. M., Hops, H., & Seeley, J. R. (1999). Cognitive-behavioral treatment of adolescent depression: efficacy of acute group treatment and booster sessions. *Journal of the American Academy of Child and Adolescent Psychiatry, 38*, 272–279.

Cobham, V. E., Dadds, R., & Spence, S. H. (1998). The role of parental anxiety in the treatment of childhood anxiety. *Journal of Consulting and Clinical Psychology, 66*, 893–905.

Cohen, P., Cohen, J., Kaasen, S., Noemi Velez, C., Hartmark, C., Johnson, J., … Streuning, E. L. (1993). An epidemiological study of disorders in late childhood and adolescence—1. Age and gender specific prevalence. *Journal of Child Psychology and Psychiatry, 34*, 851–867.

Cook, E., Wagner, K., March, J., Biederman, J., Landau, P., Wolkow, R., & Messig, M. (2001). Long-term sertraline treatment of children and adolescents with obsessive-compulsive disorder. *Journal of the American Academy of Child and Adolescent Psychiatry, 40*(10), 1175–1189.

Costello, E. J., Costello, A. J., Edelbrock, C., Burns, B. J., Dulcan, M. K., Brent, D., & Janiszewski, S. (1988). Psychiatric disorders in pediatric primary care. *Archives of General Psychiatry, 45*, 1107–1116.

Costello, E., Erkanli, A., & Angold, A. (2006). Is there an epidemic of child or adolescent depression? *Journal of Child Psychology and Psychiatry, 47*(12), 1263–1271.

Cowart, M. J. W., & Ollendick, T. H. (2010). Attentional biases in children: Implication for treatment. In J. A. Hadwin & A. P. Field (Eds.), *Information processing biases and anxiety: A developmental perspective* (pp. 297–319). Oxford: Oxford University Press.

Curry, J. F. (2001). Specific psychotherapies for childhood and adolescent depression. *Biological Psychiatry, 49*, 1091–1100.

Dadds, M. R., & Barrett, P. M. (1996). Family processes in child and adolescent anxiety and depression. *Behaviour Change, 13*, 231–239.

Dadds, M. R., Barrett, P. M., Rapee, R. M., & Ryan, S. (1996). Family processes and child psychopathology: An observational analysis of the FEAR effect. *Journal of Abnormal Child Psychology, 24*, 715–735.

Dadds, M. R., & Roth, J. H. (2001). Family processes in the development of anxiety problems. In M. W. Vasey & M. R. Dadds (Eds.), *The developmental psychopathology of anxiety disorders in children* (pp. 278–303). New York: Oxford University Press.

Davey, G. C. L. (1992). Classical conditioning and the acquisition of human fears and phobias: A review and synthesis of the literature. *Advances in Behavior Research and Therapy, 14*, 29–66.

Davidson, J., Hughes, D., George, L., & Blazer, D. (1993). The epidemiology of social phobia: Findings from the Duke Epidemiological Catchment Area Study. *Psychological Medicine: A Journal of Research in Psychiatry and the Allied Sciences, 23*(3), 709–718.

DeBaryshe, B., Patterson, G., & Capaldi, D. (1993). A performance model for academic achievement in early adolescent boys. *Developmental Psychology, 29*(5), 795–804.

Diamond, G., Reis, B., Diamond, G., Siqueland, L., & Isaacs, L. (2002). Attachment-based family therapy for depressed adolescents: A treatment development study. *Journal of the American Academy of Child and Adolescent Psychiatry, 41*(10), 1190–1196.

Duggal, S., Carlson, E. A., Sroufe, L. A., & Egeland, B. (2001). Depressive symptomatology in childhood and adolescence. *Development and Psychopathology, 13*, 143–164.

Dumas, J. E., La Freniere, P. J., & Sereketich, W. J. (1995). "Balance of power": A transactional analysis of control in mother-child dyads involving socially competent, aggressive, and anxious children. *Journal of Abnormal Psychology, 104*, 104–113.

Eley, T. C., & Stevenson, J. (1999). Exploring the covariation between anxiety and depression symptoms: A genetic analysis of the effects of age and sex. *Journal of Child Psychology and Psychiatry, 40*, 1273–1282.

Emslie, G. J., & Mayes, T. L. (2001). Mood disorders in children and adolescents: Pharmacological treatment. *Biological Psychiatry, 49*, 1082–1090.

Essau, C. A., Conradt, J., & Petermann, F. (2000). Frequency, comorbidity, and psychosocial impairment of specific phobia in adolescents. *Journal of Clinical Child Psychology, 29*, 221–231.

Feeny, N., Silva, S., Reinecke, M., McNulty, S., Findling, R., Rohde, P., … March, J. S. (2009). An exploratory analysis of the impact of family functioning on treatment for depression in adolescents. *Journal of Clinical Child and Adolescent Psychology, 38*(6), 814–825.

Flannery-Schroeder, E. C., & Kendall, P. C. (2000). Group and individual cognitive-behavioral treatments for youth with anxiety disorders: A randomized clinical trial. *Cognitive Therapy and Research, 24*, 251–278.

Goodman, S. H., & Gotlib, I. H. (1999). Risk for psychopathology in the children of depressed mothers: A developmental model for understanding mechanisms of transmission. *Psychological Review, 106*, 458–490.

Gotlib, I. H., & Hammen, C. (1992). *Psychological aspects of depression: Toward a cognitive-interpersonal integration.* Chichester: Wiley.

Gullone, E. (2000). The development of normal fear: A century of research. *Clinical Psychology Review, 20*, 429–458.

Hammen, C., & Rudolph, K. D. (1996). Childhood depression. In E. J. Mash & R. A. Barkley, (Eds.), *Child Psychopathology* (pp. 153–195). New York: Guilford.

Hankin B, Abramson L, Moffitt T, Silva P, McGee R, Angell K. Development of depression from preadolescence to young adulthood: Emerging gender differences in a 10-year longitudinal study. *Journal of Abnormal Psychology, 107*(1),128–140.

Heyman, I., Fombonne, E., Simmons, H., Ford, T., Meltzer, H., & Goodman, R. (2001). Prevalence of obsessive-compulsive disorder in the British nationwide survey of child mental health. *British Journal of Psychiatry, 179*, 324–329.

Hirshfeld, D. R., Biederman, J., Brody, L., Faraone, S. V., & Rosenbaum, J. F. (1997). Expressed emotion toward children with behavioral inhibition: Associations with maternal anxiety disorder. *Journal of the American Academy of Child and Adolescent Psychiatry, 36*, 910–917.

Hollon, S. D., Garber, J., & Shelton, R. C. (2005). Treatment of depression in adolescents with cognitive behavior therapy and medications: A commentary on the TADS Project. *Cognitive and Behavioral Practice, 12*(2), 149–155.

Horney, K. (1945). *Our inner conflicts; a constructive theory of neurosis.* New York: Norton.

Jacobs, R., Reinecke, M., Gollan, J., & Kane, P. (2008). Empirical evidence of cognitive vulnerability for depression among children and adolescents: A cognitive science and developmental perspective. *Clinical Psychology Review, 28*(5), 759–782.

Joiner, T., Coyne, J. C., & Blalock, J. (1999). On the interpersonal nature of depression: Overview and synthesis. In T. Joiner & J. C. Coyne (Eds.), *The interactional nature of depression: Advances in interpersonal approaches* (pp. 3–20). Washington, DC: American Psychological Association.

Kagan, J., Reznick, J. S., & Snidman, N. (1987). The physiology and psychology of behavioral inhibition in children. *Child Development, 58,* 1459–1473.

Kashani, J. H., Beck, N. C., Hoeper, E. W., Falahi, C., Corcoran, C. M., McAllister, J. A., … Reid, J. C. (1987). Psychiatric disorders in a community sample of adolescents. *American Journal of Psychiatry, 144,* 584–589.

Kashani, J. H., Orvaschel, H., Rosenberg, T. K., &Reid, J. C. (1989). Psychopathology in a community sample of children and adolescents: A developmental perspective. *Journal of the American Academy of Child and Adolescent Psychiatry, 28,* 701–706.

Kazdin, A. E., & Kagan, J. (1994). Models of dysfunction in developmental psychopathology. *Clinical Psychology: Science and Practice, 1,* 35–52.

Keller, M. B., Lavori, P., Wunder, J., Beardslee, W. R., Schwarts, C. E., & Roth, J. (1992). Chronic course of anxiety disorders in children and adolescents. *Journal of the American Academy of Child and Adolescent Psychiatry, 312,* 595–599.

Kendall, P. C., Brady, E. U., & Verduin, T. L. (2001). Comorbidity in childhood anxiety disorders and treatment outcome. *Journal of the American Academy of Child and Adolescent Psychiatry, 40,* 787–794.

Kendall, P. C., Cantwell, D. A., & Kazdin, A. E. (1989). Depression in children and adolescents: Assessment issues and recommendations. *Cognitive Therapy and Research, 13,* 109–146.

Kendall, P. C., Flannery-Schroeder, E., Panichelli-Mindel, S. M., Southam-Gerow, M., Henin, A., & Warman, M. (1997). Treatment of anxiety disorders in youth: A second randomised clinical trial. *Journal of Consulting and Clinical Psychology, 65,* 366–380.

Kendall, P. C., & Warman, M. J. (1996). Anxiety disorders in youth: Diagnostic consistency across DSM-III-R and DSM-IV. *Journal of Anxiety Disorders, 10,* 453–463.

Kendler, K. S., Walters, E. E., Neale, M. C., Kessler, R. C., Heath, A. C., & Eaves, L. J. (1995). The structure of genetic and environmental risk factors for six major psychiatric disorders in women: Phobia, generalized anxiety disorder, panic disorder, bulimia, major depression, and alcoholism. *Archives of General Psychiatry, 51,* 8–19.

Kessler, R. C., Avenevoli, S., & Merikangas, K. R. (2001). Mood disorders in children and adolescents: An epidemiologic perspective. *Biological Psychiatry, 49,* 1002–1014.

Kessler, R. C., McGonagle, K. A., Shanyang, Z., Nelson, C. B., Hughes, M., Eshleman, S., … Kendler, K. S. (1994). Lifetime and 12-month prevalence of DSM-III-R psychiatric disorders in the United States. *Archives of General Psychiatry, 51,* 8–19.

Kessler, R. C., Stang, P. E., Wittchen, H., Ustun, T., Roy-Burne, P. P., & Walters, E. E. (1998). Lifetime panic-depression comorbidity in the National Comorbidity Survey. *Archives of General Psychiatry, 55*(9), 801–808.

Kindt, M., Brosschot, J. F., & Everaerd, W. (1997). Cognitive processing bias of children in real life stress situation and a neutral situation. *Journal of Experimental Child Psychology, 64,* 79–97.

Kovacs, M. (1992). *Children's Depression Inventory manual.* New York: Multi-Health Systems.

Kovacs, M., Feinberg, T. L., Crouse-Novak, M., Paulauskas, S. L., & Finkelstein, R. (1984). Depressive disorders in childhood: I. A longitudinal prospective study of characteristics and recovery. *Archives of General Psychiatry, 41,* 229–237.

Krohne, H. W., & Hock, M. (1991). Relationships between restrictive mother–child interactions and anxiety of the child. *Anxiety Research, 4,* 109–124.

Labellarte, M. J., Ginsburg, G. S., Walkup, J. T., & Riddle, M. A. (1999). The treatment of anxiety disorders in children and adolescents. *Biological Psychiatry, 46,* 1567–1578.

Lang, P. J. (1979). A bio-informational theory of emotional imagery. *Psychophysiology, 6,* 495–511.

Last, C. G., Perrin, S., Hersen, M., & Kazdin, A. E. (1992). DSM-III-R anxiety disorders in children: Sociodemographic and clinical characteristics. *Journal of the American Academy of Child and Adolescent Psychiatry, 31,* 1070–1076.

Last, C. L., Strauss, C. C., & Francis, G. (1987). Comorbidity among childhood anxiety disorders. *Journal of Nervous and Mental Disease, 175,* 726–730.

Lewinsohn, P. M., Clarke, G. N., Hops, H., & Andrews, J. A. (1990). Cognitive-behavioral treatment for depressed adolescents. *Behavior Therapy, 21,* 385–401

Lewinsohn, P. M., Hops, H., Roberts, R. E., Seeley, J. R., & Andrews, J. A. (1993). Adolescent psychopathology: I. Prevalence and incidence of depression and other DSM-III-R disorders in high school students. *Journal of Abnormal Psychology, 102,* 133–144.

Lewinsohn, P. M., Zinbarg, R., Seeley J. R., Lewinsohn, M., & Sack, W. H. (1997). Lifetime comorbidity among anxiety disorders and between anxiety disorders and other mental disorders in adolescents. *Journal of Anxiety Disorders, 11*, 377–394.

Manassis, K., & Monga, S. (2001) A therapeutic approach to children and adolescents with anxiety disorders and associated comorbid conditions. *Journal of the American Academy of Child and Adolescent Psychiatry, 40*, 115–117.

March, J., Parker, J., Sullivan, K., Stallings, P., & Conners, C. K. (1997). The Multidimensional Anxiety Scale for Children (MASC): Factor structure, reliability, and validity. *Journal of the American Academy of Child and Adolescent Psychiatry, 36*, 554–565.

Markowitz, J., Weissman, M., Ouellette, R., Lish, J., & Klerman, G. L. (1989). Quality of life in panic disorder. *Archives of General Psychiatry, 46*(11), 984–992.

Mattis, S. G., & Ollendick, T. H. (2002). *Panic disorder and anxiety in adolescence*. Oxford: Blackwell.

McCarty, C., & Weisz, J. (2007). Effects of psychotherapy for depression in children and adolescents: What we can (and can't) learn from meta-analysis and component profiling. *Journal of the American Academy of Child and Adolescent Psychiatry, 46*(7), 879–886.

McClure, E. B., Brennan, P. A., Hammen, C., & Le Brocque, R. M. (2001). Parental anxiety disorders, child anxiety disorders, and the perceived parent–child relationship in an Australian high-risk sample. *Journal of Abnormal Child Psychology, 9*, 1–10.

McGee, R., Feehan, M., Williams, S., & Anderson, J. (1992). DSM-III disorders from age 11 to 15 years. *Journal of the American Academy of Child and Adolescent Psychiatry, 31*, 50–59.

McGee, R., Feehan, M., Williams, S., Partridge, F., Silvia, P. A., & Kelly, J. (1990). DSM III disorders in a large sample of adolescents. *Journal of the American Academy of Child and Adolescent Psychiatry, 29*, 611–619.

Mendlowitz, S. L., Manassis, K., Bradley, S., Scapillato, D., Miezitis, S., & Shaw, B. F. (1999). Cognitive-behavioral group treatments in childhood anxiety disorders: The role of parental involvement. *Journal of the American Academy of Child and Adolescent Psychiatry, 38*, 1233–1229.

Moreau, D., & Weissman, M. (1992). Panic disorder in children and adolescents: A review. *American Journal of Psychiatry, 149*(10), 1306–1314.

Mufson, L., Moreau, D., Weissman, M. M., & Klerman, G. L. (1993). *Interpersonal psychotherapy for depressed adolescents*. New York: Guilford.

Mufson, L., Weissman, M. M., Moreau, D., & Garfinkel, R. (1999). Efficacy of interpersonal psychotherapy for depressed adolescents. *Archives of General Psychiatry, 56*, 573–579.

Nolen-Hoeksema, S. (1995). Epidemiology and theories of gender differences in unipolar depression. In M. V. Seeman (Ed.), *Gender and psychopathology* (pp. 63–87). London: American Psychiatric Press.

Nolen-Hoeksema, S., Girgus, J. S., & Seligman, M. E. (1992). Predictors and consequences of childhood depressive symptoms: A 5-year longitudinal study. *Journal of Abnormal Psychology, 101*, 405–422.

Ollendick, T. H. (1983). Reliability and validity of the Fear Survey Schedule for Children–Revised (FSSC-R). *Behaviour Research and Therapy, 21*, 685–692.

Ollendick, T. H., & Cerny, J. A. (1981). *Clinical behavior therapy with children*. New York: Plenum.

Ollendick, T. H., Hagopian, L. P., & King, N. J. (1997). Specific phobias in children. In G. C. L. Davey (Ed.), *Phobias: A handbook of theory, research and treatment* (pp. 201–224). Oxford: Wiley.

Ollendick, T., & Hirshfeld-Becker, D. (2002). The developmental and psychopathology of social anxiety disorder. *Biological Psychiatry, 51*(1), 44–58.

Ollendick, T. H., & Horsch, L. M. (2007). Fears in children and adolescents: Relations with child anxiety sensitivity, maternal overprotection, and maternal phobic anxiety. *Behavior Therapy, 38*, 402–411.

Ollendick, T. H., & Ingman, K. (2001). Social phobia. In H. Orvaschel, J. Faust, & M. Hersen (Eds.), *Handbook of conceptualization and treatment of child psychopathology* (pp. 191–210). New York: Pergamon.

Ollendick, T. H., & Jarrett, M. A. (2009). Evidence-based treatments for adolescent depression. In C. A. Essau (Ed.), *Treatments for adolescent depression: Theory and practice* (pp. 57–80). Oxford: Oxford University Press.

Ollendick, T. H., Jarrett, M. A., Grills-Taquechel, A. E., Seligman, L. D., & Wolff, J. (2008). Comorbidity as a predictor and moderator of treatment outcome in youth with anxiety, affective, AD/HD, and oppositional/conduct disorders. *Clinical Psychology Review, 28*, 1447–1471.

Ollendick, T. H., & King, N. J. (1994). Assessment and treatment of internalizing problems: The role of longitudinal data. *Journal of Consulting and Clinical Psychology, 62*, 918–927.

Ollendick, T. H., & King, N. J. (1998). Empirically supported treatments for children with phobic and anxiety disorders. *Journal of Clinical Child Psychology, 27*, 156–167.

Ollendick, T., King, N., & Muris, P. (2002). Fears and phobias in children: Phenomenology, epidemiology, and aetiology. *Child and Adolescent Mental Health, 7*(3), 98–106.

Ollendick, T. H., Lease, C. A., & Cooper, C. (1993). Separation anxiety in young adults: A preliminary examination. *Journal of Anxiety Disorders, 7*, 293–305.

Ollendick, T. H., & March, J. S. (Eds.). (2004). *Phobic and anxiety disorders in children and adolescents: A clinician's guide to effective psychosocial and pharmacological interventions.* New York: Oxford University Press.

Ollendick, T. H., Raishevich, N., Davis, T. E. III, Sirbu, C., & Ost, L-G. (2010). Phenomenology and psychological characteristics of youth with specific phobias. *Behavior Therapy, 41*, 133–141.

Ollendick, T. H., Vasey, M. W., & King, N. J. (2000). Operant conditioning influences in childhood anxiety. In M. W. Vasey & M. R. Dadds (Eds.), *The developmental psychopathology of anxiety* (pp. 231–252). New York: Oxford University Press.

Orvaschel, H., Lewinsohn, P. M., & Seeley, R. J. (1995). Continuity of psychopathology in a community sample of adolescents. *Journal of the American Academy of Child and Adolescent Psychiatry, 34*, 1525–1535.

Orvaschel, H., & Puig-Antich, J. H. (1987). *Schedule for affective disorders and schizophrenia for school-age children* (Epidemiologic version, 4th ed.) Pittsburg, PA: Western Psychiatric Institute and Clinic.

Pfeffer, C. R., Lipkins, R., Plutchik, R., & Mizruchi, M. (1988). Normal children at risk for suicidal behavior: A two-year follow-up study. *Journal of the American Academy of Child and Adolescent Psychiatry, 27*, 34–41.

Pury, C. L., & Mineka, S. (2001). Differential encoding of affective and nonaffective content information in trait anxiety. *Cognition and Emotion, 15*, 659–693.

Rapee, R. M. (1997). Potential role of childrearing practices in the development of anxiety and depression. *Clinical Psychology Review, 17*, 47–68.

Reinecke, M., Curry, J., & March, J. (2009). Findings from the Treatment for Adolescents with Depression Study (TADS): What have we learned? What do we need to know? *Journal of Clinical Child and Adolescent Psychology, 38*(6), 761–767.

Reinherz, H. Z., Giaconia, R. M., Hauf, A., Wasserman, M. S., & Silverman, A. B. (1999). Major depression in the transition to adulthood: Risks and impairments. *Journal of Abnormal Psychology, 108*(3), 500–510.

Reiss, S. (1980). Pavlovian conditioning and human fear: An expectancy model. *Behavior Therapy, 11*, 380–396.

Reynolds, C. R., & Kamphaus, R. W. (2004). *The Behavior Assessment Scale for Children* (2nd ed.). Circle Pines, MN: Pearson Assessments.

Reynolds, C. R., & Richmond, B. O. (1985). *Revised Children's Manifest Anxiety Scale: Manual.* Los Angeles: Western Psychological Services.

Rohde, P., Clarke, G., Mace, D., Jorgensen, J., & Seeley, J. R. (2004). An efficacy/effectiveness study of cognitive-behavioral treatment for adolescents with comorbid major depression and conduct disorder. *Journal of the American Academy of Child and Adolescent Psychiatry, 43*(6), 660–669.

Rudd, D. M., & Joiner, T. E. (1998). An integrative conceptual framework for assessing and treating suicidal behavior in adolescents. *Journal of Adolescence, 21*, 489–498.

Sander, J. B. (2004, November). *CBT for depression in young adolescents: How well does it treat comorbid anxiety symptoms?* Paper presented at the Association for the Advancement of Behavior Therapy Annual Convention, New Orleans, Louisiana.

Sander, J. B., & McCarty, C. A. (2005). Youth depression in the family context: Familial risk factors and models of treatment. *Clinical Child and Family Psychology Review, 8*(3), 203–219.

Schniering, C. A., Hudson, J. L., & Rapee, R. M. (2000). Issues in the diagnosis and assessment of anxiety disorders in children and adolescents. *Clinical Psychology Review, 20*, 453–478.

Seligman, L. D., & Ollendick, T. H. (1998). Comorbidity of anxiety and depression in children and adolescents: An integrative review. *Clinical Child and Family Psychology Review, 1*, 125–144.

Seligman, L. D., & Ollendick, T. H. (2011). Cognitive behavior therapy for anxiety disorders in youth. *Child and Adolescent Psychiatric Clinics of North America, 20*(2), 217–238.

Shaw, J., Kennedy, S. H., & Joffe, R. T. (1995). Gender differences in mood disorders. In M. V. Seeman (Ed.), *Gender and psychopathology.* London: American Psychiatric Press, 89–111.

Shortt, A. L., Barrett, P. M., & Fox, T. (2001). Evaluating the FRIENDS program: A cognitive behavioral group treatment for anxiety children and their parents. *Journal of Clinical Child Psychology, 30*, 525–535.

Silverman, W. K., & Albano, A. M. (1996). *Anxiety disorders interview schedule for DSM-IV: Child version: Parent interview schedule.* San Antonio, TX: Psychological Corporation.

Silverman, W. K., Cerny, J. A., Nelles, W. B., & Burke, A. E. (1988). Behavior problems in children of parents with anxiety disorders. *Journal of the American Academy of Child and Adolescent Psychiatry, 27,* 779–784.

Silverman, W. K., Kurtines, W. M., Ginsburg, G. S., Weems, C. G., Lumpkin, P. W., & Carmichael, D. H. (1999). Treating anxiety disorders in children with group cognitive behavioural therapy: A randomised clinical trial. *Journal of Consulting and Clinical Psychology, 67,* 995–1003.

Silverman, W. K., & Ollendick, T. H. (2008). Assessment of child and adolescent anxiety disorders. In J. Hunsley & E. Mash (Eds.), *A guide to assessments that work* (pp. 181–206). New York: Oxford University Press.

Silverman, W. K., & Treffers, P. D. A. (2001). *Anxiety disorders in children and adolescents: Research, assessment and intervention.* New York: Cambridge University Press.

Siqueland, L., Kendall, P. C., & Steinberg, L. (1996). Anxiety in children: Perceived family environment and observed family interaction. *Journal of Clinical Child Psychology, 25,* 225–237.

Skinner, B. F. (1938). *The behavior of organisms.* New York: Appleton-Century-Crofts.

Stark, K. D., Sander, J. B., Yancy, M., Bronik, M., & Hoke, J. (2000). Treatment of depression in childhood and adolescence: Cognitive-behavioral procedures for the individual and family. In P. C. Kendall (Ed.), *Child and adolescent therapy: Cognitive-behavioral procedures* (2nd ed., pp. 173–234). New York: Guilford.

Stark, K. D., Schmidt, K. L., & Joiner, T. E. Jr. (1996). Cognitive triad: Relationship to depressive symptoms, parents' cognitive triad, and perceived parental messages. *Journal of Abnormal Child Psychology, 24,* 615–631.

Stark, K. D., Streusand, W., Krumholz, L. S., & Patel, P. (2010). Cognitive-behavioral therapy for depression: The ACTION treatment program for girls. In J. R. Weisz, A. E. Kazdin, J. R. Weisz, A. E. Kazdin (Eds.), *Evidence-based psychotherapies for children and adolescents* (2nd ed., pp. 93–109). New York: Guilford Press.

Strauss, C. (1994). Overanxious disorder. In T. H. Ollendick, N. J. King, & W. Yule (Eds.). *International handbook of phobic and anxiety disorders in children and adolescents* (pp. 187–206). New York: Plenum.

Strauss, C., & Last, C. (1993). Social and simple phobias in children. *Journal of Anxiety Disorders, 7*(2), 141–152.

Strauss, C., Lease, C., Last, C., & Francis, G. (1988). Overanxious disorder: An examination of developmental differences. *Journal of Abnormal Child Psychology, 11,* 433–443.

Suveg, C., Hudson, J. L., Brewer, G., Flannery-Schroeder, E., Gosch, E., & Kendall, P. C. (2009). Cognitive-behavioral therapy for anxiety-disordered youth: Secondary outcomes from a randomized clinical trial evaluating child and family modalities. *Journal of Anxiety Disorders, 23,* 341–349.

Taghavi, M. R., Neshat-Doost, H. T., Moradi, A. R., Yule, W., & Dalgleish, T. (1999). Biases in visual attention in children and adolescents with clinical anxiety and mixed anxiety-depression. *Journal of Abnormal Child Psychology, 27,* 215–223.

Thapar, A., & McGuffin, P. (1995). Are anxiety symptoms in childhood heritable? *Journal of Child Psychology and Psychiatry, 36,* 439–447.

Treatment for Adolescents With Depression Study (TADS) Team. (2004). Fluoxetine, cognitive-behavioral therapy, and their combination for adolescents with depression: Treatment for Adolescents With Depression Study (TADS) Randomized Controlled Trial. *Journal of the American Medical Association, 292*(7), 807–820.

Wagner, K., & Ambrosini, P. (2001). Childhood depression: Pharmacological therapy/treatment (pharmacotherapy of childhood depression). *Journal of Clinical Child Psychology, 30*(1), 88–97.

Wannan, G., & Fombonne, E. (1998). Gender differences in rates and correlates of suicidal behavior amongst child psychiatric outpatients. *Journal of Adolescence, 21,* 371–381.

Weisz, J., McCarty, C., & Valeri, S. (2006). Effects of psychotherapy for depression in children and adolescents: A meta-analysis. *Psychological Bulletin, 132*(1), 132–149.

Weisz, J. R., Southam-Gerow, M. A., & McCarty, C. A. (2001). Control-related beliefs and depressive symptoms in clinic referred children and adolescents: Developmental differences and model specificity. *Journal of Abnormal Psychology, 110,* 97–109.

Werry, J. S. (1991). Overanxious disorder: A review of its taxonomic properties. *Journal of the American Academy of Child and Adolescent Psychiatry, 30,* 533–544.

Wiesner, M., Kim, H., & Capaldi, D. (2005). Developmental trajectories of offending: Validation and prediction to young adult alcohol use, drug use, and depressive symptoms. *Development and Psychopathology, 17*(1), 251–270.

Williams, S., Connolly, J., & Segal, Z. V. (2001). Intimacy in relationships and cognitive vulnerability to depression in adolescent girls. *Cognitive Therapy and Research, 25*(4), 477–496.

Wolff, J. A., & Ollendick, T. H. (2006). The comorbidity of conduct problems and depression in childhood and adolescence. *Clinical Child and Family Psychology Review, 9*, 201–220.

Wood, J., Mathews, A., & Dalgleish, T. (2001). Anxiety and cognitive inhibition. *Emotion, 1*, 166–181.

World Health Organization. (1992). *The ICD-10 classification of mental and behavioral disorders: Diagnostic criteria for research*. Geneva: Author.

19
Language, Learning, and Cognitive Disorders

REBECCA S. MARTÍNEZ, STACY E. WHITE, and MICHELLE L. JOCHIM

Indiana University
Bloomington, Indiana

LEAH M. NELLIS

Indiana State University
Terre Haute, Indiana

Learning disorders represent an assorted category of generalized neurodevelopmental challenges that interfere with the ability to learn academic or social skills (Pennington, 2009). Broadly, learning disorders originate from a combination of congenital, acquired, or environmental conditions or circumstances. Congenital learning disorders include specific learning disabilities (e.g., dyslexia and dyscalculia), communication disorders (e.g., stuttering), and developmental disabilities (e.g., intellectual disabilities and autism). They are present at birth and manifest throughout the lifespan as children and adolescents engage in increasingly challenging cognitive and academic tasks. Learning disorders also can be acquired at any point in the lifespan following acute health conditions or severe injury (e.g., traumatic brain injury). Despite their organic etiology, risk and protective factors shape the developmental trajectory of both congenital and acquired learning disorders. Poor environmental conditions (e.g., not reading aloud to young children and implementing teaching methods that are not evidence based) can bring about and exacerbate learning difficulties and disorders, even when there is not a biological predisposition for them.

This chapter focuses on the three most ubiquitous learning disorders: specific learning disabilities (SLD), speech or language impairments (SLI), and intellectual disabilities (ID). Based on special education eligibility criteria, approximately 6 million (13.4%) of the total school-age population have an identified disability and receive public school special education services (U.S. Department of Education [USDOE], 2010). Roughly 2.6 million children and adolescents (5.2% of the school-age population) are identified by special education legal standards as having specific learning disabilities, representing almost half of all students who receive special education services. After SLD, the most frequently occurring learning disorders are SLIs (1.5 million or 3% of the school-age population) followed by IDs (i.e., mental retardation or cognitive impairments), representing (500,000 or 1% of the population). Although true learning disorders are present at birth, this chapter will mainly discuss malleable environmental conditions (e.g., importance of implementing excellent, research-based teaching methods) that can alter the trajectory of organic learning disorders. Protective factors that foster student resilience (e.g., teaching basic academic skills until students achieve fluency or mastery) can also prevent acquired learning disorders from manifesting in the first place. Although endogenous learning disorders have a biological origin, children and adolescents exposed to environmental risk factors (e.g., teachers who fail to teach phonics to struggling readers) may "learn to be learning disabled"

(Clay, 1987, cited in Gresham, VanDerHeyden, & Witt, 2005, p.17) and struggle academically in ways that are indistinguishable from students with endogenous learning disorders.

The first section of this chapter provides an in-depth discussion of SLD, including a description of the definition and changing identification criteria for SLD. Next, we describe a relatively recent educational paradigm applied to the prevention and early intervention of learning disorders that is rooted in the public health model commonly applied to the prevention and intervention of sickness and disease. This model, Response to Intervention (RTI), has been dubbed one of the most revolutionary manifestations in education. Response to Intervention approaches all learning disorders, regardless of their etiology or severity, from a solution-focused perspective of prevention and intervention. Proponents of RTI are less likely to focus on learning disorders as a within-student problem (i.e., nonmalleable condition) and more likely to concentrate on the instructional and environmental conditions that fail to support student learning and the ways they can be altered to help students learn (i.e., learning disorders as malleable conditions).

Next, we describe the assessment, etiology, and prevalence of communication disorders, focusing on speech and language impairments. Specifically, we provide information on the more common speech and language impairments: phonological disorders and stuttering. In the third section, we introduce intellectual disabilities (i.e., mental retardation), a less common condition but nonetheless pervasive developmental disorder that results in difficulties with learning.

This chapter concludes with specific strategies the reader can use to help students with learning disorders and their families navigate the school system, particularly within special education. We also provide suggestions for clinical psychologists and social workers who desire to work closely with staff at their clients' schools. Specifically, we recommend ways clinicians can (a) promote prevention of learning failure, (b) participate in school-wide efforts to support children and adolescents with learning disorders, and (c) partner effectively with parents and schools to improve the schooling experience of students with learning disorders.

Specific Learning Disabilities

A disability classification, such as SLD, provides a mechanism to organize a heterogeneous group of people into smaller subgroups of individuals with similar attributes who differ from other subgroups in important and observable ways. Ideally, disability classifications facilitate communication among professionals and the individuals themselves. Classification systems help inform programming and treatment efforts.

Valid disability classifications and appropriate diagnoses require clear operational definitions and identification criteria. Historically, there has been a lack of agreement about the best way to identify specific learning disabilities.[1] Despite being the most prevalent of the learning disorders, SLDs are among the least understood and most passionately debated disability categories (Bradley, Danielson, & Hallahan, 2002). Inconsistent application of identification criteria in school and clinical practice has contributed to contradictory and unstable classification, identification, and remediation procedures. Understanding the current state of the field requires a brief historical overview of the field, which is presented in the next section.

Historical Overview and Evolving Definition

Scientific, social, and political changes since the 1900s have shaped the field of learning disabilities (see Turnbull, 2009, for a recent analysis). The desire and need to identify individual

---

[1] The term *learning disability* is a broad designation for a variety of learning disorders. We use the term specific learning disability throughout this chapter to be consistent with legal language and practical consideration because learning disabilities generally manifest in specific areas, such as reading, decoding, math computation, and so forth.

differences in learning and performance have dominated scientific and clinical efforts aimed at understanding SLDs. Observations and reports of individuals with learning disabilities in one area (e.g., reading) while having otherwise average or typical performance in other areas (e.g., mathematics) first emerged in the early 19th century (Fletcher, Lyon, Fuchs, & Barnes, 2007). A hallmark of the earliest definition of learning disabilities is that it defined what learning disabilities were *not* rather than what they *were*. For example, Kirk (1963) first coined the term *learning disabilities* to describe a "group of children who have disorders in the development of language, speech, reading, and associated communication skills needed for social interaction … not includ[ing] children who have sensory handicaps such as blindness … [or] who have generalized mental retardation" (pp. 2–3). Specific exclusionary or "rule out" considerations remain in the most recent (USDOE, 2004) federal definition of a specific learning disability.

Research conducted up to and through the early 1960s had a significant impact on our modern conceptualization of learning disabilities. Collectively, evidence about individual learning disorders contributed the following to our understanding: (a) learning differences could be understood by observing how children approach tasks and process information, (b) instruction and programming should be designed in recognition of a child's specific strengths and weaknesses, (c) specific learning disabilities are associated with neurological functioning but are not a primary result of sensory impairments, and (d) specific learning disabilities occur in the context of overall average cognitive functioning (Kavale & Forness, 1985; Torgesen, 1991). Also in the 1960s, researchers, educators, and policymakers began advocating fervently and effectively for adequate educational conditions on behalf of all children with disabilities. In response, the U.S. Department of Education began the process of operationally defining the condition, specific learning disability, for legislative purposes. In 1968, the following definition, which included exclusionary factors, was adopted:

> The term "specific learning disability" means a disorder in one or more of the basic psychological processes involved in understand or in using language, spoken or written, which may manifest itself in an imperfect ability to listen, speak, read, write, spell, or to do mathematical calculations. The term includes such conditions as perceptual handicaps, brain injury, minimal brain dysfunction, dyslexia, and developmental aphasia. The term does not include children who have learning disabilities, which are primarily the result of visual, hearing, or motor handicaps, or mental retardation, or emotional disturbance, or of environmental, culturally, or economic disadvantage. (USDOE, 1968, p. 34)

This definition drew from the field's collective understanding of learning disabilities in terms of its biological etiology (Orton, 1937) and in relation to exclusionary factors (Kirk, 1963). The 1968 definition also marked the first time the term "specific learning disabilities" was used. Consequently, the 1968 definition was included in the Learning Disabilities Act of 1969 and as the statutory definition of specific learning disabilities in the landmark Education for All Handicapped Children Act of 1975 (PL 94-142), which guaranteed, for the first time in history, a free, appropriate public education to all children with disabilities, including those identified with learning disorders. The 1968 definition continues to be, with a few minor wording adjustments, the definition of SLD in the most recent federal special education regulations (Individuals With Disabilities Education Improvement Act [IDEA], 2004) that today guide school-based evaluation and eligibility decisions.

Although the federal definition and accompanying regulations were somewhat helpful in evaluation, identification, and special education program development, significant concerns remained regarding the procedures for *identifying* learning disabilities. Indeed, researchers, practitioners, and advocates continually criticize the definition for emphasizing what learning disabilities *are not* but omitting a clear description and criteria of what learning disabilities *are* (Fletcher et al., 2007) and how to identify students who have specific learning disabilities. An ongoing debate that seeks clarity regarding the definition of SLD and identification practices continues within the field and will likely continue into the foreseeable future. Although a full account of this debate is beyond the scope of this chapter, interested readers are directed to writings by Fuchs and Fuchs (2006), Kavale and Forness (2000), and Kavale and Spaulding (2008) for more information.

One of the factors contributing to the lack of shared consensus about definition and identification procedures for SLDs lies in the various definitions of SLD that have been formalized by the American Psychiatric Association (i.e., in the *Diagnostic and Statistical Manual of Mental Disorders, DSM*, 2000) and various advocacy groups such as the National Joint Committee on Learning Disabilities, and the World Health Organization (i.e., *International Classification of Diseases*, 1992). Professionals in clinical and medical practices favor the *DSM* classification system and use it to *diagnose* clients with a specific learning disability. In contrast, school personnel use the federal special education definition and identification criteria to *identify* a learning disorders (including SLD, SLI, and ID) for the purpose of providing special education services in schools. It is imperative to note that eligibility for special education services in the schools does not require a medical or clinical diagnosis of a learning disorder; likewise, a medical or clinical diagnosis of a learning disorder does not ensure special education eligibility. This may be confusing for parents and even for professionals who do not work in a school system. Legally, the purpose of special education eligibility procedures is to determine educational need and, therefore, eligibility for special education services. Federal law requires a multidisciplinary team consisting of qualified professionals to *identify* whether a student has a disability that requires special support services. The multidisciplinary team must determine whether the disorder prevents the student from learning in the general education system and if the student would benefit from specialized services offered through the local special education program.

In addition to the lack of universal consensus about the definition of a specific learning disability, an equally contentious predicament in the history of SLDs concerns identification procedures. Although PL 94-142 provided an operational definition for specific learning disabilities, as noted above, the omission of clear inclusionary criteria to help identify students with SLD immediately became problematic for multidisciplinary teams responsible for making special education eligibility decisions for children with significant learning problems.

In 1977, the USDOE published guidelines designed to facilitate the identification of students with specific learning disabilities. The guidelines included the identification criterion of a "severe discrepancy" between intelligence and academic achievement. School professionals interpreted the criterion literally to mean a significant discrepancy or difference between ability, as measured by a standardized IQ score, and academic achievement, as measured by a standardized achievement test score. Despite the widespread acceptance of the discrepancy criterion, there was limited evidence of its validity (Fletcher et al., 2002). Nevertheless school-based professionals in the fields of special education and school psychology came to consider this IQ–achievement discrepancy as *the* diagnostic criterion for the presence (or absence) of a specific learning disability.

Concerns About the IQ–Achievement Discrepancy

Since the passage of the All Handicapped Children Act of 1975, educators have expressed concern about the lack of emphasis on prevention for students with SLDs (National Association of State Directors of Special Education [NASDSE], 2005). Reschly (2003) criticized the discrepancy approach to identifying SLD as being (a) unreliable and unstable, (b) invalid (e.g., poor readers with high IQs do not substantially differ from poor readers with lower IQs), (c) neglectful of providing the necessary focus on exclusionary criteria such as mental retardation, and environmental, cultural, or linguistic diversity, and (d) harmful because it represents a "wait-to-fail" approach that delays identification and services. Gresham (2002) similarly criticized the discrepancy approach because it relied on assessment information that had restricted utility in designing, implementing, or evaluating the impact of classroom instruction and intervention. In other words, the assessment data did not drive decisions about which instructional practices or interventions would be most beneficial for the student.

In the early part of the 21st century, alternate methods for addressing learning problems at the first sign of difficulty in school and identifying SLDs began to emerge in the literature. Chief among these methods was RTI. RTI is a data-driven model for identifying and responding to the needs of students who demonstrate academic and behavioral difficulties. RTI includes school-wide universal screening, a continuum of interventions and supports, and ongoing monitoring of student growth and learning (Brown-Chidsey & Steege, 2005; Martínez & Nellis, 2008). Although RTI is relatively new to education, its conceptual origins lie in the public health model of preventing disease across a population. Response to Intervention will be discussed in greater detail later when we discuss effective ways to prevent and remediate learning disorders.

The Problem With Special Education

In the 25 years spanning 1975 to 2000, a spike in the number of students identified as having specific learning disabilities prompted great concern at the federal level. Consequently, in 2001, President George W. Bush appointed the Commission on Excellence in Special Education to report on the condition of special education broadly and propose policy for improving the educational performance and school experience of all students with disabilities. The resulting report, *A New Era: Revitalizing Special Education for Children and Their Families*, (USDOE, 2002) documented the condition of special education and shed light on fundamental systemic flaws that, at best, contributed to the overrepresentation of students identified with SLDs relative to the other disability categories and, at worst, outright failed children.

The authors of the report acknowledged that emphasis on the *process* (e.g., excessive paperwork) of providing special education services in the schools resulted too frequently in simply identifying students as eligible for special education, rather than promoting teaching practices in both general and special education that ensured effective instruction for all struggling students (regardless of an identified disability). The authors of the report did not mince words when underscoring that the education system often failed struggling learners and students with learning disorders largely because educators did not readily embrace or implement evidence-based educational and intervention practices. Indeed the authors conceded that "special education should be for those who do not respond to strong and appropriate instruction and methods provided in general education" (USDOE, 2002, p. 7). Lyon (2002) poignantly referred to students who were failed by the general education system as *instructional casualties* whose learning disorders manifested as a direct result of not being taught by teachers who used effective educational practices. The 2002 report concluded that the special education system had become obsolete because the system inadvertently facilitated a process of literally waiting for students to fail before they received help, instead of promoting prevention, early identification and hardline, evidence-based intervention approaches to help struggling learners. Finally, methods of identifying children with disabilities, particularly with respect to the category of SLDs, were sharply criticized in the 2002 federal report cited above and by Gresham (2002) as lacking validity and misidentifying, overidentifying, and, at times, underidentifying certain students for special education services.

Special Education Today

The December 2004 reauthorization of the Individuals with Disabilities Education Act of 1997 (IDEA), the United States' special education law (originally PL 94-142), was released in August 2006, and it included RTI as an alternative method (to the IQ-achievement discrepancy approach) for identifying an SLD in the schools. The regulations included language specifying that, in the identification of specific learning disabilities, state educational agencies *must not require* that local education agencies use a severe discrepancy between intellectual ability and achievement and *must permit* school districts to incorporate the use of a process based on the child's response to scientific research-based intervention or other alternative research-based procedures for determining the existence of an SLD (e.g., absolute low academic functioning irrespective of IQ) (§300.307).[2] The IDEA 2004 definition of SLD was a slightly modified version of the definition included in the first iteration of special education legislation in 1975 (PL 94-142) and reads as follows:

> §300.8(c)(10) … A disorder in one or more of the basic psychological processes involved in understanding or in using language, spoken or written, that may manifest itself in the imperfect ability to listen, think, speak, read, write, spell, or to do mathematical calculations, including conditions such as perceptual disabilities, brain injury, minimal brain dysfunction, dyslexia, and developmental aphasia. (ii) *Disorders not included.* Specific learning disability does not include learning problems that are primarily the result of visual, hearing, or motor disabilities, of mental retardation, of emotional disturbance, or of environmental, cultural, or economic disadvantage.

The eight areas in which a specific learning disability can be identified are: (1) oral expression, (2) listening comprehension, (3) written expression, (4) basic reading skill, (5) reading fluency skills, (6) reading comprehension, (7) mathematics calculation, and (8) mathematics problem solving.

Response to Intervention

Regulations in IDEA 2004 required state educational agencies to determine whether RTI would be *mandated* or simply *permitted* as a component to identify the presence of SLDs. Zirkel and Thomas (2010a) reported that 12 states require RTI, but the majority of states in the United States continue to allow schools to use the discrepancy criterion to determine presence of an SLD. Approximately 20 states also permit schools to use other research-based models that were not explicitly defined but permitted in the IDEA 2004. Zirkel and Thomas noted that while such state regulations allow for flexibility at the district and school levels, they also create the potential for confusion and foster inconsistent practice, similar to what the discrepancy model originally engendered. Zirkel and Thomas (2010b) examined state guidelines for using RTI and described and found that all elements of RTI implementation were not equally addressed across the documents. Further, the lack of explicit state or federal criteria to guide schools in determining when a student crosses the line from being a struggling student to one with a true learning disability makes it very difficult for multidisciplinary teams to make special education eligibility decisions.

What Is Response to Intervention?

RTI is a continuum of services that are available to all students based on individual needs, regardless of whether a student has been identified as eligible for special education services. The

---

[2] Under the new law, schools are still permitted to use the discrepancy approach, if their state allows it, to identifying specific learning disabilities; however, clear research evidence does not support this method to identify SLD (see Gresham, 2002; Reschly, 2003).

core RTI philosophy mirrors the public health model of prevention and early intervention in the case of disease. RTI is the application of public health in the public schools. This RTI continuum includes universal interventions, sometimes referred to as "primary prevention," which are in place for all students, including general education students, to support positive academic, behavioral, and mental health outcomes. Tier 1 (i.e., primary prevention) in an RTI model involves high-quality school and classroom environments, scientifically sound core curriculum and instruction, and intentional instructional practices. Tier 2, or secondary prevention, consists of targeted academic and behavioral services for those students who demonstrate risk for failure and for whom universal interventions are not resulting in their success. Services at Tier 2 are more intense and are focused on the specific needs of a student or group of students. Examples of educational services at Tier 2 might include small group instruction for either academic or behavioral needs, additional tutoring support, or involvement in remediation programs such as Title I. Despite the educational services at Tiers 1 and 2, some students need more intensive intervention at the tertiary or intensive level. Tier 3 services are available for those students for whom Tiers 1 and 2 services have not been sufficient. In theory, the needs of approximately 80 to 90% of all students in any given school can be met with universal educational services at Tier 1. Beyond Tier 1, 5 to 15% of the student body population may require Tier 2 intervention and 1 to 5% Tier 3 intervention (Walker & Shinn, 2002).

Response to Intervention for Identifying the Presence of a Specific Learning Disability

Eligibility for special education services for students with SLDs (as described above) are made by a multidisciplinary team, as described in §300.308. The team includes a child's parents and a team of qualified professionals, including a teacher and at least one member trained to diagnostically evaluate the student's learning (such as a school psychologist or speech-language pathologist [See Appendix A for descriptions of these roles]). As stated earlier, *eligibility* for special education services is not determined by a clinical (i.e., *DSM*) *diagnosis* of a disability. Thus, although a child or adolescent may have been diagnosed by a clinical practitioner with a specific learning disability, if the individual's impairment does not adversely affect his or her academic or functional performance, as determined by the school's multidisciplinary team, the individual may not be identified as a student with a specific learning disability and deemed eligible for special education services. For this reason, it is in a client's best interest for psychologists and social workers to work collaboratively with staff and administrators at their clients' schools to ensure that optimal educational services are provided. We provide practical suggestions for working with schools in greater detail in a later section.

As part of special education eligibility determination for an SLD, as outlined in IDEA 2004, the school-based multidisciplinary team must consider evidence that the child has *not* made sufficient progress in response to scientific, research-based intervention (e.g., RTI) *or* exhibits a pattern of strengths and weaknesses that is determined to be relevant to the identification of a SLD. Addressing longstanding concerns about the rigor and appropriateness of instruction in reading and math, the regulations also require the team to consider data that demonstrate that appropriate instruction in general education was provided prior to, or during, the referral process (§300.309 [b]). Such data might include assessments that all students in a school are taking (e.g., universal screening of core skills), tests that teachers are using in their classrooms (e.g., teacher-made assessments), and targeted assessments (e.g., progress monitoring tests) given frequently to students who are receiving additional intervention.

Despite considerable research, debate, and legislative activity regarding SLDs, and more recently the role of RTI in eligibility decisions, researchers and practitioners still cast doubt on the validity of RTI procedures for identifying SLDs (Fletcher, Morris, & Lyon, 2003; Kavale & Spaulding, 2008; McKenzie, 2009). In addition, Johnson, Humphrey, Mellard, Woods, and

Swanson (2010) cautioned that RTI, even when implemented with fidelity, may provide restricted information about *why* a student has failed to make progress over time. Thus, an explanation or hypothesis about why the student struggles is sometimes missing, which limits future education programming and planning efforts.

Speech or Language Impairment

Approximately 1.5 million school-age students in the United States have speech or language disorders. Generally, children with SLIs are identified in preschool, although some children may not be identified until early elementary school (Schuele, 2004). IDEA 2004 defines an SLI as [§300.8(c)(11)] "a communication disorder, such as stuttering, impaired articulation, a language impairment, or a voice impairment, that adversely affects a child's educational performance." Under the broad umbrella "communication disorder," there are three varieties of impairments: speech, language, and hearing (Justice, 2006); this chapter focuses on speech and language disorders or impairments. The fundamental elements of spoken communication are essential to learning, and difficulties in these areas usually negatively impact a student's educational achievement well before the student is identified as eligible for special education services. A breakdown in speech, language, or hearing can manifest as a communication disorder. As with SLDs, the earlier communication difficulties are identified, the greater the chance of improving and remediating symptoms of the disorder. The RTI model, described previously, is also applicable to the prevention, identification, and remediation of speech and language impairments, especially in the first few years of formal schooling.

Speech Disorders

A speech disorder is an impairment in the presentation of spoken language (Worster-Drought, 1968). Speech disorders are characterized by a breakdown in speech production (e.g., articulation) and include disorders of the voice. Common speech problems include stuttering or dysfluency, articulation disorders, and unusual voice quality (U.S. Preventive Services Task Force, 2006). Stuttering (i.e., stammering) is characterized by repetitions, prolongations, and long pauses in the production of speech. Stuttering affects approximately 5% of the population, and the incidence is double in boys compared to girls (Andrews, 1984). Most children recover naturally, without intervention, within 3 years of initial identification, although approximately 1% of the adult population stutters (Zebrowski, 2003).

Language Disorders

Language involves the understanding, processing, and the production of communication (U.S. Preventive Services Task Force, 2006). A language disorder is a breakdown in the linguistic system that can impact at least one of the following linguistic domains: syntax, semantics, phonology, morphology, and pragmatics (Justice, 2006). Specific language impairments encompass the largest group of children with language disorders and affect approximately 7% of all children (Ziegler, Pech-Georgel, George, Alario, & Lorenzi, 2005). Speech or language impairments are often followed by associated problems such as difficulties in reading and spelling and may generalize to include abnormalities in interpersonal relationships and emotional and behavioral disorders (Arkkila, Rasanen, Roine, & Vilkman, 2008).

Phonological disorders are considered a variety of language disorders and among the most prevalent communication disorders present in preschool and school-age children. A phonological disorder reflects an inability to articulate speech sounds (Gierut, 1998). Phonological awareness is essential to learning how to read (Adams, 1990), and deficits in phonological awareness are inextricably linked to reading disabilities (Lyon, Shaywitz, & Shaywitz, 2003). Thus, for speech-language pathologists employed in the school system, children with phonological disorders may represent as much as 91% of their average caseloads (American Speech-Language-Hearing Association, 2006).

Assessment of Speech or Language Impairments

For both articulation and phonology disorders, methods of assessment usually include a hearing screening and informal and formal procedures. Informal procedures may consist of a review of existing data, examination of the structure and function of the oral mechanism, speech sampling, and direct observation. Psychometric tests administered by licensed speech and language pathologists play a significant role in the process of identifying children with SLIs. These standardized tests allow professionals to observe different aspects of language function and to relate a child's performance to normative data (Bishop & McDonald, 2009). Generally, methods of assessing language disorders include: hearing screening, review of existing data, questionnaires, teacher/parent/student interviews, direction observation and language sampling, student work examples, and standardized tests (Sunderland, 2004).

Intellectual Disability

The third most common learning disorder is a direct result of biological, cognitive impairments present at birth. Traditionally, individuals with ID are grouped into one of four degrees of severity, based on cognitive functioning, and all levels of ID negatively impact a student's educational achievement, which is evident even before the student is identified as a special education student. As measured by most standardized assessments of cognitive ability, a standard IQ score falling within one standard deviation of the mean (85–100; mean = 100) is considered in the average range. Likewise, a score of 70, or two standard deviations below the mean, is considered the upper limit of mild ID. As of the fourth text revision edition of the *DSM* (American Psychological Association, 2000),[3] the ranges of severity of ID are: mild (55–70), moderate (40–54), severe (25–39), and profound (below 25). An IQ score as high as 75 is often considered at the borderline level of intellectual functioning. However, the DSM–5 neurodevelopmental work group (American Psychiatric Association, 2011) has recommended that the DSM–5 include only one diagnosis for ID, with severity based not only on IQ, but also on the degree of impairment in adaptive behavior. Similarly, IDEA 2004 defines intellectual disability, or mental retardation as [§300.8(c)(6)] "significantly subaverage general intellectual functioning, existing concurrently with deficits in adaptive behavior and manifested during the developmental period, that adversely affects a child's educational performance."

In 2007, the American Association on Mental Retardation officially changed its name to the American Association on Intellectual and Developmental Disabilities and has since advocated for the use of the diagnostic term *intellectual disability*. Though the term *mental retardation* remains in use in the most recent version of the *DSM*, as well as in federal educational law (IDEA, 2004), as illustrated above, it has been recommended that the upcoming publication of the *DSM* incorporate the term *intellectual developmental disorder* (American Psychiatric Association, 2011).

Assessment and Identification

Intellectual disability is characterized by three core traits: (1) significantly below average cognitive functioning, (2) limited functioning in adaptive behavior, and (3) onset prior to the age of 18. Comprehensive assessment of cognitive functioning and adaptive behavior is vital to an accurate diagnosis of ID and should take into account cultural and environmental factors that may influence performance in these areas.

---

[3] The fifth edition of the *DSM* is scheduled for publication in May 2013.

Cognitive Functioning

Several norm-referenced instruments are used to assess cognitive functioning, or intelligence. Among the most commonly used, particularly with children, are the Wechsler Intelligence Scale for Children, fourth edition (WISC-IV; Wechsler, 2003) and the Stanford-Binet Intelligence Scales, fifth edition (SB5; Roid, 2003). These instruments were created based on the theory that intelligence is a multifaceted construct that encompasses performance and ability in domains such as verbal reasoning, memory, abstract problem solving, and visual-spatial perception.

The WISC-IV is an individually administered test that consists of 10 core subtests and five supplemental subtests. The test yields a full-scale IQ, as well as four index scores: verbal comprehension, which measures verbal abilities in reasoning, comprehension, and conceptualization; perceptual reasoning, which measures perceptual reasoning and organization; working memory, which measures attention, concentration, and working memory; and processing speed, which measures the speed of mental and psychomotor processing. Similarly, the SB5 consists of 10 subtests and also yields a full-scale IQ. Each subtest in the verbal domain has a corresponding subtest in the nonverbal domain. The five domains are: fluid reasoning, knowledge, quantitative reasoning, visual-spatial processing, and working memory.

The full-scale IQ score yielded by tests such as the WISC-IV and SB5 is used as the basis for determining impaired cognitive ability. However, as both tests yield scores in verbal and nonverbal domains, if there is a significant discrepancy in an individual's performance in these areas, clinicians should closely examine the individual's pattern of strengths and weaknesses, rather than simply relying on averaging these scores to derive a full-scale IQ (American Psychiatric Association, 2000).

Adaptive Behavior

Adaptive behavior can be defined as "how effectively individuals cope with common life demands and how well they meet the standards of personal independence expected of someone in their particular age group, sociocultural background, and community setting" (American Psychiatric Association, 2000, p. 42). According to the American Association on Intellectual and Developmental Disabilities (AAIDD, 2010), adaptive behavior encompasses three types of skills: social skills (including interpersonal skills, social responsibility, social problem solving, and the ability to follow rules and avoid victimization), conceptual skills (money, time, and numerical concepts; language and literacy; self-regulation), and practical skills (including self-care and activities of daily living, occupational skills, healthcare, travel and transportation, adhering to schedules and routines, and safety). Assessment of adaptive behavior is not only a key component of the diagnostic profile of ID, but it also forms the basis from which intervention and remediation plans are typically developed.

Assessment of adaptive behavior typically consists of multi-informant rating scales, completed by parents, educators, community mental health providers, and the individual him- or herself. The most frequently used measures of adaptive behavior are the Adaptive Behavior Assessment System, second edition (ABAS-II; Harrison & Oakland, 2003) and the Vineland Adaptive Behavior Scales, second edition (VABS-II; Sparrow, Cicchetti, & Balla, 2005).

Assessments of appropriate adaptive functioning are highly subjective and heavily based on social, cultural, and other environmental norms. When selecting assessment instruments and interpreting results, therefore, the evaluator should pay attention to the suitability of the assessment tool for the individual as well as external factors that may impact his or her performance (American Psychiatric Association, 2000).

School Identification and Special Education Eligibility

In addition to community agencies, schools serve as one of the primary environments in which children with IDs are identified and receive support. Recent statistics show that students identified using special education criteria for an ID represented 9% of all students served under the IDEA, Part B (U.S. Department of Education, 2004). Educational professionals, including school psychologists, counselors, and social workers, are traditionally charged with the task of conducting valid assessments and designing educational interventions for this group of students. Though standardized assessments of cognitive ability and adaptive behavior may provide a sufficient basis for an identification of ID or for determining eligibility for special education services, results from these assessments offer little to inform the process of intervention planning in educational contexts. To help fill this void, it is recommended that school teams conduct multidisciplinary, functional, and ecologically valid assessments to inform educational planning for children with IDs (Powell-Smith, Stoner, Bilter, & Sansosti, 2008). As a starting point, detailed information on the child's developmental, medical, and social history provides important clues regarding the onset of the child's delay and possible etiologies of the condition, allowing the team to rule out other potential causes for the child's academic and behavioral difficulties (i.e., SLD). Further, information on student performance should be gathered from multiple sources in various environments, including the home, school, and community settings. Particularly important are data on functional life skills and "cues and correction procedures" that occur naturally and without planned intervention and effectively assist the individual in completing daily life tasks.

Finally, the focus of assessment and intervention should be on functional life skills that will allow for successful transition to postschool settings. Central to working with students with ID is the provision of supports that increase the individual's ability to function as independently as possible. We strongly encourage clinical professionals serving clients with ID (or specific learning disability) outside of the school system to work collaboratively with school-based identification teams and educational professionals to ensure optimal and appropriate educational and intervention supports for clients with IDs.

Working With Children Who Have Learning Disorders and Their Families

This section will provide psychologists and social workers specific suggestions for working with clients who have SLD, SLI, or ID. We contend that these and other practitioners provide optimum clinical services when they collaborate with teachers, administrators, and school personnel at their clients' schools to ensure that the full spectrum of services is provided to their clients. We believe that psychologists and social workers can be effective partners in the schooling of their clients when they (a) promote prevention and early intervention, (b) partner with school personnel to optimize the educational supports and services being provided, and (c) assist parents and families in supporting clients with learning disorders. We describe each recommendation in detail next.

Promote Prevention and Early Intervention and Encourage
Family to Become Children's First Teachers

Psychologists and other clinicians may be most helpful to their clients who have learning disorders when they promote prevention strategies at home and at school. As noted previously, environmental conditions may predispose a child without an organic learning deficit to "learn to be learning disabled" (Clay, 1987, cited in Gresham, VanDerHeyden, & Witt, 2005) such that organic and acquired learning disorders are indistinguishable. One way clinicians can promote prevention is by conducting parent education seminars, community workshops, or parent counseling sessions that emphasize the critical early role parents play in ensuring their children's subsequent academic success. In *Helping Your Child Become a Reader* (USDOE, 2005), a pamphlet available free of charge on the USDOE website, parents of young children (birth to age 6) are encouraged to (a) talk and listen to their young children even as babies, (b) spend at least 30 minutes daily reading aloud to their children, (c) bring attention to the letters and words in books and help them understand that they have meaning, and (d) foster children's innate curiosity to write, because reading and writing go hand in hand.

As consultants, psychologists can urge their clients' teachers to focus on direct, explicit instructional strategies (Carnine, Silbert, & Kame'enui, 1997). Struggling students need intense instruction in small groups for longer duration with greater frequency compared to the instruction provided to typically achieving students (Deshler, 2005). One of the best tools for being an effective consultant and recommending best practices in academic interventions is to be knowledgeable about available evidence-based academic and behavioral interventions. Appendix B lists links to helpful websites. Additionally, attending national professional conferences, such as the National Association of School Psychologist's and the American Speech-Language-Hearing Association annual conventions, can provide psychologists and other clinicians the opportunity to gain valuable knowledge about the most effective, cutting-edge instructional strategies currently available.

Participate in School Efforts to Support Clients With Learning Disorders

Another way psychologists and other clinicians can help clients who have learning disorders is by their willingness to work collaboratively with school personnel to advocate on behalf of their clients so they receive the best educational services in general and special education settings. Federal law requires that students with disabilities be educated in the least restrictive environment with typically achieving peers to the maximum extent that is deemed appropriate. Therefore, practitioners want to ensure that schools are providing their clients special education services in inclusive environments with typically achieving peers and that their clients have equal access to the curriculum and extracurricular activities. Additionally, clinicians working with children who are in special education or being considered for special education eligibility can be effective as collaborative, contributing members of the school multidisciplinary team that weighs the available evidence to make decisions about children's placement and the remedial services they receive. Collaborating with school personnel, such as school psychologists and speech-language pathologists, provides an opportunity both to give input into school programming and services and to plan direct services that seek to reinforce and generalize the school-based efforts. For students with more severe learning disabilities (i.e., ID), practitioners can also play a vital part in ensuring their clients receive the school-based services and supports they need to successfully transition into employment, supported or independent living, or further education after exiting the school system.

Assist Parents and Families to Support Clients With Learning Disorders

Psychologists can help their clients and their clients' families develop the skills and supports needed to successfully advocate in the school system. For example, they may work directly with clients on self-monitoring study strategies and on developing the social skills for asking for help when they need it. Psychologists can work with parents on skills and strategies to advocate for their children and communicate their needs and desires to school personnel successfully. Parents sometimes experience guilt or denial when their child is identified with one of the learning disorders described in this chapter. Helping parents understand the importance of consistency and routine in the home as well as following through with school recommendations for the home can help parents more effectively support their child who has a learning disorder.

Summary

This chapter has considered three specific types of learning disorders: specific learning disabilities, speech or language impairments, and intellectual disabilities. We described issues surrounding their definitions, history, identification, and intervention. Specific learning disabilities are the most prevalent of the learning disorders, occurring in 5.2% of the school-age population. Specific learning disability was first defined in 1968 and recognized in federal law in 1975. Inconsistencies in identification procedures for SLD since the disorder first appeared in federal education law have resulted in a lack of consensus about how to appropriately identify students with SLD for special education services in schools. The most promising model to date for identifying students with specific learning disabilities is Response to Intervention (RTI), which is rooted in the public health model of prevention and early intervention at the first sign of difficulty. Response to Intervention is permitted by federal law as a method for screening populations of students so that those who are not meeting important educational benchmarks can be provided intense educational interventions to remediate or reduce academic risk.

We also described SLIs, which are the second most prevalent learning disorders, occurring in 3% of all school-age children, which includes impairments in speech, language, and hearing, essential to learning in school. Finally, we described ID, the third most common learning disorder, characterized by significantly below average cognitive functioning, limited functioning in adaptive behavior, and onset before age 18.

This chapter concluded by providing the reader with specific strategies for helping clients with learning disorders and their families navigate schools generally and the special education system specifically. Specifically, we recommend strategies that psychologists in clinical practice can implement in their private practice to more effectively: (a) promote prevention of learning failure, (b) participate in school-wide efforts to support children and adolescents with learning disorders, and (c) partner effectively with parents and schools.

Appendix A: Description of School Psychologists and Speech Language Pathologists

School Psychologists

School psychologists are professionals with extensive training in both psychology and education (National Association of School Psychologists, n.d.). The main goal of the school psychologist is to help children and youth succeed academically, behaviorally, emotionally, and socially. To best achieve this goal, school psychologists collaborate with teachers, parents, administrators, and other professionals to develop healthy, safe, and supportive academic environments that emphasize and strengthen connections between school, home, and the community for all children (National Association of School Psychologists, n.d.). Some of the unique functions of the school psychologist in the schools include identifying and addressing behavior and learning problems that interfere with school success, working within a multidisciplinary team to determine student eligibility for special education services, helping teachers create positive classroom environments, and implementing school-wide prevention programs that help maintain positive school climates (National Association of School Psychologists, n.d.).

The implementation of the Response to Intervention (RTI) process creates new opportunities and a greater need for school psychologists. The training the school psychologist receives in consultation, behavior and academic interventions, research, counseling, and evaluation is called upon as districts implement new RTI procedures (National Association of School Psychologists, 2006). The roles of the school psychologist in an RTI model expand to include duties such as working with administration to obtain "buy-in" and facilitate system change, planning and conducting necessary staff training to implement RTI, developing local academic achievement norms, and consulting with both teachers and parents regarding early intervention tools for in the classroom and at home (National Association of School Psychologists, n.d.).

Speech-Language Pathologists

Speech-language pathologists (SLPs) are specialists who receive intensive training in both atypical and typical communication development and pathology (Sunderland, 2004). SLPs are often the lead service providers for individuals with speech and language disorders (Justice, 2006). An SLP has a degree or certification in speech and language pathology and is qualified to diagnose speech and language disorders and to prescribe and implement therapeutic measures for these disorders (Nicolosi, Harryman, & Kresheck, 2004). Under IDEA 2004, speech-language pathology services include the identification of children with speech or language impairments, the diagnosis and assessment of specific speech or language impairments, the referral of individuals for medical or other professional attention necessary for the treatment of speech or language impairments, the provision of speech and language services for the habilitation or prevention of communication impairments, and the counseling and guidance of children, parents, and teachers concerning speech or language impairments [§300.34(c)(15)]. The SLP plays a critical role in the identification and treatment of individuals with speech or language impairments.

SLPs working in districts where RTI procedures are being implemented are able to contribute to assessment and intervention through systemwide program design and collaboration, as well as individual work with students. SLPS are able to offer expertise in the language basis of learning and literacy, an understanding of the utilization of student outcome data in making instructional decisions, and experience with collaborative instruction and intervention approaches (Ehren, Montgomery, Rudebusch, & Whitmire, 2007). A few of the ways SLPs contribute in the RTI model include assisting in identifying systemic patterns of student need pertaining to language skills, explaining the interconnection between spoken and written language to other school professionals, and identifying, utilizing, and disseminating evidence-based practices for RTI interventions or speech and language services (Ehren et al., 2007).

Appendix B: Recommended Internet Resources

For Children

Professor Garfield: Comprehensive free website for children offering lively, interactive, and free "edutainment" games and activities that help to motivate and empower kids while addressing fundamental reading skill sets. http://www.professorgarfield.org/pgf_home.html

For Parents

Colorín Colorado: A bilingual site for families and educators. http://www.colorincolorado.org/

Star Fall: A free public service to motivate children to read with phonics. http://www.starfall.com/

Reading Rockets: Teaching kids to read and helping those who struggle. http://www.reading rockets.org/

For Professionals

Evidence Based Intervention Network. http://ebi.missouri.edu

Florida Center for Reading Research. http://fcrr.org/

Intervention Central. http://www.interventioncentral.org/

Vaughn-Gross Center for Reading and Language Arts. http://www.meadowscenter.org/vgc/

Advocacy Groups and Organizations

Centers for Disease Control and Prevention: Intellectual Disability. http://www.cdc.gov/ncbddd/dd/ddmr.htm

The International Dyslexia Association. http://www.interdys.org/

LD OnLine. http://www.ldonline.org/

National Center for Learning Disabilities. http://www.ncld.org/

National Dissemination Center for Children With Disabilities. http://www.nichcy.org

The National Research Center on Learning Disabilities (NRCLD). http://www.nrcld.org

Professional Associations

American Association on Intellectual and Developmental Disabilities. http://www.aaidd.org/

American Speech-Language-Hearing Association. http://www.asha.org/

National Association of School Psychologists. http://www.nasponline.org/

References

Adams, M. J. (1990). *Beginning to read: Thinking and learning about print*. Cambridge, MA: MIT Press.

American Association on Intellectual and Developmental Disabilities (2010). *Intellectual disability: Definition, classification, and systems of supports*. Washington, DC: Author.

American Psychiatric Association. (2000). *Diagnostic and statistical manual of mental disorders* (4th ed., text rev.). Washington, DC: Author.

American Psychiatric Association DSM-5 Development. (2011) Intellectual developmental disorder. Retrieved from http://www.dsm5.org/ProposedRevision/Pages/proposedrevision.aspx?rid=384

American Speech-Language-Hearing Association. (2006). *2006 schools survey report: Caseload characteristics*. Rockville, MD: Author.

Andrews, G. (1984). The epidemiology of stuttering. In R. F. Curlee & W. H. Perkins (Eds.), *Nature and treatment of stuttering: New directions*. San Diego, CA: College-Hill Press.

Arkkila, E., Rasanen, P., Roine, R. P., & Vilkman, E. (2008). Specific language impairment in childhood is associated with impaired mental and social well-being in adulthood. *Logopedics Phoniatrics Vocology, 33*(4), 179–189.

Bishop, D., & McDonald, D. (2009). Identifying language impairment in children: combining language test scores with parental report. *International Journal of Language and Communication Disorders, 44*(5), 600–615.

Bradley, R., Danielson, L., & Hallahan, D. P. (Eds.). (2002). *Identification of learning disabilities: Research to practice*. Mahwah, NJ: Erlbaum.

Brown-Chidsey, R., & Steege, S.M. (2005). *Response to intervention: Principles and strategies for effective practice*. New York: The Guilford Press.

Carnine, D., Silbert, J., & Kame'enui, E. (1997). *Direct instruction reading* (3rd ed.). New York: Merrill.

Clay, M. (1985). *The early detection of reading difficulties* (3rd ed.). Auckland, New Zealand: Heinemann.

Deshler, D. D. (2005). Adolescents with learning disabilities: Unique challenges and reasons for hope. *Learning Disability Quarterly, 28*, 122–124.

Ehren, B. J., Montgomery, J., Rudebusch, J., & Whitmire, K. (2007). *Responsiveness to intervention: New roles for speech-language pathologists*. Retrieved from http://www.asha.org/slp/schools/prof-consult/RtoI.htm

Fletcher, J. M., Lyon, G. R., Barnes, M., Stuebing, K., Francis, D., Olson, R., … Shaywitz, B. (2002). Classification of learning disabilities: An evidence-based evaluation. In R. Bradley, L. Danielson, & D. p. Hallahan (Eds.), *Identification of learning disabilities: Research to practice* (pp. 185–250). Mahwah, NJ: Erlbaum.

Fletcher, J. M., Lyon, R., Fuchs, L. S., & Barnes, M. A. (2007). *Learning disabilities: From identification to intervention*. New York: Guilford.

Fletcher, J. M., Morris, R. D., & Lyon, G. R. (2003). Classification and definition of learning disabilities: An integrative perspective. In H. L. Swanson, K. R. Harris, and S. Graham (Eds.), *Handbook of learning disabilities* (pp. 30–56). Guilford Publications: New York, NY.

Fuchs, D., & Fuchs, L. S. (2006). Introduction to Response to Intervention: What, why, and how valid is it? *Reading Research Quarterly, 41*(1), 93–99.

Gierut, J. (1998). Treatment efficacy: Functional phonological disorders in children. *Journal of Speech, Language and Hearing Research, 41*(1), 85–100.

Gresham, F. M. (2002). Response to treatment. In R. Bradley, L. Danielson, & D. P. Hallahan (Eds.), *Identification of learning disabilities: Research to practice* (pp. 467–519). Mahwah, NJ: Erlbaum.

Gresham, F., VanDerHeyden, A., & Witt, J. (2005). *Response to intervention in the identification of learning disabilities: Empirical support and future challenges.* Retrieved from http://www.joewitt.org/

Harrison, P., & Oakland, T. (2003). *Adaptive behavior assessment system* (2nd ed.). San Antonio, TX: Psychological Corporation.

Individuals With Disabilities Education Act. (2004). *Building the legacy: IDEA 2004.* Retrieved from http://idea.ed.gov/

Johnson, E. S., Humphrey, M., Mellard, D. F., Woods, K., & Swanson, H. L. (2010). Cognitive processing deficits and students with specific learning disabilities: A selective meta-analysis of the literature. *Learning Disability Quarterly, 33*(1), 3–18.

Justice, L. M. (2006). *Communication sciences and disorders: An introduction.* Upper Saddle River, NJ: Pearson/Merrill Prentice-Hall.

Kavale, K. A., & Forness, S. R. (1985). *The science of learning disabilities.* San Diego: College-Hill Press.

Kavale, K. A., & Forness, S. R. (2000). What definitions of learning disability say and don't say. *Journal of Learning Disabilities, 33*(3), 239–256.

Kavale, K. A., & Spaulding, L. S. (2008). Is Response to Intervention good policy for specific learning disability? *Learning Disabilities Research and Practice, 23*(4), 169–179.

Kirk, S. A. (1963). Behavioral diagnosis and remediation of learning disabilities. *Conference on Exploring Problems of the Perceptually Handicapped Child, 1,* 1–23.

Lyon, G. R. (2002, June). Testimony of Dr. G. Reid Lyon. *Learning disabilities and early intervention strategies: How to reform the special education referral and identification process. Hearing before the Subcommittee on Education Reform Committee and the Workforce United States House of Representatives.* Retrieved http://archives.republicans.edlabor.house.gov/archive/hearings/107th/edr/idea6602/lyon.htm

Lyon, G. R., Shaywitz, S. E., & Shaywitz B. A. (2003). A definition of dyslexia. *Annals of Dyslexia, 53,* 1–14.

Martínez, R. S., & Nellis, L. (2008). A school-wide approach for promoting academic wellness for all students. In B. Doll & J. Cummings (Eds.). *Transforming school mental health services* (pp. 143–164). Thousand Oaks, California: Corwin Press.

McKenzie, R. G. (2009). Obscuring vital distinctions: The oversimplification of learning disabilities within RTI. *Learning Disability Quarterly, 32*(4), 203–215.

National Association of School Psychologists. (2006). *The role of the school psychologist in the RTI process.* Retrieved from http://www.nasponline.org/advocacy/RTIrole_NASP.pdf

National Association of School Psychologists. (n.d.). *What is a school psychologist?* Retrieved from http://www.nasponline.org/about_sp/whatis.aspx

National Association of State Directors of Special Education (NASDSE) (2005). *Response to intervention: Policy considerations and implementation.* Alexandria, VA: Author.

Nicolosi, L., Harryman, E., & Kresheck, J. (2004). *Terminology of communication disorders: Speech-language-hearing.* Philadelphia: Lippincott Williams and WilkinsOrton, S. (1937). *Reading, writing, and speech problems in children: A presentation of certain types of disorders in the development of the language faculty.* New York: Norton.

Pennington, B. F. (2009). *Learning disorders: A neuropsychological framework* (2nd ed.) New York: Guilford.

Powell-Smith, K. A., Stoner, G., Bilter, K. J., & Sansosti, F. J. (2008). *Best practices in supporting the education of students with severe and low-incidence disabilities.* In A. Thomas & J. Grimes (Eds.), *Best practices in school psychology* (5th ed., pp. 1233–1248). Bethesda, MD: National Association of School Psychologists.

Public Law 94-142. *Education of All Handicapped Children Act.* Retrieved from http://www.scn.org/~bk269/94-142.html

Roid, G. H. (2003). *Stanford-Binet Intelligence Scales* (5th ed.): *Examiner's manual.* Itasca, IL: Riverside Publishing.

Reschly, D. J. (2003, December). *What if LD identification changed to reflect research findings?* Paper presented at the National Research Center on Learning Disabilities Responsiveness-to-Intervention Symposium. Kansas City, MO.

Schuele, M. (2004). The impact of developmental speech and language impairments on the acquisition of literacy skills. *Mental Retardation and Developmental Disabilities Research Reviews, 10*, 176–183.

Sparrow, S. S., Cicchetti, D. V., & Balla, D. A. (2005). *Vineland II—Vineland Adaptive Behavior Scales: Survey forms manual* (2nd ed.). Circle Pines, MN: AGS.

Sunderland, L. (2004). Speech, language, and audiology services in public schools. *Intervention in School and Clinic, 39*(4), 209–217.

Torgesen, J. K. (1991). Learning disabilities: Historical and conceptual issues. In B. Wong (Ed.), *Learning about learning disabilities* (pp. 3–39). San Diego: Academic Press.

Turnbull, H. R. (2009). Today's policy contexts for special education and students with specific learning disabilities. *Learning Disability Quarterly, 32*, 3–9.

U.S. Department of Education (USDOE), National Center for Education Statistics. (2010). *Digest of Education Statistics, 2009* (NCES 2010-013). Retrieved from http://nces.ed.gov/fastfacts/display.asp?id=64

U.S. Department of Education (USDOE), Office of Special Education and Rehabilitative Services. (2002). *A new era: Revitalizing special education for children and their families.* Washington, DC. Retrieved from http://www2.ed.gov/inits/commissionsboards/whspecialeducation/reports/index.html

U.S. Department of Education (USDOE), Office of Communications and Outreach. (2005). *Helping your child become a reader.* Retrieved from http://www2.ed.gov/parents/academic/help/reader/index.html

U.S. Department of Education, Office of Special Education Programs, Data Analysis System (DANS). (2004). *OMB #1820-0043: Children with disabilities receiving special education under Part B of the Individuals with Disabilities Education Act.* Data updated as of July 30, 2005. Retrieved from http://www2.ed.gov/about/reports/annual/osep/2006/parts-b-c/28th-vol-2.pdf

U.S. Office of Education. (1968). *First annual report of the National Advisory Committee on Handicapped Children.* Washington, DC: U.S. Department of Health, Education, and Welfare.

U.S. Preventive Services Task Force. (2006). Screening for speech and language delay in preschool children: Recommendation statement. *Pediatrics, 117*, 497–501.

Walker, H. M., & Shinn, M. R. (2002). Structuring school-based interventions to achieve integrated primary, secondary, and tertiary prevention goals for safe and effective schools. In M. R., Shinn, G. Stoner, & H. M. Walker (Eds.), *Interventions for academic and behavior problems: Preventive and remedial approaches.* Silver Spring, MD: National Association of School Psychologists.

Wechsler, D. (2003). *Wechsler Intelligence Scale for Children* (4th ed.): *Administration and scoring manual.* San Antonio: Psychological Corporation.

World Health Organization. (1992). *The ICD-10 classification of mental and behavioural disorders: Clinical description and diagnostic guidelines.* Geneva: Author.

Worster-Drought, C. (1968). Speech disorders in children. *Developmental Medicine and Child Neurology, 10*(4), 427–440.

Zebrowski, P. M. (2003, July). Developmental stuttering. *Pediatric Annals, 32*, 453–458.

Ziegler, J. C., Pech-Georgel, C., George, F., Alario, F. X., & Lorenzi, C. (2005, September 27). Deficits in speech perception predict language learning impairment. *Proceedings of the National Academy of Sciences of the United States of America, 102*, 14110–14115.

Zirkel, P. A., & Thomas, L. B. (2010). State laws and guidelines for implementing RTI. *Teaching Exceptional Children, 43*(1), 60–73.

Zirkel, P. A., & Thomas, L. B. (2010b). State laws for RTI: An updated snapshot. *Teaching Exceptional Children, 42*(3), 56–63.

20
Eating Disorders

TRACI MCFARLANE, KATHRYN TROTTIER, JANET POLIVY,
C. PETER HERMAN, and JESSICA ARSENAULT

Toronto General Hospital, University of Toronto
Toronto, Ontario, Canada

MICHELE BOIVIN

Royal Ottawa Mental Health Centre
Ottawa, Ontario, Canada

Until the 1960s and 1970s, few people had heard of anorexia nervosa (AN), but it soon started to be reported with increasing frequency in Western societies. Young females from middle- and upper-class families were voluntarily starving themselves and losing weight to the point of emaciation and sometimes death. A decade later, a new eating disorder was recognized; in bulimia nervosa (BN), young women alternate between starving and eating large amounts of food, often followed by purging. Although these eating disorders have flourished recently in Westernized societies during periods of relative affluence and enhanced social opportunities for women (Bemporad, 1996, 1997), voluntary self-starvation and periods of binge eating and purging have been reported throughout history. Eating disorders that would be recognizable today as AN and BN have existed since ancient times (Bemporad, 1997). Eating disorder not otherwise specified (EDNOS) and binge eating disorder (BED) were included in the fourth edition of the American Psychiatric Association's (APA) *Diagnostic and Statistical Manual of Mental Disorders* (*DSM–IV*; APA, 1994).

Whether the various eating disorders are fundamentally different is debatable (Fairburn, Cooper, & Shafran, 2003; Vohs & Heatherton, 2000). The transdiagnostic hypothesis cites compelling evidence of consistent core psychopathology, attitudes, and behaviors across disorders (e.g., dietary restraint, binge eating, compensation, overevaluation of eating, shape, weight, and their control) and frequent migration between diagnostic categories, considering all eating disorders different manifestations of a single disorder (Fairburn et al., 2003). Bulimic eating disorders appear to exist on a continuum of clinical severity, from BED (least severe), through nonpurging-type BN (intermediate severity), to purging-type BN (most severe; Hay & Fairburn, 1998). This chapter will discuss the major eating disorders, using the *DSM* criteria to describe the primary features of AN, BN, EDNOS, and BED, about which substantially less is known. We will review the prevalence of eating disorders and provide an overview of the main hypotheses concerning what causes them to occur in a given individual. Finally, we will discuss the principal treatment options and prognosis for eating disorders.

Diagnostic Criteria and Core Pathological Features of Eating Disorders

The *DSM–IV–TR* (APA, 2000) is the most widely accepted set of diagnostic criteria for psychological and psychiatric disorders in North America. The symptoms of eating disorders were compiled by a panel of experts who treat these problems, and the symptoms were then sent to others in the field for comments and corrections. In this edition of the *DSM*, all symptoms should be empirically supported to reflect a consensus among those who treat and study the disorders. For eating disorders, this is a difficult proposition. Not all criteria for the disorder are easy to define (for example, exactly what behaviors constitute binge eating?), and the criteria as they are listed have some ambiguities. Moreover, there are controversies concerning just how universal some symptoms are (e.g., amenorrhea). Finally, many psychologists object to the medicalization of abnormal behavior implied by a diagnosis. Despite these debates about the utility of the *DSM*, many researchers use the *DSM* criteria for eating disorders in order to facilitate communication across research settings by ensuring that all are studying the same phenomena. For clinicians treating the problems, diagnostic criteria can point to symptoms that need to be treated and methods of treating them and also can allow for assessment of successful change. We will discuss the criteria for eating disorders as set out in the *DSM* as well as point out some of the issues and concerns about the current criteria. The DSM–5 is expected in 2013 and is now considered a work in progress (APA, 2010). However, there are a number of proposed changes to the current criteria to address some of the current concerns.

The *DSM–IV* diagnostic criteria for AN are refusal to maintain body weight at or above a minimum of 85% of normal weight for age and height, accompanied by an intense fear of fatness or disturbed experience of one's body weight or shape, or self-esteem that is unduly influenced by weight and shape, and amenorrhea (for at least three consecutive menstrual cycles). In addition, AN can be subtyped into either binge-eating or purging-type anorexia, which involves regular episodes of binge eating or purging, whereas restricting-type anorexia does not involve these behaviors (both types may involve fasting and excessive exercising). Although amenorrhea has been a key diagnostic criterion for AN for some time, women with AN and women with all the features of AN except amenorrhea are otherwise indistinguishable, leading some to question the utility of amenorrhea as a diagnostic criterion (Cachelin & Maher, 1998; Garfinkel et al., 1996). In addition, this criterion cannot be applied to premenarchal females, to females taking oral contraceptives, to postmenopausal females, or to males. Therefore, deletion of this criterion has been recommended by the DSM–5 working group. Other changes proposed for the DSM–5 include removal of the example of 85% of normal weight, because it has been used as a cutoff instead of an example or guideline (to be replaced with significantly low weight), and determining the subtype based on behavior within the past 3 months, rather than the present criteria, which does not specify a timeframe.

The *DSM–IV* describes BN as recurrent episodes of binge eating (i.e., eating more food than most people would eat in a similar time period and situation and feeling out of control of one's eating during the episode) accompanied by compensatory behaviors (such as vomiting, exercising, or fasting) to prevent a corresponding weight gain. These behaviors must occur at least twice a week for at least 3 months. However, a recent literature review found that the clinical characteristics of individuals reporting bingeing and compensating once per week were similar to those meeting the current criterion of twice per week (Wilson & Sysko, 2009). Therefore, it is recommended for the DSM–5 to reduce the frequency criterion to once per week over the past 3 months. The core maladaptive cognition of BN (and AN) is reflected in the diagnostic criteria, specifically an individual's self-evaluation relies excessively on body weight and shape. If any of these symptoms occur in the context of an episode of AN, then AN becomes the diagnosis. The purging type of BN features self-induced vomiting or laxative, diuretic, or enema abuse; nonpurging BN involves fasting or excessive exercising as a means of compensating for binge eating (APA, 1994). Fasting and excessive exercise are difficult to measure and operationalize. A recent literature review indicated that those in the BN-nonpurging subtype more closely resemble individuals with BED than those with BN-purging subtype (van Hoeken, Veling, Sinke, Mitchell, & Hoek, 2009). It was proposed that the DSM–5 therefore delete subtyping of BN and categorize the current BN-nonpurging subtype as BED; however, this was met with significant criticism. As it stands now, subtyping will be removed but fasting and excessive exercising will be included as inappropriate compensatory behaviors of bulimia.

Impulsive behaviors such as sexual promiscuity, suicide attempts, drug abuse, and stealing or shoplifting are common among people with BN (Goldner, Geller, Birmingham, & Remick, 2000). Specifically, the impulsivity observed in BN patients has been associated with higher frequencies of purging behavior (Matsunaga, Kiriike, et al., 2000).

EDNOS is currently a residual category for syndromes that do not quite fit the diagnostic criteria for the other eating disorders. Interestingly EDNOS is the most common diagnostic category found in community, outpatient (Fairburn & Bohn, 2005), and tertiary care treatment settings (Rockert, Kaplan, & Olmsted, 2007). Clearly there is something amiss with the current classification system if the "residual" category captures the majority of individuals with eating disorders. One of the goals for the DSM–5 working group is to improve and expand the categories of AN, BN, and BED to reduce the number of people diagnosed with EDNOS. In the DSM–5 it is expected that EDNOS will capture a smaller number of individuals suffering from subthreshold AN, BN, and BED, purging disorder (Keel, Striegel-Moore, 2009), and night eating syndrome (Striegel-Moore, Franko & Garcia, 2009).

Binge eating disorder is described by *DSM–IV* (in the research appendix) as similar to BN in that it entails recurrent binge-eating episodes accompanied by subjective feelings of lack of control over one's eating. The difference between BN and BED is that the compensatory behaviors that occur regularly in BN are not present or are infrequent in BED (APA, 1994). The binge eating typically begins in late adolescence or the early 20s and frequently follows dieting and weight loss. Although not part of the diagnostic criteria, individuals with BED are typically overweight and do exhibit weight and shape overconcern that characterize people with AN and BN (Eldredge & Agras, 1996). Based on a comprehensive literature review, the DSM–5 plans to formally include BED as a disorder (Wonderlich, Gordon, Mitchell, Crosby, & Engel, 2009).

Despite the presence of binge eating as a diagnostic feature of BN, BED, and AN binge-eating or purging subtype, attempts to define binge eating have been unsatisfactory, and there is considerable variability in what types of eating episodes patients and professionals label as binges (Johnson, Carr-Nangle, Nangle, Antony, & Zayfert, 1997). What, for instance, is a larger than normal amount of food? Commonly noted triggers for binge eating include hunger, negative affect or stress, the presence of attractive "forbidden food," abstinence violation (i.e., having already eaten something fattening or diet-breaking), ingestion of alcohol, and being alone (Polivy & Herman, 1993). Examination of videotaped eating episodes indicates that feelings of loss of control and violation of dietary strictures are critical in leading participants to construe a particular episode as a binge (Johnson, Boutelle, Torgrud, Davig, & Turner, 2000). Laxative abuse among women with eating disorders is an indicator of greater psychopathology, irrespective of other features such as eating disorder diagnostic category, age, body weight, impulsive behaviors, or personality features (Pryor, Wiederman, & McGilley, 1996).

Course, Incidence, and Prevalence of Eating Disorders

Both AN and BN often emerge during late adolescence, with a female-to-male ratio between 10:1 and 15:1 (Bramon-Bosch, Troop, & Treasure, 2000; Braun, Sunday, Huang, & Halmi, 1999). Although these disorders are more prevalent in females, the nature of the disorders is the same in the two genders. For individuals with AN or BN, a negative body image and a variety of psychological problems appear to emerge during puberty (see Polivy & Herman, 2002, for a review). Even before the onset of their disorder, adolescents with BN report various problems such as weight-related concerns, attitudes of withdrawal and social isolation, and deterioration of body image, self-image, and relationships with siblings and peers. The prevalence of these problems among adolescents with BN suggests that early psychological distress may precede the onset of an eating disorder (Corcos et al., 2000). Binge eating disorder is radically different from AN and BN in gender distribution, with only a 3:2 ratio of women to men compared to 10:1 and 15:1 for AN and BN, suggesting possible etiological differences for this disorder (Grilo, 2006).

Hoek (2006) reviewed epidemiological studies in order to determine the incidence and prevalence of AN and BN. The incidence rates of AN and BN are 8 per 100,000 persons per year and 13 per 100,000 persons per year, respectively. The average prevalence rates for AN and BN among young females are 0.3 and 1%, respectively. As previously discussed, partial syndrome eating disorders (i.e., EDNOS) are even more common than either anorexia or bulimia, with prevalence rates of 2.37% detected in a large community sample of adolescents and young adults (Machado, Machado, Gonçalves, & Hoek, 2007). The lifetime prevalence estimates of BED are between 2 and 4% based on community samples, and 20 to 30% among individuals seeking weight-loss treatment (Hudson, Hiripi, Pope, & Kessler, 2007; Jager & Powers, 2007). With respect to ethnicity, Hoek (2006) found that AN is a common disorder among young White females, but is extremely rare among Black females. In contrast, BN and BED occur frequently among Black women, but might also be more common among White women.

There have been reports of an increase in the incidence of AN over the past century (Eagles, Johnston, Hunter, Lobban, & Millar, 1995; Moller-Madsen & Nystrup, 1992), as well as an increase in the incidence of BN since it was first described in the late 1970s (Turnbull, Ward, Treasure, Jick, & Derby, 1996). However, it is unclear to what extent these observed increases in the incidence of anorexia and bulimia are a result of increased awareness and recognition (Wakeling, 1996). Nevertheless, these incidence figures may well be significant underestimates; the disorders still often escape detection or diagnosis (Rooney, McClelland, Crisp, & Sedgwick, 1995) because dieting and the pursuit of thinness are so ubiquitous and socially acceptable in Western culture and because of the secretive nature of the disorder (Grilo, 2006). In his most recent review, Hoek (2006) concluded that even the studies with the most complete case-finding methods yield an underestimate of the true incidence of eating disorders. He found that the most substantial increase in incidence over the past century was among females aged 15–24 years, for whom a significant increase was observed from 1935 to 1999. General-practice studies show that the overall incidence rates of AN remained stable during the 1990s, compared with the 1980s. Some evidence suggests that the occurrence of bulimia nervosa is decreasing. Despite increased awareness, only about one third of those with anorexia nervosa and only 6% of those with bulimia nervosa receive mental health care. Hence, the majority of individuals with eating disorders do not receive appropriate treatment.

Concurrent Psychological Problems

As many as 80% of eating disorder patients who have been diagnosed in a clinical setting exhibit one or more other psychiatric disorders at some point, with major depression being the most common diagnosis (Grilo, 2006). People with eating disorders often engage in obsessive-compulsive behaviors such as calorie counting, body preoccupation, ruminations about food, ritualism, perfectionism, and meticulousness (Kaye, 1997). The lifetime prevalence of obsessive-compulsive disorder has been estimated to be 30% among people with eating disorders but only 2.5 to 3% among the general population. Obsessive-compulsive disorders are 3 times more common among people with AN than among people with BN (Hudson, Pope, & Jonas, 1983).

Several other disorders are frequently found in conjunction with eating disorders. Alcohol abuse is commonly found in BN, and anxiety disorders, depression, and posttraumatic stress disorder are prevalent in both AN and BN (Blinder, Cumella, & Sanathara, 2006; Dansky,

Brewerton, & Kilpatrick, 2000; Tagay, Schlegl, & Senf, 2010). A follow-up of a large sample of AN patients found that 10 years later, 51% still met the criteria for a *DSM* Axis I psychiatric disorder (especially anxiety disorder) and 23% met the criteria for a personality disorder (most often avoidant-dependent and obsessive-compulsive; Herpertz-Dahlmann et al., 2001).

Indeed, Axis II personality disorders are frequently observed among people with eating disorders (Wilfley et al., 2000; Wonderlich, 1995; Wonderlich & Mitchell, 2001). Obsessive-compulsive personality disorder, like obsessive-compulsive disorder, is especially common in AN, whereas disorders related to impulsive personality, as well as borderline personality disorders, are more often present in BN and BED (Wonderlich & Mitchell, 2001). Because malnutrition can exaggerate symptoms of personality disorders, Matsunaga, Kaye et al. (2000) studied individuals who had recovered from eating disorders for at least a year to be certain that the measurement of personality disorders was not distorted by malnutrition and eating disorder symptomatology. They found that 25% of their participants met the criteria for at least one personality disorder.

Causal Theories of Eating Disorders

Eating disorders are not uniform conditions; there is no single cause or even invariable symptoms. The etiology of eating disorders is not really understood as yet, but there seems to be multiple causes and pathways (Grilo, 2006).

Hilde Bruch, one of the first modern theorists to discuss eating disorders, described AN as "a complex condition determined by many simultaneously interacting factors" (1975, p. 159). She was the first to point out that these patients use eating or not eating to fulfill a variety of nonnutritional needs. Moreover, despite the characteristic preoccupation with food and eating accompanying eating disorders, patients are "unable to recognize hunger or distinguish it from other states of bodily tension or emotional arousal" (p. 160). Bruch posited that people with eating disorders interpret all tension states as a "need to eat" instead of identifying the correct source.

Fairburn, Welch, Doll, Davies, and O'Connor (1997) hypothesized that there are two broad classes of risk factors for eating disorders: those enhancing the general risk for psychiatric disorder and those that specifically increase the risk for dieting and eating problems. With respect to risk factors, BN patients resemble patients with other psychiatric disorders more than they resemble people without diagnosable psychological problems. Bulimia nervosa patients, however, show a distinctive pattern of exposure to factors likely to elevate the risk of dieting and negative self-evaluation, supporting the hypothesis that BN is the result of exposure to both general risk factors for psychiatric disorder and specific risk factors for dieting.

The addiction model (Davis & Claridge, 1998; Wilson, 1991) posits an addictive process operating in eating disorders. Conditioned physiological responses to food produce anticipatory secretion of insulin, which causes both craving and overeating, if only through increased tolerance to food (Booth, 1988; Wilson, 1991; Woods & Brief, 1988). Some argue that self-starvation accompanied by excessive exercising reflects an addiction to the body's endogenous opioids (Davis & Claridge, 1998). These authors cited high scores by AN and BN patients on the addiction scale of the Eysenck Personality Questionnaire as well as correlations between the addiction scale and both weight preoccupation and excessive exercising as evidence of this.

In contrast, Wilson (1991) dismissed the addiction model for three reasons. First, he claimed that compelling evidence for an addictive personality is lacking. Second, the model does not address the core clinical characteristics of eating disorders (e.g., the role of dietary restraint and abnormal attitudes about the importance of body shape) or the identified concomitant psychopathology (e.g., extremely low self-esteem, interpersonal distrust, and feelings of ineffectiveness). Third, it fails to account for psychobiological connections between dieting and eating disorders. Wilson noted that bulimic behavior does not meet the criteria for an addictive disorder (i.e., tolerance, physical dependence, or craving), and therefore he viewed the addiction model as a conceptual dead end.

Cognitive theories of eating disorders emphasize the biases in people's beliefs, expectancies, and information processing pertaining to body size and eating. Some research has supported predictions derived from these cognitive theories (Williamson, Muller, Reas, & Thaw, 1999). As discussed later in this chapter, these theories dominate current treatment strategies. Information-processing biases, such as a focus on food and weight to the exclusion of other information, may explain several psychopathological features of AN and BN, including denial, resistance to treatment, and misinterpretation of therapeutic interventions.

Personality factors are also thought to contribute to susceptibility to eating disorders. Some assessment instruments such as the eating disorders inventory (EDI; Garner, Olmsted, & Polivy, 1983) were specifically designed to measure underlying personality dispositions theoretically linked to eating disorders. Investigations using this scale found that personality factors such as perfectionism, feelings of ineffectiveness (or low self-esteem), reduced interoceptive awareness (or sensitivity to internal signals such as hunger and satiety), and interpersonal distrust are characteristic of those with eating disorders (Garner, Olmsted, Polivy, & Garfinkel, 1984; Leon, Fulkerson, Perry, & Early-Zald, 1995). Strober (1980) found evidence of obsessive personality traits, extroversion, and need for social approval before the development of the disorder in adolescents with AN who had returned to normal weight.

One investigation took the innovative step of simply asking the patients what caused the emergence of their eating disorder (Nevonen & Broberg, 2000). Interpersonal and weight-related problems were the most commonly reported causes, and dieting or dieting plus purging was the most commonly reported response to these stresses. Thus, interpersonal and weight-related distress, together with dieting behavior, are what people see as responsible for the emergence of their eating disorders. Self-report—in response to oral or written questions—is one of the main sources of data in research on eating disorders; unfortunately, self-report is notoriously unreliable (Nisbett & Wilson, 1977). Eating disorder researchers by and large are too eager to take patients' self-descriptions at face value, if only because such descriptions are easy to elicit. It is not likely that people with eating disorders would be able to identify the source of their disorder with such ease when the research of several decades has not been able to do so. A full understanding of the causes of eating disorders will require more work and more sophisticated research designs than are currently being used.

Sociocultural models suggest that the idealization of thinness and unremitting portrayals of slim role models in the media contribute to widespread body dissatisfaction, which in some susceptible individuals produces pathological dieting and ultimately eating disorders (Heatherton & Polivy, 1992; Stice, 2001; Striegel-Moore, 1993). Some research suggests that exposure to idealized models may promote dieting not by causing body dissatisfaction but rather by inspiring young women to work toward a fantasized, thinner future self (Mills, Polivy, Herman, & Tiggemann, 2002). The sociobiological position posits that eating disorders and the societal pursuit of thinness reflect sexual competition among women (Abed, 1998). Thinness may either enhance women's reproductive prospects by making them more attractive to males or, in a contrary version, delay reproduction (by impairing fertility through emaciation) until a more propitious time.

Speculation about the cause(s) of eating disorders has thus gone through many phases since the 1980s, variously favoring biological, familial, and psychosocial factors, which are hypothesized to interact in complex ways to produce the disorders (Ward, Tiller, Treasure, & Russell, 2000). Since 2000, the biopsychosocial model, positing an interplay between the organism, its past behavior, and its environment (biological, psychological, and environmental variables), has been the primary explanatory model of eating disorders (Schlundt & Johnson, 1990). For example, in binge eating, environmental (e.g., situational influences, sociorelationship systems), behavioral (e.g., previous eating or dieting, ongoing activity), cognitive (e.g., knowledge of dieting, expectations, body image), emotional (e.g., mood, psychopathology), and physiological (e.g., blood levels of nutrients, hormones, neurochemicals) antecedents affect behaviors such as binge eating, purging, and dieting, which then themselves have consequences for behavior, cognition, emotion, and physiology.

Risk Factors for Eating Disorders

Current theories of eating disorders—what causes them, why they mainly afflict women, and why there has been such an increase in recent times—range widely. The basic question of what goes wrong to produce eating disorders has been addressed at the broad level of sociocultural influences, at the narrow level of familial and environmental effects, and at the even narrower level of individual risk factors related to personality, cognition, or physiology (Leung, Geller, & Katzman, 1996; Polivy & Herman, 2002; Polivy, Herman, Mills, & Wheeler, 2003). One might expect that the research on specific risk factors would be derived from one or another of the causal theories, but this is not the case. The voluminous literature on risk factors is to a great extent independent of and uninformed by the causal theories outlined previously. Whereas some self-report questionnaires (such as the EDI) are based on theoretical models (e.g., Bruch, 1975), research on risk factors for eating disorders seems to be, for the most part, atheoretical. Many studies in this area merely report correlations among self-report inventories and make no attempt to tie the particular measures chosen to any particular theory of how eating disorders develop. In part, this situation no doubt reflects the difficulty of measuring preclinical pathological processes with paper-and-pencil self-report devices, as well as the problem of operationalizing theoretical constructs. Despite these drawbacks, literally thousands of studies have attempted to specify the risk factors for eating disorders, and numerous chapters and books have addressed these questions. It is crucial to remember, however, that the risk-factor approach is essentially correlational, and that risk factors are really just variables associated with eating disorders, usually in an unspecified fashion. Space limitations permit only a brief overview of prominent research trends examining risk factors associated with eating disorders.

Sociocultural Factors

For several decades, an unrealistically thin body shape has been the cultural ideal for women in Western society. To attain this physique, women have become increasingly likely to diet and exercise (Polivy & Herman, 1987; Stice, 2001), but are unlikely to succeed in this quest. This societal obsession with a slim female body has been blamed for women's widespread dissatisfaction with their bodies and a concomitant rise in the prevalence of eating disorders (Stice, 2001). These sociocultural pressures have long been targeted as causes of (or at least contributors to) eating disorders (Grilo, 2006; Striegel-Moore, 1993). Girls who participate in sports or professions that emphasize having a slim body such as gymnastics or ballet seem to be more at risk than usual, supporting the view that the sociocultural emphasis on slimness contributes to the disorder (Davison, Earnest, & Birch, 2002). The chief promoters of this sociocultural pressure to be thin are the media, gender-role expectations, and particular economic, racial, and ethnic contexts.

Peer and Media Influences To no one's surprise, it has been shown that adolescents watch more television, read more magazines, and in general appear to attend more to the media than any other age group and thus are bombarded with messages about thinness and dieting. These messages are directed primarily at girls, who are presented with thin, attractive models, an insistence that thinness will bring success and happiness in all spheres of life (no matter how unrelated to appearance), and a blatant derogation of fat or even normal-weight physiques (Polivy & Herman, 2002; Polivy et al., 2003). Many studies have demonstrated an increase in depression and negative self-image in young women following exposure to thin media images (Dittmar, 2005; Pinhas, Toner, Ali, Garfinkel, & Stuckless, 1999), and those with greater eating disorder symptomatology tend to expose themselves to larger doses of these media images than do most women their age (Stice & Shaw, 1994).

Some data, however, suggest that it would be premature to blame the media for the increase in eating disorder. Mills et al. (2002) found that looking at pictures of thin models actually made chronic dieters feel thinner and better about themselves, possibly by inspiring them to fantasize about emulating the models. This outcome should not be so surprising—after all, why would women voluntarily buy and read fashion magazines if looking at them induced depression and self-derogation? More important, eating disorders have been reliably documented for centuries, without the benefit of 20th-century media exposure. Media idealization of an unrealistically thin female shape may be a contributor to the increased prevalence of eating disorders, but it is clearly not the primary cause. After all, this "cause" is so prevalent in our culture that if it were as important as is sometimes claimed, we would be hard pressed to explain why fewer than 10% of young women have eating disorders.

Gender   "Why women?" and "Why now?" are the two most frequently asked questions about the recent increase in the prevalence of eating disorders (Polivy et al., 2003; Striegel-Moore, 1993). Around the time that eating disorders began to proliferate, the social role of women was undergoing drastic changes. Instead of enacting the role of homemaker and mother, women were expected to fulfill the "superwoman ideal," requiring them to be smart, beautiful, have a successful career, and still maintain a perfect house, perfect children, and a perfect relationship with the perfect man. The stress of trying to be all things to all people may drive some young women to focus on one thing that they think they can control, their weight. The societal preference for thin female shapes may provide a goal that seems more attainable than becoming a superwoman, or perhaps even a means of becoming a superwoman. This role change provides an explanation for these two questions.

In addition, the pressure to be thin makes women dissatisfied with their bodies. When dissatisfied with their bodies, men tend to turn to healthy eating (Nowak, 1998) and exercise, but women turn to dieting (Drewnowski, Kurth, & Krahn, 1995). Dieting, however, is more likely to produce eating disorder symptomatology than sustained weight loss (Polivy & Herman, 1993; Stice, 2001). The thin ideal thus produces body dissatisfaction in women, which elicits dieting, which encourages pathological eating. But if this were the whole story, all female adolescents who are unable to achieve thinness (or at least all who diet) would be eating disordered, which is clearly not the case. Therefore, we must look further for an explanation.

Race, Ethnicity, and Social Class   Until about 1990, eating disorders were restricted primarily to Western, middle- and upper-class, White adolescent females. Now, however, they have penetrated all social classes, races, and even some non-Western venues such as Japan. Although the prevalence is still lower in most non-White groups and nonindustrial countries (Polivy et al., 2003), Black women in the United States are as likely as are White women to display eating disorder symptoms (Mulholland & Mintz, 2001). In addition, they are quickly becoming comparable to their White counterparts with respect to body-image dissatisfaction (Grant et al., 1999), vomiting, and abuse of laxatives or diuretics, and they are more likely to report binge eating (Striegel-Moore et al., 2000). Among the several potential explanations for the globalization of eating disorders, the most obvious is the influence of the media (Nasser, 1997).

Young minority group females who are heavier, better educated, and who identify more closely with White, middle-class values have an increased risk of eating disorder. Assimilation into White culture thus carries with it an associated risk of developing eating disorders (Cachelin, Veisel, Barzegarnazari, & Striegel-Moore, 2000). After acculturation, non-White women appear to have eating attitudes similar to those of Western Whites, although some studies do not find this (Ogden & Elder, 1998). Black women in predominantly Black cultures, however, still seem much less likely to develop eating disorders, with a recent study in Curacao finding no cases at all in the majority Black population (Hoek et al., 2005).

The expression of eating disorders among non-White groups differs in some ways from that found with White women. Minority women with eating problems are usually truly overweight, whereas White women with disordered eating may only feel overweight, but actually tend to be normal weight (Striegel-Moore et al., 2000). Body dissatisfaction and fear of fatness occur less frequently, if at all, among non-White groups, but Black adolescents are more likely to binge and use laxatives than are Whites, who are more likely to restrict their eating (Striegel-Moore et al., 2000). Black adolescent girls may experience less pressure to conform to the thin ideal plaguing White girls and seem less inclined to derive their self-esteem, identity, and perception of self-control from their weight and appearance (Polivy et al., 2003). When eating disorder symptoms do occur among non-Whites, however, they seem to be related to the same risk factors and precipitants—including low family connectedness, perfectionism, emotional distress, body dissatisfaction, and sometimes serious depression and anxiety (e.g., Davis & Katzman, 1999)—as they are among Whites. Mixed race women (in Curacao) who experienced the identity challenge of being of mixed race and trying to fit into the wealthier White subculture and distance themselves from the Black majority were also particularly likely to develop eating disorders (Katzman, Hermans, Van Hoeken, & Hoek, 2004).

Familial and Environmental Influences

If societal values and pressures can have enough impact on an individual to constitute a risk factor for the development of an eating disorder, how much more influential are familial interactions? The family can be a source of cultural transmission of pathological values or a stressor on its own (through miscommunication, lack of emotional support, or internal conflict). It can also be a protective factor.

Family influences, such as how the family mediates cultural ideas about thinness and how family members convey these messages to one another, have been implicated as causes of eating disorders (Haworth-Hoeppner, 2000; Laliberte, Boland, & Leichner, 1999; Strober, Freeman, Lampert, Diamond, & Kaye, 2000). A critical family environment, coercive parental control, and a dominating discourse on weight in the household appear to increase the risk of eating disorders (Haworth-Hoeppner, 2000). Even during treatment, family influences are important. For example, it was found that mothers' expressed emotion (especially critical comments) predicted an adverse outcome for eating disorder patients (Vanfurth et al., 1996).

Both mothers and fathers can contribute to the development of eating disorders in their children. For example, mothers who themselves have an eating disorder transmit pathological behaviors to their daughters by the time the girls are 5 years old. Even when the mothers do not have eating disorders, one recent study identified mothers' abnormal eating attitudes as a potential risk factor for the development of an eating disorder among their adolescent daughters (Yanez, Peix, Atserias, Arnau, & Brug, 2007). Mothers of daughters with eating disorder symptoms tend to find their daughters less attractive and more in need of weight loss than do mothers whose daughters are asymptomatic. Mothers' comments about weight and shape convey their attitudes and behaviors to their daughters. Daughters of mothers who diet are more likely to do so themselves and to use more extreme weight-loss techniques if mothers encourage them to or are dissatisfied with their own bodies (Polivy & Herman, 2002; Polivy et al., 2003). Moreover, if either parent is inaccurate in estimating their daughter's body esteem, the daughter is more likely to have greater body dissatisfaction (Geller, Srikameswaran, Zaitsoff, Cockell, & Poole, 2003).

Critical comments and expression of negative emotions by either parent predict both the development of AN and worse outcome for AN patients. Parental comments that encourage weight or size control have been found to be stronger predictors of daughters' body dissatisfaction (which predicts disordered eating) than any other types of parental comments (Kluck, 2010). Mothers' complaints about a lack of family cohesion also foretell daughters' increased eating pathology 2 years later. High parental expectations for achievement that ignore the daughters' needs and goals have also been detected in girls with eating disorders; these extrinsic goals force these girls to struggle to please others at the expense of their own autonomy. Parents of both AN and BN patients appear to discourage autonomy, negating their daughters' needs and self-expression. The patients feel that their parents are overcontrolling in an affectionless manner. The fact that these types of parent–adolescent conflicts over autonomy and identity tend to be more intense among girls than among boys may help to explain why eating disorders are so much more common among females than among males (Polivy et al., 2003).

Like other psychopathologies, the environment can contribute to the etiology of eating disorders. For example, weight-related teasing has been associated with unhealthy weight control behaviors, weight-related attitudes, dietary restraint, bulimic behaviors, and clinical eating disorders (Eisenberg, 2008; Menzel et al., 2010). Also, early traumatic events are a common theme among this population, with studies reporting around 60% of individuals with eating disorders experiencing at least one trauma in their lives (Tagay et al., 2010). Examples of traumatic life events could include neglect, exposure to violence, or physical, emotional, and sexual abuse. Recent exploratory studies have found that elevated levels of perceived stress precede the onset of BED, and when compared to overweight or obese controls, more reports of neglect, emotional abuse, and higher depression levels have been observed (Allison, Grilo, Masheb, & Stunkard, 2007; Striegel-Moore & Bulik, 2007). Early experience can also have an impact on treatment outcomes in eating disorders. One South American study examined treatment response among 70 women who had unsatisfactory outcomes and 90 women with more favorable responses. They found that the poorest outcomes were observed among those who had been exposed to sexual abuse or violence. It was also noted that this group was 10 times more likely to drop out of treatment and 3 times more likely to relapse versus nonexposed patients (Rodríguez, Pérez, & García, 2005).

Again, it is important to remember that trauma is not the entire story. There is no evidence to indicate that early abuse or trauma necessarily causes eating psychopathology; not everyone who suffers a traumatic event will develop an eating disorder, and not everyone who suffers from an eating disorder has been exposed to traumatic events. In fact, once recent study showed that depression fully mediated the association between some forms of childhood trauma and disordered eating (Kong & Bernstein, 2009). This highlights the importance of not assuming causality in correlational studies, but also indicates that early intervention aimed at depression might help to create a buffer against the development of eating disorders among traumatized individuals.

Individual Factors

If sociocultural influences on pathogenesis were very powerful, AN and BN would presumably be more common than they are. In addition, the numerous clear descriptions of AN from at least the middle of the 19th century and possibly earlier suggest that factors other than our current culture cause the disorders. Moreover, although there is some evidence that the disorders may afflict more than one offspring in a family, if the family were responsible for the development of an eating disorder, we would expect to see greater concurrence among the female offspring in a family. Thus, whereas culture, family, and the environment contribute to the development of eating disorders, they are not sufficient to explain the appearance of a disorder in a given person. In light of the causal models discussed earlier, perhaps we may find the missing piece of the puzzle in factors specific to the individual, such as biological, identity, personality, or cognitive determinants.

Genetic and Physiological Factors   The reasonably stereotypic and reliable clinical presentation of AN and BN, with a consistent gender distribution and age of onset, suggests a biological substrate for the disorders. Twin studies, family studies, and recent molecular-genetic findings point to a potential genetic factor (Klump & Gobrogge, 2005), especially for AN. Females with a first-degree relative who has an eating disorder are 2 to 3 times more likely to develop one themselves (Polivy et al., 2003). Recent research has attempted to link specific genes to specific eating disorders, suggesting that AN may be linked to a different gene than BN (Grilo, 2006; Tozzi & Bulik, 2003). One interesting twin study also revealed that the role of genetics may be more important for females and the role of the environment may be of greater significance for males in the context of body satisfaction and drive for thinness (Baker et al., 2009).

A genetic predisposition to eating disorders may operate through faults in neurotransmitters, of which serotonin is the most frequently studied, possibly because it inhibits feeding, stimulus reactivity, and sexual activity. A disturbance of serotonergic activity is consistent with many accounts of patients with anorexia and is correlated with traits that are common among such populations, including higher drive for thinness and body dissatisfaction ratings (Frieling et al., 2006). Patients with BN show signs of serotonin dysregulation, which may contribute to their symptoms, including binge eating (Steiger et al., 2001, 2006). Serotonin may be associated with impulsivity, which may relate to the binge-eating behavior and other impulsive behaviors exhibited by BN patients (Steiger et al., 2001). Early research also indicates a genetic component to BED that cannot be substantially improved by including shared environment (Javaras et al., 2008). More research is needed to determine whether or not neurotransmitter abnormalities exist within BED patients as well. Because the evidence for the influence of serotonin dysregulation on eating disorders is strictly correlational, it is not possible to conclude that abnormal serotonergic activity causes eating disorders; indeed, it may instead be a consequence of the disorder.

A surge of intrauterine twin studies has recently shed light on the influence of hormones and susceptibility to eating disorders. Findings consistently demonstrate that same-sex female twins have the highest risk of developing eating disorders, followed by females of opposite-sex twins, males of opposite-sex twins, and finally same-sex male twins (Culbert, Breedlove, Burt, & Klump, 2008; Procopio & Marriott, 2007). What is particularly interesting is the fact that males of opposite-sex twins have a higher risk of developing an eating disorder than do other males, and this risk is not significantly different from that of female opposite-sex twins. These results support the notion that prenatal hormones can influence one's susceptibility for developing disordered eating in adulthood. Findings from studies by Klump et al. (2006) support this theory by showing that both lower levels of prenatal testosterone and elevated adult levels of estradiol are associated with increased eating disorder symptoms. They hypothesized that relatively low testosterone levels before birth in females predispose their brains to respond to estrogen at puberty, when the hormones activate the genes contributing to disordered eating in vulnerable individuals.

Puberty seems to be a critical period for the development of eating disorders due to genetic and hormonal influences. The tracking of changes in genetic and environmental factors has revealed that the influence of genetics seems to account for roughly half of the variance in disordered eating at ages 14 and 18 among same-sex female twins, compared to only 6% at age

11 years (Klump, Burt, McGue, & Iacono, 2007). Puberty in females is also accompanied by increased body fat and a drastically different body shape—the curves that develop in pubescent girls definitely subvert the thin ideal to which girls aspire. This new, curvy shape may give rise to the increased body dissatisfaction and accompanying dieting that become normative in adolescent females and that are themselves potential risk factors for eating disorders (Polivy et al., 2003; Striegel-Moore, 1993). At the same time, hormonal development pushes girls into heterosexual interactions, which girls appear to find more stressful than do boys (Striegel-Moore, 1993). Finally, developmental physical factors such as premature birth or birth trauma, being born between April and June, early childhood eating or digestive problems, early puberty, and having a high premorbid body mass index (BMI) all seem to increase the risk of developing an eating disorder (Touyz, Polivy, & Hay, 2008).

Self-Esteem and Identity   Among dieters who do not have eating disorders, depression scores are elevated and self-esteem scores are reduced; these scores are even more extreme among those with eating disorders (e.g., Polivy & Herman, 2002; Polivy et al., 2003) as they are in certain other psychological syndromes. Negative emotions and low self-esteem are linked to disruptive eating behaviors in a cyclic or spiral pattern (Polivy et al., 2003). Negative self-evaluation is possibly the most ubiquitous risk factor among eating disorder patients (Fairburn, Cooper, Doll, & Welch, 1999; Grilo, 2006); feelings of ineffectiveness and lack of a strong sense of self were recognized as hallmarks of eating disorders as early as the 1970s (Bruch, 1975).

The lower self-esteem among those with eating disorders also seems to be connected to a lack of a cohesive identity and distrust of one's body's ability to function on its own, both of which appear to be distinctively related to eating disorders. Self-esteem deficits may also reflect negative life experiences such as sexual or emotional abuse, which may also interfere with formation of a stable identity.

Due to already low self-esteem, individuals with eating disorders (and to a lesser extent chronic dieters) begin to connect their self-worth to their weight and shape. This connection continues to decrease overall self-esteem and can perpetuate eating disordered behaviors (McFarlane, McCabe, Jarry, Olmsted, & Polivy, 2001). For example, chronic dieters (restrained eaters), who resemble eating disorder patients in many ways, have been studied in the laboratory to learn about processes in eating disorders. Restrained eaters exposed to false feedback (from an inaccurate scale) indicating that they had gained weight reacted by overeating (McFarlane, Polivy, & Herman, 1998). Similarly, when allowed to eat after reporting about ways in which they had failed to meet their life goals, restrained eaters responded by overeating (Wheeler, Polivy, & Herman, 2002). Threats to one's identity also seem to elicit disordered eating behavior (Polivy & Herman, 2007).

Body Dissatisfaction and Dieting   The negative self-perception and low self-esteem characterizing eating disorders crystallize in negative feelings about one's body and an investment in improving it as a means of self-redemption (Polivy & Herman, 2002, 2007). The dual-pathway model posits that it is the thin ideal that produces body image dissatisfaction, which then produces dieting, and eventually eating disorder symptomatology (Stice, 2001). Adolescent girls do have greater body dissatisfaction than do boys or older women, and those who place more emphasis on their bodies and are more dissatisfied with them tend to exhibit greater eating pathology (Dittmar, 2005; Polivy et al., 2003). Moreover, dieting has been implicated as a cause of binge eating and is thought to be a primary contributor to the "dieting disorders," as eating disorders are often called (Polivy & Herman, 2002). But if all the girls who embraced the thin ideal dieted and were dissatisfied with their bodies became eating disordered, much of the adolescent female population would be incapacitated! Thus, although most models of eating disorders include a role for body dissatisfaction and dieting, it is clear that these risk factors must interact with other factors such as extremely low self-esteem and identity deficiencies, other personality factors, and the familial, environmental and cultural issues, as discussed earlier.

Personality Factors Those with eating disorders exhibit a consistent pattern of personality traits before, during, and after the disordered eating phase. Converging evidence from clinical reports, psychometric studies, and family or collateral sources presents the premorbid (i.e., before the onset of the disorder) personality of AN patients as perfectionistic, obsessive, socially inhibited, compliant, and emotionally restrained or fearful (Grilo, 2006; Wonderlich, 1995). Those with BN are not only compliant and perfectionistic, but also tend to be impulsive, emotional, lacking in interoceptive awareness, and extroverted (Lilenfeld et al., 2000; Steiger et al., 2001). Perfectionism and negative self-evaluation characterize AN and BN patients before, during, and after recovery from the disorder (Fairburn et al., 1999). Negative affect, behavioral inhibition, and obsessiveness also continue after recovery from AN (Kaye, Gendall, & Strober, 1998). Moreover, perfectionism, ineffectiveness, and interpersonal distrust are found in family members of eating disorder patients who do not themselves show symptoms of eating disorders (Lilenfeld et al., 2000). There are thus a number of personality traits linked to eating disorders. Although the evidence is correlational, the persistence of such traits before and after the disorder and their presence in nondisordered family members suggest that they could interact with adverse familial, environmental, and social experiences and render an individual more likely to develop an eating disorder (Lilenfeld et al., 2000; Strober & Humphrey, 1987).

Cognitive Factors People with eating disorders display several cognitive aberrations such as obsessive thoughts, distortions of attention and memory, and rigid, all-or-nothing thinking (Polivy & Herman, 2002). Obsessing about weight and shape and using these characteristics to determine one's self-worth are central and defining features of eating disorders. Biased attention and memory related to weight, shape, and food-related information reflect a preoccupation with these issues. Studies using the Stroop color-naming task have empirically demonstrated biased attention to weight, shape, and food-related words in patients with BN and a bias to weight and shape-related words in patients with AN (Dobson & Dozois, 2004). A memory bias for shape and weight-related words has recently been demonstrated in patients with BED, such that these patients recall less positive weight and shape-related words than an overweight control group (Svaldi, Bender, & Tuschen-Caffier, 2010).

All-or-nothing, black-and-white thinking can lead to a perception of the self as a failure if one bite of a "forbidden" food is ingested, which may promote binges (Polivy & Herman, 2002). The prominent role of cognitive features in eating disorders has encouraged the use of cognitive therapies to normalize the cognitions that are presumed to underlie the eating disorder.

Combining Risk Factors

Because risk factor research is of necessity correlational, it cannot determine cause and effect. Furthermore, no single risk factor alone is capable of producing an eating disorder, and it would be simplistic to suppose that a disorder as complex as eating disorders would have a single cause. In 1987, Johnson and Connors proposed a biopsychosocial model of eating disorder development. This model posits that biological predispositions (from genetic, hormonal, and pubertal influences), family factors, and cultural pressures to be thin and to fulfill a demanding social role interact to produce an identity-conflicted, vulnerable dieter. Those dieters with low self-esteem and affective instability are most susceptible to an eating disordered identity, particularly in response to stress or failure. Striegel-Moore (1993) suggested that the number of simultaneous life challenges faced by an individual is related to her susceptibility to eating disorders. Girls who mature early and begin dating at the same time report more disturbed attitudes about eating and shape. Striegel-Moore also suggested that early maturation is a source of adjustment difficulties, which, along with body dissatisfaction, dieting, and conflict with parents, is sufficiently stressful to increase risk for an eating disorder. A related theory proposes that the many transitions that occur in adolescence (e.g., moving to junior high or high school, puberty, dating, disruptions in friendships, increased academic and gender role demands) and the restructuring of personality and behavior demanded by these transitions may overwhelm an adolescent who is already vulnerable because of familial or personal problems (Smolak & Levine, 1996).

The combination of (a) the contextual background of sociocultural expectations to look and act a certain way, (b) familial interaction patterns that negate the individual's attempts to achieve autonomy, (c) individual vulnerabilities based on genetics and personality, self-esteem, and identity deficits, and (d) the stresses required by transitional adjustments or traumatic events offers a potential starting point for identifying individuals most likely to develop an eating disorder. Although these combinatory models attempt to incorporate the complexity of eating disorders and the many identified risk factors, they have not yet provided predictive power sufficient to identify individuals most likely to succumb to the pressures and develop eating disorders (see Jacobi, Haywood, de Zwaan, Kraemer, & Agras, 2004, for a review).

Treatment of Eating Disorders

This section reviews the basic rationale and techniques of the major therapies used in the treatment of eating disorders, as well as the effectiveness of each. We start with treatments targeting the most focal eating disorder symptoms and then discuss treatments that modify symptoms indirectly, by altering other internal or external processes. We then discuss factors that contribute to relapse.

For those with a serious eating disorder (i.e., individuals with very low body weight or intractable symptoms), intensive treatment is usually recommended. This can take the form of an inpatient or residential program (where patients are admitted for up to 5 or 6 months) or a day hospital, which is usually a shorter stay and allows patients to go home to practice their skills in the evenings and on the weekends. Ideally, intensive treatment programs utilize a step-down approach whereby patients graduate to less intense programming based on their success at interrupting their eating disorder symptoms. Intensive treatments usually involve a variety of therapeutic strategies, including cognitive-behavioral therapy (CBT) and containment for normalization of eating, symptom interruption, and weight restoration for AN, family therapy, pharmacotherapy, and group-based psychosocial programming. Although the dropout rates can be high (especially among those who are not motivated or ready to give up their eating disorder), most studies show that people who complete intensive treatment are able to experience a successful reduction of eating disorder symptoms (Olmsted et al., 2010). Unfortunately, the problem remains that 35 to 50% of people relapse within the first 2 years after intensive treatment. This speaks to the need for a long-term approach to treatment that focuses on maintenance of gains and relapse prevention.

Cognitive-Behavioral Therapy

The most widely used and presumably most effective treatment for treating eating disorders continues to be CBT. The basic ideas underlying CBT were initially described by Beck and his colleagues, who applied them to depression (see Beck, Rush, Shaw, & Emery, 1979, for a review). Soon thereafter, it was modified and extended to the treatment of the eating disorders. In 1981, Fairburn (1981) was the first to outline a cognitive-behavioral approach to the management of BN, and in 1982, Garner and Bemis applied cognitive behavior therapy to AN. This treatment has now been proposed for use with BED (Wilson & Fairburn, 2000). Although identifying, modifying, and replacing maladaptive behaviors and thoughts are central to therapy in all of these cases, the distinctive symptomatology of each disorder and individual means that treatment must be adapted accordingly. However, recently Fairburn (2008) published a CBT-enhanced (CBT-E) manual consistent with his transdiagnostic theory, aimed at treating eating disorders regardless of diagnosis, positing that eating disorders share more characteristics than they differ on. The manual recommends tailoring the treatment plan for each individual and includes optional modules on interpersonal problems, clinical perfectionism, and core low self-esteem. At 60-week follow-up of one study involving CBT-E, 61% of patients with BN and 46% of patients with EDNOS had a level of eating disorder that features less than one standard deviation above the community mean (Fairburn et al., 2009).

Cognitive-Behavior Therapy for Anorexia Nervosa   The rationale for the use of CBT for AN is that irrational and recalcitrant beliefs about the importance of body weight and shape support relentlessly pursued maladaptive behavior (especially weight loss). These patients also suffer from deficiencies of identity and self-worth, which makes treatment even more difficult. CBT for AN focuses both on specific symptoms and on underlying difficulties. According to Vitousek (1995), this therapy for AN targets four main areas. The first is the ego-syntonic nature of the disorder (i.e., seeing the disorder as positive or desirable); because individuals with AN prize slenderness, they must first acknowledge that the pursuit of slimness has a negative impact on their lives. Vitousek proposed asking the client to list both the positive and negative aspects of her anorexia; in turn, "each claimed advantage and disadvantage is cast as a hypothesis that can be examined for its validity and adaptiveness" (1995, p. 326), an exercise effectively constituting the first steps toward modifying cognitions. The second focus involves setting behavioral goals for normalized eating and weight gain and implementing cognitive coping strategies to deal with these changes. For instance, the belief that certain "forbidden" foods cause drastic weight gain may be tested by having patients eat these foods in controlled exposures. The third, related focus of treatment is modifying beliefs about weight and food. Clients are taught to challenge their self-defeating thoughts by learning to examine them rationally and replace them with more realistic possibilities (e.g., "There are no forbidden foods per se; it is excess caloric intake that leads to weight gain"). Once these most urgent aspects of the disorder have been addressed, treatment can then focus on the underlying self-concept issues that may be maintaining the disorder; ideally, other more attainable and adaptive goals may be identified to replace slenderness as the basis of identity and self-esteem.

Fairburn, Shafran, and Cooper (1998) proposed a more focused cognitive-behavioral program for AN, targeting the patient's need for control and the attempt to attain this control through dieting. Treatment involves helping the client to achieve success and fulfillment from pursuits unrelated to weight and shape. They suggested that this streamlined treatment should be used first and broadened only if other issues prove to be obstacles to change.

The data on CBT for AN are limited. There are five published randomized control studies, but none provided any evidence that CBT is more effective than the comparison treatments (i.e., treatment as usual, nutritional counseling, family therapy, and interpersonal therapy) utilized for acute AN. Unfortunately, these studies were limited by a variety of methodological issues (e.g., small sample sizes, high attrition), and future well-designed studies are needed before any conclusions can be drawn about the effectiveness of CBT for acute AN (Pike, Carter, & Olmsted, 2010). However, there are two published studies that do provide promising preliminary evidence for the effectiveness of CBT for preventing relapse and improving recovery rates in weight-restored patients (Carter et al., 2009; Pike, Walsh, Vitousek, Wilson, & Bauer, 2003).

Cognitive-Behavior Therapy for Bulimia Nervosa   Because BN is less ego-syntonic (i.e., less acceptable to one's self-image) than AN is—the binge–purge cycle is often extremely distressing to the individual—CBT for BN has a narrower focus, typically limited to eating behavior and thoughts about food, weight, and shape. Thus, as in AN, BN clients are taught to establish a normalized eating pattern consisting of regularly scheduled meals, including a variety of foods. Incorporating previous "forbidden foods" can help to prevent psychological or physiological deprivation that may foster a binge. In addition, clients work on the reduction or elimination of bingeing and associated compensatory behaviors through behavioral goal setting and the development of coping strategies. They are taught to identify the usual precipitants to eating disorder behaviors (often with the help of a daily food diary) and to use distraction techniques (alternatives to binges such as taking a walk or calling a friend) or other coping mechanisms (i.e., such as self-talk or stimulus control). Compensatory behaviors after binges—such as vomiting, laxative use, excessive exercise, or dietary restraint—are discouraged in an attempt to break the binge–purge cycle; this technique is akin to the behavioral technique of exposure with response prevention. Finally, as with AN, excessive concern with body weight and shape is challenged through cognitive restructuring (Wilson, 1996, 1999).

Cognitive-behavior therapy is considered the treatment of choice for BN (Wilson, Grilo, & Vitousek, 2007); it leads to reduction or remission of bingeing and purging in 50% of patients and improvements in dietary restraint, attitudes toward shape and weight, and associated psychopathology (Wilson, 1996). It is important to be aware of viable alternatives, however, as about half of BN patients do not see an improvement in bingeing and purging behaviors as a result of CBT.

Cognitive-Behavior Therapy for Binge Eating Disorder   Because BED involves bingeing without purging or any other form of compensatory behavior, individuals with BED are more often overweight than are those with BN. Thus, behavioral weight-loss strategies (e.g., an exercise plan) may be included, and the individual experience with weight prejudices and stigma must be addressed. Cognitive-behavior therapy seems to be effective in reducing the behavioral and psychological features of BED (i.e., binge-eating episodes and psychological distress) but not in reducing obesity (Grilo, Masheb, & Wilson, 2005; Loeb, Wilson, Gilbert, & Labouvie, 2000; Wilson & Fairburn, 2000). It has been suggested that "the treatment of choice [for BED] would appear to be cognitive behavioral self-help" (Wilson & Fairburn, 2000, p. 352). Indeed, no difference in outcome between therapist-led versus self-help format CBT has been found, and there were significant improvements over wait-list controls in the latter, suggesting that it may be a cost-effective, accessible alternative for patients with BED (Loeb et al., 2000).

These descriptions of CBT for eating disorders reflect either how it is carried out in experimental tests or in the ideal clinical setting, neither of which necessarily corresponds to clinical reality. Individual clinicians often tailor the technique as they see fit for individual clients, or they may combine CBT with other treatment strategies in an eclectic treatment plan.

Nutritional Counseling and Psychoeducation

As its name implies, nutritional or dietary counseling involves educating the patient about normal caloric needs and physiological processes. Kahm (1994) explained that while people with eating disorders may have a wealth of knowledge regarding the calorie content of most foods, this knowledge is usually used to achieve drastic weight loss rather than to maintain a healthy body. In fact, Beumont and Touyz (1995) suggested that failing to address nutritional issues in eating disorders "is as ridiculous as prohibiting the discussion of drinking behavior with patients with alcohol related disease" (p. 306). They also stated that this therapy is intended to change attitudes about food and eating, and then eating behavior, by arming people with accurate knowledge.

Psychoeducation provides accurate nutritional information but also educates patients about the nature of their disorders. Olmsted and Kaplan (1995) advocated addressing four main topics beyond dietary information: the complex etiology of eating disorders, the often serious medical consequences of severe food restriction or continual bingeing and vomiting, the sociocultural idealization of the thin female body, and cognitive and behavioral strategies that one may use to modify eating problems. Nutritional counseling and psychoeducation are rarely used as standalone therapies; it has been estimated that educational information is incorporated in 75% of treatments for BN (Olmsted & Kaplan, 1995).

Motivational Interviewing

Because CBT involves modifying problematic thoughts and behaviors related to eating disorder pathology, it is often considered an "action-oriented" approach; that is, individuals who participate in CBT are asked to take action, often within the first several days of initiating treatment, to challenge their beliefs and change their eating-disordered behavior. However, individuals with eating disorders often harbor a great deal of ambivalence about overcoming their symptoms and, as a result, may be reluctant to engage in action-oriented treatment. Motivational interviewing (MI; Miller & Rollnick, 2002) acknowledges fluctuations in motivation and readiness for change. The therapist's task is to highlight problematic aspects of symptoms and collaboratively explore and resolve ambivalence. MI is based on the transtheoretical model of change (Prochaska & DiClemente, 1992), which describes the process of behavioral change with reference to five stages: precontemplation (denial of problem existence), contemplation (acknowledgment of problem and plan to change in next 6 months), preparation (intending to change within the next month and preparing to take action), action (initiating behavioral change), and maintenance (sustaining change). The transtheoretical model posits that these stages are universal, nonlinear, and cyclical; that is, individuals are presumed to possess fluctuating insight into and motivation to change problem behaviors and may relapse often before achieving sustained behavioral modification. Research has now begun on the use of MI with individuals who have eating disorders (see Wilson & Schlam, 2004, for a review; see Treasure & Ward, 1997, for AN; see Killick & Allen, 1997, for BN). A handful of small studies suggest its potential utility with this population. Feld, Woodside, Kaplan, Olmsted, and Carter (2001) described the use of a four-session, group-based MI program conducted prior to the initiation of CBT, during which individuals were encouraged to examine the costs and benefits of their eating disorder and its consistency with their values, among other topics. Results showed that compared with patients' own baseline levels, group participation resulted in increased motivation, confidence, and readiness to change (but did not affect eating disorder symptoms). Similarly, individuals with refractory anorexia who participated in a MI program for 5 hours twice a week over 6 months displayed increased motivation for change, representing a shift from "early" to "late" contemplation (George, Thornton, Touyz, Waller, & Beumont, 2004). Studies using treatment-as-usual control groups indicate that motivational programs fostered longer engagement, increased motivation to change, and encouraged participants to continue with treatment (Dean, Touyz, Rieger, & Thornton, 2008; Wade, Frayne, Edwards, Robertson, & Gilchrist, 2009). Although MI has not been shown to reflect a change in treatment outcome, it may lead to treatment participation for many individuals who would not have otherwise been open to treatment.

It is important to note that MI is not intended as a stand-alone treatment approach, but rather as a potentially useful precursor, or adjunct to, other more action-oriented approaches. Because MI maintains a focus on an individual's readiness for change, actual symptom change is not an intended outcome of this intervention. Therefore, successful outcomes following MI presume that the individual will move on to implement the changes he or she has decided are appropriate. Further, although MI finds a natural niche among individuals whose symptoms are recalcitrant, its applicability does have limits. For instance, if an individual is medically compromised due to severe or very rapid weight loss (Killick & Allen, 1997), respect for the patient's ambivalence will necessarily be weighed against the potential consequences of inaction.

Interpersonal Therapy

In contrast to psychoeducation and CBT, which are focused on improving eating and symptom interruption, interpersonal therapy (IPT) does not touch on these issues in the treatment of eating disorders. Instead, it targets maladaptive personal relationships and relational styles because difficulties in these areas are seen as contributing to the development and maintenance of eating disorders (Birchall, 1999). Thus, the fundamental task of the interpersonal therapist is to identify one of Birchall's "problem areas—Grief, Role Transitions, Interpersonal Role Disputes (or) Interpersonal Deficits" (1999, p. 315), and to work to improve the client's functioning in that area. Improved interpersonal relationships might reduce eating disorder symptoms in a number of ways. Enhanced control in relationships may generalize to enhanced control of eating in BN or BED. Furthermore, IPT may reduce or eliminate common interpersonal triggers to bingeing. For example, depressed mood and interpersonal stress may be alleviated, and more frequent, positive social interactions may reduce boredom. Decreasing interpersonal stress may also improve anorectic behavior by providing a greater sense of control in areas of one's life other than eating. Despite the fact that CBT is considered the gold standard treatment for eating disorders, some authors view IPT as a viable alternative first-line treatment due to its conceptual similarities with etiological theories of the development of these disorders (Tantleff-Dunn, Gokee-LaRose, & Peterson, 2004).

Although CBT produces more rapid positive outcomes in BN (Birchall, 1999; Fairburn et al., 1995), IPT seems to be equally effective by the end of treatment and at follow-up (Wilson & Shafran, 2005). There has been some research to show that African American participants showed greater reductions in binge eating when treated with IPT compared to CBT, suggesting that IPT may be particularly appropriate for African American women with BN (Chui, Safer, Bryson, Agras, & Wilson, 2007). Further research on IPT for eating disorders with different racial and ethnic groups is needed.

With regard to BED, interpersonal therapy has been shown to be as effective as CBT in reducing binges (and as ineffective at producing weight loss), and the rate of improvement for BED is equal in both therapies (Tasca et al., 2006; Wilfley et al., 2002; Wilson & Fairburn, 2000). It has also been shown that those who received IPT for BED maintained their reductions in binge eating and disordered cognitions for at least 5 years (Bishop, Stein, Hilbert, Swenson, & Wilfley, 2007).

Dialectical Behavior Therapy

Dialectical behavior therapy (DBT; Linehan, 1993) was developed to treat borderline personality disorder and is now being considered in the treatment of eating disorder symptoms that have been refractory to first-line treatments (such as CBT). DBT encourages commitment to and enactment of behavioral change while validating individuals' emotions and treatment ambivalence, with a specific focus on building skills in emotional recognition and regulation. McCabe and Marcus (2002) suggested that DBT has the potential to be effective in the treatment of AN through its conceptualization of eating disorder symptoms as maladaptive emotional avoidance or regulation strategies that can be improved by increasing commitment to change and building the requisite skills to do so; although clinical experience suggests this may be the case, further empirical evidence is required to support this conclusion. Safer, Telch, and Agras (2001) found that patients with BN showed significantly fewer binge or purge episodes following 20 weeks of DBT as compared to those in the wait-list condition, though no other significant improvements were noted. Similarly, DBT appears to be effective in reducing binge eating among individuals with BED (Safer, Robinson, & Jo, 2010; Telch, Agras, & Linehan, 2000, 2001) but ineffective in producing similar gains on other indices of recovery (such as weight, mood, and affect regulation). Importantly DBT also has been shown to be superior to supportive psychotherapy in maintaining engagement in treatment (Safer et al., 2010). Given these preliminary findings, it appears that DBT may be a useful option for those with BN or BED, in particular among individuals for whom affect dysregulation is prominent (i.e., those with comorbid borderline personality disorder; Palmer et al., 2003).

Family Therapy

Family therapy focuses on interpersonal relationships, emphasizing the importance of stresses within the family as a whole rather than on individuals. It postulates that change by one member affects every other member in turn (Minuchin, Rosman, & Baker, 1978; Thode, 1990). The eating disorder patient is seen in conjunction with her parents and siblings (or with her spouse and children, as the case may be), and the goal becomes reducing family stressors and miscommunications to bring about a reduction in eating disorder symptoms. Thus, family therapy places responsibility for recovery on both the patient and her relatives. Geist, Heinmaa, Stephens, Davis, and Katzman's (2000) description of treatment provides a good example of the specific content of family therapy: (a) recruiting parents to actively engage in managing the patient's weight gain and eating, (b) ameliorating maladaptive communication within the family and particularly between the parents, and (c) elucidating the difference between normal methods of coping with family conflict and the symptoms the patient is currently exhibiting.

Because of its low prevalence and its additional medical complications, there are significantly fewer controlled treatment trials for AN than there are for BN and BED. Furthermore, very few studies directly compare various forms of treatment for AN, making differences in efficacy somewhat difficult to gauge. Despite these limitations, there is a tenuous consensus that family therapy is the first-line treatment for most cases of AN (e.g., Wilson, 1999). On the basis of five randomized controlled trials of family therapy with AN, Eisler, Lock, and le Grange (2010) concluded that family therapy is effective for AN with short duration. It may be particularly effective for adolescents because they tend to express greater denial and less desire for help (Fisher, Schneider, Burns, Symons, & Mandel, 2001), making family involvement potentially more important. Family therapy for BN has not been well studied, though Dare and Eisler (2000) reported encouraging preliminary findings for their multifamily treatment program for adolescents with BN. More recently two randomized controlled trials showed additional support for family therapy in adolescents with BN. Family therapy was shown to be superior to individual supportive psychotherapy on both behavioral and attitudinal aspects of BN (le Grange, Crosby, Rathouz, & Leventhal, 2007).

Psychoanalytic Therapy

Psychoanalytic or psychodynamic therapy may encompass a wide variety of specific techniques or foci. Herzog (1995) defined it broadly as "all long-term therapies that explicitly use the relationship between the patient and therapist as the primary treatment tool and that attend to transference and countertransference reactions" (p. 330). This therapy assumes that eating disorder symptoms are merely the overt pathological manifestations of underlying conflicts that the client has been unable to resolve adaptively. The psychoanalyst's task is to determine the unique meanings of these symptoms for each client. Many theorists suggest that establishing a strong therapeutic alliance is the first (and perhaps most crucial) step (Dare & Crowther, 1995; Gonzalez, 1988; Herzog, 1995). Establishing such an alliance may be particularly difficult and take longer in AN because the patient will perceive the therapist as someone who wants her to give up her ego-syntonic dietary restriction. Once trust has been developed, the psychoanalyst establishes a neutral stance toward the patient, who then free associates: "the hope is that the patients will project upon this 'blank screen' their characteristic thoughts and behaviors (transference)" (Johnson, 1995, p. 351). Much of therapy is then devoted to analyzing these transference reactions in the context of a thorough developmental history.

Another strategy used in identifying the roots of the eating disorder is the analysis of dreams to determine their symbolic meaning. The countertransference relationship also constitutes an important source of information about the client; therapists interpret their own reactions to the client to further elucidate the quality of the client's interpersonal relationships. A nonjudgmental relationship between the therapist and client is said to serve a further purpose, providing the patient with an opportunity to relate appropriately on an interpersonal level and allowing the patient to resolve dependent or otherwise pathological relations with others (Herzog, 1995).

Contemporary psychoanalytic writers acknowledge that psychoanalysis may not be appropriate for all eating disorder patients. Herzog (1995) maintained that the treatment is appropriate for those patients presenting with character pathology; both Herzog (1995) and Johnson (1995) recommended psychoanalysis for prior-treatment nonresponders (i.e., for those patients whose symptoms linger after a course of cognitive or interpersonal therapy). Finally, Gonzalez (1988) cautioned against using psychoanalysis for suicidal patients or for those whose extremely low weight makes hospitalization necessary; in these cases, the long-term focus of psychoanalysis would leave the patient at immediate risk of harm. Indeed, although psychoanalysis for AN has not been well studied, Herzog (1995) stated that patients often require a minimum of 1 to 2 years of psychoanalysis, and maybe as much as 8 to 10 years, for improvement to take place. One long-term outcome study (Steinhausen, Seidel, & Metzke, 2000) found that 80% of surviving AN patients recovered at 11-year follow-up, regardless of the type of therapy received. In light of this finding, it is difficult to make a case for the use of long-term psychoanalysis in the treatment of AN. Similarly, outcome data for psychodynamic treatment of BN are scarce, leading Johnson (1995) to recommend this approach only for those patients who do not respond to briefer forms of therapy. A study by Murphy, Russell, and Waller (2005) suggested that integrative and time-limited forms of psychodynamic therapy may be useful in reducing bulimic symptoms, but more research is needed.

Pharmacotherapy

Pharmacotherapy departs significantly from other treatments by postulating some sort of organic cause for the disorder—or at least that the symptoms can be controlled pharmacologically—and attempting to treat symptoms accordingly, with medications. By far the most common drugs used are antidepressants, both tricyclic and mainly selective serotonin reuptake inhibitors (SSRIs). Their use is based on the fact that depressive and anxiety symptoms are prominent in eating disorders, and that these symptoms resemble the clinical features of other disorders (i.e., major depressive disorder, anxiety disorders) that respond favorably to these medications (Kruger & Kennedy, 2000; Mayer & Walsh, 1998).

Attempts to treat AN with pharmacologic agents have not been successful. Neither antidepressants, antipsychotics, nor any other class of drugs has been found to lead to significant weight gain and improve distorted attitudes or beliefs or to enhance the effects of inpatient programs (Bulik, Berkman, Brownley, Sedway, & Lohr, 2007). In fact, most researchers recommend against the use of drugs in the acute treatment of AN (Kruger & Kennedy, 2000; Mayer & Walsh, 1998). In addition, the evidence is equivocal regarding the use of SSRIs (i.e., fluoxetine) with weight-restored AN patients and the maintenance of treatment gains. One study demonstrated better outcome related to fluoxetine versus placebo (Kaye et al., 2001); however, another larger study failed to observe any benefit of adding fluoxetine versus placebo to CBT in terms of reducing relapse and in maintaining weight (Walsh et al., 2006).

In terms of BN, the SSRI fluoxetine is the most widely studied agent with six double-blind, placebo-controlled trials (Broft, Berner, & Walsh, 2010). The results of these studies indicated that fluoxetine was superior to placebo in reducing bingeing and purging and was associated with significant improvement in other psychological symptoms (Fluoxetine BN Collaborative Study Group, 1992; Goldstein, Wilson, Thompson, Potvin, & Rampey, 1995). However, only a small minority of patients become free of eating disorder symptoms on this drug and most continue to meet diagnostic criteria (Narash-Eisikovits, Dierberger, & Westen, 2002).

Overall, treatment with antidepressants appears to be inferior to CBT at reducing frequency of bingeing and purging, depression, and distorted eating-related attitudes (Whittal, Agras, & Gould, 1999). When CBT is added to antidepressant treatment, it is better than antidepressant treatment alone (Narash-Eisikovits et al., 2002), but not better than CBT alone. Therefore, it is recommended to use pharmacotherapy (i.e., fluoxetine) only if CBT is not available or if this is the intervention the patient prefers (Broft et al., 2010). Alternatively, fluoxetine may be a viable option if psychotherapy fails, although these results are mixed (Mitchell et al., 2002; Walsh et al., 2000).

In BED, many drugs including antidepressants (McElroy, Hudson et al., 2003; McElroy et al., 2000), antiobesity medications (Wilfley et al., 2008), and anticonvulsants (McElroy et al., 2004) have demonstrated efficacy in reducing binge eating and weight. There have been three randomized controlled trials of sibutramine (antiobesity medication) and all three showed this drug to be superior to placebo in reducing the frequency of binge-eating episodes and facilitating weight loss for up to 3 months of treatment (Appolinario et al., 2003; Milano et al., 2005; Wilfley et al., 2008). An important caveat is that this weight loss is modest at best (e.g., 5% weight loss) and often does not seem to be maintained (Devlin, Goldfein, Carino, & Wolk, 2000).

There is also evidence supporting the use of anticonvulsants in the treatment of BED. Initial trials of the anticonvulsants topiramate (McElroy, Arnold et al., 2003; McElroy et al., 2007) and zonisamide (McElroy et al., 2006) resulted in significant decreases in binge-eating episodes and body weight; however, these medications also appear to be associated with a high discontinuation rate as a result of adverse events and nonadherence (McElroy et al., 2004). Also there is little evidence that any of these medications improve psychological symptoms in patients with BED (Bodell & Devlin, 2010).

Reas and Grilo (2008) conducted a review of pharmacotherapy studies for BED and concluded that pharmacologic treatments are superior to placebo in the short term for reducing binge eating and weight. There is no evidence to suggest that medication is superior to CBT or that medication enhances the effects of psychotherapy on primary outcome measures of binge eating and weight (Grilo et al., 2005). Therefore, CBT should be considered the treatment of choice for BED, whereas pharmacotherapy could be chosen for reasons of availability, cost, or preference (Bodell & Devlin, 2010).

Recent Treatment Developments

There have been a few new and exciting recent developments in treatment for eating disorders (Grilo & Mitchell, 2010). One development is cognitive remediation therapy for AN

(Tchanturia & Hambrook, 2010). This therapy draws on neuropsychology and targets the maladaptive thinking processes (not content) in AN. Patients practice cognitive flexibility, holistic processing, and metacognition in session and are then encouraged to apply these new skills into their lives. Another development is called integrative cognitive-affective therapy for BN (Wonderlich et al., 2010). This treatment retains some elements of CBT but includes an emphasis on emotional responding and exposure to emotions (i.e., emotional regulation) and strategies to identify patterns of interpersonal and self-directed behavior, which may promote the avoidance of negative affect. Given the newness of these treatments, outcome research is in its early stages.

Treatment Research Issues

Despite our poor understanding of the development of eating disorders, research into their treatment has made some progress. However, controlled trials comparing treatments may not reflect clinical reality, where therapists may sample from the available therapies and tailor treatments to specific clients. For instance, individual CBT might be paired with administration of drugs to help patients with BN, or interpersonal and family therapy might be bolstered with psychoeducation in the treatment of AN. These so-called multifaceted treatments (see Lansky & Levitt, 1992, for a review) may provide the best form of care, because the components of one therapy may enhance the effects of another or provide additional benefits beyond those available in the empirically established first-line treatment. Still, individually tailored treatments are difficult to evaluate systematically; although such tailoring makes some sense, it also makes it difficult for researchers to evaluate treatment efficacy.

Adding more complications to the study of treatment options for eating disorders is the high comorbidity rate mentioned earlier. As expressed by Harrop and Marlatt (2010), "though comorbidity rates are high, little research has been done concerning treatment" (p. 392). Substance abuse, personality disorders, and mood disorders are often severe enough to warrant treatment even when no eating disorder is present; the fact that these and many other conditions occur at elevated levels among the eating disordered population only confounds the issue of treatment. In many cases, treating an underlying condition seemingly unrelated to the eating disorder (e.g., obsessive-compulsive disorder, depression) may be enough to help alleviate symptoms or at least prepare the individual to seek and attend eating disorder treatment.

Prevention

Even if treatment is not dependent on understanding causes, the question of what causes eating disorders remains important. Most of the interventions for eating disorders are therapeutic rather than preventative; that is, we tend to focus our efforts on treating eating disorders rather than preventing them from arising in the first place. An effective public health effort—stopping eating disorders before they get started—probably would be more valuable than effective therapy; but preventative interventions require a better understanding of what causes the disorder.

Early research in prevention showed mixed results, often producing positive effects (i.e., improved attitudes and behaviors) immediately following prevention programs only to find a complete reversal of these results after 6 months and sometimes even worse effects than before participants started (Carter, Stewart, Dunn, & Fairburn, 1997). This led some to posit that prevention programs might do more harm than good; fortunately, subsequent research has helped to clarify the situation. In a 2003 review of 29 programs, Dalle Grave concluded that "school-based eating disorder prevention programs do not have harmful effects on student attitudes and behaviors" (p. 579). Negative effects were typically limited to uncontrolled programs that were run by poorly trained educators (O'Dea, 2005; O'Dea & Abraham, 2001). Recent research is much more promising, including programs such as Healthy Schools-Healthy Kids (McVey, Tweed, & Blackmore, 2007), which was successful in reducing weight-loss behaviors and the internalization of media ideals among male and female students and in reducing disordered eating among females, especially with high-risk participants. Many of these results, however, also disappeared by the 6-month follow-up. More research is needed in order to determine how to produce longer-lasting and larger-scale positive results. Early meta-analyses and review papers can offer some insight into how to effectively tailor such programs. Stice and Shaw (2004) found larger effects for programs targeting high-risk individuals, such as interactive and multisession programs, programs offered solely to females and to participants over age 15, programs without psychoeducational content, and for trials that used validated measures. Building on these findings, Yager and O'Dea (2008) confirmed that psychoeducational, information-based, and cognitive-behavioral approaches were among the least effective, while media literacy- and dissonance-based educational approaches and incorporating health education activities that build self-esteem were identified as successful elements.

Prognosis for Eating Disorders

Eating disorders are serious problems. They have the highest mortality rate of all of the psychiatric disorders (Agras et al., 2004; Licht, Mortensen, Gouliaev, & Lund, 1993). Mortality-rate estimates range from approximately 5% (Casper & Jabine, 1996; Herzog et al., 2000; Sullivan, 1995) to 8% (Steinhausen et al., 2000). The most common causes of death among individuals with eating disorders are starvation and nutritional complications (e.g., electrolyte imbalance or dehydration) and suicide (Neumärker, 2000).

With respect to longer-term outcome, relapse rates following initially successful treatment are high, with published rates ranging from approximately 20 to 60% for adults. Defining relapse and remission is difficult, however, and as a result, these rates vary considerably in the literature depending on methodological differences. Most reported rates are between 35 and 50% (Carter, Blackmore, Sutandar-Pinnock, & Woodside, 2004; McFarlane, Olmsted, & Trottier, 2008; Walsh et al., 2006), comparable to relapse rates associated with alcohol and substance use among women (Walitzer & Dearing, 2006).

Theoretically, relapse signifies a return to disordered functioning following a period of symptom amelioration. Pike (1998) defined AN relapse relative to initial treatment response, remission, and recovery. An initial satisfactory response for AN (before which relapse cannot occur) is operationalized as increasing BMI to at least 20, consuming significantly more calories (although not necessarily normalized eating), reducing fears about weight gain, a resumption of menses, and medical stabilization. Thus, complete symptom alleviation is not necessary for relapse to occur. According to Pike, relapse involves weight dropping to a BMI below 18.5, restrictive eating or bingeing with compensatory behavior, a return to overvaluing weight and shape, loss of menses, and in some cases a return of associated medical problems.

Olmsted, Kaplan, and Rockert (2005) also pointed out that relapse rates for BN are strongly influenced by definitions of remission and relapse. They recommended researchers use consensus definitions; specifically, partial remission is defined as a maximum of two symptom episodes per month for 2 months, and relapse is defined as meeting full diagnostic criteria for 3 months.

Identification of factors that predict relapse may help to advance the understanding of the psychopathology of eating disorders and also provide direction for the development of interventions aimed at relapse prevention. Previous research has identified younger age (Olmsted et al., 2005), higher frequency of vomiting (Olmsted, Kaplan, & Rockert, 1994) and restriction (McFarlane et al., 2008), longer duration of illness, and greater psychiatric comorbidity (Deter & Herzog, 1994) as predictors of relapse. These variables may represent the degree of impairment and severity of the eating disorder, indicating that those who are less well before treatment are more likely to relapse later. At the end of treatment, residual symptoms such as higher binge-eating or vomiting frequency, weight-related self-esteem (McFarlane et al., 2008), higher dietary restraint (Halmi et al., 2002), exercise aimed at weight control (Carter et al., 2004; Strober, Freeman, & Morrell, 1997), weight loss immediately following intensive treatment (Kaplan et al., 2008), and higher body dissatisfaction (Freeman, Beach, Davis, & Solyom, 1985) have also been shown to predict relapse. Finally, factors related to the process of treatment have been shown to predict continued wellness. These include a rapid response to intensive treatment (McFarlane et al., 2008) and abstinence from binge eating and vomiting during treatment (Halmi et al., 2002).

One study (Cockell, Zaitsoff, & Geller, 2004) obtained a retrospective account of self-reported factors that helped or hindered maintenance of treatment gains from 32 patients who had completed a 15-week inpatient treatment program at 6 months postdischarge. Factors identified as supporting maintenance were (a) maintaining connections with professionals (for expertise and monitoring) and nonprofessionals (for support and understanding); (b) application of the nutritional knowledge (what constitutes a normal meal, meal planning, etc.) and psychological skills (self-monitoring and emotional expression) learned in treatment; and (c) focusing beyond the eating disorder (such as on fulfilling higher order values). Factors that were believed to hinder maintenance included loss of structure and specialized support, self-defeating beliefs (e.g., need for control), and daily hassles that patients had been protected from while in treatment.

A recent study of individuals with AN found that over a 12-year follow-up period, 28% had a good outcome, 25% an intermediate outcome, 40% a poor outcome, and 8% were deceased. At the 12-year follow-up point, 19% met diagnostic criteria for AN, 10% for BN, 19% were classified as EDNOS, and 0% had BED. A total of 52% did not appear to have a *DSM–IV* eating disorder (Fichter, Quadflieg, & Hedlund, 2006). It appears that despite the fact that a substantial number of individuals relapse and continue to have clinically significant eating disorders after receiving treatment, more patients recover after receiving treatment than exhibit spontaneous recovery without treatment. For example, in a study of the natural course of bulimia nervosa, at 5-year follow-up, approximately 50% of the women had an eating disorder of clinical severity and only 35% did not show evidence of an eating disorder (Fairburn, Cooper, Doll, Norman, & O'Connor, 2000). Another study examined relapse rates following day-hospital treatment across all eating disorder diagnostic categories. Six months after completion of day-hospital treatment, the relapse rate was 38%, at 1 year it was 41%, and at 18 months it had increased to 48% (McFarlane et al., 2008).

Current estimates of relapse rates in BED are somewhat more optimistic than are those observed in AN and BN. One longitudinal study of BED to assess relapse rates found that at 6 years posttreatment, most participants did not have a diagnosable eating disorder, although approximately 15% had shifted to another diagnostic category (7.4% to BN and 7.4% to EDNOS) and approximately 6% met the criteria for BED once again (Fichter, Quadflieg, & Gnutzmann, 1998).

As is the case with both AN and BN, the severity of the disorder appears to be a prime determinant of negative outcome in BED; the more frequent bingeing is at treatment intake, the more frequent it is following treatment (Peterson et al., 2000). Negative affect also predicts poorer treatment outcome for BED (Eldredge & Agras, 1997). With respect to relapse, Safer, Lively, Telch, and Agras (2002) found that the two strongest predictors of setbacks following a successful course of DBT were earlier onset of binge eating (i.e., at or prior to age 16) and greater (cognitive) dietary restraint.

Conclusion

We still have a long way to go toward a better understanding of why and how eating disorders develop, and the obstacles to make explanatory progress are significant. The most obvious obstacle is that the vast majority of studies examine correlates (or recollected precursors) of established eating disorders. This sort of research is inevitably inconclusive about causation.

Although path-analytic strategies (e.g., Stice, 2001) attempt to extract causal patterns from correlational data, there are severe limits to the persuasiveness of such analyses. For ethical reasons, true experimentation is not likely to occur. For example, it is difficult to get permission to study the bingeing of a BN patient in the lab. Although such patients binge regularly, it is regarded as unethical for researchers to actively induce a binge. Further, although controlled experiments may provide insight into specific symptoms, the external validity of such measures would be questionable. Prospective research is more compelling than is retrospective research; but it too is correlational and therefore limited in what it can tell us.

Although many of us would certainly be most pleased with a tight, experimentally based analysis of eating disorders, there are other satisfactions to be had. Decades ago, Hilde Bruch (1975, 1978) provided us with an account of eating disorders, based on her vast clinical experience and insight. The empirical research that has been conducted since Bruch first presented her elegant formulations has done little to undermine her analysis. The reader who wants a clear understanding of eating disorders would be well advised to refer to Bruch, or if not to her, to her patients. As one of them concluded, "The main thing I've learned is that the worry about dieting, the worry about being skinny or fat, is just a smokescreen. This is not the real illness. The real illness has to do with the way you feel about yourself" (Bruch, 1978, p. 127).

References

Abed, R. T. (1998). The sexual competition hypothesis for eating disorders. *British Journal of Medical Psychology, 71*, 525–547.

Agras, W. S., Brandt, H. A., Bulik, C. M., Dolan-Sewell, R., Fairburn, C. G., Halmi, K. A., … Wilfley, D. E. (2004). Report of the National Institutes of Health workshop on overcoming barriers to treatment research in anorexia nervosa. *International Journal of Eating Disorders, 35*, 509–521.

Allison, K. C., Grilo, C. M., Masheb, R. M., & Stunkard, A. J. (2007). High self-reported rates of neglect and emotional abuse, by persons with binge eating disorder and night eating syndrome. *Behavior Research and Therapy, 45*, 2874–2883.

American Psychiatric Association. (1994). *Diagnostic and statistical manual of mental disorders* (4th ed.). Washington, DC: Author.

American Psychiatric Association. (2000). *Diagnostic and statistical manual of mental disorders* (4th ed., text rev.). Washington, DC: Author.

American Psychiatric Association DSM-5 Development. (2010). *Feeding and eating disorders.* Retrieved from http://www.dsm5.org/proposedrevision/Pages/FeedingandEatingDisorders.aspx

Appolinario, J. C., Bacaltchuk, J., Sichieri, R., Claudino, A. M., Godoy-Matos, A., & Morgan, … Coutinho, W. (2003). A randomized, double-blind, placebo-controlled study of sibutramine in the treatment of binge-eating disorder. *Archives of General Psychiatry, 60*, 1109–1116.

Baker, J. H., Maes, H. H., Lissner, L., Aggen, S. H., Lichtenstein, P., & Kendler, K. S. (2009). Genetic risk factors for disordered eating in adolescent males and females. *Journal of Abnormal Psychology, 118*, 576–586.

Beck, A. T., Rush, A. J., Shaw, B. F., & Emery, G. (1979). *Cognitive therapy of depression.* New York: Guilford.

Bemporad, J. R. (1996). Self-starvation through the ages: Reflections on the pre-history of anorexia nervosa. *International Journal of Eating Disorders, 19*, 217–237.

Bemporad, J. R. (1997). Cultural and historical aspects of eating disorders. *Theoretical Medicine, 18*, 401–420.

Beumont, P. J. V., & Touyz, S. W. (1995). The nutritional management of anorexia and bulimia nervosa. In K. D. Brownell & C. G. Fairburn (Eds.), *Eating disorders and obesity: A comprehensive handbook* (pp. 306–312). New York: Guilford.

Birchall, H. (1999). Interpersonal psychotherapy in the treatment of eating disorders. *European Eating Disorders Review, 7*, 315–320.

Bishop, M., Stein, R., Hilbert, A., Swenson, A., & Wilfley, D. E. (2007, October). *A five-year follow-up study of cognitive-behavioral therapy and interpersonal psychotherapy for the treatment of binge eating disorder.* Paper presented at the annual meeting of the Eating Disorders Research Society, Pittsburgh, PA.

Blinder, B. J., Cumella, E. J., & Sanathara, V. A. (2006). Psychiatric comorbidities of female inpatients with eating disorders. *Psychosomatic Medicine, 68*, 454–462.

Bodell, L. P., & Devlin, M. J. (2010). Pharmacotherapy for binge-eating disorder. In C. M. Grilo & J. E. Mitchell (Eds.), *The treatment of eating disorders: A clinical handbook* (pp. 402–413). New York: Guilford.

Booth, D. A. (1988). Culturally corralled into food abuse: The eating disorders as physiologically reinforced excessive appetites. In K. M. Pirke, W. Vandereycken, & D. Ploog (Eds.), *The psychobiology of bulimia nervosa* (pp. 18–32). Berlin: Springer-Verlag.

Bramon-Bosch, E., Troop, N., & Treasure, J. L. (2000). Eating disorders in males: A comparison with female patients. *European Eating Disorders Review, 8*, 321–328.

Braun, D. L., Sunday, S. R., Huang, A., & Halmi, K. A. (1999). More males seek treatment for eating disorders. *International Journal of Eating Disorders, 25*, 415–424.

Broft, A., Berner, L. A., & Walsh, B. T. (2010). Pharmacotherapy for bulimia nervosa. In C. M. Grilo & J. E. Mitchell (Eds.), *The treatment of eating disorders: A clinical handbook* (pp. 388–401). New York: Guilford.

Bruch, H. (1975). Obesity and anorexia nervosa: Psychosocial aspects. *Australia and New Zealand Journal of Psychiatry, 9*, 159–161.

Bruch, H. (1978). *The golden cage: The enigma of anorexia nervosa.* Cambridge, MA: Harvard University Press.

Bulik, C. M., Berkman, N. D., Brownley, K. A., Sedway, J. A., & Lohr, K. H. (2007). Anorexia nervosa treatment: A systematic review of randomized controlled trials. *International Journal of Eating Disorders, 40*, 310–320.

Cachelin, F. M., & Maher, B. A. (1998). Is amenorrhea a critical criterion for anorexia nervosa? *Journal of Psychosomatic Research, 44*, 435–440.

Cachelin, F. M., Veisel, C., Barzegarnazari, E., & Striegel-Moore, R. H. (2000). Disordered eating, acculturation, and treatment-seeking in a community sample of Hispanic, Asian, Black, and White women. *Psychology of Women Quarterly, 24*, 244–253.

Carter, J. C., Blackmore, E., Sutandar-Pinnock, K., & Woodside, D. B. (2004). Relapse in anorexia nervosa: A survival analysis. *Psychological Medicine, 34*, 671–679.

Carter, J. C., McFarlane, T. L., Bewell, C., Olmsted, M. P., Woodside, D. B., Kaplan, A. S., & Crosby, R. D. (2009). Maintenance treatment for anorexia nervosa: A comparison of cognitive behavior therapy and treatment as usual. *International Journal of Eating Disorders, 42*, 202–207.

Carter, J. C., Stewart, D. A., Dunn, V. J., & Fairburn, C. G. (1997). Primary prevention of eating disorders: Might it do more harm than good? *International Journal of Eating Disorders, 22*, 167–172.

Casper, R. C., & Jabine, L. N. (1996). An eight-year follow-up: Outcome from adolescent compared to adult onset anorexia nervosa. *Journal of Youth and Adolescence, 25*, 499–517.

Chui, W., Safer, D. L., Bryson, S. W., Agras, W. S., & Wilson, G. T. (2007). A comparison of ethnic groups in the treatment of bulimia nervosa. *Eating Behaviors, 8*, 485–491.

Cockell, S. J., Zaitsoff, S. L., & Geller, J. (2004). Maintaining change following eating disorder treatment. *Professional Psychology: Research and Practice, 35*, 527–534.

Corcos, M., Flament, M. F., Giraud, M. J., Paterniti, S., Ledoux, S., Atger, F., & Jeammet, P. (2000). Early psychopathological signs in bulimia nervosa. A retrospective comparison of the period of puberty in bulimic and control girls. *European Child and Adolescent Psychiatry, 9*, 115–121.

Culbert, K. M., Breedlove, S. M., Burt, A., & Klump, K. L. (2008). Prenatal hormone exposure and risk for eating disorders: A comparison of opposite-sex and same-sex twins. *Archives of General Psychiatry, 65*, 329–336.

Dalle Grave, R. (2003). School-based prevention programs for eating disorders: Achievements and opportunities. *Disease Management and Health Outcomes, 11*, 579–593.

Dansky, B. S., Brewerton, T. D., & Kilpatrick, D. G. (2000). Comorbidity of bulimia nervosa and alcohol use disorders: Results from the national women's study. *International Journal of Eating Disorders, 27*, 180–190.

Dare, C., & Crowther, C. (1995). Living dangerously: Psychoanalytic psychotherapy for anorexia nervosa. In G. Szmukler, C. Dare, & J. Treasure (Eds.), *Handbook of eating disorders* (pp. 293–308). London: Wiley.

Dare, C., & Eisler, I. (2000). A multi-family group day treatment program for adolescent eating disorder. *European Eating Disorders Review, 81*, 4–18.

Davis, C., & Claridge, G. (1998). The eating disorders as addiction: A psychobiological perspective. *Addictive Behaviors, 23*, 463–475.

Davis, C., & Katzman, M. (1999). Perfectionism as acculturation: Psychological correlates of eating problems in Chinese male and female students living in the United States. *International Journal of Eating Disorders, 25*, 65–70.

Davison, K. K., Earnest, M. B., & Birch, L. L. (2002). Participation in aesthetic sports and girls' weight concerns at ages 5 and 7 years. *International Journal of Eating Disorders, 31*, 312–317.

Dean, H. Y., Touyz, S. W., Rieger, E., & Thornton, C. E. (2008). Group motivational enhancement therapy as an adjunct to inpatient treatment for eating disorders: A preliminary study. *European Eating Disorders Review, 16*, 256–267.

Deter, H. C., & Herzog, W. (1994). Anorexia nervosa in a long-term perspective: Results of the Heidlberg-Mannheim study. *Psychosomatic Medicine, 56*, 20–27.

Devlin, M. J., Goldfein, J. A., Carino, J. S., & Wolk, S. L. (2000). Open treatment of overweight binge eaters with phentermine and fluoxetine as an adjunct to cognitive-behavioral therapy. *International Journal of Eating Disorders, 28*, 325–332.

Dittmar, H. (2005). Vulnerability factors and processes linking sociocultural pressures and body dissatisfaction. *Journal of Social and Clinical Psychology, 24*, 1081–1087.

Dobson, K., & Dozois, D. (2004). Attentional biases in eating disorders: A meta-analytic review of Stroop performance. *Clinical Psychology Review, 23*, 1001–1022.

Drewnowski, A., Kurth, C. L., & Krahn, D. D. (1995). Effects of body image on dieting, exercise, and anabolic steroid use in adolescent males. *International Journal of Eating Disorders, 17*, 381–386.

Eagles, J. M., Johnston, M. I., Hunter, D., Lobban, M., & Millar, H. R. (1995). Increasing incidence of anorexia nervosa in the female population of northeast Scotland. *American Journal of Psychiatry, 152*, 1266–1271.

Eisenberg, M. (2008). Peer harassment and disordered eating. *International Journal of Adolescent Medicine and Health, 20*, 155–164.

Eisler, I., Lock, J., & le Grange, D. (2010). Family-based treatments for adolescents with anorexia nervosa: Single-family and multifamily approaches. In C. M. Grilo & J. E. Mitchell (Eds.), *The treatment of eating disorders: A clinical handbook* (pp. 150–174). New York: Guilford.

Eldredge, K. L., & Agras, W. S. (1996). Weight and shape overconcern and emotional eating in binge eating disorder. *International Journal of Eating Disorders, 19*, 73–82.

Eldredge, K. L., & Agras, W. S. (1997). The relationship between perceived evaluation of weight and treatment outcome among individuals with binge-eating disorder. *International Journal of Eating Disorders, 22*, 43–49.

Fairburn, C. G. (1981). A cognitive behavioural approach to the management of bulimia. *Psychological Medicine, 11*, 707–711.

Fairburn, C. G. (2008). *Cognitive behavior therapy and eating disorders*. New York: Guilford.

Fairburn, C. G., & Bohn, K. (2005). Eating disorder NOS (EDNOS): An example of the troublesome "not otherwise specified" (NOS) category in DSM-IV. *Behavior Research and Therapy, 43*, 691–701.

Fairburn, C. G., Cooper, Z., Doll, H. A., Norman, P., & O'Connor, M. (2000). The natural course of bulimia nervosa and binge eating disorder in young women. *Archives of General Psychiatry, 57*, 659–665.

Fairburn, C. G., Cooper, Z., Doll, H. A., O'Connor, M. E., Bohn, K., Hawker, D. M., … Palmer, R. L. (2009). Transdiagnostic cognitive-behavioral therapy for patients with eating disorders: A two-site trial with 60-week follow-up. *American Journal of Psychiatry, 166*, 311–319.

Fairburn, C. G., Cooper, Z., Doll, H. A., & Welch, S. L. (1999). Risk factors for anorexia nervosa: Three integrated case-control comparisons. *Archives of General Psychiatry, 56*, 468–476.

Fairburn, C. G., Cooper, Z., & Shafran, R. (2003). Cognitive behavior therapy for eating disorders: A "transdiagnostic" theory and treatment. *Behavior Research and Therapy, 41*, 509–529.

Fairburn, C. G., Norman, P. A., Welch, S. L., O'Connor, M. E., Doll, H. A., & Peveler, R. C. (1995). A prospective study of outcome in bulimia nervosa and the long-term effects of three psychological treatments. *Archives of General Psychiatry, 52*, 304–312.

Fairburn, C. G., Shafran, R., & Cooper, Z. (1998). A cognitive behavioral theory of anorexia nervosa. *Behavior Research and Therapy, 37*, 1–13.

Fairburn, C. G., Welch, S. L., Doll, H. A., Davies, B. A., & O'Connor, M. E. (1997). Risk factors for bulimia nervosa—A community-based case-control study. *Archives of General Psychiatry, 54*, 509–517.

Feld, R., Woodside, D. B., Kaplan, A. S., Olmsted, M. P., & Carter, J. C. (2001). Pretreatment motivational enhancement therapy for eating disorders: A pilot study. *International Journal of Eating Disorders, 29*, 393–400.

Fichter, M. M., Quadflieg, N., & Gnutzmann, A. (1998). Binge eating disorder: Treatment outcome over a 6-year course. *Journal of Psychosomatic Research, 44*, 385–405.

Fichter, M. M., Quadflieg, N., & Hedlund, S. (2006). Twelve year course and outcome predictors of anorexia nervosa. *International Journal of Eating Disorders, 39*, 87–100.

Fisher, M., Schneider, M., Burns, J., Symons, H., & Mandel, F. S. (2001). Differences between adolescents and young adults at presentation to an eating disorders program. *Journal of Adolescent Health, 28*, 222–227.

Fluoxetine Bulimia Nervosa Collaborative Study Group. (1992). Fluoxetine in the treatment of bulimia nervosa: A multicenter, placebo-controlled, double-blind trial. *Archives of General Psychiatry, 49,* 139–147.

Freeman, R. J., Beach, B., Davis, R., & Solyom, L. (1985). The prediction of relapse in bulimia nervosa. *Journal of Psychiatric Research, 19,* 349–353.

Frieling, H., Romer, K. D., Wilhelm, J., Hillemacher, T., Kornhuber, J., de Zwaan, M., ... Bleich, S. (2006). Association of catecholamine-O-methyltransferase and 5-HTTLPR genotype with eating disorder-related behavior and attitudes in females with eating disorders. *Psychiatric Genetics, 16,* 205–208.

Garfinkel, P. E., Lin, E., Goering, P., Spegg, C., Goldbloom, D., Kennedy, S., ... Woodside, D. B. (1996). Should amenorrhoea be necessary for the diagnosis of anorexia nervosa? Evidence from a Canadian community sample. *British Journal of Psychiatry, 168,* 500–506.

Garner, D. M., & Bemis K. M. (1982). A cognitive behavioral approach to the treatment of anorexia nervosa. *Cognitive Therapy and Research, 6,* 123–150.

Garner, D. M., Olmsted, M. P., & Polivy, J. (1983). Development and validation of a multidimensional eating disorder inventory for anorexia nervosa and bulimia. *International Journal of Eating Disorders, 2,* 15–34.

Garner, D. M., Olmsted, M., Polivy, J., & Garfinkel, P. E. (1984). Comparison between weight preoccupied women and anorexia nervosa. *Psychosomatic Medicine, 46,* 255–266.

Geist, R., Heinmaa, M., Stephens, D., Davis, R., & Katzman, D. K. (2000). Comparison of family therapy and family group psychoeducation in adolescents with anorexia nervosa. *Canadian Journal of Psychiatry—Revue Canadienne de Psychiatrie, 45,* 173–178.

Geller, J., Srikameswaran, S., Zaitsoff, S. L., Cockell, S. J., & Poole, G. D. (2003). Mothers' and fathers' perceptions of their adolescent daughters' shape, weight, and body esteem: Are they accurate? *Journal of Youth and Adolescence, 32,* 81–87.

George, L., Thornton, C., Touyz, S. W., Waller, G., & Beumont, P. J. V. (2004). Motivational enhancement and schema-focused cognitive behaviour therapy in the treatment of chronic eating disorders. *Clinical Psychologist. Special Issue: Eating Disorders, 8,* 81–85.

Goldner, E. M., Geller, J., Birmingham, C. L., & Remick, H. A. (2000). Comparison of shoplifting behaviours in patients with eating disorders, psychiatric control subjects, and undergraduate control subjects. *Canadian Journal of Psychiatry—Revue Canadienne de Psychiatrie, 45,* 471–475.

Goldstein, D. J., Wilson, M., Thompson, V. L., Potvin, J., & Rampey, A. H. (1995). Long term fluoxetine treatment of bulimia nervosa. *British Journal of Psychiatry, 166,* 660–666.

Gonzalez, R. G. (1988). Bulimia and adolescence: Individual psychoanalytic treatment. In H. J. Schwartz (Ed.), *Bulimia: Psychoanalytic treatment and theory* (pp. 339–441). Madison, CT: International Universities Press.

Grant, K., Lyons, A., Landis, D., Cho, M., Scudiero, M., Reynolds, L., ... Bryant, H. (1999). Gender, body image, and depressive symptoms among low-income African American adolescents. *Journal of Social Issues, 55,* 299–315.

Grilo, C. M. (2006). *Eating and weight disorders.* New York: Psychology Press.

Grilo, C. M., Masheb, R., & Wilson, G. T. (2005). Efficacy of cognitive-behavioral therapy and fluoxetine for the treatment of binge eating disorder: A randomized double-blind placebo-controlled trial. *Biological Psychiatry, 57,* 301–309.

Grilo, C. M., & Mitchell, J. E. (2010). *The treatment of eating disorders: A clinical handbook.* New York: Guilford.

Halmi, K., Agras, W. S., Mitchell, J., Wilson, G. T., Crow, S., Bryson, S. W., & Kraemer, H. (2002). Relapse predictors of patients with bulimia nervosa who achieved abstinence through cognitive behavioral therapy. *Archives of General Psychiatry, 59,* 1105–1109.

Harrop, E. N., & Marlatt, G. A. (2010). The comorbidity of substance use disorders and eating disorders in women: Prevalence, etiology, and treatment. *Addictive Behaviors, 35,* 392–398.

Haworth-Hoeppner, S. (2000). The critical shapes of body image: The role of culture and family in the production of eating disorders. *Journal of Marriage and the Family, 62,* 212–227.

Hay, P., & Fairburn, C. (1998). The validity of the DSM-IV scheme for classifying bulimic eating disorders. *International Journal of Eating Disorders, 23,* 7–15.

Heatherton, T. F., & Polivy, J. (1992). Chronic dieting and eating disorders: A spiral model. In J. Crowther, S. E. Hobfall, M. A. P. Stephens, & D. L. Tennenbaum (Eds.), *The etiology of bulimia: The individual and familial context* (pp. 133–155). Washington, DC: Hemisphere.

Herpertz-Dahlmann, B., Muller, B., Herpertz, S., Heusen, N., Hebebrand, J., & Remschmidt, H. (2001). Prospective 10-year follow-up in adolescent anorexia nervosa—Course, outcome, psychiatric comorbidity, and psychosocial adaptation. *Journal of Child Psychology and Psychiatry and Allied Disciplines, 42,* 603–612.

Herzog, D. B. (1995). Psychodynamic psychotherapy for anorexia nervosa. In K. D. Brownell & C. G. Fairburn (Eds.), *Eating disorders and obesity: A comprehensive handbook* (pp. 330–335). New York: Guilford.

Herzog, D. B., Greenwood, D. N., Dorer, D. J., Flores, A. T., Ekeblad, E. R., Richards, A., … Keller, M. B. (2000). Mortality in eating disorders: A descriptive study. *International Journal of Eating Disorders, 28*, 20–26.

Hoek, H. (2006). Incidence, prevalence, and mortality of anorexia nervosa and other eating disorders. *Current Opinion in Psychiatry, 19*, 389–394.

Hoek, H. W., van Harten, P. N., Hermans, K. M., Katzman, M. A., Matroos, G. E., & Susser, E. S. (2005). The incidence of anorexia nervosa on Curacao. *American Journal of Psychiatry, 162*, 748–752.

Hudson, J. I., Hiripi, E., Pope, H. G., & Kessler, R. (2007). The prevalence and correlates of eating disorders in the National Comorbidity Survey Replication. *Biological Psychiatry, 61*, 348–358.

Hudson, J. I., Pope, H. G., & Jonas, J. M. (1983). Phenomenologic relationship of eating disorders to major affective disorder. *Psychiatry Research, 9*, 345–354.

Jacobi, C., Hayward, C., de Zwaan, M., Kraemer, H. C., & Agras, W. S. (2004). Coming to terms with risk factors for eating disorders: Application of risk terminology and suggestions for a general taxonomy. *Psychological Bulletin, 130*, 19–65.

Jager, J., & Powers, P. (2007). *Clinical manual of eating disorders.* Arlington, VA: American Psychiatric Publishing.

Javaras, K. N., Laird, N. M., Reichborn-Kjennerud, T., Bulik, C. M., Pope, H. Jr., & Hudson, J. I. (2008). Familiality and heritability of binge eating disorder: Results of a case-control family study and a twin study. *International Journal of Eating Disorders, 41*, 174–179.

Johnson, C. (1995). Psychodynamic treatment of bulimia nervosa. In K. D. Brownell & C. G. Fairburn (Eds.), *Eating disorders and obesity: A comprehensive handbook* (pp. 349–353). New York: Guilford.

Johnson, C., & Connors, M. E. (1987). *The etiology and treatment of bulimia nervosa.* New York: Basic Books.

Johnson, W. G., Boutelle, K. N., Torgrud, L., Davig, J. P., & Turner, S. (2000). What is a binge? The influence of amount, duration, and loss of control criteria on judgments of binge eating. *International Journal of Eating Disorders, 27*, 471–479.

Johnson, W. G., Carr-Nangle, R. E., Nangle, D. W., Antony, M. M., & Zayfert, C. (1997). What is binge eating? A comparison of binge eater, peer, and professional judgments of eating episodes. *Addictive Behaviors, 22*, 631–635.

Kahm, A. (1994). Recovery through nutritional counseling. In B. P. Kinoy (Ed.), *Eating disorders: New directions in treatment and recovery* (pp. 15–47). New York: Columbia University Press.

Kaplan, A. S., Walsh, B. T., Olmsted, M. P., Carter, J., Rockert, W., Roberto, C., & Parides, M. (2008). The slippery slope: Prediction of successful weight maintenance in anorexia nervosa. *Psychological Medicine, 39*, 1037–1045.

Katzman, M. A., Hermans, K. M., Van Hoeken, D., & Hoek, H. W. (2004). Not your "typical island woman": Anorexia nervosa is reported only in subcultures in Curacao. *Cultural Medicine and Psychiatry, 28*, 463–492.

Kaye, W. H. (1997). Anorexia nervosa, obsessional behavior, and serotonin. *Psychopharmacological Bulletin, 33*, 335–344.

Kaye, W., Gendall, K., & Strober, M. (1998). Serotonin neuronal function and selective serotonin reuptake inhibitor treatment in anorexia and bulimia nervosa. *Biological Psychiatry, 44*, 825–838.

Kaye, W. H., Nagata, T., Weltzin, T. E., Hsu, L. K. G., Sokol, M. S., McConaha, C., … Deep, D. (2001). Double-blind placebo-controlled administration of fluoxetine in restricting- and restricting-purging-type anorexia nervosa. *Biological Psychiatry, 49*, 644–652.

Keel, P. K., & Striegel-Moore, R. H. (2009). The validity and clinical utility of purging disorder. *International Journal of Eating Disorders, 42*, 706–719.

Killick, S., & Allen, C. (1997). "Shifting the balance"—Motivational interviewing to help behaviour change in people with bulimia nervosa. *European Eating Disorders Review, 5*, 33–41.

Kluck, A. S. (2010). Family influence on disordered eating: The role of body image dissatisfaction. *Body Image, 7*, 8–14.

Klump, K. L., Burt, S. A., McGue, M., & Iacono, W. G. (2007). Changes in genetic and environmental influences on disordered eating across adolescence: A longitudinal twin study. *Archives of General Psychiatry, 64*, 1409–1415.

Klump, K. L., & Gobrogge, K. L. (2005). A review and primer of molecular genetic studies of anorexia nervosa. *International Journal of Eating Disorders, 37*, 43–48.

Klump, K. L., Gobrogge, K. L., Perkins, P. S., Thorne, D., Sisk, C. L., & Breedlove, S. M. (2006). Preliminary evidence that gonadal hormones organize and activate disordered eating. *Psychological Medicine, 36*, 539–546.

Kong, S., & Bernstein, K. (2009). Childhood trauma as a predictor of eating psychopathology and its mediating variables in patients with eating disorders. *Journal of Clinical Nursing, 18*, 1897–1907.

Kruger, S., & Kennedy, S. H. (2000). Psychopharmacotherapy of anorexia nervosa, bulimia nervosa and binge-eating disorder. *Journal of Psychiatry and Neuroscience, 25*, 497–508.

Laliberte, M., Boland, F. J., & Leichner, P. (1999). Family climates: Family factors specific to disturbed eating and bulimia nervosa. *Journal of Clinical Psychology, 55*, 1021–1040.

Lansky, D., & Levitt, J. L. (1992). Multifaceted treatment of patients with severe eating disorders. In C. E. Stout, J. L. Levitt, & D. H. Ruben (Eds.), *Handbook for assessing and treating addictive disorders* (pp. 181–202). New York: Greenwood.

le Grange, D., Crosby, R. D., Rathouz, P. J., & Leventhal, B. L. (2007). A randomized controlled comparison of family-based treatment and supportive psychotherapy for adolescent bulimia nervosa. *Archives of General Psychiatry, 64*, 1049–1056.

Leon, G., Fulkerson, J. A., Perry, C., & Early-Zald, M. B. (1995). Prospective analysis of personality and behavioral vulnerabilities and gender influences in the later development of disordered eating. *Journal of Abnormal Psychology, 104*, 140–149.

Leung, F., Geller, J., & Katzman, M. (1996). Issues and concerns associated with different risk models for eating disorders. *International Journal of Eating Disorder, 19*, 249–256.

Licht, R. W., Mortensen, P. B., Gouliaev, G., & Lund, J. (1993). Mortality in Danish psychiatric long-stay patients, 1972–1982. *Acta Psychiatrica Scandinavica, 87*, 336–341.

Lilenfeld, L. R. R., Stein, D., Bulik, C. M., Strober, M., Plotnicov, K., Pollice, C., … Kaye, W. H. (2000). Personality traits among currently eating disordered, recovered and never ill first-degree female relatives of bulimic and control women. *Psychological Medicine, 30*, 1399–1410.

Linehan, M. M. (1993). *Skills training manual for treating borderline personality disorder.* Seattle, WA: Guilford.

Loeb, K. L., Wilson, G. T., Gilbert, J. S., & Labouvie, E. (2000). Guided and unguided self-help for binge eating. *Behavior Research and Therapy, 38*, 259–272.

Machado, P. P. P., Machado, B. C., Gonçalves, S., & Hoek, H. W. (2007). The prevalence of eating disorders not otherwise specified. *International Journal of Eating Disorders, 40*, 212–217.

Matsunaga, H., Kaye, W. H., McConaha, C., Plotnicov, K., Pollice, C., & Rao, R. (2000). Personality disorders among subjects recovered from eating disorders. *International Journal of Eating Disorders, 27*, 353–357.

Matsunaga, H., Kiriike, N., Iwasaki, Y., Miyata, A., Matsui, T., Nagata, T., … Kaye, W. H. (2000). Multi-impulsivity among bulimic patients in Japan. *International Journal of Eating Disorders, 27*, 348–352.

Mayer, L. E. S., & Walsh, B. T. (1998). The use of selective serotonin reuptake inhibitors in eating disorders. *Journal of Clinical Psychiatry, 59*, 28–34.

McCabe, E. B., & Marcus, M. D. (2002). Question: Is dialectical behavior therapy useful in the management of anorexia nervosa? *Eating Disorders: The Journal of Treatment and Prevention, 10*, 335–337.

McElroy, S. L., Arnold, L. M., Shapira, N. A., Keck, P. E. J., Rosenthal, N. R., Karim, M. R., … Hudson, J. I. (2003). Topiramate in the treatment of binge eating disorder associated with obesity: A randomized, placebo-controlled trial. *American Journal of Psychiatry, 160*, 255–261.

McElroy, S. L., Casuto, L. S., Nelson, E. B., Lake, K. A., Soutullo, C. A., Keck, P. E., & Hudson, J. I. (2000). Placebo controlled trial of sertraline in the treatment of binge eating disorder. *American Journal of Psychiatry, 157*, 1004–1006.

McElroy, S. L., Hudson, J. I., Capece, J. A., Beyers, K., Fisher, A. C., & Rosenthal, N. R. (2007). Topiramate for the treatment of binge eating disorder associated with obesity: A placebo-controlled study. *Biological Psychiatry, 61*, 1039–1048.

McElroy, S. L., Hudson, J. I., Malhotra, S., Welge, J. A., Nelson, E. B., & Keck, P. E. J. (2003). Citalopram in the treatment of binge-eating disorder: A placebo-controlled trial. *Journal of Clinical Psychiatry, 64*, 807–813.

McElroy, S. L., Kotwal, R., Guerdjikova, A. I., Welge, J. A., Nelson, E. B., Lake, K. A., … Hudson, J. I. (2006). Zonisamide in the treatment of binge eating disorder with obesity: A randomized controlled trial. *Journal of Clinical Psychiatry, 67*, 1897–1906.

McElroy, S. L., Shapira, N. A., Arnold, L. M., Keck, P. E. J., Rosenthal, N. R., & Wu, S., … Hudson, J. I. (2004). Topiramate in the long-term treatment of binge-eating disorder associated with obesity. *Journal of Clinical Psychiatry, 65*, 1463–1469.

McFarlane, T., McCabe, R. E., Jarry, J., Olmsted, M. P., & Polivy, J. (2001). Weight-related and shape-related self-evaluation in eating-disordered and non-eating-disordered women. *International Journal of Eating Disorders, 29*, 328–335.

McFarlane, T., Olmsted, M. P., & Trottier, K. (2008). Timing and prediction of relapse in a transdiagnostic eating disorder sample. *International Journal of Eating Disorders, 41*, 587–593.

McFarlane, T., Polivy, J., & Herman, C. P. (1998). The effects of false feedback about weight on restrained and unrestrained eaters. *Journal of Abnormal Psychology, 107*, 312–318.

McVey, G., Tweed, S., & Blackmore, E. (2007). Healthy Schools-Healthy Kids: A controlled evaluation of a comprehensive universal eating disorder prevention program. *Body Image, 4*, 115–136.

Menzel, J. E., Schaefer, L. M., Burke, N. L., Mayhew, L. L., Brannick, M. T., & Thompson, J. K. (2010). Appearance-related teasing, body dissatisfaction, and disordered eating: A meta-analysis. *Body Image, 7*, 261–270.

Milano, W., Petrella, C., Casella, A., Capasso, A., Carrino, S., & Milano, L. (2005). Use of sibutramine, an inhibitor of the reuptake of serotonin and noradrenaline, in the treatment of binge eating disorder: A placebo-controlled study. *Advances in Therapy, 22*, 25–31.

Miller, W. R., & Rollnick, S. (2002). *Motivational interviewing: Preparing people for change* (2nd ed.). New York: Guilford.

Mills, J., Polivy, J., Herman, C. P., & Tiggemann, M. (2002). Effects of media-portrayed idealized body images on restrained and unrestrained eaters. *Personality and Social Psychology Bulletin, 28*, 1687–1699.

Minuchin, S., Rosman, B. L., & Baker, L. (1978). *Psychosomatic families: Anorexia nervosa in context.* Cambridge, MA: Harvard University Press.

Mitchell, J. E., Halmi, K., Wilson, G. T., Agras, W. S., Kraemer, H., & Crow, S. (2002). A randomized secondary treatment study of women with bulimia nervosa who fail to respond to CBT. *International Journal of Eating Disorders, 32*, 271–281.

Moller-Madsen, S., & Nystrup, J. (1992). Incidence of anorexia nervosa in Denmark. *Acta Psychiatrica Scandinavica, 86*, 197–200.

Mulholland, A. M., & Mintz, L. B. (2001). Prevalence of eating disorders among African American women. *Journal of Counseling Psychology, 48*, 111–116.

Murphy, S., Russell, L., & Waller, G. (2005). Integrated psychodynamic therapy for bulimia nervosa and binge eating disorder: Theory, practice, and preliminary findings. *European Eating Disorder Review, 13*, 383–391.

Narash-Eisikovits, O., Dierberger, A., & Westen, D. (2002). A multidimensional meta-analysis of pharmacotherapy for bulimia nervosa: Summarizing the range of outcomes in controlled clinical trials. *Harvard Review of Psychiatry, 10*, 193–211.

Nasser, M. (1997). *Culture and weight consciousness.* New York: Routledge.

Neumärker, K. (2000). Mortality rates and causes of death. *European Eating Disorders Review, 8*, 181–187.

Nevonen, L., & Broberg, A. G. (2000). The emergence of eating disorders: An exploratory study. *European Eating Disorders Review, 8*, 279–292.

Nisbett, R. E., & Wilson, T. D. (1977). Telling more than we can know: Verbal reports on mental processes. *Psychological Review, 84*, 231–259.

Nowak, M. (1998). The weight-conscious adolescent: Body image, food intake, and weight-related behavior. *Journal of Adolescent Health, 23*, 389–398.

O'Dea, J. A. (2005). Prevention of child obesity: "First, do no harm." *Health Education Research, 20*, 259–265.

O'Dea, J. A., & Abraham, S. (2001). Knowledge, beliefs, attitudes, and behaviors related to weight control, eating disorders, and body image in Australian trainee home economics and physical education teachers. *Journal of Nutrition Education and Behavior, 33*, 332–340.

Ogden, J., & Elder, C. (1998). The role of family status and ethnic group on body image and eating behavior. *International Journal of Eating Disorders, 23*, 309–315.

Olmsted, M. P., & Kaplan, A. S. (1995). Psychoeducation in the treatment of eating disorders. In K. D. Brownell & C. G. Fairburn (Eds.), *Eating disorders and obesity: A comprehensive handbook* (pp. 299–305). New York: Guilford.

Olmsted, M. P., Kaplan, A. S., & Rockert, W. (1994). Rate and prediction of relapse in bulimia nervosa. *American Journal of Psychiatry, 151*, 738–743.

Olmsted, M. P., Kaplan, A. S., & Rockert, W. (2005). Defining remission and relapse in bulimia nervosa. *International Journal of Eating Disorders, 38*, 1–6.

Olmsted, M. P., McFarlane, T. L., Carter, J. C., Trottier, K., Woodside, D. B., & Dimitropoulos, G. (2010). Inpatient and day hospital treatment for anorexia nervosa. In C. M. Grilo & J. E. Mitchell (Eds.), *The treatment of eating disorders: A clinical handbook* (pp. 198–211). New York: Guilford.

Palmer, R. L., Birchall, H., Damani, S., Gatward, N., McGrain, L., & Parker, L. (2003). A dialectical behavior therapy program for people with an eating disorder and borderline personality disorder—Description and outcome. *International Journal of Eating Disorders, 33*, 281–286.

Peterson, C. B., Crow, S. J., Nugent, S., Mitchell, J. E., Engbloom, S., & Mussell, M. P. (2000). Predictors of treatment outcome for binge eating disorder. *International Journal of Eating Disorders, 28*, 131–138.

Pike, K. M. (1998). Long-term course of anorexia nervosa: Response, relapse, remission, and recovery. *Clinical Psychology Review, 18*, 447–475.

Pike, K. M., Carter, J. C., & Olmsted, M. P. (2010). Cognitive-behavioral therapy for anorexia nervosa. In C. M. Grilo & J. E. Mitchell (Eds.), *The treatment of eating disorders: A clinical handbook* (pp. 83–107). New York: Guilford.

Pike, K. M., Walsh, B. T., Vitousek, K., Wilson, G. T., & Bauer, J. (2003). Cognitive behavior therapy in the posthospitalization treatment of anorexia nervosa. *American Journal of Psychiatry, 160*, 2046–2049.

Pinhas, L., Toner, B. B., Ali, A., Garfinkel, P. E., & Stuckless, N. (1999). The effects of the ideal of female beauty on mood and body satisfaction. *International Journal of Eating Disorders, 25*, 223–226.

Polivy, J., & Herman, C. P. (1987). Diagnosis and treatment of normal eating. *Journal of Consulting and Clinical Psychology, 55*, 635–644.

Polivy, J., & Herman, C. P. (1993). Etiology of binge eating: Psychological mechanisms. In C. G. Fairburn & G. T. Wilson (Eds.), *Binge eating: Nature, assessment and treatment* (pp. 173–205). New York: Guilford.

Polivy, J., & Herman, C. P. (2002). Causes of eating disorders. *Annual Review of Psychology, 53*, 187–213.

Polivy, J., & Herman, C. P. (2007). Is the body the self? Women and body image. *Collegium Antropologicum, 31*, 43–47.

Polivy, J., Herman, C. P., Mills, J., & Wheeler, H. B. (2003). Eating disorders in adolescence. In G. Adams & M. Berzonsky (Eds.), *The Blackwell handbook of adolescence* (pp. 523–549). Oxford, UK: Blackwell.

Prochaska, J. O., & DiClemente, C. C. (1992). The transtheoretical approach. In J. C. Norcross & I. L. Goldfield (Eds.), *Handbook of psychotherapy integration* (pp. 300–334). New York: Basic Books.

Procopio, M., & Marriott, P. (2007). Intrauterine hormonal environment and risk of developing anorexia nervosa. *Archives of General Psychiatry, 64*, 1402–1407.

Pryor, T., Wiederman, M. W., & McGilley, B. (1996). Laxative abuse among women with eating disorders: An indication of psychopathology? *International Journal of Eating Disorders, 20*, 13–18.

Reas, D. L., & Grilo, C. M. (2008). Review and meta-analysis of pharmacotherapy for binge-eating disorder. *Obesity, 16*, 2024–2038.

Rockert, W., Kaplan, A., & Olmsted, M. (2007). Eating disorder not otherwise specified: The view from a tertiary care treatment center. *International Journal of Eating Disorders, 40*, 99–103.

Rodríguez, M., Pérez, V., & García, Y. (2005). Impact of traumatic experiences and violent acts upon response to treatment of a sample of Colombian women with eating disorders. *International Journal of Eating Disorders, 37*, 299–306.

Rooney, B., McClelland, L., Crisp, A. H., & Sedgwick, P. M. (1995). The incidence and prevalence of anorexia nervosa in three suburban health districts in south west London, UK. *International Journal of Eating Disorders, 18*, 299–307.

Safer, D. L., Lively, T. J., Telch, C. F., & Agras, W. S. (2002). Predictors of relapse following successful dialectical behavior therapy for binge eating disorder. *International Journal of Eating Disorders, 32*, 155–163.

Safer, D. L., Robinson, A. H., & Jo, B. (2010). Outcome from a randomized controlled trial of group therapy for binge eating disorder: Comparing dialectical behavior therapy adapted for binge eating to an active comparison group therapy. *Behavior Therapy, 41*, 106–120.

Safer, D. L., Telch, C. F., & Agras, W. S. (2001). Dialectical behavior therapy adapted for bulimia: A case report. *International Journal of Eating Disorders, 30*, 101–106.

Schlundt, D. G., & Johnson, W. G. (1990). *Eating disorders: Assessment and treatment*. Boston: Allyn and Bacon.

Smolak, L., & Levine, M. P. (1996). Adolescent transitions and the development of eating problems. In L. Smolak, M. Levine, & R. Striegel-Moore (Eds.), *The developmental psychopathology of eating disorders: Implications for research, prevention, and treatment* (pp. 210–231). Mahwah, NJ: Erlbaum.

Steiger, H., Gauvin, L., Joober, R., Israel, M., Ng Ying Kin, N. M. K., Bruce, K. R., … Hakim, J. (2006). Intrafamilial correspondences on platelet [^{3}H-]paroxetine-binding indices in bulimic probands and their unaffected first-degree relatives. *Neuropsychopharmacology, 31*, 1785–1792.

Steiger, H., Young, S. N., Kin, N. M. K., Koerner, N., Israel, M., Lageix, P., & Paris, J. (2001). Implications of impulsive and affective symptoms for serotonin function in bulimia nervosa. *Psychological Medicine, 31*, 85–95.

Steinhausen, H. C., Seidel, R., & Metzke, C. W. (2000). Evaluation of treatment and intermediate and long-term outcome of adolescent eating disorders. *Psychological Medicine, 30*, 1089–1098.

Stice, E. (2001). A prospective test of the dual-pathway model of bulimic pathology: Mediating effects of dieting and negative affect. *Journal of Abnormal Psychology, 110*, 1–12.

Stice, E., & Shaw, H. (1994). Adverse effects of the media portrayed thin-ideal on women and linkages to bulimic symptomatology. *Journal of Social and Clinical Psychology, 13*, 288–308.

Stice, E., & Shaw, H. (2004). Eating disorder prevention programs: A meta-analytic review. *Psychological Bulletin, 130*, 206–227.

Striegel-Moore, R. H. (1993). Etiology of binge eating: A developmental perspective. In C. G. Fairburn & G. T. Wilson (Eds.), *Binge eating: Nature, assessment and treatment* (pp. 144–172). New York: Guilford.

Striegel-Moore, R. H., & Bulik, C. M. (2007). Risk factors for eating disorders. *American Psychologist, 62*, 181–198.

Striegel-Moore, R. H., Franko, D. L., & Garcia, J. (2009). The validity and clinical utility of night eating syndrome. *International Journal of Eating Disorders, 42*, 720–738.

Striegel-Moore, R. H., Schreiber, G. B., Lo, A., Crawford, P., Obarzanek, E., & Rodin, J. (2000). Eating disorder symptoms in a cohort of 11- to 16-year-old Black and White girls: The NHLBI growth and health study. *International Journal of Eating Disorders, 27*, 49–66.

Strober, M. (1980). Personality and symptomatological features in young, nonchronic anorexia nervosa patients. *Journal of Psychosomatic Research, 24*, 353–359.

Strober, M., Freeman, R., Lampert, C., Diamond, J., & Kaye, W. (2000). Controlled family study of anorexia nervosa and bulimia nervosa: Evidence of shared liability and transmission of partial syndromes. *American Journal of Psychiatry, 157*, 393–401.

Strober, M., Freeman, R., & Morrell, W. (1997). The long-term course of anorexia nervosa in adolescents: Survival analysis of recovery, relapse, and outcome predictors over 10–15 years in a prospective study. *International Journal of Eating Disorders, 22*, 339–360.

Strober, M., & Humphrey, L. L. (1987). Familial contributions to the etiology and course of anorexia nervosa and bulimia. *Journal of Consulting and Clinical Psychology, 55*, 654 659.

Sullivan, P. F. (1995). Mortality in anorexia nervosa. *American Journal of Psychiatry, 152*, 1073–1074.

Svaldi, J., Bender, C., & Tuschen-Caffier, B. (2010). Explicit memory bias for positively valenced body-related cues in women with binge eating disorder. *Journal of Behavior Therapy and Experimental Psychiatry, 41*, 251–257.

Tagay, S., Schlegl, S., & Senf, W. (2010). Traumatic events, posttraumatic stress symptomatology and somatoform symptoms in eating disorder patients. *European Eating Disorders Review, 18*, 124–132.

Tantleff-Dunn, S., Gokee-LaRose, J., & Peterson, R. D. (2004). *Interpersonal psychotherapy for the treatment of anorexia nervosa, bulimia nervosa, and binge eating disorder.* Hoboken, NJ: Wiley.

Tasca, G. A., Ritchie, K., Conrad, G., Balfour, L., Gayton, J., Daigle, V., & Bissada, H. (2006). Attachment scales predict outcome in a randomized controlled trial of two group therapies for binge eating disorder: An aptitude by treatment interaction. *Psychotherapy Research, 16*, 106–121.

Tchanturia, K., & Hambrook, D. (2010). Cognitive remediation therapy for anorexia. In C. M. Grilo & J. E. Mitchell (Eds.), *The treatment of eating disorders: A clinical handbook* (pp. 130–149). New York: Guilford.

Telch, C. F., Agras, W. S., & Linehan, M. M. (2000). Group dialectical behavior therapy for binge-eating disorder: A preliminary, uncontrolled trial. *Behavior Therapy, 31*, 569–582.

Telch, C. F., Agras, W. S., & Linehan, M. M. (2001). Dialectical behavior therapy for binge eating disorder. *Journal of Consulting and Clinical Psychology, 69*, 1061–1065.

Thode, N. (1990). A family systems perspective on recovery from an eating disorder. In B. P. Kinoy (Ed.), *Eating disorders: New directions in treatment and recovery* (pp. 61–79). New York: Columbia University Press.

Touyz, S. W., Polivy, J., & Hay, P. (2008). *Eating disorders. Advances in psychotherapy: Evidence-based practice.* Ashland, OH: Hogrefe and Huber.

Tozzi, F., & Bulik, C. M. (2003). Candidate genes in eating disorders. *Current Drug Targets—CNS and Neurological Disorders, 2*, 31–39.

Treasure, J., & Ward, A. (1997). A practical guide to the use of motivational interviewing in anorexia nervosa. *European Eating Disorders Review, 5*, 102–114

Turnbull, S., Ward, A., Treasure, J., Jick, H., & Derby, L. (1996). The demand for eating disorder care. An epidemiological study using the general practice research database. *British Journal of Psychiatry, 169*, 705–712.

van Hoeken, D., Veling, W., Sinke, S., Mitchell, J. E., & Hoek, H. W. (2009). The validity and utility of subtyping bulimia nervosa. *International Journal of Eating Disorders, 42*, 595–602.

Vanfurth, E. F., Vanstrien, D. C., Martina, L. M. L., Vanson, M. J. M., Hendrickx, J. J. P., & van Engeland, H. (1996). Expressed emotion and the prediction of outcome in adolescent eating disorders. *International Journal of Eating Disorders, 20*, 19–31.

Vitousek, K. B. (1995). Cognitive behavioral therapy for anorexia nervosa. In K. D. Brownell & C. G. Fairburn (Eds.), *Eating disorders and obesity: A comprehensive handbook* (pp. 324–329). New York: Guilford.

Vohs, K. D., & Heatherton, T. F. (2000). Self-regulatory failure: A resource depletion approach. *Psychological Science, 11*, 249–254.

Wade, T. D., Frayne, A., Edwards, S., Robertson, T., & Gilchrist, P. (2009). Motivational change in an inpatient anorexia nervosa population and implications for treatment. *Australian and New Zealand Journal of Psychiatry, 43*, 235–243.

Wakeling, A. (1996). Epidemiology of anorexia nervosa. *Psychiatry Research, 62*, 3–9.

Walitzer, K. S., & Dearing, R. L. (2006). Gender differences in alcohol and substance use relapse. *Clinical Psychology Review, 26*, 128–148.

Walsh, B. T., Agras, W. S., Devlin, M. J., Fairburn, C. G., Wilson, G. T., Kahn, C., & Chally, M. K. (2000). Fluoxetine for bulimia nervosa following poor response to psychotherapy. *American Journal of Psychiatry, 157*, 1332–1334.

Walsh, B. T., Kaplan, A. S., Attia, E., Olmsted, M., Parides, M., Carter, J. C., … Rockert, W. (2006). Fluoxetine after weight restoration in anorexia nervosa: A randomized controlled trial. *Journal of the American Medical Association, 295*, 2605–2612.

Ward, A., Tiller, J., Treasure, J., & Russell, G. (2000). Eating disorders: Psyche or soma? *International Journal of Eating Disorders, 27*, 279–287.

Wheeler, H. B., Polivy, J., & Herman, C. P. (2002). *The precarious identities of restrained eaters: Effects of a threat.* Unpublished manuscript.

Whittal, M. L., Agras, W. S., & Gould, R. A. (1999). Bulimia nervosa: A meta-analysis of psychosocial and pharmacological treatments. *Behavior Therapy, 30*, 117–135.

Wilfley, D. E., Crow, S. J., Hudson, J. A., Mitchelle, J. E., Berkowitz, R. I., Blakesley, V., & Walsh, B. T. (2008). Efficacy of sibutramine for the treatment of binge eating disorder: A randomized multicenter placebo-controlled double-blind study. *American Journal of Psychiatry, 165*, 51–58.

Wilfley, D. E., Friedman, M. A., Dounchis, J. Z., Stein, R. I., Welch, R. R., & Ball, S. A. (2000). Comorbid psychopathology in binge eating disorder: Relation to eating disorder severity at baseline and following treatment. *Journal of Consulting and Clinical Psychology, 68*, 641–649.

Wilfley, D. E., Welch, R. R., Stein, R. I., Spurrell, E. B., Cohen, L. R., & Saelens, B. E., … Matt, G. E. (2002). A randomized comparison of group cognitive-behavioral therapy and group interpersonal psychotherapy for the treatment of overweight individuals with binge-eating disorder. *Archives of General Psychiatry, 59*, 713–721.

Williamson, D. A., Muller, S. L., Reas, D. L., & Thaw, J. M. (1999). Cognitive bias in eating disorders: Implications for theory and treatment. *Behavior Modification, 23*, 556–577.

Wilson, G. T. (1991). The addiction model of eating disorders: A critical analysis. *Advances in Behavior Research and Therapy, 13*, 27–72.

Wilson, G. T. (1996). Treatment of bulimia nervosa: When CBT fails. *Behavior Research and Therapy, 34*, 197–212.

Wilson, G. T. (1999). Cognitive behavior therapy for eating disorders: Progress and problems. *Behavior Research and Therapy, 37*, S79–S95.

Wilson, G. T., & Fairburn, C. G. (2000). The treatment of binge eating disorder. *European Eating Disorders Review, 8*, 351–354.

Wilson, G. T., Grilo, C. M., & Vitousek, K. M. (2007). Psychological treatment of eating disorders. *American Psychologist, 62*, 199–216.

Wilson, G. T., & Schlam, T. R. (2004). The transtheoretical model and motivational interviewing in the treatment of eating and weight disorders. *Clinical Psychology Review, 24*, 361–378.

Wilson, G. T., & Shafran, R. (2005). Eating disorders guidelines from NICE. *Lancet, 365*, 79–81.

Wilson, G. T., & Sysko, R. (2009). Frequency of binge eating episodes in bulimia nervosa and binge eating disorder: Diagnostic considerations. *International Journal of Eating Disorders, 42*, 603–610.

Wonderlich, S. (1995). Personality and eating disorders. In K. D. Brownell & C. G. Fairburn (Eds.), *Eating disorders and obesity: A comprehensive handbook* (pp. 171–176). New York: Guilford.

Wonderlich, S. A., Gordon, K. H., Mitchell, J. E., Crosby, R. D., & Engel, S. G. (2009). The validity and clinical utility of binge eating disorder. *International Journal of Eating Disorders, 42*, 687–705.

Wonderlich, S., & Mitchell, J. E. (2001). The role of personality in the onset of eating disorders and treatment implications. *Psychiatric Clinics of North America, 24*, 249–258.

Wonderlich, A. S., Peterson, C. B., Smith, T. L., Klein, M., Mitchell, J. E., Crow, S. J., & Engel, S. G. (2010). Integrative cognitive-affective therapy for bulimia nervosa. In C. M. Grilo & J. E. Mitchell (Eds.), *The treatment of eating disorders: A clinical handbook* (pp. 317–338). New York: Guilford.

Woods, S. C., & Brief, D. J. (1988). Physiological factors. In D. M. Donovan & G. A. Marlatt (Eds.), *Assessment of addictive behaviors* (pp. 296–322). New York: Guilford.

Yager, Z., & O'Dea, J. A. (2008). Prevention programs for body image and eating disorders on University campuses: A review of large, controlled interventions. *Health Promotion International, 23,* 173–189.

Yanez, A., Peix, M., Atserias, N., Arnau, A., & Brug, J. (2007). Association of eating attitudes between teenage girls and their parents. *International Journal of Eating Disorders, 53,* 507–513.

Index